GENETICS AND GENOMICS IN ONCOLOGY NURSING PRACTICE

Edited by

Kathleen A. Calzone, MSN, RN, APNG, FAAN, Agnes Masny, MSN, MPH, BS, RN, CRNP, and Jean Jenkins, PhD, RN, FAAN

Oncology Nursing Society
Pittsburgh, Pennsylvania

ONS Publishing Division
Publisher: Leonard Mafrica, MBA, CAE
Director of Publications: Barbara Sigler, RN, MNEd
Managing Editor: Lisa M. George, BA
Technical Content Editor: Angela D. Klimaszewski, RN, MSN
Staff Editor: Amy Nicoletti, BA
Copy Editor: Laura Pinchot, BA
Graphic Designer: Dany Sjoen

Copyright © 2010 by the Oncology Nursing Society. All rights reserved. No part of the material protected by this copyright may be reproduced or utilized in any form, electronic or mechanical, including photocopying, recording, or by an information storage and retrieval system, without written permission from the copyright owner. For information, write to the Oncology Nursing Society, 125 Enterprise Drive, Pittsburgh, PA 15275-1214, or visit www.ons.org/publications.

Library of Congress Cataloging-in-Publication Data
Genetics and genomics in oncology nursing practice / edited by Kathleen A. Calzone, Agnes Masny, and Jean Jenkins.
   p. ; cm.
  Includes bibliographical references and index.
  ISBN 978-1-890504-91-5 (alk. paper)
  1. Cancer–Genetic aspects. 2. Cancer–Nursing. I. Calzone, Kathleen A. II. Masny, Agnes. III. Jenkins, Jean. IV. Oncology Nursing Society.
  [DNLM: 1. Neoplasms–genetics–Nurses' Instruction. 2. Neoplasms–nursing–Nurses' Instruction. 3. Oncologic Nursing–methods–Nurses' Instruction. QZ 202 G33166 2010]
  RC268.4.G454 2010
  616.99'4042–dc22

2010006413

Publisher's Note
    This book is published by the Oncology Nursing Society (ONS). ONS neither represents nor guarantees that the practices described herein will, if followed, ensure safe and effective patient care. The recommendations contained in this book reflect ONS's judgment regarding the state of general knowledge and practice in the field as of the date of publication. The recommendations may not be appropriate for use in all circumstances. Those who use this book should make their own determinations regarding specific safe and appropriate patient-care practices, taking into account the personnel, equipment, and practices available at the hospital or other facility at which they are located. The editors and publisher cannot be held responsible for any liability incurred as a consequence from the use or application of any of the contents of this book. Figures and tables are used as examples only. They are not meant to be all-inclusive, nor do they represent endorsement of any particular institution by ONS. Mention of specific products and opinions related to those products do not indicate or imply endorsement by ONS. Web sites mentioned are provided for information only; the hosts are responsible for their own content and availability. Unless otherwise indicated, dollar amounts reflect U.S. dollars.
    ONS publications are originally published in English. Publishers wishing to translate ONS publications must contact the ONS Publishing Division about licensing arrangements. ONS publications cannot be translated without obtaining written permission from ONS. (Individual tables and figures that are reprinted or adapted require additional permission from the original source.) Because translations from English may not always be accurate or precise, ONS disclaims any responsibility for inaccuracies in words or meaning that may occur as a result of the translation. Readers relying on precise information should check the original English version.

Printed in the United States of America

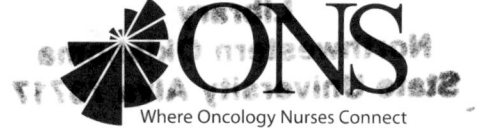

Oncology Nursing Society

Integrity • Innovation • Stewardship • Advocacy • Excellence • Inclusiveness

Contributors

EDITORS

KATHLEEN A. CALZONE, MSN, RN, APNG, FAAN
Senior Nurse Specialist (Research)
Genetics Branch
Center for Cancer Research
National Cancer Institute
National Institutes of Health
Bethesda, Maryland
Chapter 1. The Scope of Cancer Genetics and Genomics Nursing Practice; Chapter 13. Genetic/Genomic Competencies and Recommendations for Education

AGNES MASNY, MSN, MPH, BS, RN, CRNP
Nurse Practitioner
Risk Assessment Program
Fox Chase Cancer Center
Philadelphia, Pennsylvania
Preface; Chapter 6. Establishment of a Cancer Genetic Risk Assessment Program; Glossary

JEAN JENKINS, PhD, RN, FAAN
Senior Clinical Advisor
National Human Genome Research Institute
National Institutes of Health
Bethesda, Maryland
Preface; Chapter 13. Genetic/Genomic Competencies and Recommendations for Education; Chapter 16. Identifying Appropriate Referrals and Resources

AUTHORS

WALTER BROWN, PhD
Clinical Psychologist
Health Development Services
Culver City, California
Chapter 12. Multicultural Considerations in Providing Genetic and Genomic Cancer Care

SUSAN D. BRUCE, MSN, RN, OCN®
Oncology Clinical Nurse Specialist
Duke Raleigh Cancer Center
Raleigh, North Carolina
Chapter 10. Targeted Therapies

Contributors

BERNICE L. COLEMAN, PhD, ACNP-BC, FAHA
Certified Nurse Practitioner
Heart Transplant and Ventricular Assist Device Programs
Cedars-Sinai Medical Center
Los Angeles, California
Chapter 12. Multicultural Considerations in Providing Genetic and Genomic Cancer Care

YVETTE P. CONLEY, PhD
Associate Professor of Nursing and Human Genetics
School of Nursing
University of Pittsburgh
Pittsburgh, Pennsylvania
Chapter 15. Research: Making a Difference in Practice

JULIA EGGERT, PhD, APRN-BC, GNP, AOCN®
Associate Professor and Doctoral Coordinator
Clemson University
Clemson, South Carolina
Advanced Practice Nurse and Consultant
Bon Secours St. Francis Hospital–Eastside
Cancer Risk Screening Program
Greenville, South Carolina
Chapter 2. Biology of Cancer; Chapter 9. Pharmacogenomics

LORRAINE FRAZIER, PhD, RN, MS, FAHA, FAAN
Nancy B. Willerson Distinguished Professor in Nursing
Houston School of Nursing
University of Texas Health Science Center
Houston, Texas
Director
TexGen/CTSA Biobank
Houston, Texas
Executive Nurse Fellow
Robert Wood Johnson Foundation
Houston, Texas
Chapter 13. Genetic/Genomic Competencies and Recommendations for Education

MICHELE E. GAGUSKI, MSN, RN, AOCN®, CHPN, APN-C
Oncology Clincial Nurse Specialist
Ocean Medical Center
Brick, New Jersey
Chapter 10. Targeted Therapies

CATHLEEN M. GOETSCH, MSN, RN, ARNP, AOCNP®
Cancer Prevention and Hereditary Cancer Risk Specialist
Virginia Mason Medical Center Cancer Institute
Seattle, Washington
Chapter 5. Delivering Genetic Education and Counseling Services; Chapter 8. Tumor Profiling

KAREN E. GRECO, PhD, RN, MSN, ANP-BC
Nurse Specialist (Research)
Contractor
Genetics Branch
Center for Cancer Research
National Cancer Institute
Bethesda, Maryland
Chapter 1. The Scope of Cancer Genetics and Genomics Nursing Practice; Chapter 5. Delivering Genetic Education and Counseling Services

LUCIA A. HINDORFF, PhD, MPH
Epidemiologist
Office of Population Genomics
National Human Genome Research Institute
National Institutes of Health
Bethesda, Maryland
Chapter 7. Genome-Wide Association Studies and Cancer

LINDA HOWE, PhD, RN, CNS, CNE
Associate Professor and Navigator
Freshmen Nursing
Clemson University
Clemson, South Carolina
Chapter 9. Pharmacogenomics

MONICA E. KASSE, BS
Department of Microbiology
Clemson University
Clemson, South Carolina
Chapter 2. Biology of Cancer

MEREDITH K. KESSLER, MS, RN, CS
Nurse, Genetic Counselor, and Career Information and Referral Specialist
Rosenfeld Cancer Center
Abington Memorial Hospital
Abington, Pennsylvania
Glossary

DALE HALSEY LEA, MPH, RN, CGC, FAAN
Health Educator
Education and Community Involvement Branch
Genomic Healthcare Branch
National Human Genome Research Institute
National Institutes of Health
Bethesda, Maryland
Chapter 11. Handling Genetic and Genomic Information Responsibly

BRIDGET A. LEGRAZIE, MSN, RN, APNc, AOCN®, APNG
Manager, Cancer Genetics Program
Virtua Fox Chase Health Cancer Program
Mount Holly, New Jersey
Chapter 6. Establishment of a Cancer Genetic Risk Assessment Program

SUZANNE M. MAHON, DNSc, RN, AOCN®, APNG
Professor
Division of Hematology/Oncology
Department of Internal Medicine
Professor
Adult Nursing
School of Nursing
Saint Louis University
St. Louis, Missouri
Chapter 4. Common Risk Prediction Models and Cancer Risk Communication

TERI A. MANOLIO, MD, PhD
Senior Advisor to the Director for Population Genomics
National Human Genome Research Institute
National Institutes of Health
Bethesda, Maryland
Chapter 7. Genome-Wide Association Studies and Cancer

RITA BLACK MONSEN, DSN, MPH, RN, FAAN
Nursing Education Consultant
Hot Springs, Arkansas
Chapter 14. Ensuring Competence: Nursing Credentialing in Cancer Genetics

TERESA PRELLE, AS
Volunteer
Risk Assessment Program
Fox Chase Cancer Center
Philadelphia, Pennsylvania
Glossary

KAREN ROESSER, MS, RN, AOCN®
Oncology Clinical Nurse Specialist
The Thomas Johns Cancer Hospital
Chippenham and Johnston Willis Medical Center
Richmond, Virginia
Chapter 3. How to Perform a Cancer Genetic Risk Assessment

SUSAN R.M. VASQUEZ, BA
Special Assistant
National Human Genome Research Institute
National Institutes of Health
Bethesda, Maryland
Chapter 16. Identifying Appropriate Referrals and Resources

DISCLOSURE

Editors and authors of books and guidelines provided by the Oncology Nursing Society are expected to disclose to the participants any significant financial interest or other relationships with the manufacturer(s) of any commercial products.

A vested interest may be considered to exist if a contributor is affiliated with or has a financial interest in commercial organizations that may have a direct or indirect interest in the subject matter. A "financial interest" may include, but is not limited to, being a shareholder in the organization; being an employee of the commercial organization; serving on an organization's speakers bureau; or receiving research from the organization. An "affiliation" may be holding a position on an advisory board or some other role of benefit to the commercial organization. Vested interest statements appear in the front matter for each publication.

Contributors are expected to disclose any unlabeled or investigational use of products discussed in their content. This information is acknowledged solely for the information of the readers.

The contributors provided the following disclosure and vested interest information:

Michele E. Gaguski, MSN, RN, AOCN®, APNC, EUSA Pharma, speakers bureau

Contents

PREFACE: GENETICS AND GENOMICS: THE EVOLUTION OF ONCOLOGY NURSING xiii
- Where We Have Been xiii
- Genetics and Genomics in Oncology xiv
- Genetic and Genomic Advances Affect Oncology Nursing xvii
- New Discoveries, New Technology, New Content xvii
- Where We Are Going xx
- Summary xxxii
- References xxiii

SECTION I. GENETIC AND GENOMIC FUNDAMENTAL PRINCIPLES FOR ONCOLOGY NURSING 1

Chapter 1. The Scope of Cancer Genetics and Genomics Nursing Practice 3
- Introduction 3
- What Influences the Scope of Nursing Practice? 4
- Interfacing the Oncology and the Genetic and Genomic Scopes of Nursing Practice 5
- Dimensions of Cancer Genetic and Genomic Nursing Practice 5
- Incorporation of Cancer Genetics and Genomics in Various Practice Settings 7
- Scope of Oncology Nursing Practice in Genetics and Genomics 7
- Summary 11
- References 11

Chapter 2. Biology of Cancer 13
- Introduction 13
- Models of Cancer Development 13
- DNA and Chromosomes: Structure and Function 14
- Gene Expression 18
- Causes of Mutations 23
- Types of Mutations Associated With Cancer and Other Disorders 23

Gene Transmission in Cancers 26
Cancer and Genetics 29
Types of Genetic Alterations in Cancer Cells... 36
Types of DNA Repair Mechanisms 38
The Cell Cycle.. 40
Summary 43
References.. 43

SECTION II. GENETICS AND GENOMICS: IDENTIFICATION AND RISK REDUCTION   47

Chapter 3. How to Perform a Cancer Genetic Risk Assessment................................. 49
Introduction 49
Cancer Genetic Assessment 50
Purpose of a Cancer Genetic Risk Assessment.. 50
Familial Cancer Susceptibility Syndromes 52
Components of a Cancer Genetic Assessment 55
Family History 64
Psychosocial Assessment 68
Physical Examination 69
The Assessment Process 70
Common Problems of Genetic Evaluation 71
Sample Assessments 72
Summary 74
References.. 75

Chapter 4. Common Risk Prediction Models and Cancer Risk Communication 79
Introduction 79
Common Terms in Risk Assessment and Risk Communication 80
Quantifying Risks... 84
Specific Models Quantifying Cancer Risk or Mutation Probability 86
Case Study 88
Cancer Risk Communication 92
The Media's Role in Risk Information 98
The Long-Term Impact of Risk Communication.. 99
Summary 99
References.. 100

Chapter 5. Delivering Genetic Education and Counseling Services........................... 103
Introduction 103
The Role of Nurses in Genetic Counseling.. 104
Elements of Cancer Risk Assessment, Education, and Counseling........................ 108
Issues Related to Cancer Genetic Testing 109
Informed Decision Making Related to Cancer Genetic Testing............................. 110
Preparing for Genetic Testing.. 114
Pretest Education Regarding Potential Test Results... 116

    Results Disclosure and Post-Test Counseling 119
    Cancer Screening, Risk Reduction, and Follow-Up 123
    Summary 124
    References 124

Chapter 6. Establishment of a Cancer Genetic Risk Assessment Program 129
    Introduction 129
    Needs Assessment and Planning 130
    Institutional Policy Considerations 138
    Choosing a Type of Cancer Genetic Risk Assessment Program 141
    What a Cancer Genetic Risk Assessment Program Looks Like 143
    Quality Assurance 147
    Summary 148
    References 149

Chapter 7. Genome-Wide Association Studies and Cancer 151
    Introduction 151
    The Road to Genome-Wide Scans 152
    Anatomy of a Genome-Wide Association Study 159
    Identifying Promising Genomic Regions 160
    Replication in Independent Studies 164
    Fine Mapping and Beyond: Hints at Biologic Function 166
    Challenges for Genome-Wide Association Studies: Present and Future 166
    Clinical Implications and Future Directions 167
    Summary 168
    Resources 169
    References 171

SECTION III. GENOMICS AND CANCER CARE   175

Chapter 8. Tumor Profiling 177
    Introduction 177
    The Need for Tumor Profiling 177
    Beginnings of Tumor Profiling 178
    Advances in Tumor Profiling: Molecular Profiling 180
    Current Work 190
    Fast Forward Into the Future 192
    Coordination of Efforts 192
    Summary 194
    References 195

Chapter 9. Pharmacogenomics 199
    Introduction 199
    History 199
    Pharmacogenetics and Pharmacogenomics 200
    Polymorphisms in Drug-Metabolizing Enzymes 206

Contents

- Polymorphisms in Drug Transporters ... 208
- Polymorphisms in Drug Targets ... 209
- Technologic Advances Applicable to Pharmacogenomics ... 212
- Summary ... 213
- References ... 213

Chapter 10. Targeted Therapies ... 217
- Introduction ... 217
- Rationale for Targeted Therapies ... 217
- History of Targeted Therapy ... 218
- Mechanisms for Targeted Intervention ... 223
- Applying Targeted Therapies to Signaling Pathways in Cancer ... 226
- Toxicities of Targeted Therapies ... 231
- Future Direction of Targeted Therapies ... 236
- Summary ... 237
- References ... 237

SECTION IV. ETHICAL, LEGAL, AND SOCIAL ISSUES OF GENETICS AND GENOMICS 241

Chapter 11. Handling Genetic and Genomic Information Responsibly ... 243
- Introduction ... 243
- Ethical Considerations of Genetic and Genomic Information ... 244
- Facilitating Autonomous Decision Making ... 249
- Principles of Beneficence and Nonmaleficence ... 250
- Recognition of Ethnocultural Differences ... 251
- Privacy and Confidentiality ... 252
- Client Advocacy ... 254
- Emerging Ethical Issues for Oncology Nurses ... 256
- Maintaining a Current Knowledge Base in Genetic and Genomic Developments ... 260
- Summary ... 263
- References ... 263

Chapter 12. Multicultural Considerations in Providing Genetic and Genomic Cancer Care ... 267
- Introduction ... 267
- Multicultural Considerations in the Delivery of Genetic and Genomic Cancer Nursing Care ... 268
- Why Are Multicultural Considerations Important for Oncology Nurses? ... 270
- Ethnicity and Sociopolitical Factors ... 271
- Multicultural Aspects of Delivery of Genetic and Genomic Services ... 274
- Education ... 277
- Consent ... 277
- Community Healing Models ... 278
- Steps Toward Multicultural Competence ... 279
- Research Implications ... 279
- Summary ... 281
- References ... 281

SECTION V. PROFESSIONAL PRACTICE ISSUES — 285

Chapter 13. Genetic/Genomic Competencies and Recommendations for Education 287
- Introduction 287
- What Do Nurses Already Know About Genetics and Genomics? 287
- Are All Nurses the Target for Education? 288
- Education Recommendations for Oncology Nurses 289
- Exemplars 293
- Summary 294
- References 295

Chapter 14. Ensuring Competence: Nursing Credentialing in Cancer Genetics 297
- Introduction 297
- The Significance of Credentialing to Clinical Practice 298
- Establishment of Competence 300
- Certification of Nurses in Oncology 301
- Certification of Nurses in Genetics 301
- Future Directions in Licensure and Certification 303
- Summary 303
- References 304

Chapter 15. Research: Making a Difference in Practice 305
- Introduction 305
- Translational Research: Necessary to Make a Difference in Practice 305
- Molecular Genomic Tumor Profiling for Breast Cancer as an Example of Moving Basic Research Toward Clinical Utility 308
- RNA Interference as an Example of Cutting-Edge Technologies Expected to Affect Practice 309
- Highlights of Select Research Initiatives 310
- Additional Tips to Stay Current With Genomic Research 312
- Incorporating Genetics and Genomics Into Oncology Nursing Research 313
- Summary 313
- References 316

SECTION VI. RESOURCES — 317

Chapter 16. Identifying Appropriate Referrals and Resources 319
- Introduction 319
- Professional Organizations: Resources for Networking and Genetic and Genomic Information 319
- Physician Groups 326
- Resources for Continuing Education 327
- Clinical Resources: Sources for Patient Information and Referrals 329
- Family History and Other Client Resources 331
- Resources for Information Regarding Genetics Education 332
- Genetics Legislation, Guidelines, and Policies 333

Research Opportunities 335
Summary 337
References 337

GLOSSARY 339

INDEX 347

PREFACE

Genetics and Genomics: The Evolution of Oncology Nursing

Agnes Masny, MSN, MPH, BS, RN, CRNP, and Jean Jenkins, PhD, RN, FAAN

WHERE WE HAVE BEEN

Since its inception, the nursing profession has continually endeavored to evolve so that individuals and communities could benefit from the care, knowledge, and skills of practicing nurses (Ponte, 2004). Throughout the 20th century, nurses' knowledge of genetics was influenced by the findings of Gregor Mendel, who, in 1865, described how heredity is transmitted. Mendel's findings were followed by further genetic discoveries that shaped nursing practice and health care in general (see Figure 1). Many of these genetic discoveries influenced the understanding of single gene disorders, such as Huntington disease, but did not affect our understanding of the genetic mechanisms of common diseases.

The release of *Genetics in Oncology Nursing: Cancer Risk Assessment* (Tranin, Masny, & Jenkins, 2003) coincided with the completion of the Human Genome Project, and genetic discoveries have been on the fast track ever since. Our understanding of the impact of genes on health and disease has evolved beyond the notion of a single-gene approach to a genomic approach (e.g., multiple genes interacting with each other and with the environment). In the past, most nurses learned about genetic disorders caused by single genes. For example, sickle-cell disease is caused by a mutation in the beta globulin gene of hemoglobin (*HBB*). Clinical differences in patients with sickle-cell disease have long been observed with the severity of disease ranging from mild with long-term survival to severe with organ damage and early death (Genetics Home Reference, 2009). This clinical diversity in a single-gene disorder suggested that other differences affect the *HBB* mutation (Steinberg, 1996). With the mapping of the human genome (International Human Genome Sequencing Consortium, 2001; Venter et al., 2001), other genes that modify the *HBB* mutation have been identified, such as variations in coagulation genes and gene variations in specific populations (Kutlar, 2007). These newly discovered variations in other genes were found to interact with the *HBB* gene (gene-gene interactions) and accounted for the clinical differences in sickle-cell disease severity. The genomic discoveries in sickle-cell disease now are resulting in the identification of new diagnostic approaches and new targets for treatment. A genetic disorder once attributed to a single gene is now studied, diagnosed, and treated utilizing a genomic approach (i.e., looking at multiple genes and their interaction). This simplified summary

FIGURE 1. TIMELINE OF GENETIC DISCOVERIES

1902: Chromosome Theory of Inheritance—Walter Sutton observes that the segregation of chromosomes during meiosis matched the patterns of inheritance described by Mendel.
1909: The Word *Gene* is Coined—Wlihelm Johannsen coins the word *gene* to describe the Mendelian unit of heredity.
1911: Chromosomes Carry Genes—Thomas Hunt Morgan and his students study fruit fly chromosomes and show that they carry genes.
1952: Genes are Made of DNA—Alfred Hershey and Martha Chase show that only the DNA of a virus needs to enter a bacterium to infect it, supporting the idea that genes are made of DNA.
1953: DNA Double Helix—Francis H. Crick and James D. Watson describe the double helix structure of DNA.
1955: Humans have 46 Chromosomes—Joe Hin Tjio defines 46 as the exact number of chromosomes in human cells.
1956: Cause of Disease Traced to Alteration—Vernon Ingram finds a specific chemical alteration in a hemoglobin protein that causes sickle-cell disease.
1959: Chromosome Abnormalities Identified—Jerome Lejeune and colleagues discover that Down syndrome is caused by three copies of chromosome 21 (trisomy 21).
1961: First Screen for Metabolic Defect in Newborns—Robert Guthrie develops test for the metabolic defect, phenylketonuria.
1966: Genetic Code Cracked—Marshall Nirenberg and others figure out the code that allows nucleic acids (adenosine, thymine, cytosine, and guanine) to produce the 20 kinds of amino acids in proteins.
1975: Discovery of DNA Sequencing Method—Fredrick Sanger and colleagues, and Alan Maxam and Walter Gilbert developed the method to identify each of the four nucleic acids that comprise DNA.
1982: GenBank Database Started—Scientists begin submitting DNA sequence data to a National Institutes of Health database.
1983: First Disease Gene Mapped—A genetic marker for Huntington disease is found on chromosome 4.
1987: First Human Genetic Map—First comprehensive genetic map based on variations in DNA.
1990: Launch of the Human Genome Project
2003: Completion of the Human Genome Sequence

Note. From *Genetic Timeline,* by National Human Genome Research Institute, n.d. Retrieved August 4, 2009, from http://www.genome.gov/Pages/Education/GeneticTimeline.pdf.

example for one disease illustrates how the practice of genetics has evolved to genomics. Now, health professionals are elucidating the underlying genetic and genomic mechanisms for all diseases using the same genetic and genomic approach. This has resulted in the invariable evolution of nursing practice to meet the genetic and genomic healthcare needs of individuals, families, and communities.

GENETICS AND GENOMICS IN ONCOLOGY

Cancer is a genetic disease at the level of the cell. Hematologic cancers, such as leukemia, have long been known to be caused by chromosomal abnormalities (Nowell & Hungerford, 1961). DNA replication errors were later suspected as the basis for solid tumors (Loeb,

Genes are units of DNA. The genes code for normal proteins, which regulate cell growth. Normal cells respond in a controlled fashion to genes that activate the cell cycle (oncogenes) and stop cell division (tumor suppressor genes). When cells are damaged, DNA repair mechanisms can make corrections, and damaged cells that cannot be repaired signal other genes for programmed cell death (apoptosis). When the genetic regulation of normal cells goes awry via genetic mutations, the cells can continue to grow and lose their ability to stop growing and to perform apoptosis. These unregulated cells make clones of themselves and accumulate. If immune mechanisms fail to clear the body of these cells, they accumulate further mutations, which results in the initiation and progression of cancer (Brenner, 2004).

Springgate, & Battula, 1974). The 1970s through the early 1990s saw the field of cancer genetics evolving with breakthroughs such as
- Recognition of family constellations of cancers that fit hereditary patterns of transmission (Lynch et al., 1979)
- Study of genes infected by viruses leading to the discovery of genes that regulate human cell division (i.e., oncogenes and tumor suppressor genes) (Klein, 1988)
- Human Genome Project beginning in 1990 (National Human Genome Research Institute, 2009)
- Identification of the multiple genetic events needed to progress from normal colon mucosa to an adenoma to a colon cancer to a colon cancer with metastatic potential (Cho & Vogelstein, 1992)
- Discovery of the DNA sequence of the *BRCA1* gene associated with hereditary breast and ovarian cancer (Miki et al., 1994)
- Cancer therapies developed to stop cell growth: Radiation therapy caused DNA strand breaks (Olive, 1998), and chemotherapy irreparably damaged newly dividing cells (Frei, 1985). The aim of using both treatments is to kill off cancer cells that started and progressed because of genetic mutations.

The field of oncology had embraced cancer genetics, recognizing the molecular events involved in the carcinogenesis process and was, therefore, primed for the genomic era (see Figure 2).

FIGURE 2.   GENES AND CARCINOGENESIS

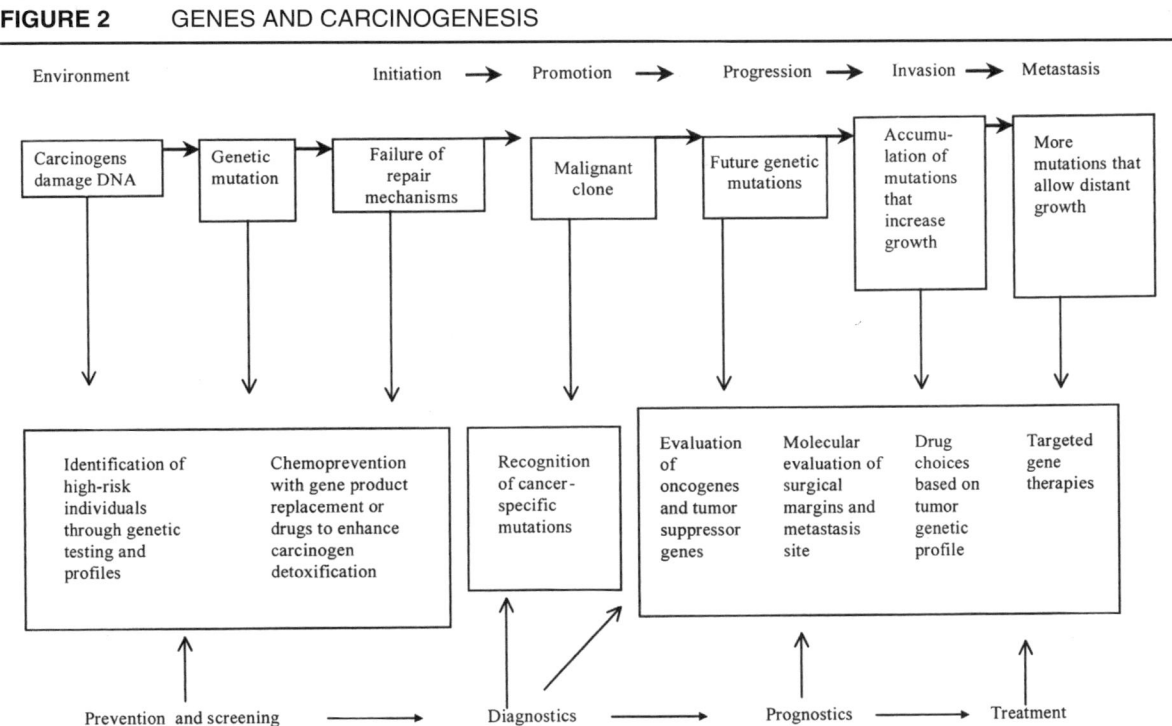

Note. Based on information from Peters et al., 1997.

In 1996, the National Cancer Institute (NCI) established the Office of Cancer Genomics (OCG) to make resources, technology, and databases available to improve the identification of normal functioning genes compared to those in tumors. The goal of OCG was to provide a technology and research infrastructure to help to identify groups of genes and how their interactions influenced cancer with the goal of "improving cancer prevention, early detection, diagnosis, and treatment of cancer" (NCI OCG, 2009). Then, the mapping of the human genome (Venter et al., 2001) catapulted oncology research and genetic technology to rapidly identify the genes and their related functions involved in the carcinogenesis process. As a result, OCG launched several research initiatives, including

- The Cancer Genome Anatomy Project (CGAP) (http://cgap.nci.nih.gov)—to identify in normal tissue which genes are active or normally turned off. Any given normal tissue (e.g., prostate tissue) has its own profile of working genes, a gene profile. Then gene changes in precancerous or cancerous tissue are identified compared to the normal tissue. All the information on normal, precancerous, or tumor profiles is stored in a database for research and clinical use (CGAP, 2008).
- The Initiative for Chemical Genetics (http://ocg.cancer.gov/programs/icg.asp)—to study the biology of cancer using small molecules (e.g., studying manmade molecules that can be used for new screening markers or targets for drug development). All the data about the small molecules are put in a data bank where they can be used for cancer research or biologic investigation (Tolliday et al., 2006).
- The Cancer Genome Atlas (http://ocg.cancer.gov/programs/tcga.asp)—to identify the normal gene activity (gene profile) and gene changes (tumor profile) in three specific cancers (brain, lung, and ovarian) to learn about the normal gene functions and what gene malfunctions affect carcinogenesis in these tissues. This research effort received a funding boost for 2010 with plans to collect more than 20,000 tissue samples from more than 20 cancer types, complete maps of the genomic changes in 10 of those cancers, and sequence and characterize at least 100 tumors of as many as 15 additional cancers. These maps will be deposited into public databases for use by the worldwide research community in research programs aimed at finding new ways to diagnose, treat, and prevent cancer.
- The Cancer Genetic Markers of Susceptibility (http://ocg.cancer.gov/programs/cgems.asp)—to scan more than 500,000 common genomic variations that may play a role in prostate and breast cancer.
- The Therapeutically Applicable Research to Generate Effective Treatments (TARGET) Initiative (http://ocg.cancer.gov/programs/target.asp)—to find the genomic changes associated with acute lymphocytic leukemia and neuroblastoma, two childhood cancers, in order to speed treatment discoveries for these cancers.

Based on these initiatives and other resulting research, staggering advances in genomic technology have emerged, which affect the detection of predisposition to cancer, diagnosis, and treatment. Two pivotal technology advances have been in DNA and proteomic microarray technology. Microarray is the use of chip technology. In DNA microarray, a chip about the size of a laboratory slide compares thousands of genes from normal and cancer tissue at the same time. The proteomic microarray examines the protein patterns activated most often in cell signals within cancer cells. Proteins in cancer cells also are examined with mass spectrometry. This microarray technology has strengthened discoveries in tumor profiles, finding gene markers for cancer screening, cancer recurrence potential or metastasis, and treatment targets. Now cancer tissue is examined not only by pathology, looking at the types of cells, but with molecular diagnosis looking at the genes and protein information from cancer tissue to aid in the diagnosis, staging, and treatment decisions in cancer (NCI, 2005).

GENETIC AND GENOMIC ADVANCES AFFECT ONCOLOGY NURSING

Genetic and genomic technology advances affect all aspects of oncology care and therefore have direct implications for the role of the oncology nurse. Oncology nurses serve as translators and mediators of scientific and medical information given to clients to facilitate referrals, services, treatment, and follow-up care. More than ever, oncology nurses are challenged to be the knowledgeable interface between their clients and the information stemming from these genomic advances (Loescher & Merkle, 2005).

Understanding the genetic and genomic mechanisms of cancer etiology, diagnosis, and treatment is now central to the role of the oncology nurse. In response to this recognition, oncology nurses collaborated with the American Nurses Association (ANA) to spearhead the development of *Essential Nursing Competencies and Curricula Guidelines for Genetics and Genomics* for all RNs regardless of academic preparation, role, or clinical specialty (Jenkins & Calzone, 2007). The competencies were designed to delineate expectations of the entire nursing workforce when delivering genetically and genomically competent health care. Oncology Nursing Society, along with 48 other professional nursing organizations, endorsed the *Essential Nursing Competencies and Curricula Guidelines for Genetics and Genomics* (Consensus Panel on Genetic/Genomic Nursing Competencies, 2006). A second edition of the competencies, which included outcome indicators, was released in 2009 (Consensus Panel on Genetic/Genomic Nursing Competencies, 2009). An action plan is in progress for the integration of the competencies into curricula, licensure and registration examinations, specialty certification processes, and continuing nursing education. These competencies provide a framework upon which oncology nurses can build their specialty knowledge to be able to provide competent care both now and in the future.

NEW DISCOVERIES, NEW TECHNOLOGY, NEW CONTENT

Since the publication of *Genetics in Oncology Nursing: Cancer Risk Assessment* (Tranin et al., 2003), new genetic and genomic discoveries have influenced the fundamental understanding of cancer development, diagnosis, prognosis, and treatment. This, in turn, has created a demand for oncology nurses who are knowledgeable and competent in genetic and genomic applications affecting practice. The focus of *Genetics and Genomics in Oncology Nursing Practice* has been broadened from risk assessment to encompass the key concepts of cancer biology, the resulting clinical applications, and the scope of oncology nursing practice. The changes include updated information in cancer genetic risk assessment and the addition of several new chapters reflecting the clinical use of genetics and genomics in oncology practice. The table of contents is organized into six sections to give the reader an overview of the principles, practice areas, clinical application, and issues related to genetics and genomics of cancer. The framework for every chapter follows the *Essentials of Genetic and Genomic Nursing: Competencies, Curricula Guidelines, and Outcome Indicators* (Consensus Panel on Genetic/Genomic Nursing Competencies, 2009). Each chapter begins with the competencies that are integral to the chapter content and practice issues. The sections and chapters are as follows.

Section I. Genetic and Genomic Fundamental Principles for Oncology Nursing

Chapter 1. "The Scope of Cancer Genetics and Genomics Nursing Practice" (**Rewritten**) provides nurses with information on how genetics and genomics influence the scope and standards and the dimensions of care at the basic and advanced levels of nursing practice.

Chapter 2. "Biology of Cancer" (**Updated**) focuses on the basic principles of genetics and the carcinogenesis process. New information in the chapter includes the role of epigenetics, oncogene classification, newly discovered mechanisms of tumor suppressor genes, and gene regulation in the cell cycle.

Section II. Genetics and Genomics: Identification and Risk Reduction

Chapter 3. "How to Perform a Cancer Genetic Risk Assessment" (**Updated**) discusses the components of cancer risk assessment to identify high-risk individuals who may benefit from further genetic evaluation or risk-reduction interventions. New information is given on developing a differential list of cancer syndromes.

Chapter 4. "Common Risk Prediction Models and Cancer Risk Communication" (**Updated**) provides the reader with information about how to evaluate and when to use risk prediction models in cancer risk assessment. New content about ways to present risk information is provided.

Chapter 5. "Delivering Genetic Education and Counseling Services" (**Updated**) covers the elements of cancer risk education and counseling, delivery modes, and psychosocial considerations.

Chapter 6. "Establishment of a Cancer Genetic Risk Assessment Program" (**Updated**) gives the reader the main components of a cancer genetic risk assessment program and points to consider when deciding when and how to start a program. New information is given on financial and billing issues and considerations for selecting laboratories for genetic testing.

Chapter 7. "Genome-Wide Association Studies and Cancer" (**New**) explains the role of single nucleotide polymorphisms in disease development. Technology used in genome-wide association studies is described and details how common genetic variants related to genetic variation across the entire human genome are identified.

Section III. Genomics and Cancer Care

Chapter 8. "Tumor Profiling" (**New**) describes gene expression profiles, molecular diagnostics, and the techniques used in tumor profiling (i.e., DNA microarray assays). The chapter also describes clinical trials that use tumor profiles for the prediction of recurrence and evaluation of the effectiveness of treatment.

Chapter 9. "Pharmacogenomics" (**New**) provides the history of pharmacogenetics and pharmacogenomics, current discoveries, and implications for nursing practice with today's oncologic treatments and regimens.

Chapter 10. "Targeted Therapies" (**New**) describes how genetic tumor profiles and other cellular factors, such as growth factors, influence tumor growth and make each cancer unique. The chapter discusses how the tumor's unique profile and cellular environment are targets for cancer treatment.

Section IV. Ethical, Legal, and Social Issues of Genetics and Genomics

Chapter 11. "Handling Genetic and Genomic Information Responsibly" (**Updated**) explores emerging ethical issues in genetics and genomics and how nurses can apply existing ethical, social, and legal principles to these issues. Some of these issues include direct-to-consumer marketing and genetic testing, pre-implantation genetic diagnosis and prenatal genetic testing for adult-onset genetic disorders, oversight of genetic testing, cancer predisposition genetic testing in children, stem cell research, and human cloning.

Chapter 12. "Multicultural Considerations in Providing Genetic and Genomic Cancer Care" (**New**) defines multicultural considerations in cancer nursing in the context of delivering genetic and genomic care to individuals, families, and communities. The chapter examines how genetics and genomics affect nurses' understanding of culture, race, and ethnicity and the implications of genetic variations on the delivery of culturally competent nursing care.

Section V. Professional Practice Issues

Chapter 13. "Genetic/Genomic Competencies and Recommendations for Education" (**Updated**) defines what all nurses should know about genetics and genomics and how the *Essentials of Genetic and Genomic Nursing: Competencies, Curricula Guidelines, and Outcome Indicators* were developed and are now being implemented into nursing training and practice.

Chapter 14. "Ensuring Competence: Nursing Credentialing in Cancer Genetics" (**New**) discusses the significance of credentialing to nursing practice and the history of certification for oncology nurses and nurses in genetics. The chapter spells out the ways nursing has validated genetic and genomic nursing competence, provides information for nurses who specialize in oncology and genetic settings, and examines methods used to demonstrate their knowledge, skills, and abilities to provide care that meets professional standards of practice.

Chapter 15. "Research: Making a Difference in Practice" (**New**) explores the current research environment with a focus on how genetic and genomic oncology research will be translated into practice. Selected research initiatives, genetic nursing initiatives, and challenges for genetic nursing research for the future are presented.

Section VI. Resources

Chapter 16. "Identifying Appropriate Referrals and Resources" (**Updated**) describes resources important for professional networking, continuing education, client education, and clinical reviews. Listings of Web sites are provided to help nurses access the resources needed to stay current in genetics and genomics.

Genetic and Genomic Glossary. **(Updated)**. An expanded glossary provides peer-reviewed definitions for related terms found bolded throughout the text.

WHERE WE ARE GOING

As evident throughout this text, advances in the understanding of the genetic and genomic contributions throughout the cancer continuum are occurring at a rapid rate. The more that is learned, the more complex the cancer process appears to be. Discoveries from new programs of research are constantly arriving on the scene that can make a difference in the care that oncology nurses provide. What is described in this text is only the tip of the iceberg, with great hopes for the future of cancer care. This creates a tremendous responsibility for oncology nurses to be able to attain, synthesize, and then explain to clients and their families the emerging research results.

Clients, appropriately so, are most interested in knowing what this genetic and genomic information means to their health and well-being. Nurses have the opportunity to use such information to personalize cancer care. Many examples of tools and resources already are available to personalize cancer care (NCI, 2009). Nurses should pay attention in the years ahead to genetic and genomic research that builds on these advances that can make a difference in the care that they provide.

Genomic Variation: What Is It? How Is It Measured? What Difference Does It Make?

Personalized genetic variation screening tests can benefit patient response, guide the drug development process, and facilitate prescriber treatment selection. The potential for reducing drug-associated morbidities or even mortalities is tremendous because of the adverse events that could be avoided when using pharmacogenetic and pharmacogenomic information. The field of pharmacogenomics has made strides in identifying inherited genetic variations associated with medication metabolism and efficacy, with the goal of tailoring treatment to an individual's genomic makeup (Weinshilboum & Wang, 2006). Newer approaches are combining multigene analysis of the individual's genetic metabolic profile, tumor profile, and drug cellular pathways. For example, molecular diagnostic tools evaluate gene expression patterns in normal versus cancerous biospecimen samples and identify targets for treatment. *Proteomics,* the study of the structure and function of proteins and how they interact with each other, is an example of ongoing genomic variation research utilizing molecular characteristics to understand a patient's predisposition for or experience with cancer. Researchers also are studying this combined genomic analysis to determine the relationship of chemotherapy toxicity with the genetic metabolic profile, drug targets, and efflux transporters (van Erp et al., 2009). Cells have efflux transporters to pump a drug in or out of the targeted cell to keep a nontoxic balance of a drug within the cells. However, some individuals have genetic variations causing increased drug transport out of the cell that decreases the drug effectiveness (Netterwald, 2009). These combined genomic evaluations are broadening pharmacogenomic approaches in oncology treatment. Understanding these genomic variations and their interaction will result in (a) the creation of new cancer screening tools, (b) the design of new targeted treatments, (c) mechanisms to determine and monitor treatment effectiveness, and (d) the ability to predict the patient's response to treatment (NCI, 2005).

Health disparities in cancer outcomes is variation in cancer treatment and prevention outcomes because of genetic and genomic reasons or a combination of inherited risk, societal factors, environmental exposures, and personal behaviors. For example, molecular profiling of breast cancers according to their gene expression has identified subtypes (Kurian et al., 2009). This study reported that the risk for a second primary breast cancer was influenced by hormonal status, age, race, and ethnicity. To study the molecular basis of cancer, researchers need adequate representation of racially and genetically diverse sources. A focus on ensuring that research participation reflects the different populations is crucial to ensuring that results can be applied to all individuals.

Do the Genetic and Genomic Changes That Occur Throughout a Lifetime, Often in Response to Something in the Environment (e.g., Stress, Drug, Toxicant), Influence Cancer Care?

Toxicogenomics is a field of research concerned with the influence of toxicants on the gene and how these may be altered for a defined health condition (Oregon Health and Science University, n.d.). Technologic advances and sensitive screening processes are important to understanding the influence of all variables that affect cancer treatment and prevention outcomes. For example, McWhinney and McLeod (2009) reported that germ line and somatic DNA samples were comparable when assessing cancer pharmacogenomic variants. This finding indicates that the utilization of either sample type will provide needed information to individualize treatment decisions. Resources and processes that standardize and improve upon the collection and interpretation of such information are essential.

How Can the Identification of Genetic and Genomic Variation Be Used to Improve Cancer Treatment?

The use of molecular disease characteristics to diagnose an individual's type of cancer can enable the selection of the best treatment for that individual (e.g., lymphoma stratification [Dave et al., 2006]). Ongoing research will provide additional results to guide targeted therapy options, such as Vectibix® (Amgen, Inc.) for those with colon cancer who are *KRAS* negative (Amgen, 2009), identify those who may best benefit from such interventions (e.g., prophylactic breast surgery [Garcia-Etienne et al., 2009]), and guide in the design of new treatment options, such as olaparib for *BRCA* mutation carriers (Fong et al., 2009). This area of research has tremendous implications for treatment morbidity and mortality.

What Resources and Tools Are Needed to Improve Access and Use of Genetic and Genomic Information in Cancer Care?

Technologic software advances, personal genome assistants, and collaborative working groups are examples of resources that are on the horizon to facilitate the clinical application of genetic and genomic research advances. Software applications that integrate genetic and genomic content into electronic health records have the potential to improve upon the collection, documentation, and use of personalized health information. However, improvements to standards and guidelines are recommended to improve the integration of genetics and genomics into clinical care (Scheuner et al., 2009).

Dr. Andras Pellionisz presented personal genome assistants (PRWeb, 2009) as a way to identify the toxic substances that an individual should avoid (e.g., specific foods) based on that individual's personal genome. This personal genome handheld applicator is available for $5,000. Other inventions to improve decision making and access to services are under way.

The potential for emerging personal and clinical applications of genomic information necessitates improved oversight of quality, cost, access, and utility of genomic applications. One collaborative effort aimed at developing processes for enhancing translation of research discoveries into clinical care is the Genomic Applications in Practice and Prevention Network (GAPPNet) (Khoury et al., 2009). Stakeholder meetings will define the activities and programs to be created for GAPPNet. Its proposed goal is to accelerate the effective integration of genomic information into clinical care.

How Do Other New Technologies, Such as Nanotechnology, Influence Personalized Healthcare Options That Integrate Genetics and Genomics?

NCI is coordinating efforts to use new technologies, materials, and devices developed through nanotechnology research (http://nano.cancer.gov) to improve upon currently available cancer care options. Applications from additional scientific and epidemiologic fields of study need to be considered.

Does Ongoing Research Address the Ethical Issues and Biobehavioral Aspects of Cancer Care That Integrate Genetic and Genomic Information?

This is an area of research that benefits from interdisciplinary collaboration and research focus. One research example reported by Clancy (2009) provides a clinical perspective on the use of prenatal or pre-implantation diagnosis for later-onset inherited cancer predisposition. Such complex issues require considerable informed discussion by all care providers to address such policy issues when explaining options to clients and their families.

SUMMARY

Nurses can anticipate that the growing knowledge of cancer genetics and genomics will serve to further the mission of the Oncology Nursing Society (n.d.): "to promote excellence in oncology nursing and quality cancer care." Oncology nurses have an opportunity to model for other nurses how to build upon this foundational scientific understanding of how the DNA structure, function, and interaction within ourselves (i.e., our body), outside ourselves (i.e., the environment and other external influences), and between ourselves (i.e., communities and populations) modifies health care. This book is only a beginning step of that lifelong, evolving journey of the learning necessary to become aware of, use, and maintain competency in the genomic era of oncology nursing.

REFERENCES

Amgen. (2009). *Vectibix® in combination with chemotherapy significantly improved progression-free survival in first-line metastatic colorectal cancer* [Press release]. Retrieved August 6, 2009, from http://wwwext.amgen.com/media/media_pr_detail.jsp?releaseID=1318284

Brenner, C. (2004). At the precarious cusp of oncogenomics. In C. Brenner & D. Duggan (Eds.), *Oncogenomics: Molecular approaches to cancer* (pp. 1–13). Hoboken, NJ: Wiley.

Cancer Genome Anatomy Project. (2008). *Cancer Genome Anatomy Project*. Retrieved September 23, 2009, from http://cgap.nci.nih.gov/

Cho, K.R., & Vogelstein, B. (1992). Genetic alterations in the adenoma-carcinoma sequence. *Cancer, 70*(Suppl. 6), 1727–1731.

Clancy, T. (2009). A clinical perspective on ethical arguments around prenatal diagnosis and preimplantation genetic diagnosis for later onset inherited cancer predisposition [Epub ahead of print]. *Familial cancer*. Retrieved July 31, 2009, from http://www.springerlink.com/content/4424685071052166/fulltext.pdf

Consensus Panel on Genetic/Genomic Nursing Competencies. (2006). *Essential nursing competencies and curricula guidelines for genetics and genomics*. Silver Spring, MD: American Nurses Association.

Consensus Panel on Genetic/Genomic Nursing Competencies. (2009). *Essentials of genetic and genomic nursing: Competencies, curricula guidelines, and outcome indicators* (2nd ed.). Silver Spring, MD: American Nurses Association.

Dave, S.S., Fu, K., Wright, G.W., Lam, L.T., Kluin, P., Boerma, E.J., et al. (2006). Molecular diagnosis of Burkitt's lymphoma. *New England Journal of Medicine, 354*(23), 2431–2442.

Fong, P., Boss, D., Yap, T., Tutt, A., Wu, P., Mergui-Roelvink, M., et al. (2009). Inhibition of poly(ADP-Ribose) polymerase in tumors from *BRCA* mutation carriers. *New England Journal of Medicine, 361*(2), 123–134.

Frei, E., III. (1985). Curative cancer chemotherapy. *Cancer Research, 45*(12, Pt. 1), 6523–6537.

Garcia-Etienne, C., Barile, M., Gentilini, O., Botteri, E., Rotmensz, N., Sagona, A., et al. (2009). Breast-conserving surgery in *BRCA1/2* mutation carriers: Are we approaching an answer [Epub ahead of print]? *Annals of Surgical Oncology*. Retrieved August 1, 2009, from http://www.springerlink.com/content/g84qj47540u4m086/fulltext.pdf

Genetics Home Reference. (2009). *HBB*. Retrieved September 23, 2009, from http://ghr.nlm.nih.gov/gene=hbb

International Human Genome Sequencing Consortium. (2001). Initial sequencing and analysis of the human genome. *Nature, 409*(6822), 860–921.

Jenkins, J., & Calzone, K. (2007). Genomics to health: Establishing the essential nursing competencies for genetics and genomics. *Journal of Nursing Scholarship, 39*(1), 10–16.

Khoury, M., Feero, W., Reyes, M., Citrin, T., Freedman, A., Leonard, D., et al. (2009). The genomic applications in practice and prevention network. *Genetics in Medicine, 11*(7), 488–494.

Klein, G. (1988). Oncogenes and tumor suppressor genes. *Acta Oncologica, 27*(4), 427–437.

Kurian, A., McClure, L., John, E., Horn-Ross, P., Ford, J., & Clarke, C. (2009). Second primary breast cancer occurrence according to hormone receptor status. *Journal of the National Cancer Institute, 101*(15), 1058–1065.

Kutlar, A. (2007). Sickle cell disease: A multigenic perspective of a single gene disorder. *Hemoglobin, 31*(2), 209–224.

Loeb, L.A., Springgate, C.F., & Battula, N. (1974). Errors in DNA replication as a basis of malignant changes. *Cancer Research, 34*(9), 2311–2321.

Loescher, L.J., & Merkle, C.J. (2005). The interface of genomic technologies and nursing. *Journal of Nursing Scholarship, 37*(2), 111–119.

Lynch, H.T., Follett, K.L., Lynch, P.M., Albano, W.A., Mailliard, J.L., & Pierson, R.L. (1979). Family history in an oncology clinic. Implications for cancer genetics. *JAMA, 242*(12), 1268–1272.

McWhinney, S., & McLeod, H. (2009). Using germ line genotype in cancer pharmacogenomic studies. *Pharmacogenomics, 10*(3), 489–493.

Miki, Y., Swensen, J., Shattuck-Eidens, D., Futreal, P.A., Harshman, K., Tavtigian, S., et al. (1994). A strong candidate for the breast and ovarian cancer susceptibility gene *BRCA1*. *Science, 266*(5182), 66–71.

National Cancer Institute. (2005, January). *Understanding cancer series: Molecular diagnostics*. Retrieved July 8, 2009, from http://www.cancer.gov/cancertopics/understandingcancer/moleculardiagnostics

National Cancer Institute. (2009, August). *NCI features: Toward personalized cancer care*. Retrieved November 10, 2009, from http://www.cancer.gov/features/personalizedcare2009

National Cancer Institute Office of Cancer Genomics. (2009). *Understanding cancer at the molecular level to improve prevention, early detection, diagnosis, and treatment*. Retrieved June 24, 2009, from http://ocg.cancer.gov/

National Human Genome Research Institute. (2009). *About the institute: A history and timeline*. Retrieved October 20, 2009, from http://www.genome.gov/10001763

Netterwald, J. (2009, September). Drug transporters: Easy as ABC? *Drug Discovery and Development*. Retrieved November 10, 2009, from http://www.dddmag.com/article-Drug-Transporters-Easy-As-ABC-090809.aspx

Nowell, P.C., & Hungerford, D.A. (1961). Chromosome studies in human leukemia. II. Chronic granulocytic leukemia. *Journal of the National Cancer Institute, 27*, 1013–1035.

Olive, P.L. (1998). The role of DNA single- and double-strand breaks in cell killing by ionizing radiation. *Radiation Research, 150*(Suppl. 5), S42–S51.

Oncology Nursing Society. (n.d.). *Vision, mission, and core values*. Retrieved November 10, 2009, from http://www.ons.org/about/vision

Oregon Health and Science University. (n.d.). *CROET Research Centers—(Neuro)toxicogenomics and Child Health Research Center: What is toxicogenomics?* Retrieved November 10, 2009, from http://www.ohsu.edu/croet/research/centers/toxicogenomics/whatis.html

Peters, J., Dimond, E., & Jenkins, J. (1997). Clinical applications of genetic technologies to cancer care. *Cancer Nursing, 20*(5), 359–377.

Ponte, P.R. (2004). The American health care system at a crossroads: An overview of the American Organization of Nurse Executives monograph. *Online Journal of Issues in Nursing, 9*(2). Retrieved September 23, 2009, from http://www.nursingworld.org/MainMenuCategories/ANAMarketplace/ANAPeriodicals/OJIN/TableofContents/Volume92004/No2May04/NurseExecutivesMonograph.aspx

PRWeb. (2009, June). *HolGenTech demonstrates first-ever PDA combination with high performance genome computing at Boston consumer genetics conference* [Press release]. Retrieved September 23, 2009, from http://www.prweb.com/releases/2009/06/prweb2549724.htm

Scheuner, M., de Vries, H., Kim, B., Meili, R., Olmstead, S., & Teleki, S. (2009). Are electronic health records ready for genomic medicine? *Genetics in Medicine, 11*(7), 510–517.

Steinberg, M.H. (1996). Modulation of the phenotypic diversity of sickle cell anemia. *Hemoglobin, 20*(1), 1–19.

Tolliday, N., Clemons, P.A., Ferraiolo, P., Koehler, A., Lewis, T.A., Xiaohua, L., et al. (2006). Small molecules, big players: The National Cancer Institute's initiative for chemical genetics. *Cancer Research, 66*(18), 8935–8942.

Tranin, A.S., Masny, A., & Jenkins, J. (Eds.). (2003). *Genetics in oncology practice: Cancer risk assessment*. Pittsburgh, PA: Oncology Nursing Society.

van Erp, N.P., Eechoute, K., van der Veldt, A.A., Haanen, J.B., Reyners, A.K.L., Mathijssen, R.H.J., et al. (2009). Pharmacogenetic pathway analysis for determination of sunitinib-induced toxicity. *Journal of Clinical Oncology, 27*(26), 4406–4412.

Venter, J.C., Adams, M.D., Myers, E.W., Li, P.W., Mural, R.J., Sutton, G.G., et al. (2001). The sequence of the human genome. *Science, 291*(5507), 1304–1351.

Weinshilboum, R.M., & Wang, L. (2006). Pharmacogenetics and pharmacogenomics: Development, science, and translation. *Annual Review of Genomics and Human Genetics, 7*, 223–245.

SECTION I

Genetic and Genomic Fundamental Principles for Oncology Nursing

CHAPTER 1 THE SCOPE OF CANCER GENETICS AND GENOMICS NURSING PRACTICE

CHAPTER 2 BIOLOGY OF CANCER

CHAPTER 1

The Scope of Cancer Genetics and Genomics Nursing Practice

Kathleen A. Calzone, MSN, RN, APNG, FAAN, and Karen Greco, PhD, RN, MSN, ANP-BC

> **Professional Responsibilities Domain:**
> - Examine competency of practice on a regular basis, identifying areas of strength as well as areas in which professional development related to genetics and genomics would be beneficial (Consensus Panel on Genetic/Genomic Nursing Competencies, 2009)

INTRODUCTION

Traditionally, knowledge of genetics has been viewed as useful but not necessary to nursing practice (Prows, Glass, Nicol, Skirton, & Williams, 2005). In the 1990s, cancer genetics emerged as a medical specialty, introducing new options to identify individuals with an inherited susceptibility to cancer (Biesecker & Garber, 1995). The influence of genetics on cancer care has continued to expand with the transition into genomics, the interaction of multiple genes and the environment and how they affect cancer development, screening, diagnosis, and treatment. With the rapid translation of genetics and genomics into the clinical arena, the implications for oncology nursing are profound and have changed the scope of oncology nursing practice (Calzone, Lea, & Masny, 2006).

Evidence for the broad implications of genetics and genomics on cancer care spans the entire cancer care continuum from conception to end of life. Genetic and genomic information is being used not just to predict risk but also to increase the understanding of the biology of the disease, develop novel screening and diagnostic modalities, characterize malignancies with greater precision, establish tumor-specific treatment regimens, develop novel therapeutic modalities, and optimize medication response through the elucidation of drug metabolism. Cancer care is in the midst of a transition from traditional disease-oriented therapies to one of personalized care secondary to genetic and genomic information and technology.

The diffusion of genetics and genomics into cancer care hinges on the ability of oncology healthcare providers, including nurses, to incorporate this information and technology into their practice (Khoury et al., 2007). The science of genetics and genomics is the foundation of oncology nursing practice because at the cellular level, cancer is a complex disease consisting of multiple genetic changes (Calzone et al., 2006). Genetics and genomics practice is no longer just a specialty limited to care of the 5%–10% of individuals with an inherited susceptibility to cancer, but also influences the care provided by nurses to all individuals at risk for or affected by any form of cancer. Oncology nurses are challenged with developing and implementing nursing interventions that take into account the influence of a person's genotype when providing care. Cancer predisposition genetic testing and tumor genotyping have become much more widespread, resulting in the availability of more tailored interventions for cancer screening, surveillance, risk reduction, and treatment.

The vast majority of oncology nurses at all levels of educational preparation have had no instruction in genetics and genomics as a basic science or preparation regarding the unique implications of genetic and genomic information (Peterson, Rieger, Marani, deMoor, & Gritz, 2001; Prows et al., 2005). As a result, oncology nurses currently are limited in their understanding of genetic and genomic concepts and their ability to incorporate genetics and genomics into their practice. Oncology nurses at both the general and advanced practice levels must be competent in a basic foundation in genetics and genomics to practice in today's oncology healthcare environment. Oncology nurses who are involved in the subspecialty of cancer genetics require extensive ongoing educational preparation, clinical experience, and credentialing by the Genetic Nursing Credentialing Commission (Cook, Kase, Middelton, & Monsen, 2003). Details of credentialing in the specialty of nursing and genetics are covered in Chapter 14.

WHAT INFLUENCES THE SCOPE OF NURSING PRACTICE?

Genetic and genomic advances applicable to oncology care have expanded the scope of oncology nursing practice and highlight the critical need for oncology nurses to have a foundational understanding of the scientific underpinning of genetics and genomics. Although nurses are bound by the scope of nursing practice as defined by the American Nurses Association (ANA), state boards of nursing, and nursing specialty organizations, few nurses understand how these documents influence their practice. Scope of nursing practice refers to the activities that an individual can perform within a specific profession, for example, whom the practitioner can treat and under what circumstances (Klein, 2007). ANA (2004) broadly defines the scope of nursing practice at the basic and advanced practice level for the entire profession. Scope of practice is further refined in the United States by individual states through each state's Nurse Practice Act, which defines the legal authority for registered nurses (RNs) and advanced practice nurses (APNs) to practice in that state. Individual state boards of nursing regulate nursing practice at the state level, define the legal requirements that must be met to practice within that state, and are responsible for enforcing the state Nurse Practice Act. Specialty organizations further refine the scope of nursing practice within a given specialty by defining additional activities that can be performed specific to that specialty. For oncology nurses, the Oncology Nursing Society defines the scope of practice (Brant & Wickham, 2004; Jacobs, 2003). For nurses practicing in genetics and genomics, the International Society of Nurses in Genetics (ISONG, 2007) defines the scope of practice. Scope and standards of specialty nursing practice in the United States are the responsibility of professional nursing organizations who use as the foundation the scope and standards of practice that apply to all nurses as defined by ANA (2004).

INTERFACING THE ONCOLOGY AND THE GENETIC AND GENOMIC SCOPES OF NURSING PRACTICE

Oncology nursing care is holistic and complex, interfacing with the scope of practice of numerous nursing specialties, especially genomics. When considering the biology of cancer, a disease that is genomic at the level of the cell, the scope of oncology nursing practice falls within the domain of the definition of genetic and genomic nursing.

> Genetics/genomics nursing is the protection, promotion, and optimization of health and abilities, prevention of illness and injury, alleviation of suffering through the diagnosis of human response, and advocacy in the care of the genetic and genomic health of individuals, families, communities, and populations. This includes health issues, genetic conditions, and diseases or susceptibilities to diseases caused or influenced by genes in interaction with other risk factors that may require nursing care. (ISONG, 2007, p. 2)

The genetics and genomics specialty is different from most other nursing specialties that interface with oncology nursing in that it affects the entire continuum of cancer care from conception to end of life (Calzone et al., 2006). The genetic and genomic influence on cancer care includes identifying at-risk individuals; using gene expression profiles to characterize disease, determine aggressiveness, and optimize therapeutic decision making; developing genetically and genomically targeted therapies; and using pharmacogenomics to more precisely predict outcomes of medications.

DIMENSIONS OF CANCER GENETIC AND GENOMIC NURSING PRACTICE

Four levels differentiate the scope of oncology nursing practice in genetics and genomics: general oncology nurses, general oncology nurses with a subspecialty in genetics, advanced practice oncology nurses, and advanced practice oncology nurses with a subspecialty in genetics (see Figure 1-1). The features that distinguish one level of practice from another include educational preparation, professional experience, practice specialty, and specific job roles and responsibilities. As an example, general oncology nurses may specialize in a particular area, such as radiation oncology or chemotherapy, and some tasks and job responsibilities may be the same as those of APNs. However, this is not equivalent to practicing at the advanced practice level, which is defined by educational preparation and overall job responsibilities.

All oncology nurses, regardless of their level of practice in genetics and genomics, are responsible for delivering care within the framework of the nursing process and the boundaries of the scope of oncology nursing practice as defined by ANA and ONS (ANA, 2004; Brant & Wickham, 2004; Jacobs, 2003). The scope of practice outlined in this chapter more clearly delineates the role of oncology nurses in cancer genetics. The cancer genetics nursing role is encompassed by the scope of practice in oncology nursing. The practice of genetics oncology nursing, as in all oncology nursing, incorporates the roles of direct caregiver, educator, consultant, administrator, and researcher. Oncology nursing practice that integrates genetics and genomics extends to all care delivery settings in which clients experiencing or at risk for developing cancer receive health care, education, and counseling for prevention, screening, early detection, treatment, and rehabilitation.

FIGURE 1-1. LEVELS OF ONCOLOGY NURSING PRACTICE IN GENETICS AND GENOMICS

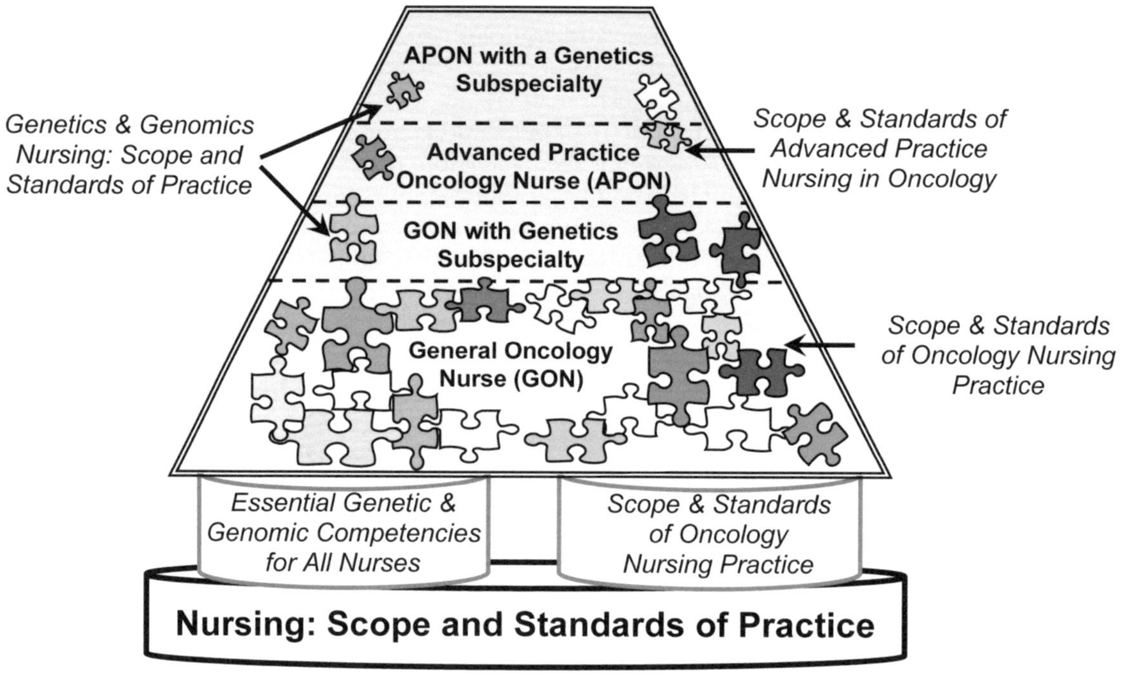

Note. Copyright 2008 by Karen E. Greco. Used with permission.

At all four practice levels, nurses incorporate theoretical knowledge of genetics and genomics into their role as direct care providers, coordinators, consultants, educators, researchers, and administrators (Middelton, Dimond, Calzone, Davis, & Jenkins, 2002). General oncology nurses and advanced practice oncology nurses use genetic and genomic information in a manner consistent with their educational preparation and the role, scope, and standards of oncology nursing as established by ONS (Brant & Wickham, 2004; Jacobs, 2003). At both levels, the genetic and genomic knowledge integrated into practice has broad applicability and limited depth. Just as all oncology nurses are expected to comprehend and incorporate into their practice the basic tenets of carcinogenesis, the same expectation is applied to cancer genetics and genomics because cancer is a genomic disease. APNs in oncology with a genetics subspecialty are prepared at the master's or doctoral level with additional training in genetics.

Scope of practice for APNs in genetics, oncology, or any other specialty depends upon basic education as a nurse combined with additional specialized training that entitles the APN to practice in areas beyond the scope of the RN. All APNs must first be trained and recognized by their state of practice with their RN license and are additionally certified in their advanced practice specialty (Klein, 2007).

INCORPORATION OF CANCER GENETICS AND GENOMICS IN VARIOUS PRACTICE SETTINGS

The incorporation of genetics and genomics into oncology nursing practice occurs in settings that encompass the entire spectrum of cancer care. This includes settings of health promotion, prevention, and detection; surgical, medical, and radiation oncology; and bone marrow transplantation. Cancer genetics and genomics is not simply a subspecialty; it is the scientific basis for understanding the process of carcinogenesis and the response of cancer to intervention. Therefore, genetics and genomics permeate all aspects of oncology nursing practice and have implications for nurses in any and all oncology practice settings. Examples of practice settings in oncology resulting from genetics and genomics advances include, but are not limited to, cancer genetics centers, laboratories offering genetic testing and tumor profiling, private industry (including clinical and biotechnology laboratories and pharmaceutical companies), and cancer genomics education programs. As genetic services continue to expand into a variety of settings, especially primary care settings, so too will genetics nursing practice.

SCOPE OF ONCOLOGY NURSING PRACTICE IN GENETICS AND GENOMICS

General Oncology Nurses

Nurses at the general level apply genetic and genomic knowledge in their practice by identifying, referring, educating, supporting, treating, and caring for clients at risk for or affected by cancer. The general oncology nurse requires knowledge of genetic and genomic principles as they relate to the assessment of cancer through screening, early-detection methods, prevention practices, and treatment. In this era of direct to consumer marketing, clients are becoming more aware of the genetic and genomic contribution to health and illness (Gray & Olopade, 2003; Wolfberg, 2006). As a consequence, general oncology nurses are addressing clients' questions about genetics and genomics as well as referring them to genetics professionals when indicated. In terms of cancer genetic and genomic practice, general oncology nurses function similar to nurses at the beginner or advanced-beginner stage (Benner, 2000). As Benner described, these stages of practice are characterized by limited practical experience in cancer genetics and genomics, functioning directed by rules and guidelines. General oncology nurses do not have the knowledge base or experience in cancer genetics and genomics to prioritize the importance of genetic and genomic information or know what to expect in certain situations regarding genetic and genomic interventions. Practice by general oncology nurses related to genetic and genomic conditions and interventions predominately focuses on the accomplishment of tasks. However, many of these tasks will have a genetic and genomic component. For example, general oncology nurses will collect family histories, educate clients on and administer genetically and genomically targeted therapies, collect biospecimens for clinical or research purposes that include evaluation of genetic or genomic information, and assess clients for medications or other substances that may affect drug metabolism that is regulated by genes such as the cytochrome P450 system. As such, general oncology nurses must achieve the basic competencies in genetics and genomics to practice in today's oncology healthcare environment (Consensus Panel on Genetic/Genomic Nursing Competencies, 2009). For example, the ability to identify a client who needs a cancer genetics referral and refer them to an appropriate genetics professional is one of the core competencies.

General Oncology Nurses With a Subspecialty in Genetics

Nurses at this level are oncology nurses whose education and clinical training in genetics and genomics extends beyond that of general oncology nurses. The additional training is in the form of continuing education and experience specific to genetics and genomics or cancer genetics and genomics. However, this additional training does not fulfill the requirements for an advanced academic degree. General oncology nurses with a subspecialty in genetics and genomics are prepared to
- Perform genetics-specific assessments
- Monitor clients' and patients' status from the genetic and genomic perspective
- Educate and counsel clients about genetic and genomic issues
- Consult, collaborate with, and refer clients to other providers in the provision of genetic and genomic services.

General oncology nurses in cancer genetics and genomics have at minimum met the following criteria:
- Completion of an accredited baccalaureate program in nursing
- Continuing education in genetics
- Clinical experience as a basic genetic nurse with a greater than 50% genetic practice component.

Among the factors that distinguish general oncology genetic nursing practice from basic oncology nursing practice are expanded practice skills and knowledge in cancer genetics and genomics (ISONG, 2007).

Advanced Practice Oncology Nurses

Because advanced practice nursing requires substantial theoretical knowledge and proficient use of this knowledge in providing care, APNs understand the role of genetics and genomics in cancer care to a greater degree than do general practice nurses. Although APNs may work at the advanced practice level in oncology, in terms of genetics and genomics they may be at the beginner or advanced-beginner stage (Benner, 2000). Advanced practice oncology nurses may be faced with using theoretical knowledge uncoupled with practical experience when aspects of genetic and genomic information must be incorporated into care. Similar to general oncology nurses, when presented with an atypical case, advanced practice oncology nurses may not fully know the significance of genetic and genomic information and may not completely see the implications of a situation or know when action is needed (Benner). Nurses at both levels need genetics practitioners to help them identify what they cannot recognize. For instance, advanced practice oncology nurses may recognize that an individual with multiple primary cancers is a red flag for an inherited susceptibility to cancer. However, working with the genetic practitioner would provide expertise to determine what, if any, cancer syndrome could be associated with the individual's multiple primary cancers and whether genetic testing for a specific gene or genes is an option.

Oncology nursing practice in genetics and genomics at the advanced practice level builds on the scope of practice described for general oncology nurses. For example, advanced practice oncology nurses will interpret a family history and refer for further evaluation if indicated, educate clients and other nurses on the administration of genetically and genomically targeted therapies, interpret the results of analysis performed on biospecimens for clinical or research purposes that include evaluation of genetic or genomic information, and assess and manage clients experiencing drug toxicities that may be the result of variations in genes such as the cytochrome P450 system. As such, advanced practice oncology nurses also must achieve a basic competency in genetics and genomics to practice in today's oncology healthcare environment.

Advanced Practice Oncology Nurses With a Subspecialty in Genetics

Nurses at this level are APNs whose education and clinical training in genetics and genomics extends beyond that of advanced practice oncology nurses. The additional training in the form of an academic degree, continuing education, and experience specific to genetics and genomics or cancer genetics and genomics prepares nurses to
- Perform genetics-specific assessment and diagnosis
- Conduct a physical examination from a genetic perspective
- Develop and implement genetic and genomic–specific treatment plans
- Monitor clients' and patients' status from the genetic and genomic perspective
- Educate and counsel clients about genetic and genomic issues
- Consult, collaborate with, and refer clients to other providers in the provision of genetic and genomics services.

APNs in cancer genetics and genomics have at minimum met the following three criteria:
- Completion of an accredited graduate (masters or doctoral) program in nursing
- Completion of graduate-level genetic course work, which includes content about human, molecular, biochemical, and population genetics and genomics, technologic applications, and therapeutic modalities
- Participation in genetic and genomic clinical training supervised by any combination of the following: genetics APN, clinical geneticist, and genetic counselor.

Among the factors that distinguish advanced genetics nursing practice from basic genetics nursing practice are the complexity of decision making, leadership skills, ability to negotiate complex organizations, and expanded practice skills and knowledge in nursing and cancer genetics and genomics (ISONG, 2007). Advanced practice oncology nurses with a subspecialty in genetics and genomics:
- Ascertain which individuals, families, and populations need cancer genetic and genomic services.
- Provide and manage comprehensive care, which includes state-of-the-art cancer genetic counseling, screening, diagnosis, and therapy.
- Develop, evaluate, and improve cancer genetic and genomic services.
- Educate individuals, families, the general public, and healthcare professionals about cancer genetics and genomics.
- Assess, deliberate on, and develop recommendations about the ethical, legal, and social consequences of new and existing genetic and genomic services and technology.

Advanced practice oncology nurses with a subspecialty in genetics practice at the proficient or expert stage (Benner, 2000). At this level of practice, genetics and genomics are integrated into every aspect of oncology nursing care. Advanced practice oncology nurses with a subspecialty in genetics are able to establish the relevancy of information, rely on extensive practical knowledge from both oncology and genetics and genomics, and in specific clinical situations, understand the significance of the client's history, grasp the current situation, and modify plans in response to events. The skills of advanced practice oncology nurses with a subspecialty in genetics include, but are not limited to, those described in Table 1-1.

TABLE 1-1. Scope of Oncology Nursing Practice in Genetics: Advanced Practice Oncology Nurse With a Subspecialty in Genetics

Role	Competency
Direct care	• Conducts an in-depth personal and family assessment based on personal, medical, occupational, environmental, and family risk factors • Performs an assessment based on prior understanding of genetic conditions and practical knowledge of what ordinarily would be expected • Constructs a detailed pedigree expanded to the degree of reliable information but a minimum of three generations, including confirmation with medical records • Establishes the relevancy of genetic information • In collaboration with the cancer genetics healthcare team, uses genetic assessment data to contribute to the diagnosis of genetic risk or illness for the client and his or her family • Evaluates eligibility for genetic testing or therapeutics • Provides genetic counseling, which enhances voluntary and autonomous decision making • Provides the education necessary for informed consent for genetic testing or therapeutics • Remains sensitive to the ability of individuals and families to receive and understand genetic information • Evaluates and monitors the impact of genetic conditions, therapeutics, or testing on the client and his or her extended family and intervenes as needed • Identifies events typical of a suspected or actual genetic condition or situation and modifies the nursing plan in response to these events • Responds to the needs of the client and his or her extended family • Provides psychological support to the client and his or her extended family and facilitates successful adaptive responses
Coordinator	• Coordinates and initiates the cancer genetics healthcare team's plan, including submission of genetic samples for testing, interpretation of test results, and delivery of results to the client and his or her family • Administers and/or supervises the administration of genetic therapeutics
Consultant	• Provides consultative cancer genetic expertise to staff, the client, and the client's extended family
Educator	• Conducts an assessment of the learning and psychosocial needs of the client and his or her immediate family regarding genetic services and responds to needs that are both identified and anticipated • Delivers genetic counseling services, answers complex genetic questions, and addresses concerns • Develops further interventions based on typical expectations in regard to the suspected or actual genetic condition and the current situation • Evaluates psychosocial and physical responses to genetic testing, diagnosis, and treatment • Integrates the evaluation of responses into all aspects of care
Researcher	• Coordinates genetic clinical trials and uses research findings in care implementation • Participates in the development of cancer genetic research trials
Administrator	• Develops and monitors cancer genetic programs and services

Note. Based on information from Calzone et al., 2002.

SUMMARY

Regardless of their practice setting, oncology nurses have a role in the delivery of genetic and genomic services and the management of genetic information. All nurses at every level of academic preparation, role, or clinical specialty require genetic and genomic knowledge to identify, refer, support, and care for individuals at risk for or affected by cancer (Consensus Panel on Genetic/Genomic Nursing Competencies, 2009). Because lack of competence in a particular area by definition excludes it from a nurse's scope of practice (Klein, 2007), proficiency in the core competencies in genetics and genomics is critical for oncology nurses. A foundation in genetics and genomics currently is considered an essential part of baccalaureate nursing education in the United States (American Association of Colleges of Nursing, 2008), and the scope of this requirement has expanded with the publication of this latest edition of the *Essentials of Baccalaureate Education for Professional Nursing Practice*.

Genetics and genomics offer oncology nurses the opportunity to utilize new knowledge and technologies to improve health outcomes. Oncology nurses need to understand the biologic, ethical, and psychosocial impact of genetics and genomics on their nursing practice in order to effectively serve individuals, families, and communities in such areas as determining if a client is a carrier of a cancer-predisposing gene mutation, providing risk-based cancer screening, and administering standard cancer therapy or individualized pharmacogenomic therapy. The four phases of translating research into practice require that nurses appropriately and adequately integrate human genome variables into health care (Khoury et al., 2007). Oncology nurses are pivotal providers of quality healthcare services and are at the front line of closing the gap between research discoveries that are efficacious to cancer care and their successful adoption to optimize health.

REFERENCES

American Association of Colleges of Nursing. (2008). *The essentials of baccalaureate education for professional nursing practice*. Washington, DC: Author. Retrieved August 10, 2009, from http://www.aacn.nche.edu/Education/pdf/BaccEssentials08.pdf

American Nurses Association. (2004). *Nursing: Scope and standards of practice*. Washington, DC: Author.

Benner, P.E. (2000). *From novice to expert: Excellence and power in clinical nursing practice* (Commemorative ed.). Upper Saddle River, NJ: Prentice Hall Health.

Biesecker, B.B., & Garber, J. (1995). Testing and counseling adults for heritable cancer risk. *Journal of the National Cancer Institute Monographs, 1995*(17), 115–118.

Brant, J.M., & Wickham, R.S. (Eds.). (2004). *Statement on the scope and standards of oncology nursing practice*. Pittsburgh, PA: Oncology Nursing Society.

Calzone, K., Jenkins, J., & Masny, A. (2002). Core competencies in cancer genetics for advanced practice oncology nurses. *Oncology Nursing Forum, 29*(9), 1327–1333.

Calzone, K., Lea, D.H., & Masny, A. (2006). Non-Hodgkin's lymphoma as an exemplar of the effects of genetics and genomics. *Journal of Nursing Scholarship, 38*(4), 335–343.

Consensus Panel on Genetic/Genomic Nursing Competencies. (2009). *Essentials of genetic and genomic nursing: Competencies, curricula guidelines, and outcome indicators* (2nd ed.). Silver Spring, MD: American Nurses Association.

Cook, S.S., Kase, R., Middelton, L., & Monsen, R.B. (2003). Portfolio evaluation for professional competence: Credentialing in genetics for nurses. *Journal of Professional Nursing, 19*(2), 85–90.

Gray, S., & Olopade, O.I. (2003). Direct-to-consumer marketing of genetic tests for cancer: Buyer beware. *Journal of Clinical Oncology, 21*(17), 3191–3193.

International Society of Nurses in Genetics. (2007). *Genetics/genomics nursing: Scope and standards of practice*. Silver Spring, MD: American Nurses Association.

Jacobs, L.A. (Ed.). (2003). *Statement on the scope and standards of advanced practice nursing in oncology* (3rd ed.). Pittsburgh, PA: Oncology Nursing Society.

Khoury, M.J., Gwinn, M., Yoon, P.W., Dowling, N., Moore, C.A., & Bradley, L. (2007). The continuum of translation research in genomic medicine: How can we accelerate the appropriate integration of human genome discoveries into health care and disease prevention? *Genetics in Medicine, 9*(10), 665–674.

Klein, T.A. (2007). Scope of practice and the nurse practitioner: Regulation, competency, expansion, and evolution. *Topics in Advanced Practice Nursing eJournal, 7*(3). Retrieved December 7, 2009, from http://www.medscape.com/viewarticle/495161

Middelton, L., Dimond, E., Calzone, K., Davis, J., & Jenkins, J. (2002). The role of the nurse in cancer genetics. *Cancer Nursing, 25*(3), 196–206.

Peterson, S.K., Rieger, P.T., Marani, S.K., deMoor, C., & Gritz, E.R. (2001). Oncology nurses' knowledge, practice, and educational needs regarding cancer genetics. *American Journal of Medical Genetics, 98*(1), 3–12.

Prows, C.A., Glass, M., Nicol, M.J., Skirton, H., & Williams, J. (2005). Genomics in nursing education. *Journal of Nursing Scholarship, 37*(3), 196–202.

Wolfberg, A. (2006). Genes on the web—direct-to-consumer marketing of genetic testing. *New England Journal of Medicine, 355*(6), 543–545.

CHAPTER 2
Biology of Cancer

Julia Eggert, PhD, APRN-BC, GNP, AOCN®, and Monica Kasse, BS

Professional Practice Domain:
Nursing Assessment: Applying/Integrating Genetic and Genomic Knowledge
- Demonstrate an understanding of the relationship of genetics and genomics to health, prevention, screening, diagnostics, prognostics, selection of treatment, and monitoring of treatment effectiveness

(Consensus Panel on Genetic/Genomic Nursing Competencies, 2009)

INTRODUCTION

Learning about **genes** and their function means learning a new language. To help to build your genetics vocabulary, note the terms presented in boldface in this chapter. These are key terms, and their definitions appear in the glossary. Other ways to improve your genetics language skills are to continue reading about cancer genetics, visit Web sites about genetics, and join professional groups that have genetics as their focus. (See the resources listed in Chapter 16.) Remember that immersion—reading, practicing, and speaking—is the best way to learn any language. The language of cancer genetics may seem overwhelming at first. Do not be discouraged if the concepts are not clear after one reading. Comprehension of the language will increase as you build your vocabulary.

Clinically, cancer includes more than 200 diseases that vary in regard to age of the patient at onset and disease growth rate, differentiation, detectability, invasiveness, metastatic potential, response to treatment, and prognosis. On the molecular and cellular levels, however, cancer actually may be just a few diseases caused by similar genetic alterations and defects in **cell** function (Ward, Brueggemeier, Caligiuri, Gahbauer, & Kraut, 2005). Ultimately, cancer results from **abnormal gene expression**, which can include abnormal activation of a gene that is largely attributable to alterations in deoxyribonucleic acid (DNA) and gene **transcription** or **translation**. This chapter will present an overview of cancer biology, focusing on genetic mechanisms that may transform a normal cell into a cancer cell.

MODELS OF CANCER DEVELOPMENT

The two well-known models for the development of a malignancy are the random hit model (also known as the stochastic model) and the cancer stem cell model. In the random hit model, each cancer cell has the ability to proliferate and form new tumors. In the cancer stem cell model, cells have limited ability to proliferate, with a few rare cells identified as cancer stem cells that have the ability to form new tumors (Buchstaller, Quintana, & Morrison, 2008; Schinazi, 2006).

A few small subpopulations of cancer cells are believed to be cancer stem cells. This depends on the type of cancer where the ratio of cancer stem cells can range from 1:10,000 to 1:100. Similar to normal stem cells, cancer stem cells have the ability to self-renew; differentiate; express telomerase (the **enzyme** responsible for making **telomeres** [end of **chromosomes**] longer); prevent programmed cell death, which allows immortalization of the cell; migrate; and metastasize. One of these factors, expression of telomerase, an enzyme that prevents the destruction of the telomere, is known to be associated with longevity of cell life. Short telomeres are associated with a shorter life span. Thus, the cancer stem cells have an extended life enhanced by the protected telomere at the ends of the chromosome and the inability of the cell to have programmed cell death. Of note are the cancer stem cells that remain in the G_0 resting phase of the cell cycle. Because they are not rapidly dividing cancer stem cells, they are not sensitive to chemotherapy and radiation (Wicha, Liu, & Dontu, 2006).

DNA AND CHROMOSOMES: STRUCTURE AND FUNCTION

The human **genome**, or "master blueprint" of human genetic material, consists of 23 pairs of chromosomes. A chromosome is a single double-helix DNA molecule with a continuous string of millions of **base pairs** that is long, intricately coiled, and composed of tightly interspersed **proteins**, called **histones** (see Figure 2-1).

Histones are like spools that control the long threads of DNA and package them into a tight coil so DNA can fit into the **nucleus** of the cell. The coiling is important because if all the strands of DNA in a person's body were unwound and set end to end, they would stretch almost six feet but would be only 50 trillionths of an inch wide. This long but thin physical structure would cause the DNA to be extremely fragile, hence the need for tight packaging to protect the DNA message. Once the DNA is coiled around the histones, it continues twisting until it is tightly wound (much like continual twisting of a rope which will coil back upon itself) until it forms a **chromatid**, which enables the chromosomes to be seen for karyotyping, during the metaphase of cell division (Klug & Cummings, 2005; U.S. Department of Energy Office of Science Office of Biological and Environmental Research, n.d.).

The 23 pairs of chromosomes consist of 22 pairs of **autosomes**, or nonsex chromosomes, and one pair of sex chromosomes (XX for female, or XY for male) that reside within the nucleus of every human cell (National Cancer Institute [NCI], 2005). People inherit one chromosome of the pair from their father and the other from their mother. A chromosome has a short arm ("p" for "petite") and a long arm ("q" follows "p" in the alphabet) with a unique banding pattern that identifies specific regions. These regions are numbered from the **centromere** (a constricted region of the chromosome where the p and q arms meet) to the end of each arm (see Figure 2-2).

For example, a gene that defines susceptibility to breast and ovarian cancer, *BRCA1*, is on chromosome 17q, and band position 21 on the long arm of chromosome 17. If the position of the gene is uncertain, a range might be noted, such as 17q21–24 (Genetics Home Reference, 2009a).

Chapter 2. Biology of Cancer   15

FIGURE 2-1   PACKAGING OF DNA

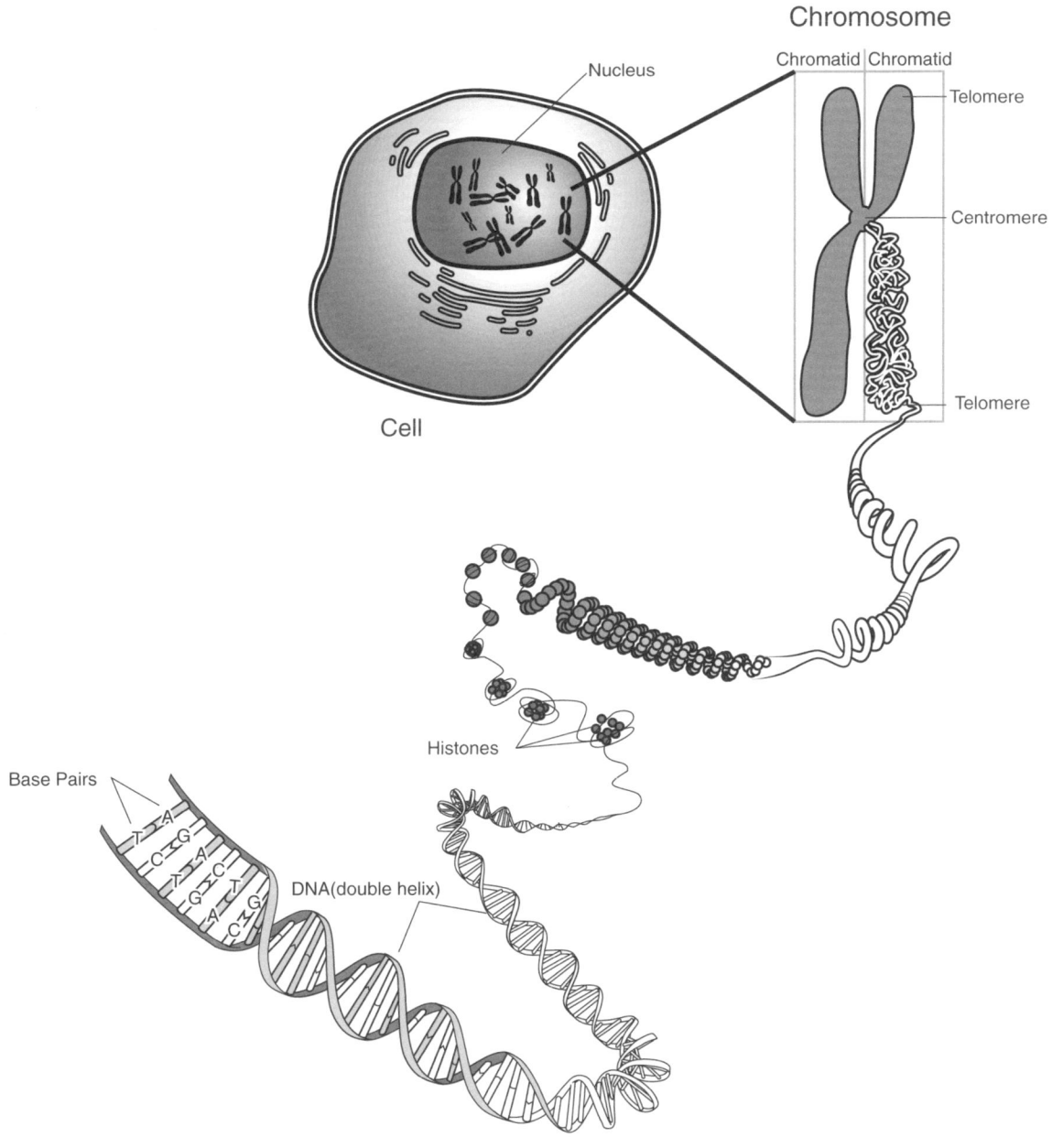

Note. From *Chromosome,* by National Human Genome Research Institute, n.d. Retrieved November 9, 2009, from http://www.genome.gov/Pages/Hyperion/DIR/VIP/Glossary/Illustration/Pdf/chromosome.pdf.

FIGURE 2-2 CHROMOSOME

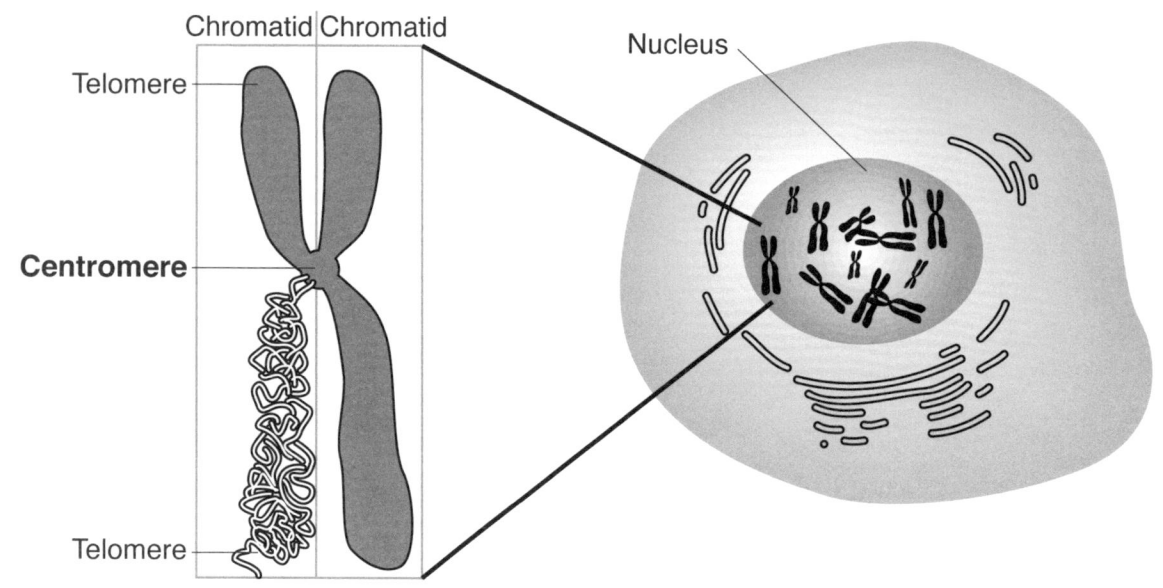

The p arm is above the centromere; the q arm is below the centromere.

Note. From *Centromere,* by National Human Genome Research Institute, n.d. Retrieved November 9, 2009, from http://www.genome.gov/Pages/Hyperion/DIR/VIP/Glossary/Illustration/Pdf/centromere.pdf.

Each DNA molecule consists of anti-parallel double strands wound around each other to resemble a twisted staircase (see Figure 2-3). The side strand is an arrangement of units called **nucleotides**, consisting of one sugar, one phosphate, and a nitrogenous base. The nucleotides are linked together in a chain consisting of an alternating series of sugar and phosphate molecules. The 5′ (5 prime) position of one pentose sugar ring, composed of five carbon atoms connected in a ring of sugar, is connected to the 3′ (3 prime) position of the next pentose sugar ring via a phosphate group. As a result, this "backbone" consists of 5′–3′ phosphodiester linkages. The nitrogenous bases stick out from this repetitive backbone and form the "steps" of the staircase (Klug & Cummings, 2005).

The steps of the double helix consist of four DNA bases: the pyrimidine bases (**cytosine** and **thymine**) and the purine bases (**guanine** and **adenine**). These bases form the genetic alphabet and are abbreviated C, T, G, and A, respectively. The specific order of the bases arranged along one strand of the sugar-phosphate backbone is the **DNA sequence**. By means of weak hydrogen bonds, one strand of DNA pairs with the other strand. C on one strand always pairs with G on the other strand; similarly, T always pairs with A. This phenomenon is called **complementary base pairing**, and each resulting twosome is a base pair. The human genome contains approximately three billion base pairs. Base pairing is critical for the storage, retrieval, and transfer of genetic information, whether DNA is being copied or read (D'Andrea, 2008). In double-stranded DNA, the nucleotide sequence of the upper strand is always written and read in the 5′ to 3′ direction; the lower strand is written and read in the

3′ to 5′ direction: 5′ GCA would be "read" as complementary pairing with 3′ CGT (Klug & Cummings, 2005).

> Complementary DNA base pairing (A-T and G-C) is critical for the storage, retrieval, and transfer of genetic information.

In summary, DNA is a molecule that comes in the form of a twisted ladder-like strand, called the double helix. The ladder's rungs are built with four letters of the DNA alphabet: A-C-T-G. On the strand, A always pairs with T (A-T) and C with G (C-G). The order of the paired letters is called the DNA sequence. A section of the ordered, paired letters on the strand makes words (genes), and the words make sentences (the proteins reading out how the cells and body function).

Complementary base pairs not only ensure the structural integrity of DNA but also are essential for its accurate replication. Each time a cell divides into two daughter cells, its full genome is duplicated in the nuclei of the new cells (Klug & Cummings, 2005).

Cell division in **somatic cells** (**mitosis**) results in two daughter cells with the same number of chromosomes as the parent cell (46 chromosomes). During cell division, the DNA unwinds down the middle, causing the weak hydrogen bonds between the base pairs to break. Each strand serves as a template and directs synthesis of a new complementary strand (daughter strand), with free nucleotides matching up with their complementary bases on each of the separated strands. This process allows the dividing cell to pass on its entire genetic content to its progeny (Klug & Cummings, 2005).

Germ cells, also called gametes or ovum and sperm, form during **meiosis**, a two-stage process of reduction and division. A reduction of the chromosome number by half (to 23) during meiosis is necessary so the original number of chromosomes (46) is restored following fertilization. Without this process, the number of chromosomes in offspring would be doubled (Klug & Cummings, 2005).

Genes are the smallest functional units of **inherited** information in DNA. They are segments, or regions, of DNA that occupy specific sites, or loci, on particular chromosomes. Genes consist of DNA sequences (nucleotides) that code for specific proteins. The human genome packs approximately 20,600 protein-coding genes into the 46 chromosomes (U.S.

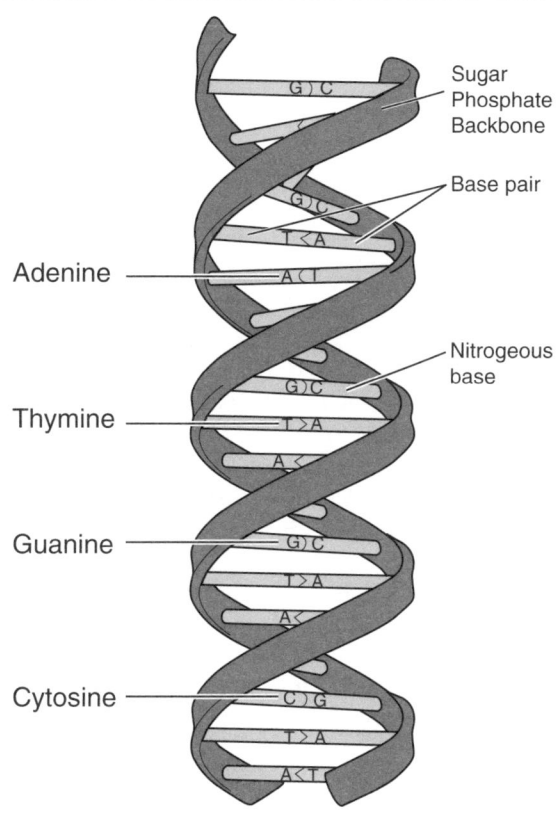

FIGURE 2-3 BASE PAIR

Note. From *Deoxyribonucleic Acid (DNA),* by National Human Genome Research Institute, n.d. Retrieved November 9, 2009, from http://www.genome.gov/Pages/Hyperion/DIR/VIP/Glossary/Illustration/Pdf/dna.pdf.

National Institutes of Health [NIH], 2004). Although each human gene often extends over thousands of bases, only about 10% of the genome includes protein-coding sequences of genes. These protein coding sequences of DNA are called **exons**. Sequences of genes with no coding function are called **introns** (see Figure 2-4). One gene can code for multiple proteins depending on where the splicing occurs. **Splicing** refers to the process of removing the introns from the **messenger ribonucleic acid** (mRNA).

Because each child inherits a set of paired chromosomes from each parent, alternate forms of genes, called **alleles**, may be present in the pair. A person with the same allele on both parent chromosomes of a chromosome pair is said to be homozygous for a particular trait; someone who has two different alleles is said to be heterozygous (National Center for Biotechnology Information [NCBI], 2004). One common example of this is the ABO blood group. One chromosome could have a Type A allele and the other chromosome a type B allele. That person would be heterozygous, or blood type AB. If both alleles are identical for type O, then that person is homozygous, or blood type O. The three possible alleles are A, B, and O, but only one is present on a chromosome at a time. Each individual would normally have two chromosomes, one from each parent with one allele for a blood type on each chromosome.

Mendel's **wild-type** genes are "typical" forms of genes found in nature, meaning that the base pairs and nucleotide sequences are in the proper order (Genetics Home Reference, 2009e). Although wild-type genes are the most common forms, small changes in the DNA code called polymorphisms can still produce normal proteins with a different DNA template from the wild-type. Polymorphisms are changes in the DNA found in at least 1% of the **population**. Most frequently, these are changes in multiple nucleotide base pair sequences that distinguish identity of families or differences between individuals. Simply, polymorphisms are what make humans different from each other. An example is shown in Figure 2-5.

Single changes in base pairs, which occur in greater than 1% of the population, are identified as **single nucleotide polymorphisms** (SNPs, pronounced "snips"). For example, a DNA sequence might change from CCG to CAG, with one nucleotide change. Mutant genes are rare, occurring in less than 1% of the population (Human Genome Project, 2008). A simple example is using a cake recipe analogy to compare polymorphisms and **mutations**. Many different flavors of cake recipes are available (polymorphisms). In rare circumstances, an ingredient is misread and replaced with another ingredient. This might result in a very flat cake that is still edible (benign mutation). Sometimes, a misread ingredient in the recipe will result in something inedible. This type of mutation might be the example for cancer. Typically, changes in the DNA recipe are not a problem for the protein outcome. Remember that many of the proteins have multiple nucleotide recipes that result in the same protein as seen in Figure 2-6. In rare circumstances, the nucleotide alterations create products that cause changes to a cell that result in the molecular distortions of malignancy.

GENE EXPRESSION

DNA has one function: to store genetic information used for the synthesis of proteins or enzymes. DNA stores this genetic information as a **genetic code**. The code consists of

FIGURE 2-4 CODING AND NONCODING REGIONS FOR PROTEINS

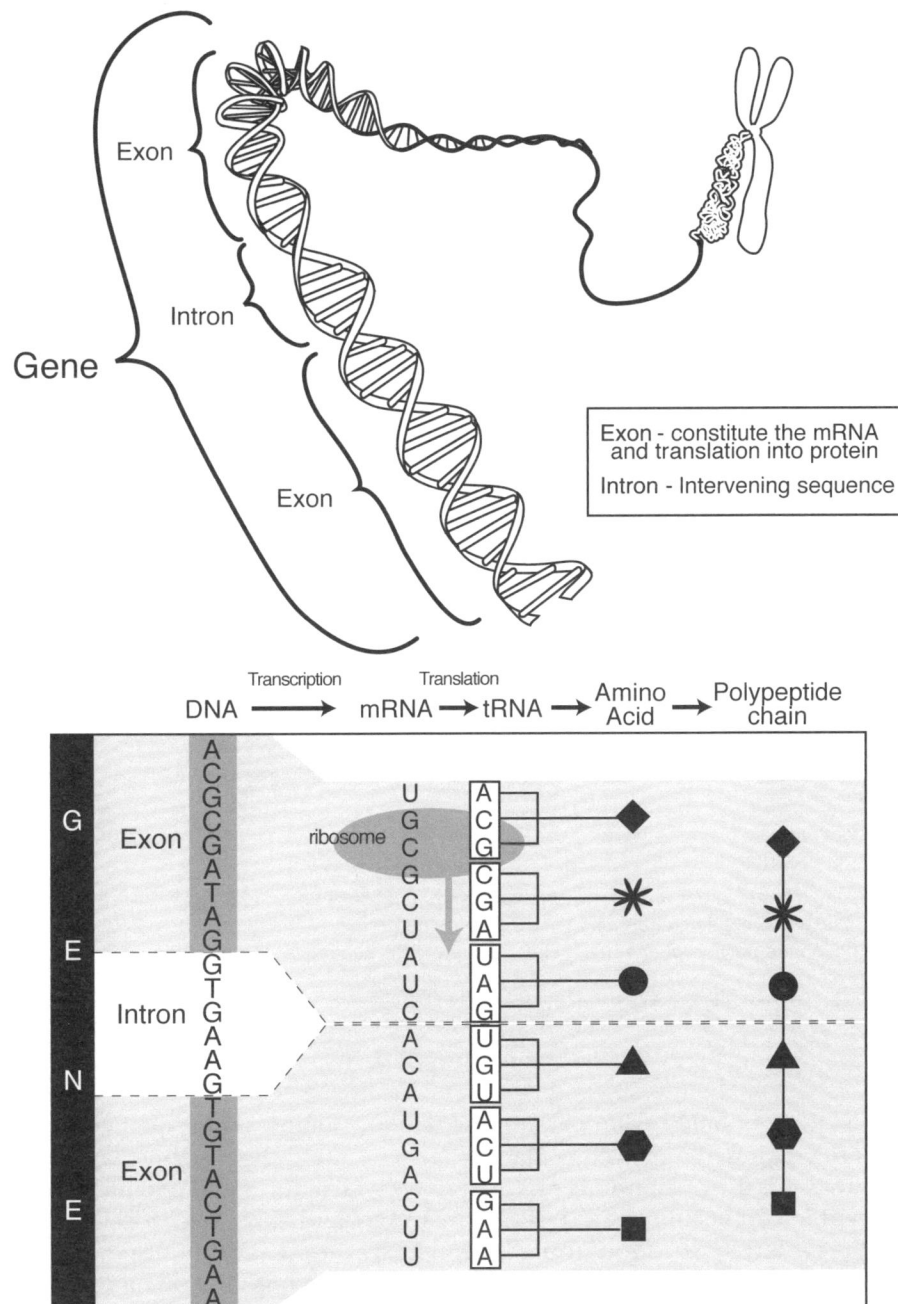

Note. From *Intron*, by National Human Genome Research Institute, n.d. Retrieved November 9, 2009, from http://www.genome.gov/Pages/Hyperion/DIR/VIP/Glossary/Illustration/Pdf/intron.pdf.

FIGURE 2-5. POLYMORPHISM

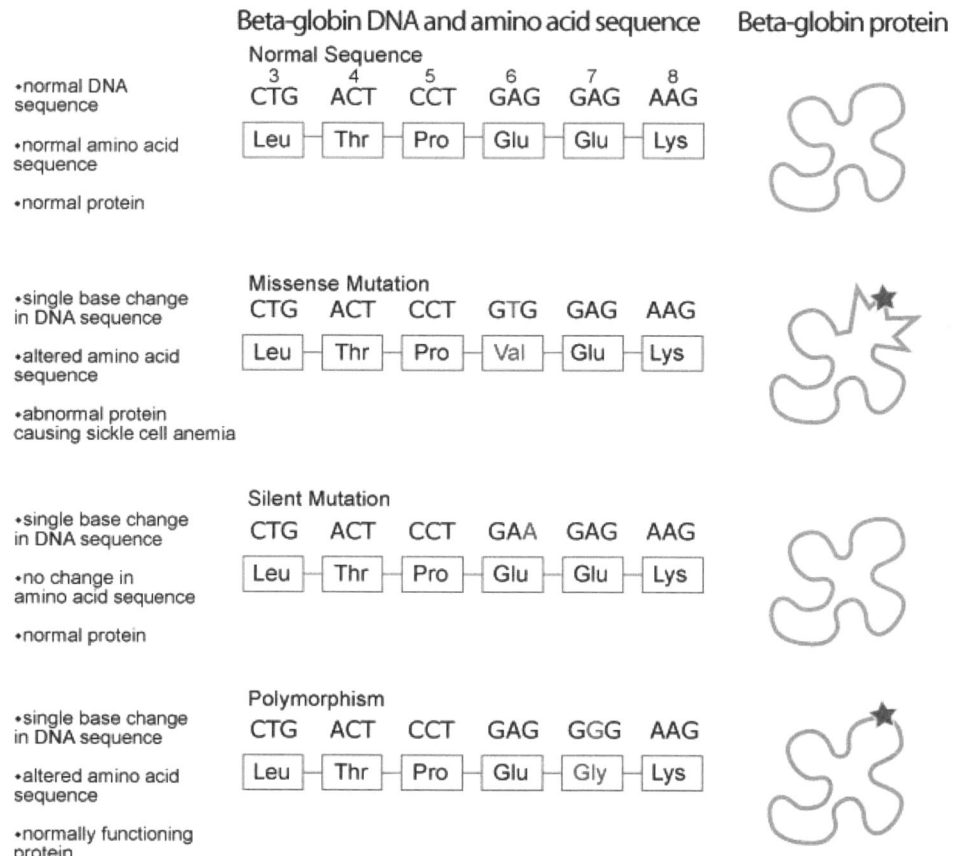

This figure compares the difference between polymorphisms and mutations in the beta-globin DNA and amino acid sequence. Note how a missense mutation changes the structure of the protein whereas a silent mutation yields the same protein in position 6. Although the polymorphism has a change in the DNA sequence, the resulting amino acid does not change the structure of the protein.

Note. This information was provided by Clinical Tools, Inc. and is copyrighted by Clinical Tools, Inc. Used with permission.

triplets of bases called **codons**, which specify the **amino acid** sequence of a protein. Proteins are composed of amino acids. Amino acids are called the body's building blocks because they are the compounds essential to body structures and chemical reactions. Of the 64 possible codons, one is a start codon (ATG) and three are stop codons (TAG, TAA, and TGA). The start codon initiates protein synthesis, and the stop codons direct termination of this synthesis. Each of the other 61 codons codes for an amino acid. Twenty amino acids are naturally occurring; more than one codon can code for the same amino acid. This overlap may protect against the detrimental effects that could occur if a mutation in a codon changed the code, thereby forming the wrong amino acid. If that happened, another codon could still code for the same amino acid as seen in Figure 2-6 (Klug & Cummings, 2005).

> Genes are regions of DNA that occupy specific locations (loci) on chromosomes. Specific DNA nucleotide sequences in genes encode specific proteins, which are the primary products of gene expression.

The primary product of **gene expression** is a protein, commonly called gene product. Protein synthesis occurs in the cytoplasm of the cell, so genetic information must travel from the cell nucleus to the cytoplasm (see Figure 2-7). This is accomplished in a process called transcription, in which **RNA** is synthesized from the genetic information encoded by DNA. In RNA, the base **uracil** (U) substitutes for T. The DNA nucleotides T, A, G, and C are used to transcribe the RNA complementary nucleotides of A, U, C, and G, respectively (Klug, Cummings, & Spencer, 2005).

FIGURE 2-6 TRANSLATION CHART OF RNA CODONS AND THEIR CORRESPONDING AMINO ACIDS OR START/STOP DESIGNATION

		Second base of codon				Third base of codon
		U	C	A	G	
First base of codon	U	UUU Phenylalanine phe / UUC / UUA Leucine leu / UUG	UCU / UCC Serine ser / UCA / UCG	UAU Tyrosine tyr / UAC / UAA STOP codon / UAG	UGU Cysteine cys / UGC / UGA STOP codon / UGG Tryptophan trp	U / C / A / G
	C	CUU / CUC Leucine leu / CUA / CUG	CCU / CCC Proline pro / CCA / CCG	CAU Histidine his / CAC / CAA Glutamine gln / CAG	CGU / CGC Arginine arg / CGA / CGG	U / C / A / G
	A	AUU / AUC Isoleucine ile / AUA / AUG Methionine met (start codon)	ACU / ACC Threonine thr / ACA / ACG	AAU Asparagine asn / AAC / AAA Lysine lys / AAG	AGU Serine ser / AGC / AGA Arginine arg / AGG	U / C / A / G
	G	GUU / GUC Valine val / GUA / GUG	GCU / GCC Alanine ala / GCA / GCG	GAU Aspartic acid asp / GAC / GAA Glutamic acid glu / GAG	GGU / GGC Glycine gly / GGA / GGG	U / C / A / G

Note. This information was provided by Clinical Tools, Inc. and is copyrighted by Clinical Tools, Inc. Used with permission.

FIGURE 2-7 PROTEIN TRANSLATION

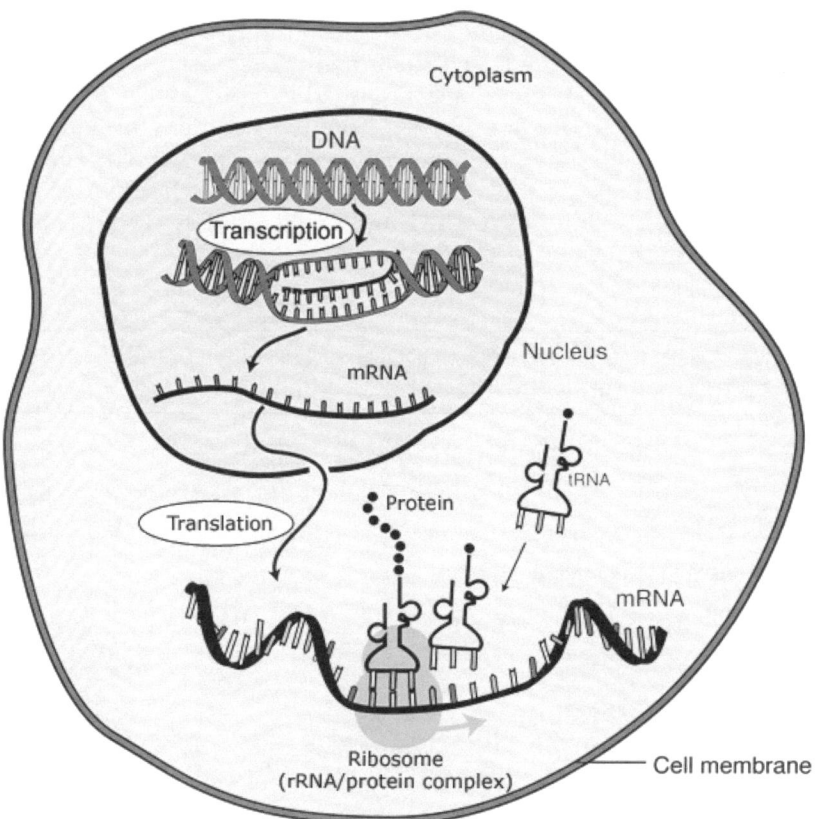

This figure emphasizes the Central Dogma of DNA→ RNA→ Protein. It specifically shows the transcription of DNA to RNA and then mRNA in the nucleus. Translation of mRNA to amino acids and protein occurs outside of the nucleus on the ribosome in the cytoplasm.

Note. This information was provided by Clinical Tools, Inc. and is copyrighted by Clinical Tools, Inc. Used with permission.

The enzymes that carry out transcription are called RNA **polymerases**. Certain DNA sequences (see the **promoter** regions discussion later in this chapter) tell RNA polymerase where to start transcription. During the course of transcription, one strand of DNA (the template) is copied into mRNA. After additional processing in the nucleus, mRNA carries the genetic message into the cytoplasm to the **ribosomes**, molecular machines in which RNA directs the assembly of the amino acids that constitute proteins. The process of amino acid assembly is called translation (Klug & Cummings, 2005).

In the translation process, each amino acid is carried to the ribosome by transfer RNA (tRNA). The tRNA docks onto a specific coding region of mRNA. For mRNA, amino acid chains are arranged in the same order as the codons of the DNA strand (Klug & Cummings, 2005). For example, the DNA sequence 5′ATGGGTGGATATCCCTAG 3′ is transcribed into the mRNA sequence 5′AUGGGUGGAUAUCCCUAG 3′. This mRNA is read as codons AUG GGU GGA UAU CCC UAG and then translated into the amino acid chain methionine-glycine-glycine-tyrosine-proline.

Amino acid chains go through post-translational changes, such as folding upon the nucleus, assembling with other chains, or dropping off a part of a chain to form the mature protein complexes that participate in specific cellular functions. These functions include directing the duplication, replacement, and differentiation of cells (Klug et al., 2005).

> Transcription copies one strand of DNA into mRNA. During translation, RNA catalyzes the assembly of amino acids for building proteins. The Central Dogma is DNA→ RNA→ Protein

As noted, SNPs, polymorphisms, and mutations occur because of change(s) in the nucleotide sequence of DNA. Everyone has cells that have harmless alterations in at least one gene, creating individual differences between human beings. Mutations occur infrequently and can alter gene structure and regulatory sites (e.g., exons). A mutation is of concern only if it gives rise to a **clonal population** of cells (see Tumorigenesis later in this chapter) or affects a cell that is particularly sensitive to mutations (Klug et al., 2005).

CAUSES OF MUTATIONS

Mutations may be inherited if they are present in the **germ line** (cells stemming from the sperm or ova), arise during **DNA replication** and **recombination** (the exchange of DNA between two parental chromosomes during meiosis), may be caused by mutagens (environmental agents that prompt mutations), or may arise spontaneously. See Figure 2-8 for an example of recombination.

> Mutations may be caused by mutagens. They occur during DNA replication or recombination, or arise spontaneously.

Errors that occur during the exact duplication of the DNA template (replication) are rare, occurring in only 1 of 100 million bases. More frequently, **DNA** rearranges itself by recombination, a process whereby DNA is lost or may be inserted into the gene. Recombination may result in loss of control of gene expression or may disrupt the coding sequence of the gene. Mutagens that damage DNA may be made by humans (e.g., pesticides, organic chemicals, alkylating agents), occur naturally (e.g., plant toxins), or be generated during normal cellular metabolism. Chemically damaged DNA can cause incorrect base pairing during replication, resulting in a mutation being passed to daughter strands. Radiation—including gamma rays, x-rays, and ultraviolet radiation—can damage and distort DNA, impairing transcription and replication. DNA spontaneously may undergo alterations that result in self-damage (Campbell & Reece, 2005). For example, one base spontaneously can change into another base, causing abnormal base pairing during subsequent replication (NCBI, 2004).

TYPES OF MUTATIONS ASSOCIATED WITH CANCER AND OTHER DISORDERS

Point Mutations

Single-base substitutions, in which a single base is substituted for another base creating a harmful effect, are called point mutations. Point mutations are the most common types of mutations. Point mutations in DNA sequences that encode proteins are classified as silent, missense, or nonsense mutations as included in Table 2-1 (Klug & Cummings, 2005).

Silent Point Mutations

A silent point mutation is a base substitution in the third position of a codon, which usually results in the generation of a synonymous codon. In other words, the amino acid encoded by the gene does not change. Thus, the protein product of the gene is unaltered (Klug & Cummings, 2005). One example is phenylalanine as seen in Figure 2-6.

Missense Point Mutations

A base substitution that results in the generation of a codon specifying a different amino acid is a missense point mutation. In a missense point mutation, an amino acid change in the sequence of the gene product substitutes the amino acid. This may or may not result in a deleterious gene product, depending on the amino acid that has been substituted. If the structure and properties of the normal and substituted amino acids are similar, no deleterious gene products will result. If the structure and properties of the two amino acids are very different, causing major variation, a deleterious gene product may result (Klug & Cummings, 2005).

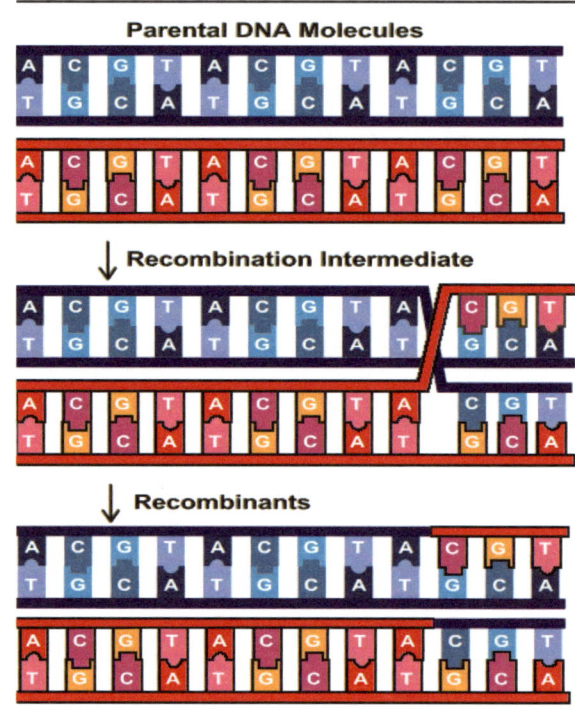

FIGURE 2-8 RECOMBINATION AS CAUSE OF MUTATION

This figure demonstrates how two strands of DNA can crossover and recombine to create a new mutation.

Note. From *A Science Primer: What Is a Genome?* by National Center for Biotechnology Information, 2004. Retrieved November 9, 2009, from http://www.ncbi.nlm.nih.gov/About/primer/genetics_genome.html.

Nonsense Point Mutations

A **nonsense point mutation** occurs when a base substitution results in the generation of a stop codon, meaning that the gene protein product will be truncated (shortened) and, possibly, nonfunctional. Nonsense point mutations may be harmful (deleterious) depending on the resultant protein (Klug & Cummings, 2005).

The previously described types of point mutations are provided to simplify the explanation of how one nucleotide change in the triplet "spelling" for an amino acid can cause a variation in the protein. Remember that missense and nonsense mutations also can be caused by several changes in the nucleotide sequence (except for multiples of three), not just one nucleotide alteration (Klug & Cummings, 2005).

TABLE 2-1. Examples of DNA Codons With Point Mutations and Effect on Amino Acid Formation

Types of mutations	Position 1 DNA Codon and Amino Acid (a.a.)	Position 2	Position 3	Position 4	Position 5	Position 6
Mendel's wild-type protein (normal, most common form in nature)	ATG (Start message and a.a.) Met	GCC Ala	TGC Cys	AAA Lys	CGC Arg	TGG Trp
Silent point mutation (protein product unchanged)	ATG Met	GC**T** (Alternate codon for Ala) Ala	TGC Cys	AAA Lys	CGC Arg	TGG Trp
Missense point mutation (results in a different protein product)	ATG Met	GCT Ala	**G**GC (Change in codon causes different a.a. and protein) Arg	AAA Lys	GCG Arg	TGG Trp
Nonsense point mutation (results in stop codon)	ATG Met	GCC Ala	TG**A** (Stop codon) –	AAA –	GCG –	TGG –

The top rows in each set are DNA bases: A (adenine), T (thymine), C (cytosine), and G (guanine). The bottom rows in each set are amino acids encoded by the bases: Ala (alanine), Arg (arginine), Asn (asparagine), Cys (cysteine), Gln (glutamine), Leu (leucine), Lys (lysine), Met (methionine), Ser (serine), Thr (threonine), and Trp (tryptophan). Each codon represents an amino position in a wild-type protein that develops a point mutation, designated as a bolded base.

Note. Based on information from the Universal Codon Chart.

Deletions and Insertions

A base **deletion** occurs when one or more base pairs are lost from DNA. Three DNA bases (codons) constitute each amino acid. One way to think of reading an amino acid sequence is to think of a "reading frame," a window through which three, and only three, bases are always seen. Deletion of one or two bases changes the reading frame of the sequence; the frame grows to allow a view of three bases, but they may not be the same three that the frame held before the deletion (see Figure 2-9). The result is an altered message called a frameshift mutation. The gene product of such a mutation usually is nonfunctional. If a deletion of three or a multiple of three in frame base pairs occurs, the reading frame remains intact. **Insertion** of additional base pairs also may lead to a frameshift mutation, depending on whether multiples of three base pairs are inserted (Klug & Cummings, 2005).

Combinations of insertions and deletions are possible. They can range from single bases to entire exons being inserted, deleted, or even a combination of insertions in deletions. In some cases, in fact, an insertion restores the reading frame of a gene with a deletion mutation (or vice versa). The gene product would contain a garbled amino acid sequence between the insertion and deletion, but it is otherwise correct (Klug & Cummings, 2005).

GENE TRANSMISSION IN CANCERS

All cancers have a genetic component. Cancers can be categorized simplistically as two different types of genetic conditions: somatic genetic disorders and inherited genetic diseases. Earlier in the chapter, somatic cells were described as any cells in the body that are not germ line cells. Most cancers are sporadic (or acquired) and fall under the category of somatic genetic disease because they arise from any cell in the body except an ovum or sperm. Therefore, these sporadic cancers would not be inherited. Sporadic cancers are caused by the new appearance and accumulation of multiple abnormal forms of a variety of genes (i.e., an acquired mutation) in a somatic cell (Cancer Research UK, 2009).

FIGURE 2-9   TYPES OF MUTATIONS

Types of mutations frequently associated with cancers are point mutations (silent, missense, and nonsense mutations) and insertion and deletion mutations (frameshift mutations). Mutations can be described as "reading" errors similar to misspelled words, for example:
Normal: The fat cat sat for the rat
Missense: The fit cat sat for the rat
Nonsense: The fat cat sat for
Insertion: The fea tca tsa tfo rth era
Deletion: The ftc ats atf ort her at

Acquired mutations occur throughout a lifetime and generally are not inherited. A single-gene disorder occurs when an allele is mutated at a **single locus** on one or both chromosomes in a pair. If the predisposition to develop a cancer is inherited, this predisposition is thought to result from the alteration of a single gene. This means that an individual is born with a mutation in one allele arising from germ line. The mutated allele has an alternate pair that functions. In order for the function of the gene to be lost, both alleles will need to mutate before the loss occurs. Therefore, additional acquired mutations are required for cancer to develop. Examples of cancers associated with the inheritance of a single defective gene are *BRCA1*, which is associated with breast and ovarian cancer, and *RB1*, which is associated with retinoblastoma. Cancers that develop in the context of a known inherited genetic defect account for approximately 5%–10% of all cancers (D'Andrea, 2008).

> Most cancers are sporadic, caused by a series of somatic mutations acquired over a lifetime. A small percentage of cancers are caused by mutations transmitted from one generation to the next via the germ cells (sperm and ova). Cancer is a multifactorial disease in that environmental factors and genes interact to effect its development.

Although some cancers are inherited and associated with the germ line loss of one allele, most require that the function of both alleles be lost. Usually this bilateral loss has multifactorial influences caused by an interaction of genetics, age, diet, and environmental sources. Examples of cancers associated with multifactorial influences include lung, kidney, colon, and cervical. (See the section on tumor suppressor genes later in this chapter.)

Tumorigenesis

Tumorigenesis, the process of tumor development, is a complex process that has been best studied in colorectal cancer. Researchers chose colorectal cancer to study genetic mutations because most colorectal tumors arise from preexisting benign tumors (adenomas); because colorectal tumors in various stages of development, ranging from small adenomas to large metastatic lesions, can be easily accessed for study; and because colorectal cancer allowed the study of both inherited and somatic mutations. Fearon and Vogelstein (1990) proposed a model that showed the genetic basis of colorectal cancer. Their model was among the first to suggest that tumorigenesis is a multistep process. The researchers concluded that colorectal cancers probably arise from mutational activation of oncogenes coupled with mutational inactivation of tumor suppressor genes, although the latter mutations predominate. Fearon and Vogelstein proposed that mutations in at least four genes are necessary for tumor development. In addition, Fearon and Jones (1992) suggested that the total accumulation of mutations, not their specific sequence, is responsible for tumor formation. Figure 2-10 shows the accumulation of mutations that may occur.

Fearon and Vogelstein's (1990) multistep model is based on the theory that all cells in all stages of tumorigenesis have a particular genetic makeup and that this similarity is necessary for identifying specific genes. This theory, called clonal evolution (Nowell, 1976), supports the idea that the origin of cancer lies in a single cell or a small number of cells. Initiation of clonal evolution likely involves a stem cell that already is dividing but increases the proportion of daughter cells in mitosis rather than proceeding to differentiation. Unrestrained proliferation may be accompanied by morphologic and biochemical changes or altered gene expression in early-stage neoplastic cells. Over time, proliferation may increase and show further evidence of escape from growth-control mechanisms. Increasingly malignant biologic characteristics during tumor progression result from acquired genetic instability in neoplastic cells and variant subpopulations produced as a result of genetic instability (Murga & Fernandez-Capetillo, 2007).

Some tumors do not behave according to the theory of clonal evolution. These include tumors of viral etiology, which may involve whole populations of infected cells, and genet-

---

FIGURE 2-10 MODEL OF COLORECTAL CANCER SHOWING MULTIPLE GENETIC CHANGES IN CARCINOGENESIS

		Normal	Dysplasia	Adenoma	Carcinoma in situ	Invasive Carcinoma	Metastasis
Chromosomal changes	LOH:		5q21, 18q, 17p, 15q24		4p, 5p, 8p, 10q, 15q, 16p, 22q, 4q		4q32-34, 9p, 10p13-14, 12q24.1
	Gain:				Xp, Xq, 4q11-13, 5q, 7p, 7q, 8q, 12q, 13q, 20q		6p
Epigenetic effects (methylation)			HPP1, hMLH1, SFRP1				
Gene expression changes			APC, AMACR, KRAS, p16, CTNNB, GAS, TGFβ, CCKBR, ECAD, SMAD4, hMSH2, DCC, p53, COX2, BCL2				BAX

Note. From "Genetic Alteration and Gene Expression Modulation During Cancer Progression," by C. Garnis, T.P.H. Buys, and W.L. Lam, 2004, *Molecular Cancer, 3*(9). Retrieved July 7, 2009, from http://www.molecular-cancer.com/content/3/1/9.

© 2004 Garnis et al.; licensee BioMed Central Ltd. This is an Open Access article; verbatim copying and redistribution of this article are permitted in all media for any purpose, provided this notice is preserved along with the article's original URL.

ically predisposed cancers, in which an inherited genetic defect involves every cell and increases susceptibility to neoplastic change (Dayaram & Marriott, 2008).

In reality, cancer is a multifactorial disease in which gene-environment interactions play a key developmental role. These interactions are complex but can be viewed simplistically as genes acting in a specific cellular environment to generate a malignant phenotype (presence of disease) and the environment (e.g., mutagens) acting on genetic material to produce a specific phenotype.

Epigenetics

The study of epigenetics looks at heritable changes in gene expression of somatic cells that alter the **phenotype** (e.g., developing a cancer) without altering the **genotype** (e.g., having a somatic or germ line mutation): an observable change occurs, but the DNA template remains the same. Instead of changes in the primary base sequence of DNA, epigenetic-related changes target the nuclear packaging of DNA, such as the histones or chromatin. One mechanism to modify the nuclear package is methylation of the DNA at cytosines located 5′ to guanines, and known as the CpG dinucleotide. When the nucleotides are "read," the cytosine (C) can be interpreted, but if it has the methyl group attached ($C\text{-}CH_3$), it is skipped.

This is a similar to taking the scenic route on a trip versus the interstate highway. Taking the scenic route yields much different information about an area versus riding along the interstate highway, and important directions for the trip might even be missed. The big problem with the CpG "scenic route" is that important nucleotides are skipped. As noted previously, skipping a segment of nucleotides can lead to altered proteins that cause a change in the shape of histones. For example, a change in histone shape could cause a skip in the segment of DNA responsible for activation of a tumor suppressor gene. This "skip" would alter the transcription and translation and ultimately result in a change to the protein responsible for activating the tumor suppressor gene. "Turning off" a tumor suppressor gene would allow proliferation of cells, including those with a malignant lineage.

Typically, the genome has few of these epigenetic areas with CpG dinucleotides known as "CpG islands." Many of these islands are located in promoter regions of the DNA that are responsible for starting transcription of DNA to RNA, enabling rapid protein production. If a promoter region for a DNA repair gene contains long segments of CpG islands, the normal transcription can be skipped, producing a protein that turns off the DNA repair gene. Because of proximity to a promoter region, transcription and translation of the "off" message occurs quickly, thus allowing rapid proliferation of cells, which are accumulating genetic errors, and promoting growth of malignant cells (Baylin, 2008; Klug & Cummings, 2005).

When methylation occurs in the areas of transcription, it interrupts the message leading to inactivation and silencing of genes, causing absence of normal protein function. For example, if the DNA repair genes *MLH1* and *MGMT* are hypermethylated, they become inactivated, which results in microsatellite instability and increased frequency of mutations of those genes. This breakdown of the repair genes can result in colon cancer or glioma, respectively. Methylation also can enhance DNA binding of carcinogens and increase ultraviolet absorption by DNA, thereby promoting the mutation rate and DNA adduct formation, which ultimately results in inactivation of genes and loss of gene product (protein). Some sporadic cancers associated with hypermethylation are listed in Table 2-2 (Baylin, 2005; NCBI, 2009b).

CANCER AND GENETICS

Studies have identified three groups of genes that mutate frequently and whose mutations cause cancer: **oncogenes**, **tumor suppressor genes**, and **mutator genes** (Besaratinia & Pfeifer, 2006).

Proto-Oncogenes

Genes that participate in normal proliferation of tissue, such as tissue repair, are referred to as **proto-oncogenes**. Almost all proto-oncogenes participate in normal transduction pathways that can be thought of as molecular "bucket brigades." These brigades relay "buckets" with different types of growth-stimulating signals (growth factors), via growth factor receptors, from outside to inside the cell and to the nucleus (Hanahan & Weinberg, 2000; Zhivotovsky & Orrenius, 2006). Figure 2-11 illustrates how these path-

TABLE 2-2 Selected Genes Hypermethylated in Some Cancers

Gene or Gene Product	Function	Tumor Type
Rb	Cell cycle regulation	Retinoblastoma
APC	Wnt signal transduction	Colorectal and other cancers
P14/ARF	Cell cycle regulation	Colorectal cancer
P15/CDKN2B	Cell cycle regulation	Leukemias
P16/CDKN2A	Cell cycle regulation	Various cancers
BRCA1	DNA repair	Breast and ovarian cancers
VHL	Tumor suppressor	Renal cell cancers
hMLH1	DNA mismatch repair	Colorectal, gastric, and endometrial cancers
MGMT	DNA repair	Non-small cell lung, esophageal, and other cancers
ER-α	Estrogen receptor-alpha	Breast, colorectal, and other cancers

APC—adenomatosis polyposis coli; *ARF*—alternative reading frame; *BRCA1*—breast cancer 1, early onset; *CDKN2A*—cyclin-dependent kinase inhibitor 2A (p16k inhibits CDK4); *CDKN2B*—cyclin-dependent kinase inhibitor 2B (p1, inhibits CDK4); *ER-α*—estrogen receptor-alpha; *hMLH1*—human mutL homolog 1; *MGMT*—O-6-methylguanine-DNA methyltransferase; *Rb*—retinoblastoma; *VHL*—von Hippel-Landau tumor suppressor

Note. Based on information from Baylin, 2005; National Center for Biotechnology Information, 2009a.

FIGURE 2-11   SIGNAL TRANSDUCTION

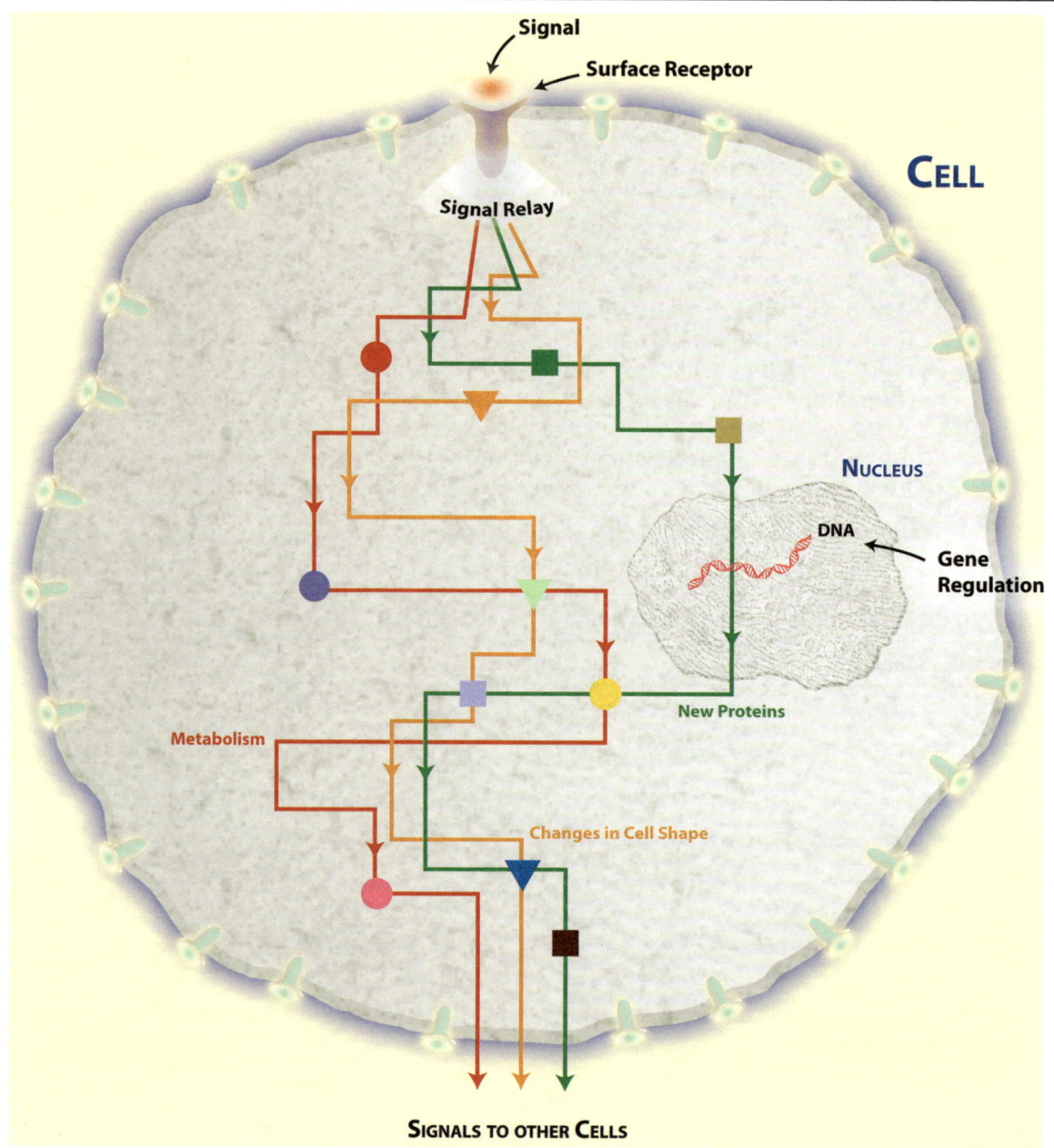

The transduction pathways are molecular signal brigades that deliver growth factors to receptors on the cell membrane, promoting signal transduction and transcription of genes.

Note. From *Biological Pathways,* by National Human Genome Research Institute, 2009. Retrieved November 9, 2009, from http://www.genome.gov/images/illustrations/Biological_Pathways.pdf.

ways transmit information to signal-transduction proteins and then to transcription factors in the nucleus. Inside the nucleus, the transcription factors affect growth factor genes, which regulate cell behavior. Because the pathways control such essential functions as cell division, death, and motility, signaling is highly regulated. Signaling regulation is achieved through alterations in the enzymatic activity of key components in the pathways and through the assembly of large multimolecular signaling complexes within discrete cellular locations (Bafico, Grumolato, & Aaronson, 2008; Pawson & Jorgensen, 2008).

The complexity of these pathways results in two important implications for tumor development. First, the large number of components involved provides many potential targets that can activate cancer-causing genes. Second, because of the redundancy and "cross talk" within the pathways, human cancers rarely result from activation of only one cancer-causing gene (Bafico et al., 2008).

Oncogenes

> Proto-oncogenes are normal genes that become oncogenes when mutated. Oncogenes cause uncontrolled cell proliferation. An oncogene requires only one gene of a pair to mutate for it to be activated.

Similar to proto-oncogenes, oncogenes encode proteins (oncoproteins) whose action causes cell proliferation. However, oncogenes are excessively or inappropriately active versions of normal cellular genes (proto-oncogenes) (Mishra, Pandey, & Nong, 2007). Consider an analogy to a car. A cell containing oncogenes is like a car in high gear that has its accelerator stuck to the floor; cell growth is moving at top speed. Oncogenes require only one allele of each pair to mutate for the gene to be activated. Oncogene activation results in a gain of function. In a gain of function, protein products become excessively active without appropriate regulation by the cell. Gain-of-function events increase cell proliferation and decrease cellular differentiation or maturation (Zhivotovsky & Orrenius, 2006).

Usually, activating mutations in oncogenes is the result of somatic events. An oncogene that can be inherited is the rearranged during transfection (*RET*) gene, which is associated with multiple endocrine neoplasia type 2A, 2B, and familial medullary thyroid carcinoma. It causes a gain-of-function mutation, which codes for a member of the receptor tyrosine kinase family. These hereditary syndromes are characterized by a markedly increased **incidence** of medullary thyroid carcinoma, pheochromocytoma, and hyperparathyroidism (Cancer Genetics Web, 2003c).

Oncogene Classification

Oncogenes are classified according to their overall function. Broad classes of oncogenes include secreted growth factors, cell-surface growth-factor receptors, nonreceptor tyrosine kinases, membrane-associated G proteins, cytoplasmic serine threonine kinases, and transcription factors (Bafico et al., 2008). MicroRNAs (miRNAs) also can be included in this category.

MicroRNAs

A new area of research targets miRNAs. These are small, about 21–25 nucleotides in length, and are negative regulators of gene expression (Meltzer, 2005). These newly identified players in the development of cancer are thought to target mRNA and either downregulate their translation to protein or degrade the RNA messenger. Either way, interference occurs in the ability to produce protein. The miRNAs have important functions, including signaling pathways for metabolism, **apoptosis**, cell differentiation, and development. They also have been linked to the initiation and development of cancer, including cancers of the prostate and breast (Ma, Teruya-Feldstein, & Weinberg, 2007; Wang & Wu, 2007). Some miRNAs have been identified as oncogenes or tumor suppressor genes (Greene, Long-Cheng, Okino, & Carroll, 2008; Meltzer).

Growth Factor Receptors

Oncogenic growth factor receptors release proliferative signals into the cytoplasm. Most growth factor receptors possess tyrosine kinase activity. Activation of tyrosine kinase receptors leads to biochemical reactions that stimulate mitotic cell division. As a result, tyrosine kinases play a key role in regulating cell proliferation (Chan & Feng, 2007; Zhivotovsky & Orrenius, 2006). Increased tyrosine kinase activity can cause clonal expansion of cells, a topic that will be discussed later in this chapter.

Examples of growth factor receptors that are oncogenic when overexpressed are **epidermal growth factor receptor** (EGFR), erythroblastic leukemia viral oncogene homolog 2 (HER2/neu/ERBB2), and **transforming growth factor-beta** (TGF-β). A variety of cancers express EGFR, including non-small cell lung, breast, ovarian, and colorectal cancers. Head and neck cancers exhibit about 80%–100% overexpression of EGFR. Overexpression of EGFR in these tumors correlates with low survival. Overexpression of ERBB2 coincides with an aggressive clinical course of certain cancers, including ovarian and breast cancers. Expression of EGFR and TGF-β together is a prognostic marker for tumor relapse and decreased survival (Baficio et al., 2008; Pawson & Jorgensen, 2008).

Growth Factors

Most growth factors act outside of the cell as chemical signals that regulate cellular behavior. Growth factors affect cell growth, differentiation, and survival, as well as help to determine tissue architecture and morphology. In signaling pathways, growth factors initiate **signal transduction** across the cell membrane.

As Figure 2-11 suggests, growth factors must interact with specific receptors to accomplish signaling (Baficio et al., 2008; Pawson & Jorgensen, 2008).

The binding of a growth factor to a receptor initiates a signal that activates other proteins in the cytoplasm, causing transmission of a signal to the cell nucleus. The end result of transmission is a change in the expression of certain genes that help to usher the cell through its growth cycle (Zhivotovsky & Orrenius, 2006). Several growth factors, when overproduced, are associated with cancers. Vascular endothelial growth factor (VEGF) plays an important role in tumor neoangiogenesis (i.e., the growth of new vessels in a tumor). Tumor cells induce hypoxia through the hypoxia inducible factor-1 alpha pathway. This leads to transcription of various factors, including VEGF-A, which bind to cell surface receptors and ultimately cause increased blood vessel permeability, angiogenesis, and the proliferation of cells (Nguyen, Tran, Lipkin, & Fruehauf, 2006). VEGF is overexpressed in metastatic breast and colorectal cancers.

Endothelial cells overexpress **fibroblast** growth factor in hemangiomas. Overexpression of platelet-derived growth factor has been reported in sarcomas and gliomas. Other growth factors implicated in cancer development include epidermal growth factor, transforming growth factor, and colony-stimulating factor (Pawson & Jorgensen, 2008).

Nonreceptor Tyrosine Kinases

Some oncogenes do not require a receptor to initiate tyrosine kinase activity at the cell membrane. One example is the *SRC* gene family. It initiates tyrosine kinase activity at the C terminus where biosynthesis is supposed to end, allowing continuation of the protein and continued growth signaling. Such *SRC*-initiated activity is increased in neuroblastoma, small cell lung cancer, colon cancer, breast adenocarcinoma, and rhabdomyosarcoma (Okutani, Lodyga, Han, & Liu, 2006).

Membrane-Associated Guanine Nucleotide-Binding Proteins

Membrane-associated guanine nucleotide-binding proteins (G proteins) act as on-off switches for cell-surface growth factor receptors. These changes disrupt part of the signal cascade that occurs in the cell cytoplasm. G proteins are members of the *ras* superfamily of oncogenes, which comprises more than 50 members. The ras proteins are known to act at the cell membrane to cause malignant transformation. Normally, proteins encoded by normal *ras* genes transmit stimulatory signals from growth factor receptors to other proteins. Mutant *ras* genes activate signaling pathways, even when unprompted by growth factor receptors. Mutant *ras* is found in virtually all types of human cancer and occurs in approximately two-thirds of all malignant tumors (Bos, Rehmann, & Wittinghofer, 2007).

Serine Threonine Kinases

Oncoproteins with serine threonine protein kinase activity are important components of intracellular signal transduction. The prototype serine threonine kinase in the cytoplasm, RAF1, is activated by tyrosine kinase–associated receptors in the signal transduction pathway. RAF1 acts as an intermediary between RAS on the cell membrane and the cell nucleus by activating a series of other kinases known as mitogen-activated protein kinases. These kinases are critical for regulating the onset of cell division (Barbash & Diehl, 2008).

Transcription Factors

Proteins that bind to DNA and cause changes in gene expression are called transcription factors. Mutation of the transcription factors that regulate genes involved in growth and survival drives malignant transformation in many tumors. Transcription factors have specific structures that "recognize" specific DNA sequences. Examples of oncogenic transcription factors are proteins with activator protein-1 (AP-1) activity (e.g., JUN, FOS), which are implicated in signal-dependent processes that control cell growth and, hence, carcinogenesis. Oncogenic transcription factors are associated with Ewing sarcoma, clear-cell sarcoma, alveolar rhabdomyosarcoma, and many kinds of leukemia. All these conditions are characterized by chromosomal translocations (see Chromosomal Abnormalities later in this chapter) (Aplan, 2006). The gene **TP53** is considered a tumor suppressor gene (see the next section) and also acts as a transcription factor. In this role, *TP53* "senses" DNA damage and halts cell division by controlling expression of other genes that directly regulate the cell cycle (Ozanne, Spence, McGarry, & Hennigan, 2007).

Tumor Suppressor Genes

Tumor suppressor genes (also called anti-oncogenes) normally suppress or negatively regulate cell proliferation by encoding proteins that block the action of growth-promoting proteins. Using a car as a comparison, with out-of-control cell growth caused by a stuck accelerator, tumor suppressor genes are the brakes that can suppress oncogenesis. At the cellular level, tumor suppressor genes have loss of function of both alleles, caused by mutations, in the cell. In other words, loss of function or mutations of both copies of the gene are required for uncontrolled cell growth leading to tumorigenesis (NCBI, n.d.-c).

> Tumor suppressor genes normally block the action of growth-promoting proteins. In cancer cells, both alleles of a pair are mutated, or lost. Mutated tumor suppressor genes cause loss of function.

Discovery and Mechanisms of Tumor Suppressor Genes

Studies of retinoblastoma provided initial clinical evidence of the existence and behavior of tumor suppressor genes and information about their behavior. Retinoblastoma is a rare malignant eye tumor that occurs in children. The tumor can be either hereditary or nonhereditary. In the hereditary form, multiple tumors occur in early childhood and frequently involve both eyes. In the sporadic form, a single tumor forms usually when the individual is older. A careful analysis by Knudson (1971) of families with retinoblastoma led to the "two-hit" hypothesis of cancer development.

In the "two-hit" theory, Knudson (1971) proposed that a first mutation is transmitted in the germ line, causing that chromosome in all cells of the body to lack one normal allele. When the remaining normal allele on the second chromosome is lost or inactivated by a new mutation in a body cell (somatic mutation), tumors will occur. This second event could be relatively common, leading to the multifocal appearance of the hereditary form. In the sporadic form, Knudson hypothesized that all cells contain two functional copies of the gene, meaning that tumors could arise only when both copies are lost or inactivated within the same target cell.

When researchers cloned the *RB1* gene, they found that its mutations were highly associated with retinoblastoma. The frequent and reproducible inactivation of *RB1* provided strong circumstantial evidence that an actual tumor suppressor gene had been isolated. The loss of function of *RB1* is now known to play a role in the development of osteosarcoma as well as in some common malignancies of adults, including lung, breast, and bladder cancers (Lohmann & Gallie, 2007).

Loss of Heterozygosity

When both alleles of any gene are capable of functioning, it is labeled as **homozygous**. Commonly, the first inherited mutation of a tumor suppressor gene is a small change confined to the actual gene. Because the other allele has not mutated, the function of the gene and its product is maintained. With one normal allele and one mutated or changed, the gene is labeled as **heterozygous**. Once the functioning allele becomes mutated, this gene and its product will lose function. The heterozygosity has been changed and is now termed *loss of heterozygosity*. Thus, if a patient with cancer is heterozygous for a specific genetic marker located close to the tumor suppressor gene, and the function is lost, the tumor tissue loses this heterozygosity. Cells can experience loss of heterozygosity with the loss of an entire chromosome, the translocation of a piece of the chromosome, the reduplication of a piece of chromosome that already has an abnormal gene, or the development of a point mutation in the second functioning allele. Loss of heterozygosity commonly is described in association with cancer susceptibility genes such as oncogenes and tumor suppressor genes. One example is allelic loss in the short arm of chromosome 3 (3p) with non-small cell lung cancer (NCI, 2005). Investigators examining loss of heterozygosity have been able to identify and clone an increasing number of tumor suppressor genes that, when mutated, are critical to the development of human cancers.

TP53 (located on 17p13) is one of the well-studied tumor suppressor genes. Deletions and mutations of *TP53* are common in a wide variety of cancers, including lung, breast, esophageal, liver, bladder, and ovarian carcinomas; brain tumors; sarcomas; lymphomas; and leukemias. Overall, *TP53* mutations may contribute to approximately 50% of all sporadic human cancers, making *TP53* the most common target for genetic mutations leading to cancers (Levine, Hu, & Feng, 2008). Germ line mutations of *TP53*, transmitted in an **autosomal dominant** fashion, are a hallmark of Li-Fraumeni syndrome. This syndrome is a rare disorder causing multiple types of cancers, including soft-tissue sarcomas, osteosarcomas, adrenal and breast cancers, and different types of leukemias (Genetics Home Reference, 2009b; Levine et al.).

Specific Functions of Tumor Suppressor Genes

Some normal tumor suppressor gene products are localized in the cell nucleus and act as transcription factors (see Figure 2-12). For example, *MTS1*, which encodes the p16 protein, also contributes to deregulation of the cell cycle, which results in excess cell proliferation. The *TP53* gene can halt cell division and induce programmed cell death, or apoptosis (see Apoptosis later in this chapter).

Tumor suppressor genes also can encode for proteins in the cytoplasm. The *NF1* (neurofibromatosis) gene encodes a protein that is similar to the proteins that modulate *ras* oncogene function. Loss of *NF1* may keep *ras* activated and prolong the signal for cell proliferation. Loss of other tumor suppressor genes, such as *NF2* and *APC* (adenomatous polyposis coli), may cause cellular disorganization that leads to abnormal cell proliferation (Schindeler & Little, 2008). The breast-ovarian cancer genes, *BRCA1* and **BRCA2**, are known to be associated with an elevated lifetime risk of developing breast-ovarian syndrome. Research results suggest *BRCA2* is important in DNA repair (see Homologous Recombination Repair). However, *BRCA1* has multiple roles as an E3 ubiquitin ligase (an enzyme associated with protein degradation) that has an impact on DNA repair, transcriptional regulation, cell cycle progression, and meiotic sex chromosome inactivation (Boulton, 2006).

Mutator Genes

Unlike oncogenes or tumor suppressor genes, mutator genes (DNA repair genes) are not part of cell regulatory

FIGURE 2-12 TUMOR SUPPRESSOR GENE FUNCTION

Normal tumor suppressor gene function
- Tells the cell when to stop growing (called deactivation or downregulation)
- Plays a key role in cell cycle activity (when to move on or stop cell cycle activity)
- Helps abnormal cells to die (apoptosis).

Loss of function or mutation of the tumor suppressor gene results in
- Cells that do not stop growing (increase in clonal proliferation)
- Abnormal cells that lose apoptosis function.

pathways. Instead, mutator genes prevent genetic instability. Mutator genes can be either oncogenes or tumor suppressor genes. They encode error-correction systems that check DNA for damaged or mismatched base pairs (see Defects in Mismatch Repair: Microsatellite Instability later in this chapter). Mutations in these genes lead to inefficient replication or repair of DNA. Colon cancer studies have provided clues to the identity of genes important in stability at the DNA level (Genetics Home Reference, 2009d; Jenkins et al., 2007).

TYPES OF GENETIC ALTERATIONS IN CANCER CELLS

Other than mutations, the genetic alterations associated with cancer include chromosomal abnormalities, amplification, and defects in mismatch repair. Defects in mismatch pair, including microsatellite instability, will be discussed in the Types of DNA Repair Mechanisms section of this chapter.

Chromosomal Abnormalities

Cancer cells typically have a bizarre, unstable chromosomal structure composed of many gains, losses, or rearrangements of chromosomes. Chromosomal instability is linked to both germ line and somatic mutations indicating potential for malignancies. Germ line mutations include the cancer syndromes associated with the *NBS1* (Nijmegen breakage syndrome 1 and non-Hodgkin lymphoma) and *ATM* (ataxia telangiectasia mutated with lymphatic, leukemias, and other malignancies) genes (Cancer Genetics Web, 2003a, 2003b). Somatic mutations include the *MRE11* and *Ding* in colorectal tumors (Carter, Eklund, Kohane, Harris, & Szallasi, 2006; Wang et al., 2004). The most common gene found to be altered in cancers with chromosomal instability is the *APC* tumor suppressor gene, commonly inactivated in colon and rectal cancer (Bommer & Fearon, 2008).

Recurrent structural chromosomal rearrangements are a common feature of most cancers. How these rearrangements develop may be attributed to genetic weak points or chromosomal fragile sites. Chromosomal fragile sites are regions on chromosomes that are particularly sensitive to forming nonrandom gaps or breaks when DNA synthesis is disturbed. Fragile sites are highly sensitive to low folic acid. They can be induced by a wide variety of mutagens and carcinogens that are known to act through different molecular mechanisms. Fragile sites have been implicated in a wide variety of cancers, including multiple myeloma (Smith, Zhu, McAvoy, & Kuhn, 2006) and chronic lymphocytic leukemia (Gollin, 2007).

Translocations

Chromosomal translocations are structural abnormalities that primarily affect oncogenes. **Translocations** cause oncogene deregulation (overexpression) and the fusion of oncogenes at the points in the chromosome where abnormal breaks occur (breakpoints). **Reciprocal translocations** involve exchange of genetic material between two chromosomes or within the same chromosome. Translocations are the hallmarks of leukemias and lymphomas (NCBI, 2008). For example, in chronic myeloid leukemia, the reciprocal translocation between the q arm of chromosome 9, band 34 and the q arm of chromosome 22, band 11 causes the *ABL* proto-oncogene to translocate to chromosome 22 (the Philadelphia chromosome). This produces the *BCR-ABL* fusion gene, which dysregulates tyrosine kinase activity (NCBI, n.d.-b). The abbreviated method of describing this translocation is t(9;22)(q34;q11), which identifies in the first parentheses the two chromosomes involved in the translocation, in this case chromosomes 9 and 22. Information in the second set of parentheses specifies the exact location on each chromosome where the breakpoints occur. Eighty percent of Burkitt lymphoma cases have a translocation of t(8;14)(q24;q32). This translocation deregulates expression of the transcription factor encoded by the *MYC* proto-oncogene, causing activation of the *MYC* oncogene (Hartmann, Ott, & Rosenwald, 2008; NCBI, n.d.-a).

Deletions

Chromosomal deletions occur when pieces of DNA are lost from a chromosome. If the section is close to a tumor suppressor location, suppression of cancer could be lost thus allowing cell proliferation and the development of malignant tumors. Recently, a study identified that certain chromosomal deletions are associated with increased risk for leukemia and cancers of the renal system, eye, and female genitalia. The most common deletions were on chromosomes 22q, 15q, 7q, 5p, and 17p. Study results reinforced previously known data that deletions of 11p and 13q increase the risk of retinoblastoma and Wilms tumor, respectively. However, a new finding suggests an increase of anogenital cancers with an 11q24 deletion (Swerdlow, Schoemaker, Higgins, Wright, & Jacobs, 2008).

Aneuploidy

Aneuploidy is an abnormal chromosome number. The term can refer to a gain or a loss of a chromosome. Aneuploidy is associated with malignant transformation in that gross changes in chromosome number usually occur as tumorigenesis progresses. In most colorectal cancers, for example, aneuploidy is associated with genetic instability. Aneuploidy may be random or nonrandom. In random aneuploidy, the change in chromosome number has no association with tumor type; rather, it happens late in tumor development and reflects the genetic instability of the tumor. Nonrandom aneuploidy involves a specific change in a given chromosome associated with a specific tumor. Nonrandom aneuploidy tends to occur earlier than the random form (Barber et al., 2008).

Amplification

Amplification, an increase in the number of gene copies, results in overexpression of the gene product without modification of the gene itself. Amplifications can be extrachromosomal—in this case, as minichromosomes called double minutes. Amplifications also can be intrachromosomal, appearing as homogenously stained regions in the chromosome—areas where chromosome regions have increased length, are stable, and remain amplified. Amplification of certain genes may be related to carcinogenesis, as in the enhancement of amplification by ultraviolet light. As tumor cells progress, they gain the ability to amplify genes as they lose cell cycle control and tumor suppressor gene activity. Oncogenes such as *MYC* and *ERBB2* (*HER2/neu*) often have amplified gene sequences, which may be related to tumor progression (Myllykangas, Bohling, & Knuutila, 2007).

TYPES OF DNA REPAIR MECHANISMS

An understanding of the six repair mechanisms is enhanced by considering the range of DNA-damaging events that can occur within a cell. These events include spontaneous damage caused by chemicals, mismatched bases from error-prone enzymes during the S phase of the cell cycle, or attack by reactive oxygen species. Damage also can occur from ultraviolet light or ionizing radiation leading to mutagenesis. Also, DNA damage can be caused by the antineoplastic agents used to treat malignancies (D'Andrea, 2008).

As a group, the six DNA repair pathways are highly regulated and often activated only at distinct and separate times within the cell cycle. In addition, the repair pathways may be differentially active in various tissues and cell types. Furthermore, absence of a particular DNA repair pathway may distort the growth and survival of some normal tissues and cancers (D'Andrea, 2008).

Base Excision Repair

Base excision repair is used by cells throughout the cell cycle to correct damage to DNA bases or single-strand DNA breaks caused by environmental alkylating agents or spontaneous injury. The problem base is tagged, nicked, and repaired, and the DNA is filled in or "sealed" by a variety of enzymes with personalized activity for each step in base excision repair. Transitional cell and lung cancers have been associated with problems in this DNA repair system (D'Andrea, 2008).

Mismatch Repair: Microsatellite Instability

In normal DNA synthesis, specific repair proteins recognize and bind to mismatched DNA relying on a back-up signal within DNA to distinguish between the parental strand and a daughter strand containing a replication error. The result is a process that essentially unwinds DNA in the direction of the mismatch, degrades the DNA strand with the error, and seals the nick that degradation causes in the strand. Sometimes, however, the wrong nucleotide incorporates into the strand during DNA-strand synthesis and DNA's normal editing system fails to correct the error, causing a mismatch of the bases that are repaired.

Defects in genes that encode the repair proteins most often have been associated with hereditary nonpolyposis colorectal cancer, also called Lynch syndrome. Six genes have been associated with Lynch syndrome; four of them involve mismatch repair. These include *MSH2*, *MSH6*, *MLH1*, and *MLH3*. Because these genes are involved in DNA repair occurring prior to replication, defects in these genes can allow rapid accumulation of mutations throughout the genome resulting in the development of colorectal and other cancers. Most patients with Lynch syndrome show alterations in the DNA-base sequences, or microsatellite sequences, distributed throughout the genome. These sequences may be associated with defects in mismatch repair (Genetics Home Reference, 2009c; Klug et al., 2005).

Microsatellite DNA sequences consist of two nucleotides repeated in tandem. For example, a segment of DNA may have tandem repeats of cytosine (C) and adenine (A), CACACACACA. In normal tissue, these tandem repeats also are defined as polymorphisms and help to identify differences between individuals. They may consist of coding (exon) or noncoding (intron) DNA (Clamp et al., 2007). Because of the repetitions, the segment is highly unstable or fragile and prone to single-nucleotide deletion or insertion (Klug & Cummings,

2005). With this instability, the length of microsatellite DNA repetitions becomes different in tumors than in normal tissue. Microsatellite instability is a characteristic of autosomal-dominant Lynch syndrome, and the genes *MSH2* and *MLH1* are thought to account for most mutations of the mismatch repair genes found in families with Lynch syndrome. Microsatellite instabilities are not always associated with germ line tumors. Approximately 15%–20% of sporadic colorectal, gastric, and endometrial cancers have identifiable microsatellite instability (Ahuja & Baylin, 2007; Söreide, Janssen, Söiland, Körner, & Baak, 2006).

Nucleotide Excision Repair

Nucleotide excision repair primarily acts on bulky lesions that distort the helix of the DNA. These areas of single-strand damage typically are caused by damage from ultraviolet light. To repair, the length of single-strand DNA is removed, resynthesized by an enzyme "reading" the corresponding DNA template, and then sealed or filled by another enzyme (ligase). Testicular germ cell tumors have been associated with a loss of nucleotide excision repair (D'Andrea, 2008).

Homologous Recombination Repair

Double-strand breaks to the DNA are caused by multiple environmental factors, including antineoplastic drugs such as bleomycin, anthracyclines, or topoisomerase inhibitors. Reactive oxygen species also can cause damage to both strands of the DNA. Sometimes, endogenous factors cause both strands of the DNA to break during normal progression of the cell cycle through the S phase. If these are not repaired, mutations, chromosomal rearrangements, and aberrations can result, leading to carcinogenesis and cellular death. This type of defective repair is associated with *BRCA*-deficient breast and ovarian tumors (McCabe et al., 2006). Also, lung and prostate cancers are associated with problems in this DNA repair pathway. Simply, **homologous recombination repair** is achieved by resecting the double-strand DNA with an enzyme (exonuclease), identifying an undamaged piece of replicated sister chromosome (sister chromatid) for use as a template, synthesis of the new strands of DNA, disengagement of the sister chromatid, and filling the disconnected double strand of DNA (D'Andrea, 2008).

Nonhomologous End Joining

Another type of repair for double-strand DNA breaks is nonhomologous end joining (NHEJ). Although similar to homologous recombination repair, the NHEJ type of DNA repair is error-prone. Because it does not use a sister chromatid, the blunt ends of the double-strand break are covered by a binding protein. NHEJ may allow the insertion or deletion of new nucleotides to be fused at the break. This type of error-prone repair is used in the immunoglobulin gene and associated with the diversity of the *Ig* gene and its resultant antibodies. Problems with this pathway of DNA repair are associated with cervical, rectal, and colon cancers (D'Andrea, 2008; Lieber, Ma, Pannicke, & Schwarz, 2003).

Translesion DNA Synthesis

The sixth type of DNA repair, translesion DNA synthesis, is another way to handle thymine dimers and bases with bulky additions because of damage. These bulky DNA adducts may cause stalling of a replicative enzyme (polymerase). Although human cells have at least 15 DNA polymerases, one error-prone translesion DNA synthesis polymerase is known to cause high rates of mutagenesis. Errors in this DNA pathway are associated with cancers of the breast, uterus, ovary, prostate, and stomach (D'Andrea, 2008).

THE CELL CYCLE

Normally, a complex molecular process in the cell nucleus, the cell cycle, regulates cell division. The cell cycle integrates the various growth-regulating signals received by the cell and decides to allow the cell to replicate (McCance, 2006). In a malignancy, ineffective DNA repair leads to an accumulation of genetic errors that affect cell cycle control mechanisms. The cell cycle operates autonomously without control of cell proliferation.

Normal Functioning of the Cell Cycle

The cell cycle consists of four active phases, seen in Figure 2-13. In the first phase, gap 1 (G_1), the cell readies itself to copy DNA. Late in G_1 is a restriction point (R); this is the point at which the cell "decides" to commit itself to replication. Once committed, the cycle cannot be stopped. During the synthesis (S) phase, DNA replication occurs and the cell duplicates its complement of chromosomes. Following chromosomal replication, the cell proceeds to the gap 2 (G_2) phase and prepares itself for mitosis (M). During the M phase, chromosome segregation occurs and culminates in cytokinesis (division into two daughter cells, each with a full complement of chromosomes). The daughter cells immediately enter G_1. The cell cycle begins again, or it may stop cycling and enter a resting (G_0) state (McCance, 2006).

FIGURE 2-13 THE CELL CYCLE

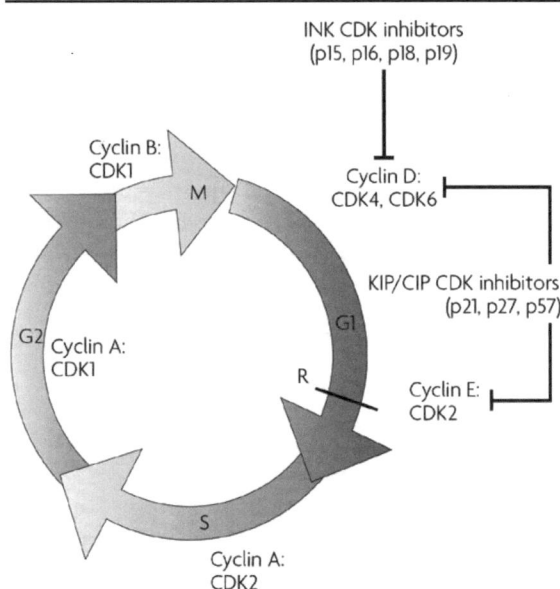

The cell cycle consists of four active stages (G1, S, G2, M) that are controlled by proteins called cyclins. The cyclins (D, E, A, B) activate upon forming complexes with enzymes called cyclin-dependent kinases (CDKs). Upon activation, the cyclin-CDK complexes allow the cell to progress through each specific cell cycle stage. Present throughout the cell cycle, the cyclin-CDK complexes serve as checkpoints, or monitors, of the cell cycle. Inhibitory proteins—such as p21, p27, and p53—prevent progression through the cell cycle if DNA damage is present or if the nutrients or oxygen necessary to support cellular proliferation is in short supply. Inhibitory proteins, in turn, are regulated by inhibitory growth factors and *TGFB*. Cyclin-CDK complexes and pRb ("the master brake") tightly regulate the R (restriction) point. Once past R, the cell cycle "turns on," and progression through the cell cycle is inevitable. The stability of the inhibitory proteins and cyclin-CDK complexes are altered in cancer. Normal cell cycle controls are absent and uncontrolled cellular proliferation prevails.

Note. From "Cell-Cycle Control and Cortical Development," by C. Dehay and H. Kennedy, 2007, *Nature Reviews Neuroscience, 8*(6), p. 443. Retrieved November 9, 2009, from http://www.nature.com/nrn/journal/v8/n6/images/nrn2097-i1.jpg. Copyright 2007 by Nature Publishing Group. Reprinted with permission.

Proteins called cyclins combine with and activate enzymes called cyclin-dependent kinases (CDKs). The transient activation of various cyclins and CDKs, at specific points in the cell cycle, regulates the intricate series of cell cycle events. For example, CDK1 is involved primarily in control of mitosis. CDK2 is involved in G_1 and in G_1–S transition points. CDK1, -2, and -3 are thought to carry out the start function of the cell cycle (McCance, 2006).

Checkpoints in the Cell Cycle

Checkpoints, specific gene products in the cell cycle, ensure that events occur in correct sequence and that one event terminates before the other begins (NCBI, 2009a). For example, checkpoints govern entrance into the S phase and the M phase and exit from the M phase (Deng, 2006). Defects in the checkpoint surveillance of DNA could account for chromosomal deletions, amplifications, and translocations. The checkpoint controlling entry into the S phase prevents replication of DNA damage. Therefore, checkpoint surveillance plays an integral role in maintaining the integrity of the human genome (Deng). Cancer cells probably have weak or deficient cell cycle checkpoints (Deng).

Currently, genetic instability in the G_1/S checkpoint in human cancers is best understood. Loss of the G_1/S checkpoint leads to the instability of the human genome, survival of genetically damaged cells, and clonal evolution (see Tumorigenesis). For example, mutations of *TP53* commonly are associated with several cancers, suggesting that abnormalities in the G_1/S checkpoint are important in tumorigenesis (see Table 2-3).

TABLE 2-3   Selected Cell Cycle Checkpoint Genes

Checkpoint Genes	Checkpoint Gene Function
G_1/S checkpoint	
ATM	Detects DNA damage; maintains normal telomere length
CCND1, CCNE1, CDC25A, CDK4, CDK6, CDKN1A, CDKN1B, CDKN2A, CDKN2B, E2F1, HDAC1, MADH3, MADH4, RB1, SKP2, and *TFDP1*	Multiple factors that participate in pathways to signal that the cell needs to make ready for duplication, specifically prior to the G_1 checkpoint
CHEK2	Stabilizes *p53* and prevents movement into G_1
p53	Blocks activity of certain cellular factors, which prevents movement of the cell through the G_1 checkpoint.
S-phase checkpoint	
BRCA1	Responsible for DNA repair
MDC	Mediates DNA damage checkpoint
G_2 checkpoint	
RAD17, RAD1, and *HUS1*	Proteins of these genes have tyrosine kinase activity and act as tumor suppressors to prevent movement through the G_2 phase if there is DNA damage.

Note. Based on information from Weizmann Institute of Science, n.d.

Apoptosis

In some cases, *TP53*-induced DNA damage triggers apoptosis rather than G_1 arrest. Apoptosis is "programmed" cell death—in other words, cell death occurs as a result of an active process that involves a distinct series of biochemical and cellular changes. Apoptosis allows an organism to remove old, dead, or unwanted cells as seen in Figure 2-14. This type of programmed cell death often is a response to DNA damage in order to prevent movement through the cell cycle and duplication of two cells with DNA damage. Cell cycle progression can be arrested following externally induced damage, such as damage resulting from chemotherapeutic drugs (Zhivotovsky & Orrenius, 2006).

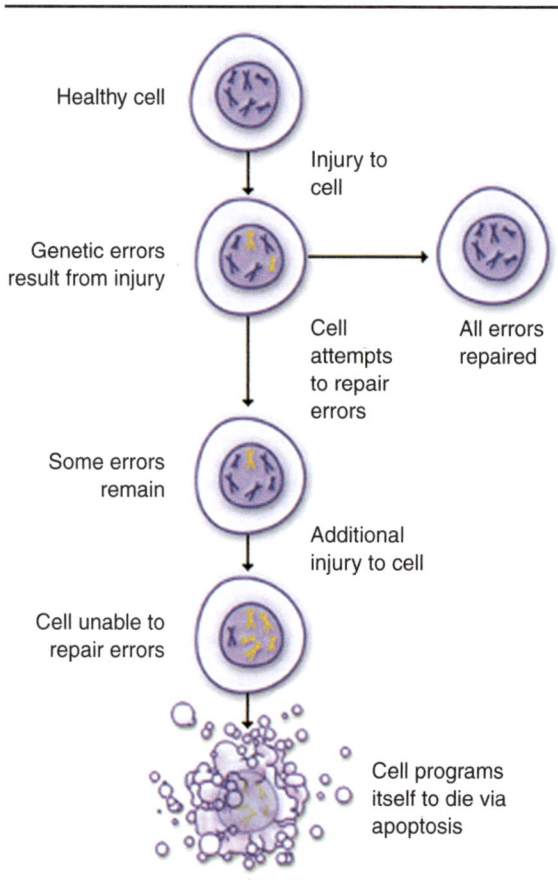

FIGURE 2-14   APOPTOSIS

Note. From *The Process of Apoptosis,* by Genetics Home Reference, 2009. Retrieved November 9, 2009, from http://ghr.nlm.nih.gov/handbook/illustrations/apoptosisprocess.

> The types of genetic alterations commonly found in cancer cells include mutations; chromosomal translocations, deletions, and aneuploidy; gene amplification; and defects in mismatch repair, including microsatellite instability.

Loss of apoptotic signals may contribute to early tumorigenesis because of the inability to eliminate genetically damaged cells, or later in tumorigenesis with survival of damaged cells (Zhivotovsky & Orrenius, 2006). Apoptosis that is dependent on *TP53* activity, in response to abnormal cell proliferation, inhibits the growth of a developing tumor. Inactivation of the *TP53* gene leads to a decrease of apoptosis and rapid tumor progression. The loss of *TP53* function may indirectly contribute to tumor development by permitting the proliferation of mutated cells. Therefore, reduced susceptibility to apoptosis may be a direct consequence of loss of *TP53* function rather than an accumulation of secondary mutations (Levine et al., 2008).

Another example is follicular lymphoma, a type of indolent (slow-growing) non-Hodgkin lymphoma. This form accounts for approximately 20% of all non-Hodgkin lymphomas and commonly has a rearrangement of the *BCL-2* gene. The overexpression of the bcl-2 protein inhibits apoptosis, allowing continued cellular proliferation, making it difficult to destroy this lymphoma (NCI, 2009). These examples suggest that restoration of apoptosis may provide an approach to cancer therapy.

SUMMARY

> Several genes play a critical role in normal regulation of the cell cycle. If those genes are damaged, the cell cycle malfunctions and uncontrolled cell proliferation can occur. For apoptosis to function properly, for example, *TP53* must function properly.

Genetic abnormalities and instability in various forms are key features of all cancers. This chapter summarized how cancers can be traced to molecular defects in DNA, chromosomal abnormalities, and specific genes that interfere with signal transduction, enzymatic pathways, and the cell cycle. Tumorigenesis at the molecular level appears to be a complex, multistep process characterized by the accumulation of multiple genetic defects.

Through the process of clonal evolution, these defects lead to the development of the fully malignant phenotype characteristic of clinical cancer. In other words, a single mutation may initiate a process leading to cancer, but more mutations are needed for cancer to progress. As the steps involved in cancer development are clarified, risk assessment, diagnosis, treatment, and prognostic predictions are becoming rational responses to specific cellular mechanisms.

> Cancer is the result of a complex, multistep process characterized by the accumulation of multiple genetic defects. A single genetic mutation may initiate a process leading to cancer, but more mutations are needed for cancer to progress.

REFERENCES

Ahuja, N., & Baylin, S.B. (2007). Subclassification of microsatellite-unstable tumors in colorectal cancer. *Current Colorectal Cancer Reports, 3*(4), 212–219.

Aplan, P.D. (2006). Causes of oncogenic chromosomal translocation. *Trends in Genetics, 22*(1), 46–55.

Bafico, A., Grumolato, L., & Aaronson, S.A. (2008). Oncogenes and signal transduction. In J. Mendelsohn, P. Howley, M. Israel, J. Gray, & C. Thompson (Eds.), *The molecular basis of cancer* (3rd ed., pp. 17–30). Philadelphia: Elsevier Saunders.

Barbash, O., & Diehl, A. (2008). Regulation of the cell cycle. In J. Mendelsohn, P. Howley, M. Israel, J. Gray, & C. Thompson (Eds.), *The molecular basis of cancer* (3rd ed., pp. 177–188). Philadelphia: Elsevier Saunders.

Barber, T.D., McManus, K., Yuen, K.W., Reis, M., Parmigiani, G., Shen, D., et al. (2008). Chromatid cohesion defects may underlie chromosome instability in human colorectal cancers. *Proceedings of the National Academy of Sciences, 105*(9), 3443–3448.

Baylin, S. (2008). Epigenetics and cancer. In J. Mendelsohn, P. Howley, M. Israel, J. Gray, & C. Thompson (Eds.), *The molecular basis of cancer* (3rd ed., pp. 57–65). Philadelphia: Elsevier Saunders.

Baylin, S.B. (2005). DNA methylation and gene silencing in cancer. *Nature Clinical Practice Oncology, 2*(Suppl. 1), S4–S11.

Besaratinia, A., & Pfeifer, G.P. (2006). Investigating human cancer etiology by DNA lesion footprinting and mutagenicity analysis. *Carcinogenesis, 27*(8), 1526–1537.

Bommer, G., & Fearon, E. (2008). Molecular abnormalities in colon and rectal cancer. In J. Mendelsohn, P. Howley, M. Israel, J. Gray, & C. Thompson (Eds.), *The molecular basis of cancer* (3rd ed., pp. 409–422). Philadelphia: Elsevier Saunders.

Bos, J.L., Rehmann, H., & Wittinghofer, A. (2007). GEFs and GAPs: Critical elements in the control of small G proteins. *Cell, 129*(5), 385.

Boulton, S.J. (2006). Cellular functions of the *BRCA* tumour-suppressor proteins. *Biochemical Society Transactions, 34*(Pt. 5), 633–645.

Buchstaller, J., Quintana, E., & Morrison, S. (2008). Cancer stem cells. In J. Mendelsohn, P. Howley, M. Israel, J. Gray, & C. Thompson (Eds.), *The molecular basis of cancer* (3rd ed., pp. 141–154). Philadelphia: Elsevier Saunders.

Campbell, N., & Reece, J. (2005). *Biology* (7th ed.). San Francisco: Pearson Education.

Cancer Genetics Web. (2003a). *Ataxia telangiectasia mutated.* Retrieved June 6, 2009, from http://www.cancerindex.org/geneweb/ATM.htm

Cancer Genetics Web. (2003b). *Nijmegen breakage syndrome 1.* Retrieved June 6, 2009, from http://www.cancerindex.org/geneweb/NBS1.htm#summary

Cancer Genetics Web. (2003c). *RET.* Retrieved June 6, 2009, from http://www.cancerindex.org/geneweb/RET.htm#summary

Cancer Research UK. (2009). *Causes and cancer: Your environment and cancer.* Retrieved June 6, 2009, from http://www.cancerhelp.org.uk/help/default.asp?page=121&order=18

Carter, S.L., Eklund, A.C., Kohane, I.S., Harris, L.N., & Szallasi, Z. (2006). A signature of chromosomal instability inferred from gene expression profiles predicts clinical outcomes in multiple human cancers. *Nature Genetics, 38*(9), 1043–1048.

Chan, R.J., & Feng, G. (2007). PTPN11 is the first identified proto-oncogene that encodes a tyrosine phosphatase. *Blood, 109*(3), 862–867.

Clamp, M., Fry, B., Kamal, M., Xie, X., Cuff, J., Lin, M.F., et al. (2007). Distinguishing protein-coding and noncoding genes in the human genome. *Proceedings of the National Academy of Sciences, 104*(49), 19428–19433.

Consensus Panel on Genetic/Genomic Nursing Competencies. (2009). *Essentials of genetic and genomic nursing: Competencies, curricula guidelines, and outcome indicators* (2nd ed.). Silver Spring, MD: American Nurses Association.

D'Andrea, A.D. (2008). DNA repair pathways and human cancer. In J. Mendelsohn, P. Howley, M. Israel, J. Gray, & C. Thompson (Eds.), *The molecular basis of cancer* (3rd ed., pp. 39–56). Philadelphia: Elsevier Saunders.

Dayaram, T., & Marriott, S.J. (2008). Effect of transforming viruses on molecular mechanisms associated with cancer. *Journal of Cellular Physiology, 216*(2), 309–314.

Deng, C. (2006). BRCA1: Cell cycle checkpoint, genetic instability, DNA damage response and cancer evolution. *Nucleic Acids Research, 34*(5), 1416–1426.

Fearon, E.R., & Jones, P.A. (1992). Progressing toward a molecular description of colorectal cancer development. *FASEB Journal, 6*(10), 2783–2790.

Fearon, E.R., & Vogelstein, B. (1990). A genetic model for colorectal tumorigenesis. *Cell, 61*(5), 759–767.

Genetics Home Reference. (2009a). *How do geneticists indicate the location of a gene?* Retrieved June 6, 2009, from http://ghr.nlm.nih.gov/handbook/howgeneswork/genelocation

Genetics Home Reference. (2009b). *Li-Fraumeni syndrome.* Retrieved June 6, 2009, from http://ghr.nlm.nih.gov/condition=lifraumenisyndrome

Genetics Home Reference. (2009c). *Lynch syndrome.* Retrieved June 6, 2009, from http://ghr.nlm.nih.gov/condition=lynchsyndrome

Genetics Home Reference. (2009d). *Mutator gene.* Retrieved June 6, 2009, from http://ghr.nlm.nih.gov/glossary=mutatorgene

Genetics Home Reference. (2009e). *Wild-type.* Retrieved June 6, 2009, from http://ghr.nlm.nih.gov/glossary=wildtypeallele

Gollin, S.M. (2007). Mechanisms leading to nonrandom, nonhomologous chromosomal translocations in leukemia. *Seminars in Cancer Biology, 17*(1), 74–79.

Greene, K.L., Long-Cheng, L., Okino, S.T., & Carroll, P.R. (2008). Molecular basis of prostate cancer. In J. Mendelsohn, P. Howley, M. Israel, J. Gray, & C. Thompson (Eds.), *The molecular basis of cancer* (3rd ed., pp. 431–440). Philadelphia: Elsevier Saunders.

Hanahan, D., & Weinberg, R.A. (2000). The hallmarks of cancer. *Cell, 100*(1), 57–70.

Hartmann, E.M., Ott, G., & Rosenwald, A. (2008). Molecular biology and genetics of lymphomas. *Hematology/Oncology Clinics of North America, 22*(5), 807–823.

Human Genome Project. (2008, September). *SNP fact sheet.* Retrieved June 6, 2009, from http://www.ornl.gov/sci/techresources/Human_Genome/faq/snps.shtml

Jenkins, M., Hayashi, S., O'Shea, A.M., Burgart, L.J., Smyrk, T.C., Shimizu, D., et al. (2007). Pathology features in Bethesda guidelines predict colorectal cancer microsatellite instability: A population-based study. *Gastroenterology, 133*(1), 48–56.

Klug, S., & Cummings, M. (2005). *Genetics: A molecular perspective.* Prentice Hall.

Klug, S., Cummings, M., & Spencer, C. (2005). *Concepts of genetics* (8th ed.). Prentice Hall.

Knudson, A.G., Jr. (1971). Mutation and cancer: Statistical study of retinoblastoma. *Proceedings of the National Academy of Sciences, 68*(4), 820–823.

Levine, A., Hu, W., & Feng, Z. (2008). Tumor suppressor genes. In J. Mendelsohn, P. Howley, M. Israel, J. Gray, & C. Thompson (Eds.), *The molecular basis of cancer* (3rd ed., pp. 31–38). Philadelphia: Elsevier Saunders.

Lieber, M., Ma, Y., Pannicke, U., & Schwarz, K. (2003). Mechanism and regulation of human non-homologous DNA end-joining. *Nature Reviews Molecular Cell Biology, 4*(9), 712–720.

Lohmann, D.R., & Gallie, B.L. (2007). *Gene reviews: Retinoblastoma.* Retrieved June 6, 2009, from http://www.ncbi.nlm.nih.gov/bookshelf/br.fcgi?book=gene&part=retinoblastoma

Ma, L., Teruya-Feldstein, J., & Weinberg, R.A. (2007). Tumour invasion and metastasis initiated by microRNA-10b in breast cancer. *Nature, 449*(7163), 682–688.

McCabe, N., Turner, N.C., Lord, C.J., Kluzek, K., Bialkowska, A., Swift, S., et al. (2006). Deficiency in the repair of DNA damage by homologous recombination and sensitivity to poly (ADP-ribose) polymerase inhibition. *Cancer Research, 66*(16), 8109–8115.

McCance, K. (2006). Cellular biology. In K. McCance & S. Huether (Eds.), *Pathophysiology: The biologic basis for disease in adults and children* (5th ed., pp. 1–44). St. Louis, MO: Elsevier Mosby.

Meltzer, P.S. (2005). Cancer genomics: Small RNAs with big impacts. *Nature, 435*(7043), 745–746.

Mishra, A., Pandey, A., & Nong, X. (2007). Head and neck squamous cell cancer: Biology (1). *Indian Journal of Otolaryngology and Head and Neck Surgery, 59*(1), 28–32.

Murga, M., & Fernandez-Capetillo, O. (2007). Genomic instability: On the birth and death of cancer. *Clinical and Translational Oncology, 9*(4), 216–220.

Myllykangas, S., Bohling, T., & Knuutila, S. (2007). Specificity, selection and significance of gene amplifications in cancer. *Seminars in Cancer Biology, 17*(1), 42–55.

National Cancer Institute. (2005). *Understanding cancer series: Cancer genomics.* Retrieved June 6, 2009, from http://www.cancer.gov/cancertopics/understandingcancer/cancergenomics/allpages

National Cancer Institute. (2009). *Adult non-Hodgkin lymphoma treatment (PDQ®): Cellular classification of adult non-Hodgkin lymphoma.* Retrieved June 6, 2009, from http://www.cancer.gov/cancertopics/pdq/treatment/adult-non-hodgkins/HealthProfessional/page3

National Center for Biotechnology Information. (2004, March). *A science primer: What is a genome?* Retrieved June 6, 2009, from http://www.ncbi.nlm.nih.gov/About/primer/genetics_genome.html

National Center for Biotechnology Information. (2008). *Cancer chromosomes.* Retrieved June 6, 2009, from http://www.ncbi.nlm.nih.gov/sites/entrez?db=cancerchromosomes

National Center for Biotechnology Information. (2009a). *Entrez Gene: DDC1 DNA damage checkpoint protein, part of a PCNA-like complex required for DNA damage response, required for pachytene checkpoint to inhibit cell cycle in response to unrepaired recombination intermediates; potential Cdc28p substrate [Saccharomyces cerevisiae].* Retrieved June 6, 2009, from http://www.ncbi.nlm.nih.gov/sites/entrez?Db=gene&Cmd=ShowDetailView&TermToSearch=855907&ordinalpos=3&itool=EntrezSystem2.PEntrez.Gene.Gene_ResultsPanel.Gene_RVDocSum

National Center for Biotechnology Information. (2009b). *Entrez Gene: MGMT O-6-methylguanine-DNA methyltransferase [Homo sapiens].* Retrieved August 11, 2009, from http://www.ncbi.nlm.nih.gov/sites/entrez?db=gene&cmd=retrieve&list_uids=4255

National Center for Biotechnology Information. (n.d.-a). *Genes and disease: Burkitt Lymphoma.* Retrieved June 6, 2009, from http://www.ncbi.nlm.nih.gov/books/bv.fcgi?rid=gnd.section.92&ref=sidebar

National Center for Biotechnology Information. (n.d.-b). *Genes and disease: Leukemia, chronic myelogenous.* Retrieved June 6, 2009, from http://www.ncbi.nlm.nih.gov/books/bv.fcgi?rid=gnd.section.93&ref=sidebar

National Center for Biotechnology Information. (n.d.-c). *Genes and disease: The p53 tumor suppressor protein.* Retrieved June 6, 2009, from http://www.ncbi.nlm.nih.gov/books/bv.fcgi?rid=gnd.section.107

Nguyen, H., Tran, A., Lipkin, S., & Fruehauf, J.P. (2006). Pharmacogenomics of colorectal cancer prevention and treatment. *Cancer Investigation, 24*(6), 630–639.

Nowell, P.C. (1976). The clonal evolution of tumor cell populations. *Science, 194*(4260), 23–28.

Okutani, D., Lodyga, M., Han, B., & Liu, M. (2006). Src protein tyrosine kinase family and acute inflammatory responses. *American Journal of Physiology: Lung Cellular and Molecular Physiology, 291*(2), 129–141.

Ozanne, B.W., Spence, H.J., McGarry, L.C., & Hennigan, R.F. (2007). Transcription factors control invasion: AP-1 the first among equals. *Oncogene, 26*(1), 1–10.

Pawson, T., & Jorgensen, C. (2008). Signal transduction by growth factor receptors. In J. Mendelsohn, P. Howley, M. Israel, J. Gray, & C. Thompson (Eds.), *The molecular basis of cancer* (3rd ed., pp. 155–168). Philadelphia: Elsevier Saunders.

Schinazi, R.B. (2006). A Stochastic model for cancer risk. *Genetics, 174*(1), 545–547.

Schindeler, A., & Little, D.G. (2008). Recent insights into bone development, homeostasis and repair in Type 1 neurofibromatosis (NF1). *Bone, 42*(4), 616–622.

Smith, D.I., Zhu, Y., McAvoy, S., & Kuhn, R. (2006). Common fragile sites, extremely large genes, neural development and cancer. *Cancer Letters, 232*(1), 48–57.

Söreide, K., Janssen, E., Söiland, H., Körner, H., & Baak, P. (2006). Microsatellite instability in colorectal cancer. *British Journal of Surgery, 93*(4), 395–406.

Swerdlow, A.J., Schoemaker, M.J., Higgins, C.D., Wright, A.F., & Jacobs, P.A. (2008). Cancer risk in patients with constitutional chromosome deletions: A nationwide British cohort study. *British Journal of Cancer, 98*(12), 1929–1933.

Wang, V., & Wu, W. (2007). MicroRNA: A new player in breast cancer development. *Journal of Cancer Molecules, 3*(5), 133–138.

Wang, Z., Cummins, J.M., Shen, D., Cahill, D.P., Jallepalli, P.V., Wang, T.L., et al. (2004). Three classes of genes mutated in colorectal cancers with chromosomal instability. *Cancer Research, 64*(9), 2998–3001.

Ward, D., Brueggemeier, R., Caligiuri, M., Gahbauer, R., & Kraut, E. (2005, February). Cancer—one name, many diseases. *NetWellness.* Retrieved June 6, 2009, from http://www.netwellness.org/healthtopics/cancer/introduction.cfm

Weizmann Institute of Science. (n.d.). *The GeneCards human gene database.* Retrieved November 28, 2009, from http://www.genecards.org/index.shtml

Wicha, M., Liu, S., & Dontu, G. (2006). Cancer stem cells; an old idea—a paradigm shift. *Cancer Research, 66*(4), 1883–1890.

U.S. Department of Energy Office of Science Office of Biological and Environmental Research. (n.d.). *Human Genome Project Information.* Retrieved June 6, 2009, from http://www.ornl.gov/sci/techresources/Human_Genome/project/info.shtml

U.S. National Institutes of Health. (2004). *International Human Genome Sequencing Consortium describes finished human genome sequence.* Retrieved June 6, 2009, from http://www.genome.gov/12513430

Zhivotovsky, B., & Orrenius, S. (2006). Carcinogenesis and apoptosis: Paradigms and paradoxes. *Carcinogenesis, 27*(10), 1939–1945.

SECTION II

Genetics and Genomics: Identification and Risk Reduction

CHAPTER 3 HOW TO PERFORM A CANCER GENETIC RISK ASSESSMENT

CHAPTER 4 COMMON RISK PREDICTION MODELS AND CANCER RISK COMMUNICATION

CHAPTER 5 DELIVERING GENETIC EDUCATION AND COUNSELING SERVICES

CHAPTER 6 ESTABLISHMENT OF A CANCER GENETICS RISK ASSESSMENT PROGRAM

CHAPTER 7 GENOME-WIDE ASSOCIATION STUDIES AND CANCER

CHAPTER 3

How to Perform a Cancer Genetic Risk Assessment

Karen Roesser, MS, RN, AOCN®

Professional Practice Domain:
Nursing Assessment: Applying/Integrating Genetic and Genomic Knowledge
- Demonstrate ability to elicit a minimum of three-generation family health history information
- Construct a pedigree from collected family history information using standardized symbols and terminology
- Collect personal, health, and developmental histories that consider genetic, environmental, and genomic influences and risks
- Conduct comprehensive health and physical assessments that incorporate knowledge about genetic, environmental, and genomic influences and risk factors
Identification
- Identify clients who may benefit from specific genetic and genomic information and/or services based on assessment data

(Consensus Panel on Genetic/Genomic Nursing Competencies, 2009)

INTRODUCTION

All oncology nurses are aware of the importance of patient assessments. Assessments are a key component to providing comprehensive cancer care. An assessment typically includes collecting information on physical, environmental (diet, exercise, exposures), and psychosocial factors to develop a thorough plan of care. To fully assess the client for an inherited cancer predisposition, a comprehensive assessment includes the evaluation of genetic and genomic factors. The mapping of the human genome has changed the view of genetics from a specialty focused on single-gene disorders to recognition that everyone has genetic and genomic contributions to their health (Consensus Panel on Genetic/Genomic Nursing Competencies, 2009). Because cancer is influenced by biologic, medical, environmental, genetic, and genomic factors, a comprehensive cancer assessment includes evaluation of all these elements.

Information obtained through a genetic and genomic assessment may reveal that an individual has a higher-than-average risk of developing cancer or that an individual with cancer has a higher-than-average risk for developing a second primary cancer. Accurately predicting cancer risk provides the rationale for risk-reducing interventions. In addition, risk identification provides valuable information for family members who are at increased risk. Thus, the oncology nurse has the responsibility to identify high-risk individuals, to begin to provide education on identified risks, and to refer those high-risk individuals for cancer-risk evaluation, education, and counseling. Although risk assessment occurs across the cancer continuum, this chapter will focus on genetic cancer risk assessment to identify high-risk individuals who may benefit from further genetic evaluation or risk-reduction interventions.

CANCER GENETIC ASSESSMENT

A genetic assessment for cancer evaluates multiple **risk factors** to determine the likelihood that an individual will develop cancer or has an inherited predisposition to an existing cancer. A genetic cancer risk assessment includes evaluation of evidence of known cancer syndromes along with risk factors identified for cancer. Other nongenetic risk factors remain important because a single genetic mutation is not enough to cause a malignancy (National Cancer Institute [NCI], 2008). Although an individual may be born with a gene mutation that predisposes him or her to cancer, it does not mean that the person inevitably will develop the disease. The complex interaction between cancer-predisposing genes and other genes in the body, as well as the interactions with endogenous and exogenous factors, may initiate or modify the carcinogenic process (NCI, 2008). Identifying a likely familial cancer susceptibility syndrome and detecting an inherited predisposition to cancer makes possible the initiation of risk-management measures to decrease the risk of cancer development and facilitates early detection.

PURPOSE OF A CANCER GENETIC ASSESSMENT

The main purposes of a cancer genetic risk assessment are to collect and evaluate personal, medical, and family information; to identify high-risk individuals who could benefit from genetic testing, cancer risk reduction, or early detection strategies; and to improve the quantity and quality of life. This process of collecting and evaluating personal, medical, and family history aims to assist the multidisciplinary team to estimate the client's cancer risk, to identify familial cancer susceptibility syndromes, and to determine the associated probability of finding a genetic mutation. The graphic representation of the family history compiled in a pedigree (described later in this chapter) is evaluated to find patterns of cancer that may be suggestive of sporadic, familial, or hereditary cancer. These patterns help to categorize the family history as follows.

- Hereditary: A family has a known genetic predisposition for cancer.
- Assumed or putative hereditary: The family history has the hallmarks and features of a hereditary cancer syndrome.
- Familial: Several cancers that do not clearly fit a hereditary cancer syndrome are present in a family. The cancers may be related to gene-environment interactions shared in a family.
- Sporadic: Family members have cancers that are caused by acquired mutations or environmental exposures.

The patterns of Mendelian inheritance (autosomal dominant [AD], autosomal recessive [AR], or X-linked) displayed in the family history give further clues to the type of cancer syndrome (see Table 3-1). For example, knowing the presence of an AR pattern of inheritance in a family with early-onset colon cancers and adenomatous polyps would guide the healthcare provider to include *MYH*-associated polyposis as a possible cancer syndrome because *MYH* mutations are inherited in an AR fashion (Lipton & Tomlinson, 2004). The client's medical and surgical history as well as health information from the family may yield further features suggestive of a specific cancer syndrome. For example, the existence of multiple family members with colon polyps is suggestive of several polyposis cancer syndromes. Use of risk tools to quantify the probability of a cancer predisposition gene mutation in the fam-

family also may be helpful. (See Chapter 4 for a more detailed discussion of cancer risk prediction models.) With all this information, a differential list of possible cancer syndromes is compiled that may account for the cancers in a given family having a familial or hereditary pattern of cancer. The differential list is evaluated systematically to either rule out or select the most likely cancer syndrome based on the cancers in the family, the malignant or benign features present, and the Mendelian pattern of inheritance. The identification of the most likely cancer syndrome guides the plan for genetic testing, medical management, and risk reduction strategies. The knowledge of cancer risk factors, patterns of cancer, and familial cancer syndromes drives the cancer genetic risk assessment, identifies the most likely familial cancer syndromes that are present, and guides the plan for genetic testing.

TABLE 3-1. Characteristics of Mendelian Transmission

Characteristic	Autosomal Dominant	Autosomal Recessive	X-Linked
Cluster of affected members	Vertical transmission; seen in successive generations. The condition may appear to skip a generation because of incomplete penetrance, early death because of other causes, older age at onset, small family size, or few females or males when the target organ is sex-specific.	Horizontal transmission (i.e., seen in one generation only); not seen in successive generations. Affected individuals usually cluster within one sibship.	Females are rarely affected, and when they are, the effects are usually milder than they are in males.
Side of family or sex usually affected	Usually seen on only one side of the family. Male-to-male transmission may be seen.	Mutated genes must come from both sides of the family; biparental inheritance	Males in the maternal lineage (brothers and maternal uncles) are affected.
Percentage of offspring affected	Males and females may inherit and transmit the disorder to offspring. Offspring have a 50% chance of inheriting a mutation and a 50% chance of inheriting the normal allele.	Parents are heterozygous carriers; each carries one mutated copy of the gene and one functional copy. Heterozygous parents have a 25% recurrence risk for future offspring being affected.	No father-to-son transmission of the mutation occurs because the father cannot transmit an X-linked condition to his son because he gives the son his Y chromosome and not his X. 50% of males will be affected when mother is a carrier. 50% of females will be a carrier when mother is a carrier.
Examples of disorders characterized by Mendelian inheritance pattern	Hereditary breast/ovarian cancer syndrome, Lynch syndrome, familial adenomatous polyposis (FAP), von Hippel-Lindau disease, and multiple endocrine neoplasia	Bloom syndrome, ataxia telangiectasia, *MYH* mutations in FAP, and Fanconi anemia	Hemophilia

Note. Based on information from Hartl & Jones, 2008; Ringo, 2004; Schneider, 2002.

Another purpose of cancer genetic risk assessment is to provide information to help individuals and families to make an informed decision about proceeding with genetic testing, consider the impact of testing, and determine what risk-reduction measures can be undertaken with or without genetic testing. In 2003 and again in 2010 (Robson et al., 2010), the American Society of Clinical Oncology (ASCO) updated its policy statement on the indications for genetic testing for cancer susceptibility:

> ASCO recommends that genetic counseling and testing be offered when 1) the individual has personal or family history features suggestive of a genetic cancer susceptibility condition, 2) the genetic test can be adequately interpreted, and 3) the test results will aid in diagnosis or influence the medical or surgical management of the patient or family members at hereditary risk of cancer. ASCO recommends that genetic testing only be done in the setting of pre- and post-test counseling, which should include discussion of possible risks and benefits of cancer early detection and prevention modalities. (ASCO, 2003, p. 2397)

Chapter 5 provides an in-depth discussion of the education and counseling that is provided in cancer genetic risk assessment.

Having a process for the collection of the personal, medical, and family history enables the risk assessment team to evaluate potential cancer risks and presence of hereditary cancer syndromes in order to plan for individualized screening and risk-reduction strategies.

FAMILIAL CANCER SUSCEPTIBILITY SYNDROMES

The discovery of multiple germ line cancer susceptibility genes along with their identified clinical characteristics has made the nursing evaluation of family history information challenging. Learning the types of cancer constellations along with associated clinical features that are suggestive of a predisposition to cancer is essential to oncology nursing proficiency in cancer genetic risk assessment. Several cancer syndromes may be suspected for cancers seen in a given family. Knowing about cancer syndrome resources will help the healthcare team to review pedigrees for potential cancer syndromes and develop a cancer syndrome differential list. The central resource is the Online Mendelian Inheritance in Man® (OMIM), a comprehensive database with referenced reviews of all known Mendelian disorders (National Center for Biotechnology Information, n.d.).

A key resource based on the OMIM data is the *Concise Handbook of Familial Cancer Susceptibility Syndromes* (Lindor, McMaster, Lindor, & Greene, 2008). This monograph presents more than 50 cancer syndromes with a description of their associated OMIM number related to the cancer syndrome and genotype, the inheritance pattern, gene and chromosome location, the mutations and their incidence, diagnosic and laboratory features, the associated malignant and benign neoplasms, and risk management. For ease of clinical use and to facilitate the development of a differential list, the Lindor et al. resource provides a table of 55 cancer syndromes that can be matched to associated malignancies seen in each syndrome. A separate table also summarizes the nonmalignant and clinical features associated with each syndrome. These tables are a handy and concise resource to have in a clinical setting when compiling a differential list of cancer syndromes. Table 3-2 shows selected cancer syndromes by cancer type.

TABLE 3-2 Selected Hereditary Cancer Syndromes by Cancer Type

Syndrome	Gene	Inheritance Mode	Associated Cancers	Other Clinical or Distinguishing Features
Breast				
Hereditary breast/ovarian cancer (HBOC)	BRCA1 and BRCA2	AD	Female and male breast, ovarian, fallopian tube, primary peritoneal, pancreatic, prostate, melanoma	Ductal carcinoma institu is part of HBOC. Ovarian tumors and primary peritoneal cancer are epithelial type.
Cowden syndrome	PTEN	AD	Endometrial, female and male breast, follicular and papillary thyroid	Mucocutaneous: oral mucosa papillomatosis, facial trichilemmomas, acral or palmoplantar keratosis. Hamartomatous polyps of the stomach, small bowel, and colon. Fibrocystic breast disease, uterine fibroids, macrocephaly.
Li-Fraumeni syndrome	TP53	AD	Osteogenic and chondrosarcoma, rhabdomyosarcoma, breast, brain (especially glioblastoma), leukemia, lymphoma, and adrenocortical carcinoma	Classically, sarcomas and cancers of the breast, brain, and adrenal glands comprise 80% of cancers in Li-Fraumeni syndrome.
Peutz-Jeghers syndrome	STK11	AD	Breast, colorectal, endometrial, cervical, gastric, lung, pancreatic, ovarian	Ovarian tumors are sex cord tumors; cervical cancers are primarily adenoma malignum type. Menorrhagia or precocious puberty secondary to ovarian sex cord tumors. For more gastrointestinal characteristics, see Peutz-Jeghers syndrome in GI section.
Gastrointestinal (GI)				
Lynch syndrome	MLH1 MSH2 PMS2 MSH6	AD	Colorectal, endometrial adenocarcinoma, gastric, biliary tract, urinary tract, ovarian, small bowel, pancreatic	Gliomas and polyps, colonic adenomas, keratoacanthomas, sebaceous adenomas
Familial adenomatous polyposis (FAP)	APC	AD	Gastric, duodenal, colon, pancreatic	Colonic, gastric, and duodenal (primarily ampulla of Vater) polyps; desmoid tumors. Osteomas of the jaw. Dental abnormalities: absent or supernumerary teeth. Brain tumors, primarily medulloblastoma.
MYH-associated polyposis	MYH	AR	Colon, duodenal	Tumors show stable microsatellites. Colonic and duodenal adenomas, gastric fundic gland polyps, osteomas and sebaceous gland adenomas, pilomatricomas

(Continued on next page)

TABLE 3-2   Selected Hereditary Cancer Syndromes by Cancer Type *(Continued)*

Syndrome	Gene	Inheritance Mode	Associated Cancers	Other Clinical or Distinguishing Features
Peutz-Jeghers syndrome	STK11	AD	Stomach, small intestines, colon, pancreatic, breast, lung, uterine, ovarian	GI cancers are the most common group of cancers in Peutz-Jeghers syndrome. Multiple polyps throughout the GI tract; having first polypectomy from age 13–22 years. Sertoli cell tumors of the testis. For more breast and reproductive characteristics, see Peutz-Jeghers syndrome in Breast section.
Hereditary diffuse gastric cancer	CDH1	AD	Diffuse gastric and lobular breast carcinoma	None known.
Pancreatic				
Hereditary pancreatic	PALLD	AD	Adenocarcinoma of pancreas	See also HBOC, Lynch syndrome, FAP, hereditary melanoma, and Peutz-Jeghers syndrome.
Prostate				
Hereditary prostate	HPC1 HPC2 HPCX	AD X-linked	Prostate	No clear single gene explains all familial prostate cancer. See also HBOC.
Skin				
Basal cell nevus syndrome or Gorlin syndrome	PTCH	AD	Multiple basal cell carcinoma, medulloblastoma (children younger than 2 years old), ovarian fibrosarcoma	Fibromas or dermoid tumors of the ovary; juvenile polyps of the small or large bowel; odontogenic keratocysts of the jaw mean number = 5), epidermal cysts, palmoplantar pits
Hereditary melanoma	CDKN2A	AD	Melanoma, pancreatic	Dysplastic nevi
Endocrine				
Multiple endocrine neoplasia type 1 (MEN type 1)	MEN1	AD	Adrenal cortical, carcinoid, islet cell pancreatic, parathyroid, malignant schwannoma	Hepatic, adrenal cortex, parathyroid, pituitary and pancreatic adenomas. Cutaneous epidermoid and sebaceous cysts. Multiple lipomas.
MEN type 2	RET	AD	Medullary thyroid, bilateral pheochromocytomas	Hyperparathyroidism, benign pheochrom cytomas

AD—autosomal dominant; AR—autosomal recessive
Note. Based on information from Lindor et al., 2008.

GeneTests (www.genetests.org) is an online resource that provides peer-reviewed summaries on a variety of genetic disorders along with diagnosis, clinical descriptions, and differential diagnoses. Using the *GeneTests* Web site requires some foundational knowledge of cancer syndromes because the user needs to submit the name of a cancer syndrome or the principal cancer seen in a syndrome to drive the search. Continued use of these resources will help to build knowledge of familial cancer susceptibility syndromes and associated clinical features. This, in turn, helps to familiarize the nurse with the range of information that needs to be collected for the cancer genetic risk assessment.

COMPONENTS OF A CANCER GENETIC RISK ASSESSMENT

The components of cancer genetic risk assessment include gathering and evaluating information about the client's medical and psychosocial health history, lifestyle, cognition and beliefs of the individual, the medical history of his or her family, tumor features of identified cancers in the client and family members, findings from a physical examination, prior surgeries, and his or her motivation for seeking risk assessment (see Figure 3-1).

FIGURE 3-1 COMPONENTS OF A CANCER GENETIC ASSESSMENT

- A three-generation family history
- Any features related to the identified cancers or benign findings in the client and family members suggestive of familial cancer syndromes
- Client's health history
- Current health status
- Medical, surgical, reproductive, and cancer screening history
- Lifestyle factors and environmental exposures
- Assessment of cultural and religious beliefs
- Information about race and ethnicity
- Assessment of client's psychosocial state, history, support, and coping mechanisms
- Motivation for seeking risk assessment and risk perception
- Evaluation of cognitive style and preferences for learning
- Physical examination, as indicated
- Analysis of the personal, medical, and family history information
- Constellation of cancers and any significant clinical features
- Mendelian pattern of inheritance: autosomal dominant, autosomal recessive, X-linked
- Pattern of cancer (e.g., sporadic, familial, hereditary)
- Likely familial cancer susceptibility syndromes
- Estimated cancer risk and carrier probability
- Communication and education regarding the risk information

The Client's Health History

The interplay of health behaviors such as tobacco use with genetic factors that influence the development of cancer is growing (Schwartz, Prysak, Bock, & Cote, 2007; Yeo et al., 2009). Information about known personal and medical cancer risk factors along with new information related to polymorphisms with corresponding cancer risk will be important to perform a comprehensive cancer risk assessment. The impact of findings from genome wide-association studies (see Chapter 5) will elucidate the interaction of inherited polymorphisms, health behaviors, and exposures in cancer risk estimations. Therefore, nurses cannot overlook the importance of the client's health history.

The cancer genetic risk assessment begins with the client seeking risk information and evaluation. The client's medical history includes a review of medical history, including birth defects, genetic disorders, and benign or malignant conditions, as well as current medical conditions, medications, lifestyle and exposure history, reproductive history, and cancer screening with abnormal findings, if applicable.

Medical History

Obtaining a detailed medical history of birth defects, genetic disorders, and benign or malignant conditions helps with the potential identification of familial cancer syndromes or a higher risk of cancer. For example, birth defects such as aniridia (a congenital, hereditary, bilateral condition characterized by the underdevelopment of the eyes' irises) increase the risk for familial Wilms tumor (van Heyningen, Hoovers, de Kraker, & Crolla, 2007) or undescended testicles for testicular cancer. Having Turner syndrome, a cytogenetic disorder with complete or partial loss of the X chromosome, is seen in females presenting with short stature and premature ovarian failure. Turner syndrome increases the risk for central nervous system tumors or uterine cancer (Schoemaker et al., 2008). Other benign conditions such as multiple adenomatous polyps may indicate a colon cancer syndrome (Lindor et al., 2008) or multiple dysplastic nevi for melanoma (Tucker et al., 2002). Past radiation treatment for Hodgkin lymphoma increases the risk for breast cancer (American Cancer Society [ACS], 2008k). Women who received ionizing radiation of the chest (particularly mantle radiation) in the treatment of Hodgkin lymphoma at a young age (prepubertal years of 10–14) have been particularly vulnerable to develop cancer with almost all cases in or at the margin of the radiation field (Guibout et al., 2005). The presence of adenomatous colon polyps, particularly those larger than 1 cm and those with villous or tubulovillous histology, will increase the risk of colorectal cancer. In colorectal cancer syndromes, a rapid progression from polyp to cancer may occur (Levine & Ahnen, 2006).

Reproductive History

Information about reproductive history is an important component of a health history. Such information is useful in evaluating a woman's risk of breast, endometrial, and ovarian cancers. Document a woman's age at menarche and menopause. Ask about infertility, findings from any workup for infertility, and the use of donor egg or donor sperm. Record the total number of pregnancies and note whether the results were live births, if any children were born with birth defects, and if any pregnancies were terminated or if spontaneous abortions occurred. If the patient terminated the pregnancy, was this for personal reasons or because of an abnormality in the fetus? Note the woman's age when her first child was born and whether she breast-fed and for how long. Record whether she ever used exogenous hormones (e.g., oral contraceptives, fertility drugs, hormone replacement therapy) and if so, which ones, age at use, and duration of use. This information is important because the risk of breast, ovarian, or endometrial cancer is associated with features such as early menarche, late age at first pregnancy, nulliparity, and the use of exogenous hormones (ACS, 2008b, 2008c, 2008d). Also, include any gynecologic surgery that the client or her family members have had, such as tubal ligation, total abdominal hysterectomy, and bilateral salpingo-oophorectomy, and the reason for these procedures.

In males, ask about infertility problems if they have not had any children. For men with infertility and male breast cancer, consider a workup for Klinefelter syndrome. Most males with this syndrome have an extra X chromosome in all of their cells. Instead of the XY chromosome pattern normally seen, men with Klinefelter syndrome have XXY. This condition also is associated with delayed muscular development in infancy, small testes that do not produce enough testosterone, and in adulthood, autoimmune disorders, enlarged breasts, and osteoporosis (Genetics Home Reference, 2008a).

Environmental Exposures

Note if the client has had unusual exposures to radiation, chemicals, or industrial processes. Exposure to ionizing radiation or various chemicals such as benzene, asbestos, or alkylating agents is associated with increased rates of some cancers, including leukemia, breast cancer, lung cancer, mesothelioma, multiple myeloma, and thyroid cancer (ACS, 2008a, 2008g, 2008h, 2008j).

Lifestyle Assessment

A comprehensive assessment of an individual's lifestyle may provide important information about factors contributing to or modifying cancer risk. Characteristics to consider include weight, diet, exercise, tobacco use, alcohol use, and sun exposure. For the majority of Americans who do not smoke cigarettes, dietary choices and physical activity are important modifiable determinants of cancer risk (Danaei et al., 2005).

Weight

In the assessment, include the client's current height and weight. These measurements are important because of the relationship between obesity and certain cancers. According to the World Health Organization, obesity, defined by a body mass index greater than 30 kg/m^2, has been associated with an increased risk for a variety of cancers. NCI (2004) and ACS noted an increased risk of cancers of the colon, breast (postmenopausal), esophagus, uterus, and kidney in obese individuals (Kushi et al., 2006). The Million Women Study (Reeves et al., 2007) found an association with various hematologic cancers, including multiple myeloma, non-Hodgkin lymphoma, and leukemia, along with colorectal cancer in premenopausal obese women.

Diet

Ask about dietary intake related to the amounts of fat, fiber, fruits, and vegetables. A diet high in red meat and fat may increase a person's risk of developing colorectal cancer (Doyle, 2007). In addition to their link to colorectal cancer, high-fat diets have been associated with an increased risk of cancers of the prostate and endometrium (Byers et al., 2002). Little evidence supports that the total amount of fat consumed affects cancer risk. However, diets high in fat tend to be high in calories and may contribute to obesity, which in turn is linked with an increased risk of cancers. With regard to fiber intake, a dose-response relationship exists with higher intake of dietary fiber showing a protective effect for colorectal cancer (World Cancer Research Fund & American Institute of Cancer Research, 2007).

Exercise

Assessment of the client's exercise patterns may be helpful to plan risk reduction measures. ACS (2009) reported that people who engage in physical activity are at a lower risk for developing colon and breast cancer. These guidelines recommend 45–60 minutes of moderate to vigorous physical activity at least five days per week for adults. Healthful dietary patterns in combination with regular physical activity have been shown to reduce cancer risk. Exercise decreases the risk of some cancers either by reducing obesity or through other mechanisms, some of which are specific to particular cancer types, such as colon, breast, and prostate cancer. The biologic mechanisms include the effects of exercise on fat and sugar metabolism;

immune function; levels of several hormones, including insulin and estradiol; factors that regulate cell proliferation and growth, apoptosis, differentiation, and angiogenesis such as insulin-like growth factor, insulin-like growth factor binding protein, and prostaglandins; and proteins that make hormones more or less available to tissues such as sex hormone–binding globulin (Bardia et al., 2006; Neilson, Friedenreich, Brockton, & Millikan, 2009; Wolin & Colditz, 2008). The association between physical activity and decreased risk of breast and colon cancer has been demonstrated across levels of obesity, suggesting that the protective effect of activity goes beyond its effect on body weight (Bardia et al.; Hu et al., 2004). Another biologic mechanism related to exercise and colon cancer suggests that reducing the amount of time colon cells are exposed to biliary acids, dietary toxins, or carcinogens decreases mucosal damage that can lead to abnormal cell growth and cancer. Exercise increases the transit time of food through the digestive tract. More research is needed on whether an individual needs to participate in high-intensity exercise to reduce food transit time or if moderate-intensity exercise is enough (ASCO, 2007).

Tobacco Use

Note whether the client has used or currently uses tobacco and alcohol and, if so, how much and for how long. Smoking accounts for at least 30% of all cancer deaths (U.S. Department of Health and Human Services, 2004). Tobacco is associated with a greater risk of cancers of the lung, head and neck, bladder, and esophagus; however, it is linked to at least 15 different cancers (ACS, 2008i). Although smoking has long been associated with the development of lung cancer, data show that multiple genes and gene-environment interactions have influence on the development of lung cancer with even low levels of smoke exposure conferring increased risk (Schwartz et al., 2007). These gene-environment interactions related to smoking also have been associated with risk for familial and sporadic pancreatic cancer (Yeo et al., 2009). Individuals may benefit from having recommendations about smoking cessation as part of risk-reduction measures because smokers are more likely to quit if a healthcare professional advises them to do so (ACS, 2008i).

Alcohol Consumption

Alcohol is associated with a greater risk of cancers of the oral cavity, esophagus, larynx, liver, and breast (Kushi et al., 2006). ACS recommends that individuals who drink alcohol limit their intake to no more than two drinks per day for men and one drink per day for women (Kushi et al.).

Sun Exposure

Record whether the client is exposed to the sun on a regular basis. Ultraviolet (UV) radiation is thought to be the main risk factor for most skin cancers and sunlight is the main source of UV radiation. The effects of the sun on the risks for melanoma and nonmelanoma cancers of the skin are well established. Also assess the use of tanning lamps and booths, another source of UV radiation. Caucasians with fair (light-colored) skin that freckles or burns easily, blond or red hair, and light eyes are at especially high risk. People who live in areas with year-round, bright sunlight or those people who spend a lot of time outdoors for work or recreation without protective clothing and sunscreen have an increased risk. Do not forget to ask about childhood sun exposure and sunburns. Cumulative sun exposure causes mainly basal cell and squamous cell skin cancers, whereas episodes of severe burns in childhood present a great risk for melanoma (ACS, 2008e, 2008f). Whiteman, Whiteman, and Green (2001) calculated an observed melanoma risk of 1.8 (95% confidence interval [CI], 1.6–2.2) for childhood sunburns compared to 1.5 (95% CI, 1.3–1.8) sunburns in adulthood. Counsel clients to practice sun protective behaviors such as midday sun avoidance and the use of protective clothing as effective primary risk-reducing strategies against the development of skin cancers.

Vitamins and Supplements

List the medications the client uses, including over-the-counter agents such as vitamins and supplements, along with the quantities and duration of use. Studies are ongoing in regard to the relationship between the use of medications, vitamins, and supplements and cancer; some show negative results. The long-term use of vitamin E and selenium did not reduce the risk of prostate cancer (Peters et al., 2008), and the use of supplemental multivitamins, vitamin C, vitamin E, and folate was not associated with a decreased risk of lung cancer (Slatore, Littman, Au, Satia, & White, 2008). Several studies have shown protective associations of calcium and the development of polyps, thus decreasing the risk of developing colorectal cancer (Grau et al., 2007; McCullough et al., 2003). Grau et al. found that clients with a history of polyps who took 1,200 milligrams of supplemental calcium for four years had a significant reduction in colon polyp recurrence that persisted for as long as five years after treatment ended. Further research about supplements and cancer risk is being conducted; however, ensuring that information about medication and vitamins is in the client's history for reference in the future may be helpful if established correlations are identified.

Healthcare Practices and Screening Tests

Include in the lifestyle assessment a description of the client's healthcare practices and beliefs. Assess compliance with the recommended early-detection screening tests, including the dates of the client's most recent screening examinations and self-tests, note how frequently the client undergoes such screenings and performs self-tests, and document unusual findings (see Table 3-3 for recommended screening tests). If the client has had these tests, try to validate self-reports with medical records or test reports when possible. Relying on the client's self-report of the test results may lead to false assumptions in care. If the client is not using the recommended early-detection cancer screening methods, find out why. This will allow the healthcare team to clarify misperceptions, identify barriers to use of screening, and provide useful information that will help the client to understand the importance of early detection.

Surgical History

Documenting past surgeries using official records is important. The surgical history includes the organs removed, location, and pathology findings on biopsies and surgical resections. The client may not be able to provide this information immediately. Most people who have had biopsies report a growth was benign and do not know the pathologic features. The same holds true for surgical resection for a cancer. Clients may not remember or know the details of what was removed in their surgery. Obtaining pathologic reports whenever possible can verify the location and the organs removed, confirm the cancer diagnosis, and help to determine if the pathologic features suggest the presence of an inherited cancer syndrome. In addition, individuals often report multiple cancers such as colon and

TABLE 3-3 American Cancer Society Guidelines for the Early Detection of Cancer

Type of Cancer	Screening Measure	Age	Recommendations
Breast	Clinical breast examination	20s–30s	For all women every three years
		40 and older	For all women every year
	Breast self-examination	20s	Option for all women
	Mammography	40	For all women who are in good health every year
	Breast magnetic resonance imaging	Based on lifetime risk of breast cancer	
		Greater than 20% risk	Women should get annually along with mammogram.
		15%–20% risk	Women should talk with physicians about risk/benefits.
		Less than 15% risk	Not recommended
Colon and rectal	Flexible sigmoidoscopy[a]	50	For both men and women every five years (colonoscopy should be performed if test results are positive)
	Colonoscopy[a]	50	For men and women every 10 years
	Double-contrast barium enema[a]	50	For men and women every five years (colonoscopy should be done if test results are positive)
	Computed tomography colonography[a] (virtual colonoscopy)	50	For men and women every five years (colonoscopy should be done if test results are positive)
	Fecal occult blood test[b,c] (FOBT)	50	For men and women every year[b]
	Fecal immunochemical test[b,c] (FIT)	50	For men and women every year[b]
	Stool DNA test[b]	50	Interval uncertain (colonoscopy should be done if test results are positive)
Cervical	Pap test	Begin three years after starting vaginal intercourse or at least by age 21	For all women every one to two years (based on type of Pap test used)
		30–69	Screening may be changed to every two to three years for women ≥ 30 years who have three normal Pap tests.
		70 or older	If ≥ 70 years with three or more normal Pap tests in a row plus no abnormal Pap test results in last 10 years, may choose to stop cervical screening.

(Continued on next page)

TABLE 3-3	American Cancer Society Guidelines for the Early Detection of Cancer *(Continued)*		
Type of Cancer	Screening Measure	Age	Recommendations
	Human papillomavirus (HPV) DNA test plus conventional or liquid-based Pap test	30–69	Another option for women ≥ 30 years is screening every three years with either conventional or liquid-based Pap test plus the HPV DNA test.
Endometrial (uterine)	Endometrial biopsy	35 and older	Yearly for all women who have Lynch syndrome or are at high risk for it
Prostate	Prostate-specific antigen (PSA) + digital rectal examination	50	ACS does not support routine testing, but recommends discussion of benefits and limitations of early detection testing. If testing is requested, it should be yearly for all men who have at least a 10-year life expectancy.
		45 for African American men and men with positive family history (one or more first-degree relatives diagnosed before age 65)	Discussion of potential benefits and limitations of early detection testing If testing is requested, it should be yearly.
		40 for men with several first-degree relatives with prostate cancer at an early age	Discussion of potential benefits and limitations of early detection testing If testing is requested, it should be yearly.

[a] Tests that find polyps and cancer are preferred if they are available and the client is willing to undergo them.
[b] Tests that mainly find cancer
[c] For FOBT or FIT used as a screening test, the take-home multiple sample method should be used. A FOBT or FIT done during a digital rectal examination in the physician's office is not adequate for screening.

Note. Based on information from American Cancer Society, 2009.

ovarian when it was a primary cancer with metastasis to another organ. Accurate surgical and pathology information may help to identify potential cancer syndromes and who may benefit from genetic testing or other risk-reduction options.

Past surgeries may have been part of risk-reduction measures. Knowing the type of surgery and what organs were removed is equally important in order to assess further risk and to plan for medical management. For example, it is important to know what was removed when a woman reports having her ovaries removed. *BRCA1* and *BRCA2* mutations increase the risk for ovarian and fallopian tube cancer, with recent data showing dysplastic changes and occult cancers in the fimbriae of surgically removed fallopian tubes (Rabban, Crawford, Chen, Powell, & Zaloudek, 2009). If this same woman is planning to take either tamoxifen or raloxifene to reduce breast cancer risk, then knowing if the uterus was removed will help with planning chemoprevention, as a side effect of tamoxifen is uterine cancer (Wickerham et al., 2009). Therefore, the surgical report of the organs removed gives clarification for how much risk-reduction was achieved with surgery and if further surgical consideration is needed.

Surgical and pathology information may provide genotype-phenotype correlations suggestive of hereditary cancer. The phenotype is the observable characteristics of an organism, such as its shape or biologic properties, determined by the organism's genes or genotype. Pathology findings may have phenotypic characteristics that suggest an underlying genetic cause for cancer. For example, multiple endocrine neoplasia type 2A (MEN2A), MEN2B, or familial medullary thyroid cancer often is first suspected after the diagnosis of medullary thyroid carcinoma (Gertner & Kebebew, 2004; Raue & Frank-Raue, 2007). If a person had a colonoscopy and reported having polyps, pathology reports can clarify cancer risk. Hyperplastic polyps carry a lower risk for cancer, whereas villous adenomatous polyps are associated with a higher risk of cancer (Levine & Ahnen, 2006).

Other Distinguishing Surgical Features

The occurrence of specific precursor lesions has been associated with hereditary cancer syndromes. The client or family members may manifest precursor lesions, that is, lesions that can evolve into invasive cancers. Obtaining information about the location, the number, and the pathology features of precursor lesions is helpful in determining if the lesion fits a cancer syndrome. For example, the colon and rectum of an individual with familial adenomatous polyposis typically are carpeted with hundreds or thousands of polyps. A number of cancer syndromes are characterized by the occurrence of hamartomatous polyps in the gastrointestinal tract, including Peutz-Jeghers syndrome, juvenile polyposis, and neurofibromatosis (Lindor et al., 2008). In some cases, precursor lesions are considered a premalignant syndrome, such as familial dysplastic nevus syndrome.

Other benign findings may be associated with a cancer syndrome. For example, individuals with Peutz-Jeghers syndrome have multiple pigmented spots on the lips and buccal mucosa. These pigmented spots typically present in infancy or childhood and occur in more than 95% of cases of Peutz-Jeghers syndrome (Schneider, 2002). A client with a history of multiple hamartomatous polyps of the colon and pigmented spots on the lips and buccal mucosa may point the clinician toward the diagnosis of Peutz-Jeghers syndrome.

Other Pathology Features

Tumors in *BRCA1* mutation carriers are predominantly of basal cell–like subtype, which includes the triple negative (estrogen receptor negative, progesterone receptor negative, and human epidermal growth factor receptor 2 [*HER2*] negative) features (Kandel et al., 2006). Basal cells are derived from the basal epithelial layer of the mammary gland and are thought to represent the breast stem cells. These cells give rise to cells with the same high-grade features seen in *BRCA1*-related cancers that are often triple negative (Roukos & Briasoulis, 2007; Sasa, Bando, Takahashi, Hirose, & Nagao, 2007). A diagnosis of breast cancer can be assessed to determine the presence or absence of these features. Triple-negative breast cancer is associated with aggressive behavior and distinct patterns of metastasis (Anders & Carey, 2008). The triple-negative, basal cell–like phenotype of *BRCA1*-related tumors show an excess of medullary histopathology and are of higher histologic grade (Foulkes et al., 2004; Lacroix & Leclercq, 2005). The biology of *BRCA1* and *BRCA2* breast cancers with distinctive DNA double-strand breaks makes them sensitive to newer treatment with poly adenosine diphosphate-ribose polymerase (commonly known as PARP) inhibitors (Rubinstein, 2008). Knowing the pathologic features that have an association with a hereditary cancer syndrome may help to identify a client who needs a genetic risk assessment at the time of diagnosis in order to individualize treatment.

Histopathologic features may be associated with risk for hereditary cancer syndromes. Serous adenocarcinomas of the ovary have been observed in women with *BRCA1* and *BRCA2* mutations. More than 90% of ovarian tumors in women with *BRCA* mutations are serous, compared to 50%–60% in women without a *BRCA* cancer-predisposing mutation (Piek et al., 2003). Mucinous or endometrioid ovarian cancers in women younger than 40 years old may be suggestive of Lynch syndrome (Domanska, Malander, Masback, & Nilbert, 2007).

Some tumors, such as colon and uterine, are tested after surgery for microsatellite instability (MSI). Microsatellites are stretches of DNA with a repetitive sequence of nucleotides (e.g., CGCGCGCGCGCGCG) that are unstable and particularly susceptible to acquiring errors when the mismatch repair gene function is impaired. Cells with a high number of nucleotide repeats when compared to normal tissue are referred to as microsatellite instability high (MSI-H). Although only 15% of colon cancers show evidence of MSI, approximately 85% of clients with Lynch syndrome have tumors that show MSI (Hampel et al., 2008; Jenkins et al., 2007). The presence of MSI-H can help to identify clients who may be appropriate for genetic testing for Lynch syndrome.

Immunohistochemistry (IHC) of tumor tissue detects the presence or absence of the protein products expressed by the mismatch repair genes (*MLH1*, *MSH2*, *MSH6*, and *PMS2*) associated with Lynch syndrome. The absence of protein expression by these mismatch repair genes is highly correlated with MSI status (Lindor et al., 2008). The absence of protein expression especially in conjunction with MSI-H would suggest the need for genetic counseling and testing for Lynch syndrome. The identification of loss of protein expression by a given mismatch repair gene (e.g., no protein product expressed by *MLH1*) has been shown to have equal **sensitivity** compared to MSI in the identification of Lynch syndrome with significantly less cost (Hampel et al., 2008).

The surgical and pathologic features described previously underscore the need for a thorough review of the client and family member's surgical history. These surgical features will continue to be expanded as new tumor markers and molecular tumor profiles are developed (Douglas-Jones & Woods, 2009). Routine screening of tumors for molecular markers will be used for determining prognosis and treatment decisions. MSI and IHC testing for colon tumors has been suggested to determine the most effective treatment for stage II and III colon cancers (Bertagnolli et al., 2009). These molecular markers will have an impact on individualized treatment and the identification of patients and families who may be at higher risk for recurrence or new cancer. The information from surgical and pathology records currently provides critical information for cancer genetic risk assessment. As the knowledge of tumor profiles expands (see Chapter 8), the surgical and molecular pathology may offer a cost-effective method to facilitate cancer genetic risk assessment (Hampel at al., 2008).

Ethnicity, Culture, and Religious Beliefs

Awareness of a client's cultural background, religion, and ethnicity provides a deeper understanding of how the individual may perceive and utilize information provided. Ethnicity and health beliefs are therefore an important part of a health history because they may affect patterns of decision making, ability to cope with risk information, willingness to share risk information with other family members, and compliance with screening measures and risk management options. People from each culture assume that their own behavior is correct, so clinicians need to have some awareness of the variations they may encounter in different cultures (Haydon, 2007a). Detailed information about ethnicity and culture is found in Chapter 12.

Assessment of ethnicity may facilitate the identification of a hereditary cancer syndrome associated with particular populations. Mutations specific to a certain ethnic group may be the result of a founder effect. A founder mutation is suspected when a given population has a greater-than-expected frequency of a specific mutation in common descendants of an ancestor. The founder effect begins when one individual in an isolated community develops a mutation that is rare to the population as a whole. If the community is small and isolated from other areas, the mutation stays within the given community and is passed down from one generation to the next. The mutation is then seen among the progeny of the founder, typically in homogeneous ethnic groups (e.g., Ashkenazi Jewish heritage) or geographic isolate (e.g., Iceland) that results in a high frequency of a specific genotype (National Comprehensive Cancer Network, 2009). *BRCA* founder mutations have been associated with several European and non-European populations (Ferla et al., 2007). An American founder mutation of *MSH2* in Lynch syndrome also has been identified (Clendenning et al., 2008). Therefore, recording ethnicity or the family's country of origin may provide further information related to a suspected cancer syndrome.

FAMILY HISTORY

Approximately 5%–10% of all cancers develop because of a highly penetrant cancer susceptibility gene mutation, with many following an AD inheritance pattern (Genetics Home Reference, 2008b). Many clients who have experienced cancer in their families do not have a hereditary cancer syndrome. Complex gene-environment interactions and less-penetrant gene mutations may be associated with the cancers in these families. Individuals usually are considered to be candidates for genetic counseling if they have a strong family history of cancer. In general, this means a family history that includes several relatives affected with cancer, with at least some affected at atypically early ages (see Figure 3-2).

Early Age of the Client at Onset of the Disease

Cancers associated with a hereditary cancer syndrome usually occur earlier than in the general population. The 2001–2005 Surveillance,

FIGURE 3-2 HALLMARKS OF HEREDITARY CANCERS

- Early age at disease onset
- Multiple affected family members
- Transmission across three generations
- Specific tumor-site clusters
- Multiple primary cancers in the same individual
- Bilateral disease or multifocal disease
- Presence of rare cancers in multiple family members
- Evidence of autosomal dominant inheritance
- Precursor lesions
- Specific locations of lesions and findings
- Specific pathologic features

Note. Based on information from Hampel et al., 2004; Lynch & de la Chapelle, 2003; Sifri et al., 2004.

Epidemiology, and End Results (SEER) program reported that the mean age for the occurrence of breast cancer is 61 years and 64 years for colon cancer (Horner et al., 2008). Therefore, the occurrence of most common cancers before the age of 50 is suggestive of a hereditary cancer syndrome, and collecting the age at which primary diagnosis of cancer occurred (not the age at metastasis) is important when obtaining a family history.

Bilateral Disease

In a hereditary cancer syndrome, paired organ sites often are involved. Bilateral ovarian cancer with both ovaries having cancer or bilateral breast cancer with both breasts having a cancer diagnosis and representing two different primary sites of cancer are examples.

Multiple Affected Members and Transmission in Multiple Generations

If several individuals in the same biologic family are affected with the same cancer or a cluster of certain cancers known to be associated with a specific hereditary cancer syndrome, this may indicate of a hereditary cancer syndrome. For example, a 30-year-old woman with endometrial cancer and 40-year-old brother with colon cancer indicate the possibility of Lynch syndrome (Lindor et al., 2008). Typically, cancers associated with a hereditary cancer syndrome are present in multiple generations of a family. For example, a family with a mother, daughter, and grandmother of the same lineage demonstrate transmission across three generations.

Unique Tumor Site Combinations

Certain types of hereditary cancers tend to cluster within a family. For example, if a person has hereditary nonpolyposis colorectal cancer, also known as Lynch syndrome, he or she has a greater-than-average risk for cancers of the colon, uterus (endometrium), ovary, small bowel, hepatobiliary system, kidney, and ureter (Garber & Offit, 2005). Individuals with a mutated *BRCA2* gene may have family members with cancers of the breast, ovary, pancreas, prostate, and melanoma (Lindor et al., 2008). See Table 3-2 for malignancies associated with common cancer syndromes.

Multiple Primary Cancers in Same Individual

Hereditary cancer syndromes also are suspected when two or more primary cancers occur in the same individual. For example, if a patient develops a primary colon cancer and later develops a second primary colon cancer (not a recurrence of the first one), if a patient has two primary colon cancers diagnosed at the same time (synchronous), or if a patient develops colon cancer and endometrial cancer, this raises the suspicion of Lynch syndrome.

Rare Cancers

Certain cancers (e.g., retinoblastoma, medullary thyroid carcinoma, pheochromocytoma, adrenocortical carcinoma, paraganglioma, Wilms tumor) are so rare that a single case requires a cancer genetics consultation (Hampel, Sweet, Westman, Offit, & Eng, 2004). Other cancers that have low incidence in the general population, such as ovarian cancer with a 1.7% incidence rate, are considered rare cancers (Hayat, Howlader, Reichman, & Edwards, 2007).

Key Elements in Taking a Family History

In collecting or reviewing a family history, keep in mind those essential competencies on nursing assessment related to applying and integrating genetic and genomic knowledge that pertain to taking and assessing a family history. The documentation will vary, depending on whether a family history is taken to identify a family in need of further evaluation or for the purpose of cancer genetic risk assessment. When taking or evaluating the family history for cancer genetic risk assessment, information about family includes

- At least a three-generation family history, including both maternal and paternal relatives (hereditary cancer syndromes can be inherited from either the mother or the father), as well as current individuals both affected and unaffected by cancer
- Family members' ages or ages at death, history of benign or malignant tumors, any hospitalizations or surgeries, especially if they may have reduced the risk for cancer
- Notation of adoption, nonpaternity, consanguinity, and use of assisted reproductive technology (e.g., donor egg or sperm), when appropriate
- Information about all medical and surgical histories even if it may seem initially to be an unrelated condition, such as birth defects or other nonmalignant conditions of children and adults, that may aid in the diagnosis of a cancer susceptibility syndrome
- Race, ancestry, and ethnicity of the family.

When possible, obtaining pathology reports of benign or malignant conditions will help to confirm cancers or determine the presence of lesions that may be associated with cancer syndromes. Other pertinent physical findings associated with inheritable diseases, major illnesses, environmental exposures, and cancer screening or surveillance measures may be collected if the information is known. Information about family members' illnesses may indicate the presence of other familial conditions and potential for early intervention, as in the case of cardiovascular disease (Miller, Ridker, Libby, & Kwiatkowski, 2007).

Information on Genetic Testing for Other Family Members

Inquire about other family members having had genetic testing. Some relatives may not readily share their genetic test results, whereas others inform the entire family. A family member with genetic test results may be willing to share their results if these results could help another relative who is pursuing testing. Documentation of the official result can be obtained directly from the relative who had testing or from the laboratory that did the testing with informed consent. If a family member's test results are positive for a known mutation, other family members can be tested for the same mutation. This is referred to as site-specific testing (i.e., testing the same gene and mutation). However, site-specific testing may not be appropriate if a hereditary cancer risk on both maternal and paternal sides is suggested, if different cancers are in the branch of the family already tested, or if the known mutation is in a more distant relative, such as to the

third or fourth degree. In more distant relatives, clarifying their family history may indicate that their genetic mutation was inherited from someone who is not a blood relative to the person who is seeking testing. The closer the degree of the relative, the more genetic information shared.
- First-degree relatives share 50% of the client's genes (including parents, siblings, and children).
- Second-degree relatives share 25% of the client's genes (including aunts, uncles, grandparents, nieces, and nephews).
- Third-degree relative share 12.5% of the client's genes (including cousins, great-aunts, great-uncles, and great-grandparents).

The Pedigree

The family history can be recorded in the form of a pedigree, a symbolic representation of family members, social and biologic relationships, lines of descent, and reproductive scenarios. A pedigree facilitates analysis of possible hereditary patterns of transmission suggestive of specific hereditary cancer syndromes and determination of the best methods for risk assessment (NCI, 2008). Factors that may suggest inherited cancer risk are found in Figure 3-2.

Standardized nomenclature for human pedigrees was developed in 1995 and updated in 2008 to facilitate correct interpretation of the pedigree and communication between healthcare professionals (Bennett, French, Resta, & Doyle, 2008; Bennett et al., 1995). Figure 3-3 presents selected pedigree symbols and their definitions. Pedigrees can be hand drawn or constructed using computer software programs. Many of the pedigree software programs available for purchase also have data management functions (see Table 3-4).

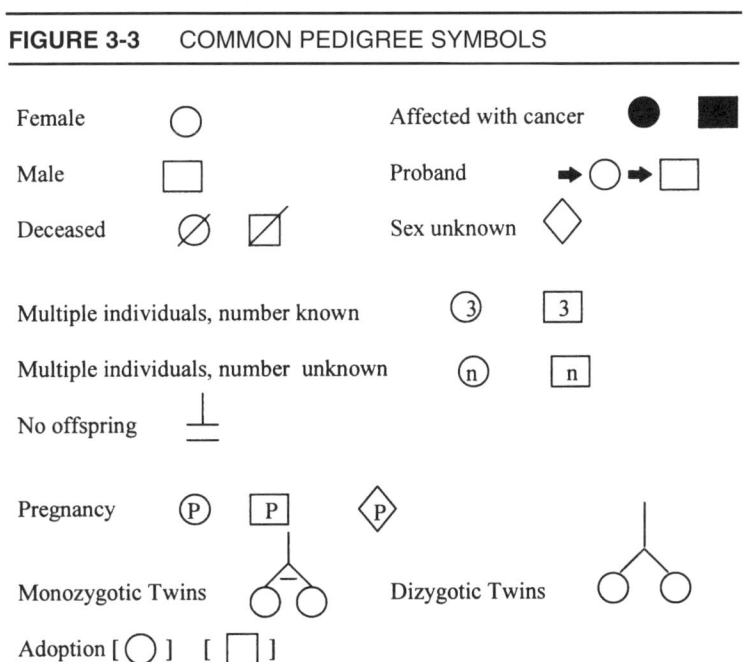

FIGURE 3-3   COMMON PEDIGREE SYMBOLS

Review the preliminary pedigree with the client to verify that the family history is properly represented. Clients can mistakenly provide inaccurate information; seeing the mistake on the pedigree often prompts them to identify and correct the error. Be particularly careful to verify biologic relationships. Confirm whether anyone in the pedigree was adopted and whether siblings in the pedigree share the same mother and father. Do not make assumptions about paternity. If biologic relationships are documented inaccurately, the result could be a misdiagnosis.

TABLE 3-4. Resources for Pedigree Drawing Software and Data Management

Resource	Contact	Description
American Medical Association: Family History Tools	www.ama-assn.org/ama/pub/category/2380.html	Tools for gathering family history and links to resources
Centers for Disease Control and Prevention	www.cdc.gov/genomics/fhix.htm	Family history resources and tools
Cyrillic	www.cyrillicsoftware.com	Pedigree drawing software for genetic counselors and clinicians; links to genetic sites
Pedigree-Draw	www.pedigree-draw.com	Pedigree drawing software for Macintosh
Progeny	www.progenygenetics.com	Genetic data management and pedigree drawing software
U.S. Surgeon General's Family History Initiative: "My Family Health Portrait"	www.hhs.gov/familyhistory/	Client-completed pedigree drawing software

Note. From *Essentials of Genetic and Genomic Nursing: Competencies, Curricula Guidelines, and Outcome Indicators* (2nd ed., p. 65), by Consensus Panel on Genetic/Genomic Nursing Competencies, 2009, Silver Spring, MD: American Nurses Association. Copyright 2009 by American Nurses Association.

PSYCHOSOCIAL ASSESSMENT

Assessment of psychosocial issues provides the clinician with insight on factors that affect risk perception and adaptation to cancer genetic information (Haydon, 2007b). Using a formal questionnaire can be helpful to ensure consistent collection of the needed information; however, these tools have limitations. Although questionnaires may be very sensitive, they are neither specific nor diagnostic in nature and do not replace the individual assessment. Include in the assessment these psychosocial features: the client's current emotional well-being, mental health history, emotional response to family history of cancer, coping strategies, and reactions during the counseling session (Schneider, 2002). Keep in mind that clients with cancer who are undergoing genetic risk assessment may have many concerns. For example, they may be undergoing cancer treatment or coping with a fear of cancer recurrence. The psychosocial assessment should include evaluation of

- Present emotional state
- History of psychological conditions such as anxiety or depression
- Perception of cancer risk
- Cancer worries
- Issues related to personal or family history of cancer such as guilt or grief
- Coping strategies
- Social and financial support.

Further psychosocial counseling issues are discussed in depth in Chapter 5.

Motivation for Assessment

As part of the psychosocial assessment, assess the client's motivation for seeking cancer risk information. Why does the client want to know about his or her cancer risk, and in what form does he or she want risk information? Clarifying the client's goals for the consultation by determining what information he or she hopes to gain will help in determing how to deliver information in the session (Trepanier et al., 2004).

If genetic testing is an option, assess the client's interest in genetic testing and the reasons for this interest. Prior to genetic testing, determine how the client thinks the genetic test results will affect him or her or the family. Explore how the cancer genetic information will alter health behaviors, risk-management strategies, or treatment of an existing malignancy. Identify barriers to recommended health behaviors and explore methods to promote compliance (Trepanier et al., 2004). Role playing may be a way to help the client express anticipated reactions to testing results and may prompt discussion of pertinent issues.

In the psychosocial assessment, identify the primary support person and any other social relationship factors such as marital status, living as married, and any children. Keep in mind that this support person may not be a spouse, partner, or family member. The client may be interested in having this support person attend any counseling sessions. This may be beneficial; however, be aware that having others present during a counseling session may interfere with the client's ability to fully disclose information related to his or her family (e.g., a child who has a different father than the other children).

Cognitive Assessment

The cognitive assessment begins with an evaluation of how much the client knows about cancer, risk factors, the effectiveness and limitations of screening measures, risk management and reduction options, and the influence of family history on cancer risk. Assess the client's literacy level, cultural background, primary language, language skills, learning style, and the resources the client has used in the past to obtain cancer and cancer genetic information (e.g., written materials, audio or visual aids, the Internet). Understanding misperceptions, knowledge gaps, and in what form information will be most effective helps the nurse to tailor education to the client's needs.

To facilitate comprehensive holistic cancer care, ask the client if the referring healthcare provider should be informed of any recommendations about cancer screening and surveillance and risk management options as a result of a cancer risk assessment. For example, the healthcare practitioner's knowledge of this information may facilitate ordering of recommended screening or surveillance tests for all cancers associated with a given hereditary cancer syndrome.

PHYSICAL EXAMINATION

The physical examination focuses on those areas that are relevant to a particular hereditary cancer syndrome. For example, examination of the skin or oral mucosa to look for hyperpigmentation is important if the patient may have Carney complex type 1 (formerly known as NAME [nevi, atrial myxoma, myxoid neurofibroma, and ephelides]) or Peutz-Jeghers syndrome (Lindor et al., 2008). With Cowden syndrome, a hallmark feature is facial and oral mucocutaneous lesions that often are trichilemmomas (benign follicular epithelial neoplasms). In addition, clients with Cowden syndrome may have macrocephaly, usually dolichocephaly (an abnormally long and narrow head) (Lindor et al.). Thus, a physical examination may yield further findings that are helpful to the genetic assessment. Refer to Table 3-2 for clinical features associated with hereditary cancer syndromes.

THE ASSESSMENT PROCESS

A genetic assessment may take several visits to complete. As reviewed previously, a comprehensive cancer assessment includes a medical, surgical, personal, and family history. People seeking genetic cancer risk assessment are informed that multiple pieces of information are required in order to provide the most accurate information about cancer risk. Helping clients to understand the steps of the assessment process facilitates the gathering of medical, surgical, and family history.

The Questionnaire

A questionnaire can aid in the collection of medical and surgical health information, including any risk factors for cancer and the family's health history. This can facilitate the process by helping the client to gather and submit information before the first consultation. Upon making an appointment for consultation, the client can be asked to complete the questionnaire prior to the consultation. Completing the questionnaire at home allows the client the opportunity to find answers to questions that he or she does not know and provides the client time to contact family members or check family records. If the completed questionnaire is submitted before the first visit, the healthcare provider who will complete the genetic assessment is able to use the information on the questionnaire to prepare a preliminary pedigree or family tree. However, validation and clarification are important during the appointment to correct, clarify, and expand the pedigree.

Many clients may not know medical information about relatives with whom they have had little or no relationship; therefore, obtaining an accurate family history may necessitate contacting family members who have not been in contact with the client for a prolonged period of time.

Education and Counseling Environment

Preferably, the environment for conducting a genetic assessment is private and conducive to client interaction, typically an area such as a small conference room or consultation room. Such a setting provides a therapeutic environment for counseling, as opposed to a clinical atmosphere, such as that of an examination room. A table facilitates the discussion of family history because it enables the nurse and client to see the pedigree as it is developed. Keep interruptions to a minimum—they are distracting and may upset the client, who may be talking about confidential and personal matters.

Sequence

The assessment often begins with a discussion of the client's motivation for seeking cancer risk counseling. Ask the client to describe his or her expectations of the consultation. The client's expectations often help to identify questions or concerns that need to be addressed in the process. Describe the assessment process, and clarify that often several steps are involved in the process, including the evaluation of the client's medical and family history. Tell the client how the pedigree will be used for the assessment and underscore the importance of having as much confirmed family and medical information as possible.

A genetic assessment does not proceed in any standard format. Collecting the family data is the most time-consuming task; therefore, it is very helpful if the client completes this task prior to the visit. The consultation time is then used to verify and clarify the family history. In addition, psychosocial evaluations can be made throughout the genetic assessment as the client shares information about family dynamics, cancer experiences, and the impact of these experiences.

Solicitation and Verification of Family History

One way to prompt accurate responses is to ask the client specific questions. For example, when questioning the client about family members, ask about specific symptoms experienced or treatment received. Direct questions may help the client to remember. Clients can become frustrated when they cannot provide information. Offer reassurance and explain that many clients have limited information, particularly if family members are estranged, are uncomfortable discussing family medical issues, or are lost to contact. For clients who have family contact, explore the feasibility of obtaining needed information or official records, including

- Pathology reports (discussed in surgical history)
- Death certificates
- Medical records
- Autopsy reports.

These documents may or may not be helpful to confirm a type of cancer. Freedman, Sigurdson, Doody, Love-Schnur, and Linet (2006) found that 28.5% of cancers identified in state cancer registries were not captured by self-report, death certificate, or other medical records. Self-reports failed to identify 12.2% of total cancer diagnoses, although respondents failed to report only 2.6% of female breast cancers and less than 5% each of prostate and colon cancers. Ascertainment was less complete for death certificates, which did not identify 35.2% of cancers recorded in cancer registries. If family members are deceased, the next of kin with legal authority signs the authorization papers to permit release of the necessary documents. If cancer information is included in these reports, verify that the client has supplied accurate information about the family members' ages at cancer onset, the types of cancer in the family, and biopsy results and surgeries.

COMMON PROBLEMS OF GENETIC EVALUATION

Missing or inaccurate client-supplied information can be problematic in a comprehensive genetic assessment. One of the best defenses against misinformation is thorough knowledge of the cancers being reported: the usual age at onset, the natural history of the disease, treatment methods, and survival rates. This knowledge may lead a nurse to question the **accuracy** of a client's report. For example, if a client reports that her father had pancreatic cancer in his 40s and lived to his 60s, question the report or the diagnosis because survival rates for pancreatic cancer are poor (Hayat et al., 2007). Similarly, if a client reports that her mother had ovarian cancer in her 30s and is still alive at 90, seek verification because the ovarian pathology may show that the tumor was a different type of gynecologic cancer or was a germ cell and not an epithelial ovarian cancer, which typically has poorer survival (Hayat et al.).

Family characteristics may prove to be limitations. The following factors may complicate the recognition of basic inheritance patterns.
- Small family
- Deaths at particularly early ages from other causes (e.g., accidental death)
- Removal of target organ either for risk reduction or as a result of a medical condition (e.g., total abdominal hysterectomy with bilateral salpingo-oophorectomy because of a history of uterine fibroids or endometriosis)
- Male dominance in predominantly female hereditary cancer syndrome or vice versa
- Misidentified parentage
- Consanguinity
- Adoption with no knowledge of birth family history

Paternal transmission of an inherited cancer predisposition involving predominantly female cancers can complicate the risk assessment, such as a woman with breast cancer in her 40s who has only sons. Even if the woman had a deleterious *BRCA* mutation and her sons also were positive for the mutation, the risk of the son's developing breast cancer is 1.2% for *BRCA1* male carriers (Tai, Domchek, Parmigiani, & Chen, 2007) and 6% for *BRCA2* carriers (Fentiman, Fourquet, & Hortobagyi, 2006). Therefore, breast cancer in the sons will be less likely, and this family will not appear to have a higher risk for a hereditary cancer syndrome until female offspring develop cancer.

SAMPLE ASSESSMENTS

Case 1

Marie, a 40-year-old woman, is seeking genetic cancer risk assessment after her recent diagnosis of unilateral infiltrating ductal carcinoma, which was triple-negative (estrogen receptor, progesterone receptor, and *HER2* negative) breast cancer. She is married and has a 14-year-old daughter. One sister was diagnosed with serous-type ovarian cancer at age 50 and is now 52. Her mother had breast cancer at 43 and died at age 47. A maternal uncle developed prostate cancer at age 65 and died at age 72. Her maternal grandmother developed breast cancer at age 45 and died at age 49. She is of Ashkenazi Jewish heritage both maternally and paternally. Figure 3-4 shows Marie's pedigree.

Cancer genetic risk assessment shows the following.
- Suspected side at risk: Maternal
- Mendelian pattern of inheritance: AD
- Cancer pattern: Suggestive of hereditary pattern with vertical transmission across multiple generations

- Hereditary cancer syndrome and rationale: Hereditary breast/ovarian cancer syndrome (HBOC)
  - Early-onset cancer, multiple family members with the same cancer
  - Clusters of cancer associated with a hereditary cancer syndrome
  - Rare cancer (ovarian cancer)
  - Ethnic background associated with a population having a known founder mutation
  - Pathologic features of cancers suggestive of *BRCA* phenotype (triple-negative breast cancer and serous-type ovarian cancer)

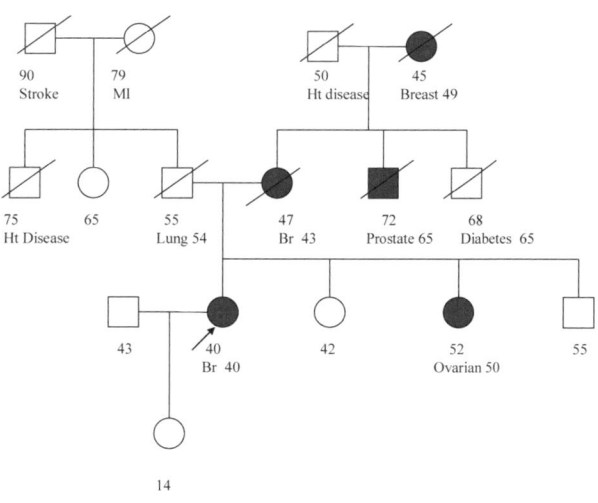

FIGURE 3-4   SAMPLE PEDIGREE, MARIE

This assessment shows that the most likely cancer syndrome present is HBOC. The client is offered the option to begin with genetic testing for the three common mutations seen in Ashkenazi Jewish individuals. If she is not interested in testing, she would still be considered at high risk for HBOC, and appropriate screening, surveillance, and risk reduction measures should be considered.

Case 2

Kevin is seeking genetic counseling upon the advice of his surgeon. He is 46 years old and underwent a colorectal resection and was found to have synchronous colon cancer (two separate primary colonic tumors separated by normal tissue). He had a stage II adenocarcinoma of the proximal colon and a stage I colon cancer in the transverse colon. Further pathologic testing revealed that this was a poorly differentiated, mucinous cancer with MSI-H. He is married, and an evaluation of his lifestyle reveals that he does not eat red meat more than twice per week, eats more than three servings of vegetables per day, does not smoke or drink more than one alcoholic beverage per day, and is not obese. He also runs one to two miles per day. The only significant family history was that his mother had endometrial cancer at age 62 and is still alive. Figure 3-5 shows Kevin's pedigree.

Kevin's cancer genetic risk assessment shows the following.
- Suspected side at risk: Maternal
- Personal history and lifestyle factors are not contributory to colon cancer.
- Mendelian pattern of inheritance: AD
- Cancer pattern: Maternal side suggestive of familial pattern with vertical transmission across multiple generations; paternal side shows sporadic pattern.
- Hereditary cancer syndrome and rationale: Lynch syndrome
  - Early-onset synchronous colorectal cancer, two primary sites

- Clusters of cancers associated with Lynch syndrome (colon and endometrial)
- Tumor features of cancer suggestive of Lynch syndrome (MSI-H and mucinous histology)

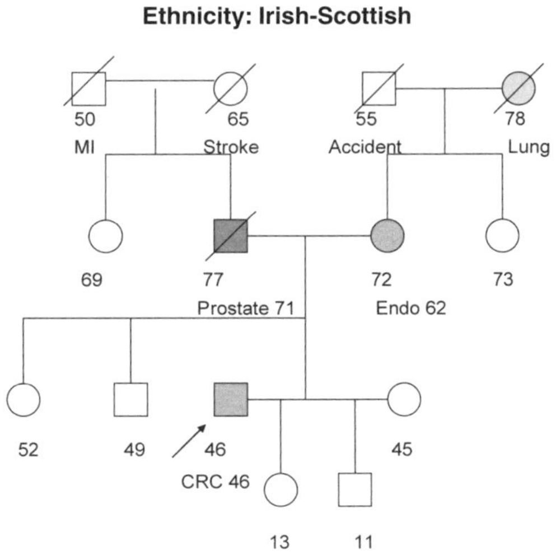

Kevin's personal and family history suggest Lynch syndrome based on features that meet revised Bethesda criteria (i.e., diagnosis of colorectal cancer at younger than 50 years, synchronous hereditary nonpolyposis colorectal cancer–associated tumors regardless of age, MSI histology diagnosed before age 60) (Umar et al., 2004). The mucinous histology of his colon cancer is also a specific histologic feature suggestive of MSI-H and Lynch syndrome (Truta et al., 2008). Although his mother's endometrial cancer was diagnosed at a later age (62 years), endometrial cancer is considered one of the related Lynch syndrome cancers (Lindor et al., 2008). Kevin could proceed directly to genetic testing for Lynch syndrome or first have IHC tumor testing to determine the loss of protein expression by a given mismatch repair gene (e.g., *MLH1*, *MSH2*, *MSH6*, and *PMS2*) and then proceed with site-specific testing for the gene having loss of protein expression (Robinson et al., 2009).

FIGURE 3-5   SAMPLE PEDIGREE, KEVIN

Ethnicity: Irish-Scottish

SUMMARY

Cancer risk assessment is an integral nursing competency to identify individuals who could benefit from genetic and genomic information. Specifically, cancer genetic risk assessment will identify those who might benefit from genetic testing, cancer risk reduction, or early detection strategies to improve cancer morbidity and mortality. The field of cancer genetic risk assessment will grow as more healthcare providers integrate cancer risk assessment into their roles and cancer risk assessment services expand (Zon et al., 2009). The use of family history tools in the community and medical practices will abound, thus increasing the need for health professionals who have the ability to evaluate and interpret the constellations of cancers that present in families. Molecular screening of tumors and gene expression profiles used for determining prognosis and treatment decisions will identify features suggestive of hereditary cancer syndromes. These molecular pathology features will provide opportunities for identifying individuals who are at higher risk for new cancers because of an inherited genetic mutation. The genetic mutations, in turn, provide information for corresponding targeted therapies. Subsequently, this genetic and genomic information will affect family members who may be at risk for the same hereditary cancer syndrome. Therefore, cancer genetic risk assessment will continue to affect oncology nursing across the continuum of care by reducing risk before cancer occurs, detecting cancers early, and providing genetic and genomic information to patients that can affect treatment and prognosis. Cancer genetic and genomic risk assessment is furthering the reality of targeted and personalized cancer care for clients.

REFERENCES

American Cancer Society. (2008a). *American Cancer Society guidelines for the early detection of cancer.* Retrieved October 26, 2008, from http://www.cancer.org/docroot/PED/content/PED_2_3X_ACS_Cancer_Detection_Guidelines_36.asp?sitearea=PED&viewmode=print&

American Cancer Society. (2008b). *Detailed guide: Breast cancer—What are the risk factors for breast cancer?* Retrieved October 20, 2008, from http://www.cancer.org/docroot/CRI/content/CRI_2_4_2X_What_are_the_risk_factors_for_breast_cancer_5.asp

American Cancer Society. (2008c). *Detailed guide: Endometrial cancer—What are the risk factors for endometrial cancer?* Retrieved October 20, 2008, from http://www.cancer.org/docroot/CRI/content/CRI_2_4_2X_What_are_the_risk_factors_for_endometrial_cancer.asp

American Cancer Society. (2008d). *Detailed guide: Ovarian cancer—What are the risk factors for ovarian cancer?* Retrieved October 20, 2008, from http://www.cancer.org/docroot/CRI/content/CRI_2_4_2X_What_are_the_risk_factors_for_ovarian_cancer_33.asp

American Cancer Society. (2008e). *Detailed guide: Skin cancer—basal and squamous cell.* Retrieved October 26, 2008, from http://www.cancer.org/docroot/CRI/CRI_2_3x.asp?dt=51

American Cancer Society. (2008f). *Detailed guide: Skin cancer—melanoma. What are the risk factors for melanoma?* Retrieved October 26, 2008, from http://www.cancer.org/docroot/CRI/content/CRI_2_4_2X_What_are_the_risk_factors_for_melanoma_50.asp?sitearea=

American Cancer Society. (2008g). *Prevention and early detection: Asbestos.* Retrieved October 21, 2008, from http://www.cancer.org/docroot/PED/content/PED_1_3X_Asbestos.asp?sitearea=PED

American Cancer Society. (2008h). *Prevention and early detection: Benzene.* Retrieved October 21, 2008, from http://www.cancer.org/docroot/PED/content/PED_1_3X_Benzene.asp?sitearea=PED

American Cancer Society. (2008i). *Prevention and early detection: Cigarette smoking.* Retrieved October 26, 2008, from http://www.cancer.org/docroot/PED/content/PED_10_2X_Cigarette_Smoking.asp?sitearea=PED

American Cancer Society. (2008j). *Prevention and early detection: Radiation exposure and cancer.* Retrieved October 21, 2008, from http://www.cancer.org/docroot/PED/content/PED_1_3X_Radiation_Exposure_and_Cancer.asp?sitearea=PED

American Cancer Society. (2008k). *Second cancers caused by cancer treatment.* Retrieved October 21, 2008, from http://www.cancer.org/docroot/MBC/content/MBC_2X_Second_Cancers_Caused_By_Cancer_Treatment.asp

American Cancer Society. (2009, May 21). *Guidelines for the early detection of cancer.* Retrieved November 14, 2009, from http://www.cancer.org/docroot/ped/content/ped_2_3x_acs_cancer_detection_guidelines_36.asp?sitearea=PED&viewmode=print&

American Medical Association. (2008, June 25). *Family history.* Retrieved November 9, 2008, from http://www.ama-assn.org/ama1/pub/upload/mm/464/adult_history.pdf

American Society of Clinical Oncology. (2003). American Society of Clinical Oncology policy statement update: Genetic testing for cancer susceptibility. *Journal of Clinical Oncology, 21*(12), 2397–2406.

American Society of Clinical Oncology. (2007, August 9). *Physical activity and cancer risk.* Retrieved November 25, 2008, from http://prostateca.asco.org/patient/Learning+About+Cancer/Prevention/Physical+Activity/Physical+Activity+and+Cancer+Risk

Anders, C., & Carey, L.A. (2008). Understanding and treating triple-negative breast cancer. *Oncology, 22*(11), 1233–1239.

Bardia, A., Hartmann, L.C., Vachon, C.M., Vierkant, R.A., Wang, A.H., Olson, J.E. et al. (2006). Recreational physical activity and risk of postmenopausal breast cancer based on hormone receptor status. *Archives of Internal Medicine, 166*(22), 2478–2483.

Bennett, R.L., French, K.S., Resta, R.G., & Doyle, D.L. (2008). Standardized human pedigree nomenclature: Update and assessment of the recommendations of the National Society of Genetic Counselors. *Journal of Genetic Counseling, 17*(5), 424–433.

Bennett, R.L., Steinhaus, K.A., Uhrich, S.B., O'Sullivan, C.K., Resta, R.G., Lochner-Doyle, D., et al. (1995). Recommendations for standardized human pedigree nomenclature. *American Journal of Human Genetics, 56*(3), 745–752.

Bertagnolli, M.M., Niedzwiecki, D., Compton, C.C., Hahn, H.P., Hall, M., Damas, B., et al. (2009). Microsatellite instability predicts improved response to adjuvant therapy with irinotecan, fluorouracil, and leucovorin in stage III colon cancer: Cancer and Leukemia Group B Protocol 89803. *Journal of Clinical Oncology, 27*(11), 1814–1821.

Byers, T., Nestle, M., McTiernan, A., Doyle, C., Curie-Williams, A., Gansler, T., et al. (2002). American Cancer Society guidelines on nutrition and physical activity for cancer prevention: Reducing the risk of cancer with healthy food choices and physical activity. *CA: A Cancer Journal for Clinicians, 52*(2), 92–119.

Clendenning, M., Baze, M.E., Sun, S., Walsh, K., Liyanarachchi, S., Fix, D., et al. (2008). Origins and prevalence of the American Founder Mutation of *MSH2*. *Cancer Research, 68*(7), 2145–2153.

Consensus Panel on Genetic/Genomic Nursing Competencies. (2009). *Essentials of genetic and genomic nursing: Competencies, curricula guidelines, and outcome indicators* (2nd ed.). Silver Spring, MD: American Nurses Association.

Danaei, G., Vander Hoorn, S., Lopez, A.D., Murray, C.J., Ezzati, M., & Comparative Risk Assessment Collaborating Group (Cancers). (2005). Causes of cancer in the world: Comparative risk assessment of nine behavioural and environmental risk factors. *Lancet, 366*(9499), 1784–1793.

Domanska, K., Malander, S., Masback, A., & Nilbert, M. (2007). Ovarian cancer at young age: Contribution of mismatch-repair defects in a population-based series of epithelial ovarian cancer before age 40. *International Journal of Gynecological Cancer, 17*(4), 789–793.

Douglas-Jones, A.G., & Woods, V. (2009). Molecular assessment of sentinel lymph node in breast cancer management. *Histopathology, 55*(1), 107–113.

Doyle, V.C. (2007). Nutrition and colorectal cancer risk: A literature review. *Gastroenterology Nursing, 30*(3), 178–183.

Fentiman, I.S., Fourquet, A., & Hortobagyi, G.N. (2006). Male breast cancer. *Lancet, 367*(9510), 595–604.

Ferla, R., Calò, V., Cascio, S., Rinaldi, G., Badalamenti, G., Carreca, I., et al. (2007). Founder mutations in *BRCA1* and *BRCA2* genes. *Annals of Oncology, 18*(Suppl. 6), vi93–vi98.

Foulkes, W.D., Metcalfe, K., Sun, P., Hanna, W.M., Lynch, H.T., Ghadirian, P., et al. (2004). Estrogen receptor status in *BRCA1*- and *BRCA2*-related breast cancer: The influence of age, grade, and histological type. *Clinical Cancer Research, 10*(6), 2029–2034.

Freedman, D.M., Sigurdson, A.J., Doody, M.M., Love-Schnur, S., & Linet, M.S. (2006). Comparison between cancers identified by state cancer registry, self-report, and death certificate in a prospective cohort study of U.S. radiologic technologists. *International Journal of Epidemiology, 35*(2), 495–497.

Garber, J.E., & Offit, K. (2005). Hereditary cancer predisposition syndromes. *Journal of Clinical Oncology, 23*(2), 276–292.

Genetics Home Reference. (2008a, July). *Klinefelter's syndrome*. Retrieved April 22, 2009, from http://ghr.nlm.nih.gov/condition=klinefeltersyndrome

Genetics Home Reference. (2008b, October). *Your guide to understanding genetic conditions*. Retrieved November 1, 2008, from http://ghr.nlm.nih.gov/conditionCategory=cancers

Gertner, M.E., & Kebebew, E. (2004). Multiple endocrine neoplasia type 2. *Current Treatment Options in Oncology, 5*(4), 315–325.

Guibout, C., Adjadi, E., Rubino, C., Shamsaldin, A., Grimaud, E., Hawkins, M., et al. (2005). Malignant breast tumors after radiotherapy for a first cancer during childhood. *Journal of Clinical Oncology, 23*(1), 197–204.

Grau, M.V., Baron, J.A., Sandler, R.S., Wallace, K., Haile, R.W., Church, T.R., et al. (2007). Prolonged effect of calcium supplementation on risk of colorectal adenomas in a randomized trial. *Journal of the National Cancer Institute, 99*(2), 129–136.

Hampel, H., Frankel, W.L., Martin, E., Arnold, M., Khanduja, K., Kuebler, P., et al. (2008). Feasibility of screening for Lynch syndrome among patients with colorectal cancer. *Journal of Clinical Oncology, 26*(35), 5783–5788.

Hampel, H., Sweet, S., Westman, J.A., Offit, K., & Eng, D. (2004). Referral for cancer genetics consultation: A review and compilation of risk assessment criteria. *Journal of Medical Genetics, 41*(2), 81–91.

Hartl, D.L., & Jones, E.W. (2008). *Genetics: Analysis of genes and genomes* (7th ed.). Sudbury, MA: Jones and Bartlett.

Hayat, M.J., Howlader, N., Reichman, M.E., & Edwards, B.K. (2007). Cancer statistics, trends, and multiple primary cancer analyses from the Surveillance, Epidemiology, and End Results (SEER) Program. *Oncologist, 12*(1), 20–37.

Haydon, J. (2007a). Ethnicity. In J. Haydon (Ed.), *Genetics in practice: A clinical approach for healthcare practitioners* (pp. 205–219). Hoboken, NJ: Wiley.

Haydon, J. (2007b). Risk perception and options available. In J. Haydon (Ed.), *Genetics in practice: A clinical approach for healthcare practitioners* (pp. 65–83). Hoboken, NJ: Wiley.

Horner, M.J., Ries, L.A.G., Krapcho, M., Neyman, N., Aminou, R., Howlader, N., et al. (2008). *SEER cancer statistics review, 1975–2006*. Bethesda, MD: National Cancer Institute. Retrieved November 1, 2008, from http://seer.cancer.gov/cgi-bin/csr/1975_2005/search.pl#results

Hu, F.B., Willett, W.C., Li, T., Stampfer, M.J., Colditz, G.A., & Manson, J.E. (2004). Adiposity as compared with physical activity in predicting mortality among women. *New England Journal of Medicine, 351*(26), 2694–2703.

Jenkins, M.A., Hayashi, S., O'Shea, A.M., Burgart, L.J., Smyrk, T.C., Shimizu, D., et al. (2007). Pathology features in Bethesda guidelines predict colorectal cancer microsatellite instability: A population-based study. *Gastroenterology, 133*(1), 48–56.

Kandel, M.J., Stadler, Z., Masciari, S., Collins, L., Schnitt, S., Harris, L., et al. (2006). Prevalence of *BRCA1* mutations in triple negative breast cancer (BC) [Abstract]. *Journal of Clinical Oncology, 24*(Suppl. 18), 508.

Kushi, L.H., Byers, T., Doyle, C., Bandera, E.V., McCullough, M., Gansler, T., et al. (2006). American Cancer Society guidelines on nutrition and physical activity for cancer prevention: Reducing the risk of cancer with healthy food choices and physical activity. *CA: A Cancer Journal for Clinicians, 56*(5), 254–281.

Lacroix, M., & Leclercq, G. (2005). The "portrait" of hereditary breast cancer. *Breast Cancer Research and Treatment, 889*(3), 297–304.

Levine, J.S., & Ahnen, D.J. (2006). Adenomatous polyps of the colon. *New England Journal of Medicine, 355*(24), 2551–2557.

Lindor, N.M., McMaster, M.L., Lindor, C.J., & Greene, M.H. (2008). Concise handbook of familial cancer susceptibility syndromes (2nd ed.). *Journal of the National Cancer Institute Monographs, 2008*(38), 1–93.

Lipton, L., & Tomlinson, I. (2004). The multiple colorectal adenoma phenotype and *MYH*, a base excision repair gene. *Clinical Gastroenterology and Hepatology, 2*(8), 633–638.

Lynch, H.T., & de la Chapelle, A. (2003). Hereditary colorectal cancer. *New England Journal of Medicine, 348*(10), 919–932.

McCullough, M.L., Robertson, A.S., Rodriguez, C., Jacobs, E.J., Chao, A., Carolyn, J., et al. (2003). Calcium, vitamin D, dairy products, and risk of colorectal cancer in the cancer prevention study II nutrition cohort (United States). *Cancer Causes and Control, 14*(1), 1–12.

Miller, D.T., Ridker, P.M., Libby, P., & Kwiatkowski, D.J. (2007). Atherosclerosis: The path from genomics to therapeutics. *Journal of the American College of Cardiology, 49*(15), 1589–1599.

National Cancer Institute. (2004). *Obesity and cancer: Questions and answers.* Retrieved December 4, 2007, from http://www.cancer.gov/cancertopics/factsheet/Risk/obesity/print?page=&keyword=

National Cancer Institute. (2008). *Element of cancer genetics risk assessment and counseling (PDQ®)* [Health professional version]. Retrieved November 8, 2008, from http://www.cancer.gov/cancertopics/pdq/genetics/risk-assessment-and-counseling/HealthProfessional

National Center for Biotechnology Information. (n.d.). *OMIM—Online Mendelian Inheritance in Man®.* Retrieved May 27, 2009, from http://www.ncbi.nlm.nih.gov/sites/entrez?db=omim

National Comprehensive Cancer Network. (2009). *NCCN Clinical Practice Guidelines in Oncology™: Genetic/familial high-risk assessment: Breast and ovarian* [v.1.2009]. Retrieved October 19, 2008, from http://www.nccn.org/professionals/physician_gls/PDF/genetics_screening.pdf

Neilson, H.K., Friedenreich, C.M., Brockton, N.T., & Millikan, R.C. (2009). Physical activity and postmenopausal breast cancer: Proposed biologic mechanisms and areas for future research. *Cancer Epidemiology, Biomarkers and Prevention, 18*(1), 11–27.

Peters, U., Littman, A.J., Kristal, A.R., Patterson, R.E., Potter, J.D., & White, E. (2008). Vitamin E and selenium supplementation and risk of prostate cancer in the vitamins and lifestyle (VITAL) study cohort. *Cancer Causes and Control, 19*(1), 75–87.

Piek, J.M., Torrenga, B., Hermsen, B., Verheijen, R.H., Zweemer, R.P., Gille, J.J., et al. (2003). Histopathological characteristics of *BRCA1*- and *BRCA2*-associated intraperitoneal cancer: A clinic-based study. *Familial Cancer, 2*(2), 73–78.

Rabban, J.T., Crawford, B., Chen, L.M., Powell, C.B., & Zaloudek, C.J. (2009). Transitional cell metaplasia of fallopian tube fimbriae: A potential mimic of early tubal carcinoma in risk reduction salpingo-oophorectomies from women with *BRCA* mutations. *American Journal of Surgical Pathology, 33*(1), 111–119.

Raue, F., & Frank-Raue, K. (2007). Multiple endocrine neoplasia type 2: 2007 update. *Hormone Research, 68*(Suppl. 5), 101–104.

Reeves, G.K., Pirie, K., Beral, V., Green, J., Spencer, E., & Bull, D. (2007). Cancer incidence and mortality in relation to body mass index in the million women study: Cohort study. *BMJ, 335*(7630), 1134.

Ringo, J. (2004). *Fundamental genetics.* New York: Cambridge University Press.

Robson, M.E. Storm, C.D., Weitzel, J., Wollins, D.S., Offit, K., & American Society of Clinical Oncology. (2010). American Society of Clinical Oncology policy statement update: Genetic and genomic testing for cancer susceptibility. *Journal of Clinical Oncology, 28*(5), 893–901.

Robinson, K.L., Liu, T., Vandrovcova, J., Halvarsson, B., Clendenning, M., Frebourg, T., et al. (2009). Lynch syndrome (hereditary nonpolyposis colorectal cancer) diagnostics. *Journal of the National Cancer Institute, 99*(4), 291–299.

Roukos, D.H., & Briasoulis, E. (2007). Individualized preventive and therapeutic management of hereditary breast ovarian cancer syndrome. *Nature Clinical Practice Oncology, 4*(10), 578–590.

Rubinstein, W.S. (2008). Hereditary breast cancer: Pathobiology, clinical translation, and potential for targeted cancer therapeutics. *Familial Cancer, 7*(1), 83–89.

Sasa, M., Bando, Y., Takahashi, M., Hirose, T., & Nagao, T. (2007). Screening for basal marker expression is necessary for decision of therapeutic strategy for triple-negative breast cancer. *Journal of Surgical Oncology, 97*(1), 30–34.

Schneider, K. (2002). *Counseling about cancer: Strategies for genetic counseling* (2nd ed.). New York: Wiley-Liss.

Schoemaker, M.J., Swerdlow, A.J., Higgins, C.D., Wright, A.F., Jacobs, P.A., & UK Clinical Cytogenetics Group. (2008). Cancer incidence in women with Turner syndrome in Great Britain: A national cohort study. *Lancet Oncology, 9*(3), 239–246.

Schwartz, A.G., Prysak, G.M., Bock, C.H., & Cote, M.L. (2007). The molecular epidemiology of lung cancer. *Carcinogenesis, 28*(3), 507–518.

Sifri, R., Gangadharappa, S., & Acheson, L.S. (2004). Identifying and testing for hereditary susceptibility to common cancers. *CA: A Cancer Journal for Clinicians, 54*(6), 309–326.

Slatore, C.G., Littman, A.J., Au, D.H., Satia, J.A., & White, E. (2008). Long-term use of supplemental multivitamins, vitamin C, vitamin E, and folate does not reduce the risk of lung cancer. *American Journal of Respiratory and Critical Care Medicine, 177*(5), 470–471.

Tai, Y.C., Domchek, S., Parmigiani, G., & Chen, S. (2007). Breast cancer risk among male *BRCA1* and *BRCA2* mutation carriers. *Journal of the National Cancer Institute, 99*(23), 1811–1814.

Trepanier, A., Ahrens, M., McKinnon, W., Peters, J., Stopfer, J., Grumet, S.C., et al. (2004). Genetic cancer risk assessment and counseling: Recommendations of the National Society of Genetic Counselors. *Journal of Genetic Counseling, 13*(2), 83–114.

Truta, B., Chen, Y.Y., Blanco, A.M., Deng, G., Conrad, P.G., Kim, Y.H., et al. (2008). Tumor histology helps to identify Lynch syndrome among colorectal cancer patients. *Familial Cancer, 7*(3), 267–274.

Tucker, M.A., Fraser, M.C., Goldstein, A.M., Struewing, J.P., King, M.A., Crawford, J.T., et al. (2002). A natural history of melanoma and dysplastic nevi: An atlas of lesions in melanoma prone families. *Cancer, 94*(12), 3192–3209.

Umar, A., Boland, C.R., Terdiman, J.P., Syngal, S., de la Chapelle, A., Rüschoff, J., et al. (2004). Revised Bethesda Guidelines for hereditary nonpolyposis colorectal cancer (Lynch syndrome) and microsatellite instability. *Journal of the National Cancer Institute, 96*(4), 261–268.

U.S. Department of Health and Human Services. (2004, May 27). *The health consequences of smoking: A report from the surgeon general.* Retrieved November 14, 2009, from http://www.surgeongeneral.gov/library/smokingconsequences/

van Heyningen, V., Hoovers, J.M., de Kraker, J., & Crolla, J.A. (2007). Raised risk of Wilms tumour in patients with aniridia and submicroscopic WT1 deletion. *Journal of Medical Genetics, 44*(12), 787–790.

Whiteman, D.D., Whiteman, C.A., & Green, A.C. (2001). Childhood sun exposure as a risk factor for melanoma: A systematic review of epidemiologic studies. *Cancer Causes and Control, 12*(1), 69–82.

Wickerham, D.L., Costantino, J.P., Vogel, V.G., Cronin, W.M., Cecchini, R.S., Ford, L.G., et al. (2009). The use of tamoxifen and raloxifene for the prevention of breast cancer. *Recent Results in Cancer Research, 181,* 113–119.

Wolin, K.Y., & Colditz, G.A. (2008). Can weight loss prevent cancer? *British Journal of Cancer, 99*(7), 995–999.

World Cancer Research Fund & American Institute of Cancer Research. (2007). *Food, nutrition, physical activity, and the prevention of cancer: A global perspective.* Washington, DC: American Institute of Cancer Research.

Yeo, T.P., Hruban, R.H., Borody, J., Brune, K., Fitzgerald, S., & Yeo, C.J. (2009). Assessment of "gene-environment" interaction in cases of familial and sporadic pancreatic cancer. *Journal of Gastrointestinal Surgery, 13*(8), 1487–1494.

Zon, R.T., Goss, E., Vogel, V.G., Chlebowski, R.T., Jatoi, I., Robson, M.E., et al. (2009). American Society of Clinical Oncology policy statement: The role of the oncologist in cancer prevention and risk assessment. *Journal of Clinical Oncology, 27*(6), 986–993.

CHAPTER 4
Common Risk Prediction Models and Cancer Risk Communication

Suzanne M. Mahon, DNSc, RN, AOCN®, APNG

Professional Practice Domain:
Nursing Assessment: Applying and Integrating Genetic and Genomic Knowledge
- Critically analyze the history and physical assessment finding for genetic, environmental, and genomic influences and risk factors
- Assess client's knowledge, perceptions, and responses to genetic and genomic information
- Develop a plan of care that incorporates genetic and genomic assessment information

Provision of Education, Care, and Support
- Provide clients with interpretation of selective genetic and genomic information services
- Provide clients with credible, accurate, appropriate, and current genetic and genomic information, resources, services, and technologies that facilitate decision making
- Use health promotion and disease prevention practices that
  – Consider genetic and genomic influences on personal and environmental risk factors
  – Incorporate knowledge of genetic and/or genomic risk factors

(Consensus Panel on Genetic/Genomic Nursing Competencies, 2009)

INTRODUCTION

By collecting and interpreting cancer risk information, healthcare professionals can help clients to make informed decisions about participation in cancer risk-reduction and screening programs as well as to decide if genetic testing is of value. Great strides have been made in the past decade in developing both cancer risk prediction models and models to predict the risk of carrying a hereditary cancer mutation. Older models have been refined and newer models have been developed (Freedman et al., 2005; Parmigiani et al., 2007).

Genetic testing has brought new prominence to cancer risk assessment. Many people seek cancer risk assessment to determine if they are a candidate for genetic testing, but much can be gained from the assessment process regardless of whether genetic testing is ever done. Genetic testing is just one of the tools used in comprehensive cancer risk assessment. Risk assessment is as important for people who decline genetic testing as for those who decide to have it. People who decline testing are instructed on their risk of developing cancer and the inherent strengths and weaknesses associated with screening tests and risk-reduction measures. Because families share a pool of genes and therefore similar risks, genetic risk assessment includes not only individuals but also entire biologic families. This offers particular challenges in both risk assessment and risk communication.

Applied research about communicating cancer risk information is sparse, and little is known about effective communication strategies when multiple risks exist (Finkel, 2008).

The goal of risk communication is not limited to helping people to understand the risks they face, options for cancer risk management, and providing informed consent for testing (Akobeng, 2008). Other goals include building trust, influencing public policy, and fulfilling legal obligations. In addition to guiding screening and cancer risk management decisions, risk assessment can guide treatment decisions. Issues regarding risk communication that oncology nurses need to consider include methods of communicating risk information to clients, psychosocial and ethical concerns in risk factor assessment, documentation, and concerns regarding follow-up procedures.

Many groups have published guidelines on who should provide genetic cancer risk assessment services to high-risk individuals (American Society of Clinical Oncology [ASCO], 2003; National Comprehensive Cancer Network [NCCN], 2009b; Oncology Nursing Society, 2006a, 2006b; Robson et al., 2010; Trepanier, 2004). The consensus is that individuals with expertise in cancer genetics should provide the cancer genetics services, and that genetic testing should be offered when a reasonable expectation of finding a genetic mutation exists and results of genetic testing will influence healthcare management (ASCO; Robson et al.). For more detailed information on the role of the nurse in cancer genetics and genetic counseling, see Chapter 1.

This chapter will discuss types of risk and common genetic risk prediction models, how a case is evaluated for an individual's risk of cancer, and the likelihood that the family has an inherited predisposition cancer gene. Once a risk assessment is complete, it is critical to choose the appropriate strategies to communicate risk so that each individual and family has balanced information about the potential risks, benefits, and limitations of a particular genetic test, screening modality, or risk-reduction strategy. Clinical examples will clarify discussions of risk model use and how to determine which risk model or models will be most valuable and appropriate. These concepts and examples are applicable to the other cancers for which genetic and cancer risk assessment and risk communication commonly is performed.

COMMON TERMS IN RISK ASSESSMENT AND RISK COMMUNICATION

Literature about cancer genetic risk assessment and communication typically uses a variety of epidemiologic and statistical terms. Nurses who provide genetics services that integrate genetic and genomic information use many of these terms when educating and counseling families. A working knowledge of these terms facilitates effective patient and family education.

A *risk factor* is a trait or characteristic associated with a statistically significant increased likelihood of developing a disease. Of great importance in risk communication is the concept that having a risk factor does not mean that a person will develop the disease, such as a malignancy, nor does the absence of a risk factor make the person immune to developing the disease.

Basic elements of a *cancer risk assessment* include a review of medical history, a history of exposures to carcinogens in daily living, and a detailed family history. See Chapter 3 for more details on the elements of cancer risk assessment. The goals of risk factor assessment and counseling for the client and family are to provide accurate information about the genetic, biologic, and environmental factors related to an individual's and family's risk of developing cancer, to formulate appropriate recommendations for risk reduction, to offer emotional and psychosocial support to facilitate adjustment to the risk information, and to promote adherence to recommendations for risk reduction.

Several types of risk management and reduction strategies exist. All are implemented in people with genetic risk. **Primary cancer prevention** includes measures to avoid carcinogen exposure and improve health practices and, in some cases, includes the use of chemopreventive agents. Primary prevention also may include the use of risk-reducing surgery to significantly reduce the risk of malignancy development in people with genetic susceptibility. **Secondary cancer prevention** includes cancer screening measures in asymptomatic people with the aim of detecting cancer in its earliest stages when treatment is less complex and more likely to be effective. These strategies may be implemented at an earlier age or at more frequent intervals in people with genetic susceptibility. **Tertiary cancer prevention** is aimed at people with a history of malignancy. This includes monitoring for and reducing the risk for recurrence of the originally diagnosed cancer and screening for second primary cancers. Genomic tests such as tumor expression profiles are now used for prognosis and treatment decisions are discussed (see Chapter 8). In some cases, those who have been diagnosed with cancer may carry a mutated cancer susceptibility gene placing them at significantly higher risk for developing a second malignancy. Tertiary cancer prevention is particularly important for this group of individuals.

Population is the number of people in a defined group who are capable of developing a disease. It may refer to the general population or a specific group of people defined by geographic, physical, or social characteristics. For example, nurses who provide genetic risk assessment and counseling about cancer collect a client's maternal and paternal ethnicity. Certain ethnic groups, such as the Ashkenazi Jewish population, have a greater **prevalence** of certain genetic conditions. This specific group is at high risk for three specific mutations associated with hereditary breast/ovarian cancer secondary to a founder effect (Antoniou et al., 2005). *Founder effect* is when a mutation gene has a high frequency in a population of people that have a common ancestry and had periods when the population was isolated because of geographic proximity or culture. Because the risk of having a hereditary susceptibility mutation may be higher in ethnically distinct populations, such as the Western or Central Europeans, Dutch, Newfoundlanders, or Australians, genetic professionals inquire about ancestry (Green et al., 2007; Mantelli, Barile, & Ciotti, 2002).

The *prevalence* of cancer is the actual number of cancers in a defined population at a given time. The prevalence rate commonly is expressed as the number of cancers per 100,000 individuals in the population. Estimates of the prevalence of various cancers are available from the American Cancer Society (ACS) (Jemal et al., 2009) and the National Cancer Institute Surveillance, Epidemiology, and End Results (Program SEER) database (Ries et al., 2008). The prevalence of a particular mutation in a specific population is less clearly understood, but data continue to accumulate, especially in specific populations (John et al., 2007; Risch et al., 2006; Simard et al., 2007; Weitzel et al., 2005). The second edition of the *Concise Handbook of Familial Cancer Susceptibility Syndromes* provides a review of 55 hereditary cancer syndromes (Lindor, McMaster, Lindor, & Greene, 2008).

Prevalence data also are available from some of the laboratories that perform genetic testing. Such data will include information about how many people test positive for a certain mutation with specific family and personal histories of cancer (Frank et al., 2002). Prevalence data do not predict whether a person will have a mutation or a cancer; it is an estimate of the number of individuals who have a particular cancer or mutation within a defined population.

The *incidence* of cancer is the number of cancers that develop in a population during a defined period, such as a year. For example, ACS estimated that 192,370 women would be be diagnosed with breast cancer in the United States in 2009 (Jemal et al., 2009). Incidence numbers can be helpful when trying to understand cancer risks for the general population or in a specific subpopulation. The pool of data regarding incidence of mutations in specific subpopulations is increasing. Lindor et al. (2008) provided a summary of various incidence data for 55 hereditary cancer syndromes.

The **mortality rate** is the number of people who die of a particular cancer during a defined period. The estimated mortality for breast cancer for women was 40,170 deaths in 2009 (Jemal et al., 2009). Compare that mortality estimate to the mortality estimate for small intestine cancer for the same year (1,110 deaths) (Jemal et al., 2009). Mortality rates provide insight into the strengths of risk-reduction measures for a particular cancer and the effectiveness of current standard therapy.

Outcomes include health and economic results that occur related to screening or genetic testing. Outcomes also may include the benefits, harms, and costs of screening or testing and the diagnostic evaluations that result from screening or genetic testing (Domchek & Antoniou, 2007). Short-term outcomes include the number of people screened or tested, the number of cancers detected, or the cost per cancer detected. Because genetic testing can cost thousands of dollars, patients and insurers want assurance that testing is based on a solid assessment and that it will provide useful information. Long-term outcomes often are not seen for at least a decade and may include measurements such as a decrease in the incidence or mortality of a cancer or a shift toward detection of cancers at an earlier stage. Also, outcomes specifically are associated with cancer in carriers of a cancer susceptibility mutation. For example, some mutations are associated with better overall survival than that in people without a mutation (Stigliano et al., 2008; Tan et al., 2008).

Validity is a measure of whether a test measures its intended purpose. Analytic validity refers to how well the genetic test performs in measuring the property or characteristic it is intended to measure. In the case of family history, analytic validity refers to the accuracy and reliability of the disease in reported family history information (Yoon et al., 2002). In mutation prediction models, analytic validity refers to the accuracy of the model in predicting the presence of a gene mutation (Parmigiani et al., 2007). In genetic testing for a specific mutation, analytic validity refers to the accuracy of a genetic test in identifying the presence or absence of the mutation.

In the case of genetic testing, analytic validity considers both the analytic sensitivity, which is the measure of the probability that a test will be positive when a particular genetic sequence is present, and analytic **specificity**, which is the probability that the test will be negative when no sequence abnormality is present. The analytic validity of a genetic test is affected by the technical accuracy and reliability of the testing procedure and by the quality of the laboratory processes, including specimen handling (Kristoffersson, 2008).

Clinical validity refers to the predictive value of a test to identify a clinical condition within a given population (Constantin, Faucett, & Lubin, 2005). Sensitivity and specificity data for types of genetic tests are available from both the laboratory where the test is performed and, depending on the test, in published reports (Antoniou et al., 2005). In genetic testing, clinical validity is the likelihood that cancer will develop in someone with a positive test result. Clinical validity is affected by heterogeneity and penetrance. *Heterogeneity* occurs when the same genetic disease might result from the presence of any of several different variants (alleles) of the same gene or of different genes. Currently, all disease-related alleles cannot always be identified, particularly when many of them are present, which is typically the case. This failure to detect all disease-related mutations reduces a test's clinical sensitivity. *Penetrance* is the probability that disease will appear when a disease-related genotype is present. In families with a high risk for colon cancer caused by Lynch syndrome, 20% or more of men and women with mutations in the *MLH1* or *MSH2* genes never will develop colon cancer (Aarnio et al., 1999; Jenkins et al., 2006; Lin et al., 1998). Environmental factors and possibly other inherited factors affect penetrance.

The *clinical utility* of a test also refers to the likelihood that the test will result in an improved health outcome by prompting an intervention. The clinical utility of a genetic test is based on the health benefits related to the interventions offered to people with positive test results (Potter et al., 2008). Benefits might include a reduction of uncertainty and, in those who are negative for a documented deleterious mutation in the family, escape from frequent monitoring for signs of disease, the need for risk-reducing surgery, and the fear of insurance or employment discrimination. However, in the absence of definitive interventions for improving outcomes in those with positive test results, the benefits will be limited, and not everyone will choose to be tested. Before a genetic test can be generally accepted in clinical practice, evidence is needed that demonstrates the benefits and risks that accrue from both positive and negative results and related risk-reduction recommendations.

Absolute risk is a measure of the occurrence of cancer, either incidence (new cases) or mortality (deaths), in the general population. Absolute risk can be expressed either as the number of cases for a specified denominator (e.g., 50 cases per 10,000 people annually) or as a cumulative risk up to a specified age (e.g., one in three women who live to age 85 will develop some form of cancer [Jemal et al., 2009]). When describing genetic risk, individuals often need to understand the risk of a particular cancer in the general population as well as the absolute risk if they have a mutation. For example, the absolute risk of developing kidney cancer is 4% in the general population but can be up to 40% in people with a *VHL* mutation (Jemal et al., 2008; Lindor et al., 2008).

The term **relative risk** refers to a comparison of the incidence of a risk factor or the number of deaths among those with a risk factor compared to those without the risk factor. Relative risk often is confused with absolute risk. Absolute risk is calculated on the basis of all individuals in the population, regardless of risk.

By using risk factors, nurses can determine a client's risk by using relative risk figures and thus gain a better understanding of the client's personal chances of developing a particular cancer as compared to people without such risk factors. When looking at relative risk figures, the reference point is 1.0. A relative risk greater than 1.0 indicates a risk factor associated with disease. A relative risk less than 1.0 is not a risk factor in that population. The risk of developing breast cancer is higher in male *BRCA1* and *BRCA2* mutation carriers, compared with noncarriers, but *BRCA2* mutation carriers had the highest risk. The relative risk was greatest for men in their 30s and 40s and decreased with age. For example, the estimated relative risk for breast cancer for a 70-year-old male *BRCA2* mutation carrier is 6.8, compared with 1.2 for *BRCA1* mutation carriers (Tai, Domchek, Parmigiani, & Chen, 2007).

Relative risk factors can be confusing to some clients. When providing information about relative risk, healthcare professionals need to specify exactly what comparison is being made. Percentages also can be the basis of confusion. If a news report states that breast cancer risk increased 30%–50% because of a particular hormone therapy used after menopause, the report means, in numeric terms, that 0.3–0.5 more cases of breast cancer per 100 women will occur. The only way to be able to accurately convert the percentage figure to an absolute risk is by looking at the actual study data.

Relative risk sometimes is expressed as a ratio. Ratios can create problems because people fail to consider the relevant sample size. For example, individuals may respond differently to a ratio when it is expressed as 1:10 rather than 10:100, even though both ratios express the same probability (Grimes & Schulz, 2008). People may rate a health problem as riskier if informed that it kills 1,275 of 10,000 people (12.75%) when compared with 12.75 of 100 people (12.75%). Relative risk statistics are helpful when everyone understands what the baseline group is. If the baseline is unclear, a relative risk statement can be misleading.

Attributable risk is the amount of disease within a population that could be prevented by altering a risk factor. Although historically this component of risk assessment has not received much attention, attributable risk carries important implications for public health policy. A risk factor could convey a very large relative risk but be restricted to a few individuals; changing it would benefit a small group only. Conversely, altering a risk factor such as cigarette smoking could decrease cancer-related morbidity and mortality across the population. For example, 85% of lung cancer cases diagnosed among current and never smokers can be attributed to cigarette smoking (Jemal et al., 2008). This concept also can be applied to individuals with genetic risk; an increased risk of colon cancer is possible among *MLH1* carriers associated with smoking (Watson, Ashwathnarayan, Lynch, & Roy, 2004).

QUANTIFYING RISKS

Identifying and quantifying cancer risks is important for several reasons. The identification of risk factors contributes to the understanding of the biology of cancer, and when identified, such risk factors may be altered to decrease the number of new cases or deaths from cancer (Bradbury & Olufumilayo, 2006). The quantification of risk also guides public policy for the allocation of funds for screening and for utilization of costly services (e.g., genetic testing). Genetic testing most likely will be recommended for cancer sites in which reasonable risk-reduction measures exist, incidence is substantial, risks are understood, and risk-reduction measures directly affect the morbidity and mortality associated with the disease.

Every cancer risk assessment involves comprehensive assessment of the family and medical and personal risk factors. For more detailed information about performing cancer risk assessments, see Chapter 3. Not all risk factors are amenable to change. An individual cannot change his or her sex, age, family history, or history of predisposing risk lesions (Jemal et al., 2008). In such a case, secondary cancer prevention efforts are recommended.

Methods for Quantifying Risk

Risk models have multiple uses in cancer genetics and can help healthcare providers to (Freedman et al., 2005)
- Identify individuals at high risk for an inherited predisposition to cancer
- Estimate the risk of developing cancer both in the present and over time
- Estimate the probability of carrying an inherited cancer predisposition gene

- Support the option for genetic testing
- Guide clinical recommendations for medical management, screening, and chemoprevention.

A variety of strategies can be used to perform these calculations, and all have varying levels of performance, usability, optimal application, and limitations (Freedman et al., 2005). Methods for risk calculations include prevalence study data from specific mutated genes in select populations and Mendelian inheritance when a family mutation has been identified, as well as Bayesian analysis, statistical models, and clinical information such as tumor features (Freedman et al.). Most often, risk assessment utilizes two primary types of risk quantification: (a) the probability of harboring a deleterious mutation in a cancer susceptibility gene, and (b) the risk of developing a specific form of cancer (Domchek & Antoniou, 2007).

Evaluating Risk Prediction Models

The primary limitation of risk assessment relates to the assessment models themselves. Many models were constructed based on assumptions and epidemiologic studies in select populations, so they may not be applicable to every individual or family. Carefully evaluating a model helps the user to establish the strengths, limitations, and best use for a given model. The key questions to consider when evaluating models and methods for risk calculations include the following (Freedman et al., 2005).

- Has the model been peer reviewed?
- How was the model constructed?
  - Study population
    * What kinds of patients were included and excluded, including age, race, and ethnicity?
    * What is the sample size?
  - Methods of statistical calculations
    * What findings were used to construct the model? What factors were found to correlate with cancer or a mutation depending on the type of model?
    * If the model includes confidence intervals, how wide are the intervals?
  - What are the calculation requirements?
    * Is a computer program required?
    * How detailed of a health history or pedigree is necessary for accurate calculations?
- What validation studies have been performed on the model?
  - What is the documented reliability and validity of the model?
  - Were the studies designed to accurately assess the model? What were the study weaknesses?
- Have updates to the model been incorporated based on current evidence?

Careful review of the model helps the user to determine the population best suited for use of a given model in practice and what precisely is being calculated. Some models for calculating prior probability of a gene mutation calculate the probability for the family, whereas others will calculate the probability for the individual.

Selecting Risk Prediction Models

Genetic heterogeneity affects model selection because different cancer syndromes and therefore different genes may correlate with a single type of cancer, and each model is syndrome, gene, and cancer specific. Genetic heterogeneity occurs with many cancers. For example, prostate cancer is definitely or strongly associated with hereditary breast/ovarian cancer syndrome (HBOC) (*BRCA1* and *BRCA2* genes) and hereditary prostate cancer (multiple **candidate genes**) and has been reported, though the significance is not definitely established to be associated with hereditary diffuse gastric cancer (*CDH1* gene), Li-Fraumeni syndrome (*TP53* gene), and Nijmegen breakage syndrome (*NBS1* gene) (Lindor et al., 2008). Knowledge of differentiating clinical features is important in identifying the correct syndrome. Such significant overlap highlights the need for using assessment information to establish an accurate differential list (Katki, 2007). All suspected cancer syndromes, associated genes, and their respective risk assessment models are considered when establishing and prioritizing the differential list to determine whether and for what purpose gene testing would be of value.

In the end, comprehensive methods are not available for predicting risk or establishing the prior probability for a gene mutation. Furthermore, individual risk factors and probability calculations are not additive but need to be considered as independent calculations. Models are never a substitute for clinical judgment but are used to validate clinical decision making, such as indications for enhanced cancer screening and genetic testing (ASCO, 2003).

Factors That Influence Model Calculations

The etiology of cancer is multifactorial, with endogenous and exogenous risk factors contributing to risk. Most models are designed with the assumption that cancer is a homogenous disease, although many variations are possible. Many models are not constructed to account for other modifying factors. Current models usually can only account for a few factors. Therefore, no model completely and accurately explains an individual's risk (Freedman et al., 2005).

Several family history variables can affect risk calculations, which may or may not be incorporated into a given model. Having a limited number of family members in a given lineage can greatly affect the accuracy of a model calculation. Limited numbers of family members have been compared to "missing values" in research studies, so calculations may be an underestimate (Weitzel et al., 2007). Other family history variables that can affect calculation accuracy include early deaths in family members from unrelated causes, removal of the at-risk organ, consanguinity, presence of a de novo mutation (a new mutation that arose during embryogenesis), nonpenetrance in key family members, misattributed paternity, family dominate for opposite sex in sex-specific cancers (e.g., prostate, ovarian), adoption, and inaccurately reported family history (Domchek & Antoniou, 2007). In addition, many models have been developed in predominantly Caucasian North American and Northern European populations, and validation in other populations may not have been performed (Domchek et al., 2003).

SPECIFIC MODELS QUANTIFYING CANCER RISK OR MUTATION PROBABILITY

The National Cancer Institute maintains a list of risk model resources at http://riskfactor.cancer.gov/cancer_risk_prediction. Models are organized by peer reviewed versus non–peer reviewed and by organ site. A wide range of cancers are represented, including models on breast cancer, colorectal cancer, lung cancer, melanoma, ovarian cancer, prostate cancer, cervical cancer, pancreatic cancer, bladder cancer, and multiple sites. Publications for each model are provided, as well as a list of publications that cite the model. Table 4-1 provides an overview of some selected models available for use.

Individual Risk for Developing Cancer

Quantifying an individual's chance of developing a particular cancer will vary depending on the context. When a deleterious gene mutation has been identified in an individual, cancer risk estimates are based on penetrance data in combination with risk modifiers such as mutation type, position, risk-reducing surgeries, and environmental variables such

TABLE 4-1   Selected Models for Cancer Risk and Mutation Risk Assessment

Model	Purpose	Target	Validation Sample	Advantages	Disadvantages
Pedigree Assessment Tool (Hoskins et al., 2006)	Identify women at increased risk for hereditary breast/ovarian cancer	Women being seen in primary care settings with multiple family members diagnosed with breast and/or ovarian cancer	3,609 women of varying risks	Simple point scoring system based on family history with points weighted according to male and female breast cancer and ovarian cancer	May over-refer some women for risk assessment
Melanoma Risk Assessment Tool (Fears et al., 2006)	Predict the absolute risk of developing melanoma	People with melanoma risk factors	718 non-Hispanic people with melanoma	Can be easily calculated online	May underestimate risk in people with a strong family history
BRCAPRO (Berry et al., 1997; Parmigiani et al., 1998, 2007)	Estimate risk of carrying a *BRCA1* or *BRCA2* mutation	Women with a family history of breast and/or ovarian cancer	3,364 women with a history of breast and/or ovarian cancer and at least one relative with a history of breast and/or ovarian cancer	Considers first- and second-degree relatives, age at diagnosis of breast and/or ovarian cancer, and risk reduction secondary to bilateral salpingo-oophorectomy	Has limited utility in some ethnic groups. Requires a computer program and precise ages to do an accurate calculation
PREMM$_{1,2}$ (Prediction of Mutations in *MLH1* and *MSH2*) Model (Balmaña et al., 2006)	Estimate the risk of a *MSH2* or *MLH1* mutation	People with a family history of colorectal and gynecologic cancer	1,914 unrelated probands with a history of colorectal or other Lynch syndrome cancer	Considers both colorectal and gynecologic cancers as well as personal risk factors. Tool is easy to complete with a Web-based model.	Cannot incorporate complex combinations of diagnoses

as smoking or hormone use. In the context of no genetic testing or an uninformative test result, calculations of the absolute, relative, and cumulative risk for the cancer or cancers can be utilized. These figures are based on epidemiologic information such as personal, lifestyle, and family history information and are estimates over a defined time period, which is model dependent but can be defined as the next five years, at 10-year intervals, and lifetime to a given age.

Risk for Carrying a Hereditary Susceptibility Mutation

For a client with a family history that suggests hereditary susceptibility, the chance of carrying a mutation in a particular cancer-susceptibility gene is calculated based on the differential list established from assessment information. This is referred to as the prior probability of carrying a gene mutation. This risk figure is important for those who are considering genetic testing, helps to determine the likelihood that genetic testing would reveal a mutation, and helps to prepare the client and family for the possibility of a positive result. The models themselves may be more heavily weighted for specific risk factors (e.g., early-onset cancer) or exclude the evaluation of specific types of cancers.

Communicating Model Information

Models will generate a risk profile, but it is the clinician's responsibility to interpret it to the family. In most cases, a range of risk figures will be generated because different models and methods can produce different risk figures for the same individual based on the variation in model constructs. For this reason, no model can completely explain prior probability and disease risk. To minimize confusion, those providing genetic risk assessment and counseling explain why these calculations are estimates and the limitations of these risk figures. Distinguishing between risk models that produce information about risk of disease and those that produce information about the risk of carrying a gene mutation is important. Giving a range of risk based on several models as opposed to a single figure can help to avoid calculations being interpreted as more accurate than these estimates actually are.

CASE STUDY

The pedigree in Figure 4-1 provides a case study for model selection and clinical application. Examination of the pedigree shows that autosomal dominant transmission appears to be in the family because multiple individuals are affected over three generations. Determining the risk for developing cancer and which cancer syndromes correspond with the cancers seen in this family is a challenge. Cases of early-onset breast, colon, ovarian, and endometrial cancer have occured within this family, and the genetic professional needs to consider several hereditary cancer syndromes. These include HBOC, Cowden syndrome, and Lynch syndrome (Lindor et al., 2008). The family has multiple cases of early-onset breast cancer, a case of ovarian cancer, and a case of bilateral breast cancer spread over multiple generations, which is suggestive of HBOC. The family also has multiple cases of early-onset colon cancer over multiple generations, as well as ovarian and endometrial cancers, which can be associated with Lynch syndrome. Also, one individual had both breast and endometrial cancer, which could be Cowden syndrome that is associated mutation in the *PTEN* gene. The clinician would need to gather more information about Cowden phenotype, including history of thyroid cancer, brain tumors, skin findings, and unusual kidney problems to better understand the risk for a *PTEN* mutation. For the purposes of this example, further assessment has resulted in Cowden syndrome being eliminated from the differential list.

The proband (represented by the arrow) is the consultant shown in Figure 4-1. Because the proband has not had cancer, care needs to be taken when utilizing cancer probability models to ascertain whether the calculations are for this individual or whether they are calculated for the closest relative affected with cancer. Therefore, the prior probabilities for the family carrying a mutation as well as for the proband carrying a mutation are calculated. Beginning with the first syndrome remaining on the differential list, HBOC, prior probability calculations are undertaken using the BRCAPRO probability model. These calculations are reflected in Figure 4-2 for the proband and in Figure 4-3 for the individual affected

FIGURE 4-1   CASE EXAMPLE PEDIGREE

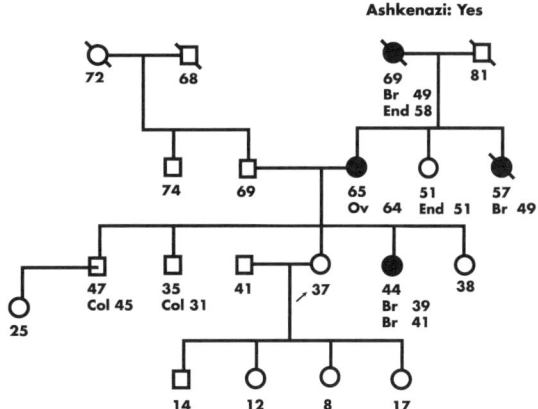

The proband (spokesperson for the family) is represented by the arrow. Multiple generations are reflected. The age at diagnosis is provided for all cancer cases. Slashes represent individuals who are deceased.

FIGURE 4-2   *BRCA* PREDICTION MODELS FOR UNAFFECTED FAMILY MEMBER

BRCA1	Proband Probability
Couch (U. Penn)	0.286
Shattuck-Eidens (Myriad I)	0.390
BRCAPRO	0.310
BRCA2	
BRCAPRO	0.182
BRCA1 or *2*	
NCI CART	0.058
Myriad.com (Myriad II)	0.286
BRCAPRO	0.485

Pedigree Information
Ashkenazi family: **YES**
Number of family members: **20**
Number with breast cancer only: **3**
Number with ovarian cancer only: **1**
Number both breast and ovarian cancer: **0**
Number with bilateral breast cancer: **1**

Ontario FHAT: 29

Values expressed as probabilities, not percents

"none" means no calculation possible

This demonstrates the range of risk estimates for having a germ line mutation for the same woman depending on the model used.

FIGURE 4-3 *BRCA* PREDICTION MODELS FOR FAMILY MEMBER WITH CANCER

BRCA1	**Proband Probability**
Couch (U. Penn)	0.572
Shattuck-Eidens (Myriad I)	0.779
BRCAPRO	0.658
BRCA2	
BRCAPRO	0.360
BRCA1 or 2	
NCI CART	0.265
Myriad.com (Myriad II)	0.569
BRCAPRO	0.999

Pedigree Information
Ashkenazi family: **YES**
Number of family members: **19**
Number with breast cancer only: **3**
Number with ovarian cancer only: **1**
Number both breast and ovarian cancer: **0**
Number with bilateral breast cancer: **1**

Ontario FHAT: 29

Values expressed as probabilities, not percents

"none" means no calculation possible

These are the mutation risk calculations for the sister with bilateral breast cancer. Note the difference in risk when testing an affected person.

---

with early-onset breast cancer. By calculating the risk for the affected individual with bilateral early-onset breast cancer, the numbers change because of the greater probability of finding a mutation in an affected individual (see Figure 4-3).

Lynch syndrome also is considered in the differential diagnosis for this family. Hereditary colorectal cancer syndromes require a careful review of the family history, presentation of malignancy, and cumulative polyp count. Familial adenomatous polyposis syndromes are considered in the presence of 20 or more cumulative polyps; other syndromes, such as Lynch syndrome, are considered when the patient has fewer polyps and other malignancies (e.g., uterine, ovarian, other gastrointestinal malignancies) are present.

Decisions about whether to test for a mutation that suggests a hereditary predisposition to developing Lynch syndrome usually are based on clinical criteria, such as the revised Bethesda guidelines or the *NCCN Clinical Practice Guidelines in Oncology*™: *Colorectal Cancer Screening* (NCCN, 2009a; Umar et al., 2004). Initially published in 1997 and revised in 2004, the revised Bethesda Guidelines (see Figure 4-4) consider clinicopathologic factors and can be used to help to identify families at highest risk of Lynch syndrome who might benefit from further evaluation (Umar et al.). Either of the brothers of the proband would meet the criteria for the Bethesda Guidelines. These criteria can be considered separately or in conjunction with computer risk models.

Although this family meets the criteria to go directly to mutation testing for Lynch syndrome, models are available that provide probability ranges for the risk of carrying a *MSH2* or *MLH1* mutation, which represent two of the most common genes associated with Lynch syndrome. *MSH2* mutations account for about 30% of all cases of Lynch syndrome, and *MSH1* mutations account for about 40% (Lynch et al., 2007). Calculation of these models for the proband and her brother with early-onset colorectal cancer are shown in Figures 4-5 and 4-6, respectively. Once again, the risk changes depending on the family member for whom the estimate is calculated.

FIGURE 4-4 2004 REVISED BETHESDA GUIDELINES FOR CONSIDERATION OF TESTING FOR LYNCH SYNDROME

Tumors from individuals should be tested for MSI in the following situations:
1. Colorectal cancer diagnosed in a patient who is less than 50 years of age.
2. Presence of synchronous, metachronous colorectal, or other HNPCC-associated tumors,* regardless of age.
3. Colorectal cancer with the MSI-H† histology‡ diagnosed in a patient who is less than 60 years of age.§
4. Colorectal cancer diagnosed in one or more first-degree relatives with an HNPCC-related tumor, with one of the cancers being diagnosed under age 50 years.
5. Colorectal cancer diagnosed in two or more first- or second-degree relatives with HNPCC-related tumors, regardless of age.

*Hereditary nonpolyposis colorectal cancer (HNPCC)-related tumors include colorectal, endometrial, stomach, ovarian, pancreas, ureter and renal pelvis, biliary tract, and brain (usually glioblastoma as seen in Turcot syndrome) tumors, sebaceous gland adenomas and keratoacanthomas in Muir–Torre syndrome, and carcinoma of the small bowel.

†MSI-H = microsatellite instability–high in tumors refers to changes in two or more of the five National Cancer Institute-recommended panels of microsatellite markers.

‡Presence of tumor infiltrating lymphocytes, Crohn's-like lymphocytic reaction, mucinous/signet-ring differentiation, or medullary growth pattern.

§There was no consensus among the Workshop participants on whether to include the age criteria in guideline 3 above; participants voted to keep less than 60 years of age in the guidelines.

Note. From "Revised Bethesda Guidelines for Hereditary Nonpolyposis Colorectal Cancer (Lynch Syndrome) and Microsatellite Instability," by A. Umar, C.R. Boland, J.P. Terdiman, S. Syngal, A. de la Chapelle, J. Rüschoff, et al., 2004, *Journal of the National Cancer Institute, 96*(4), p. 266. Copyright 2004 by Oxford University Press. Reprinted with permission.

FIGURE 4-5 PROBABILITY OF LYNCH SYNDROME GERM LINE MUTATION IN PROBAND

Gene	Proband Probabilty
MLH1	
CRCAPRO	0.163
MSH2	
CRCAPRO	0.309
Either *MLH1* or *MSH2*	
CRCAPRO	0.472
Weijnen	0.250

This shows the probability of a Lynch syndrome mutation in the same 37-year-old woman.

In conjunction with prior probability information, tumor-specific information may be used to determine the value of genetic testing. Identifying Lynch syndrome often begins with a colon cancer tumor assessment consisting of microsatellite instability or immunohistochemistry testing (Hampel et al., 2005). The advantage of immunohistochemistry testing is that it may direct mutation analysis to a specific gene because the pattern of staining is suggestive of the underlying gene defect (Vasen et al., 2007).

The case in Figure 4-1 represents the complexity of gene mutation prior probability calculations. The proband is not the ideal person to test initially for a hereditary susceptibility mutation because she is not affected. Ideally, testing begins with an affected person, preferably with a younger age of onset when the cancer is most likely to be caused by a germ line mutation. If an unaffected individual is tested first and no mutation is identified, whether the family has a germ line mutation is unclear because no mutation was detected based on the limitations of the testing techniques used, or because the family has another germ line mutation for which testing was not done. Because of the striking family history and these calculations, it is reasonable to offer the family testing for mutations in genes associated with both HBOC and Lynch syndromes. Keep in mind, more than one syndrome is possible, and therefore more than one gene mutation may be associated with the cancer in any given family.

CANCER RISK COMMUNICATION

Transmitting risk information is a central component of all screening and cancer risk assessment and genetic counseling programs. The science of risk assessment receives little attention in most basic nursing programs, and even in advanced practice programs, content is often limited. Healthcare professionals often fail to understand the complexity of risk assessment; the lay public understands it even less (Akobeng, 2008). Healthcare professionals may have difficulty educating and counseling clients because they do not have the epidemiology and statistics background needed to interpret data and understand the epidemiologic reports published in scientific journals. The difficulty is compounded by the fact that at the technical level, professionals are in a continual debate about terminology and techniques. Moreover, not all the ways of reporting risk clearly show the benefits or risks of risk-management strategies in a clinically useful way. This is particularly crucial when the management decision confronting the client is an emotionally charged decision (Fagerlin, Ubel, Smith, & Zikmund-Fisher, 2007).

Most healthcare professionals agree that clients need enough information to make an informed decision about a risk-reduction or risk-management strategy. Risk cannot be separated from choice (Tucker & Ferson, 2008). Thus, the importance of accurate cancer and genetic risk communication cannot be underestimated. To communicate information about risk to clients, healthcare professionals consider the strengths and limitations of the methods used to generate the information.

The primary premise of cancer genetic risk assessment is to provide enough information in understandable terms for an individual to make an informed decision (Rimer, Briss, Zeller, Chan, & Woolf, 2004). Collecting, interpreting, and communicating risk information to a client and family takes time, is labor intensive, and may involve more than one visit, especially in the case of genetic testing (Kausmeyer et al., 2006; Lipkus, 2007).

Americans in general have poor numeracy skills, find it difficult to recall and interpret probabilities, and have limited knowledge about the modifiable causes of cancer (Fagerlin et al., 2007; Nelson, Reyna, Fagerlin, Lipkus, & Peters, 2008). A hierarchy of numerical skills as well as literary skills are needed to comprehend and use information about the likelihood of risks and benefits of a risk-management maneuver (Nelson et al.). Furthermore,

FIGURE 4-6 PROBABILITY OF LYNCH SYNDROME IN AN AFFECTED RELATIVE

Gene	Proband Probability
MLH1	
CRCAPRO Model	0.350
MSH2	
CRCAPRO	0.643
Either *MLH1* or *MSH2*	
CRCAPRO	0.993
Weijnen	0.198
Myriad	0.272

This figure shows the probability of a germ line mutation in the proband's 47-year-old brother with early-onset colorectal cancer.

risk factors do not necessarily increase in a simple mathematical fashion. For example, if one risk factor gives a woman a 12% risk of developing breast cancer and another gives the same woman an 18% risk, the two numbers cannot be assumed to mean the woman now has a 30% chance of developing breast cancer, as they are independent predictors that are not additive. In addition, clients must be able to remember information both for a short period (for decisions made quickly) as well as for an extended period (in the case of a lifetime program of screening), and memory ability differs. Finally, clients need to be able to weigh factors to match their needs and values and to understand that they are making trade-offs, either minor or emotionally and physically devastating, to ultimately arrive at a health decision (Rimer et al., 2004).

Consideration also should be given to the client's ability to understand risk information. An individual's likelihood of seeking cancer risk assessment may be related, in part, to his or her education level and ability to understand complex technical concepts (Nelson et al., 2008). Timing also may be important. Messages suggesting increased susceptibility to a specific form of cancer may be less effective if delivered too soon after the diagnosis of that cancer in a close relative. Accurate assessment of perceptions of risk is important to determine the best way and time to deliver risk information.

What Is the Best Format for Presenting Risk Data?

A numeric result such as an absolute or relative risk figure can appear highly scientific and may be difficult for many clients to understand. Conversely, using verbal terms, such as *high risk* or *low risk*, can be equally confusing. A high risk to one man might mean a 100% chance of developing cancer; for another, it might mean a 25% chance (Carey & Burgman, 2008). Numerical data alone are not sufficient in communicating risk because people vary widely in their affective response to the same probability estimates (O'Doherty & Suthers, 2007). Personal risk perceptions are influenced by whether the exposure is considered voluntary, controllable, and socially desirable (Klein & Stefanek, 2007). Tailored communication strategies also are considered a promising approach for enhancing cancer risk communication (Matloff, Moyer, Shannon, Niendorf, & Col, 2006).

What Is the Best Way to Frame Information?

The manner in which the information is communicated, in terms of attitude and context, is called *framing*. Framing can have a significant effect on how the client perceives the information (O'Doherty & Suthers, 2007). If risk information is presented in a negative fashion, the client may assume the risk is more than it actually is. If the discussion is too positive, the client may underestimate or minimize risk. The same is true in discussions of risk-management options.

Statistical context can constitute framing. If a healthcare professional tells a client that he or she has a 1.3 in 10,000 chance of developing a particular cancer, compared to the general population's risk of 1 in 10,000, the client may not be concerned. If the professional communicates the same risk by saying that the client's risk is 30% higher than average, the client may be more concerned. People's reactions to identical risk information, however, can vary by the size of the denominator used to describe the risk statistic (Zikmund-Fisher, Fagerlin, Roberts, Derry, & Ubel, 2008).

Clearly framing statistical information is one of the most challenging aspects of cancer risk communication. What the client really needs to understand is how much more or less risk they face (Fagerlin et al., 2007; O'Doherty & Suthers, 2007). Suggested practice includes framing the same information in both a positive and negative fashion (O'Doherty & Suthers). The goal is not to frighten a client unnecessarily; however, if the risk is underplayed too much, the client may not see the value in recommended cancer risk-management measures.

Visual Aids

Graphics can be a very effective means to communicate risk—especially in communicating numeric risk (Lipkus, 2007). They often can reveal data patterns that may otherwise go undetected and can communicate magnitude of risk, relative risk, cumulative risk, uncertainty, and interactions among risk factors (Edwards et al., 2008; Lipkus). Literature is emerging on the impact of graphic displays of risk information. Many nurses use a combination of formats to present numeric, visual, and explanatory data.

Pictorial Elements

A *bar graph* may decrease the number of mathematical computations that the user must make. A high data-to-ink ratio is optimal—that is, the graph does not contain extra pictures, busy backgrounds, and patterned fills (see Figure 4-7). Graphs are not optimal to communicate a low-probability event, such as an event with a 0.0003 chance (Lipkus, 2007). Although most people can understand the probability that accompanies a high-probability event, such as the probability of a flipped coin coming up heads (which represents a 0.50 or 50% chance), understanding a low-probability event, such as a 0.0003 chance, is much more difficult. A solution to this problem is to change the probability to a frequency (e.g., 3 out of 10,000).

Line graphs (see Figure 4-8) communicate trends and changes in data. They commonly are used to show changes in incidence or mortality over time, and most clients have experience reading them.

Pie charts communicate information about proportions. Pie charts can be combined to explain subcategories of data (see Figure 4-9).

Risk ladders can be used to portray the relative risk associated with environmental hazards. The higher up the ladder the hazard is, the greater the risk it represents (see Figure 4-10). The position on the ladder helps the viewer to conceptualize risks in relation to each other, "anchoring" risk perception to highest and lowest reference points.

Stick figures often are used to communicate relative risk or to show how many people out of a certain number may develop a particular disease (see Figure 4-11). When a small number of figures are used, the viewer may perceive the risk to be higher (Lipkus, 2007). If the number of figures is increased, the impact may not be as strong, though some will find the presentation busy and difficult to understand.

Figure 4-12 presents a *histogram*, a type of representation that most clients have some experience reading. Lipkus (2007) noted that histograms often convey the magnitude of the risk more clearly than numbers alone do.

FIGURE 4-7   CONFUSING GRAPH WITH LOW DATA-TO-INK RATIO

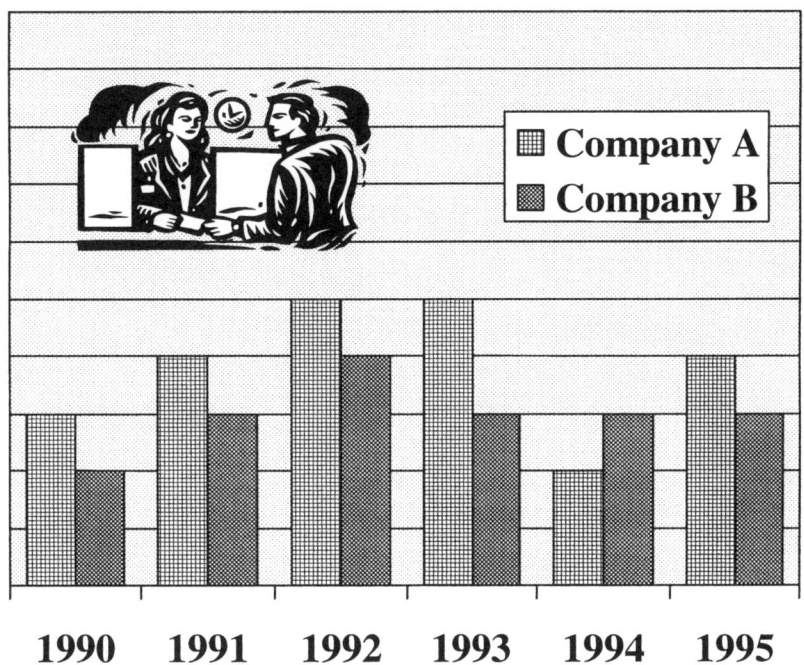

This bar graph is difficult to read because of the distracting background fill and graphic.

FIGURE 4-8   LINE GRAPH

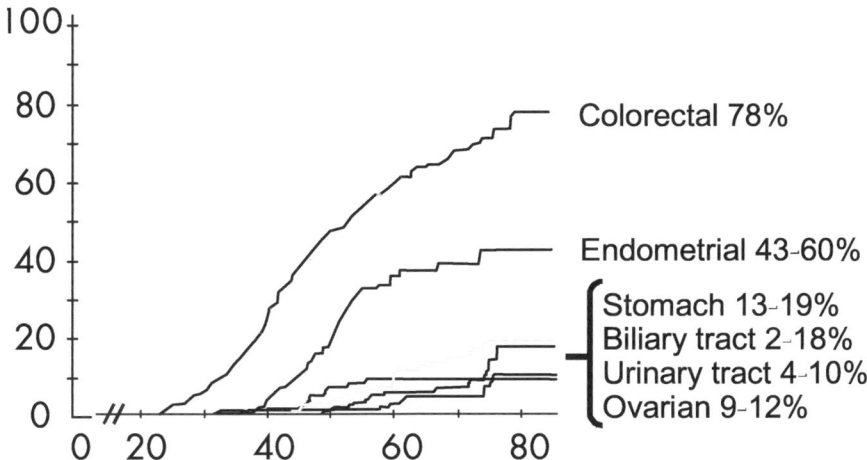

This is a typical line graph that demonstrates risk of developing various cancers in those with Lynch syndrome over time.

FIGURE 4-9 A PIE CHART

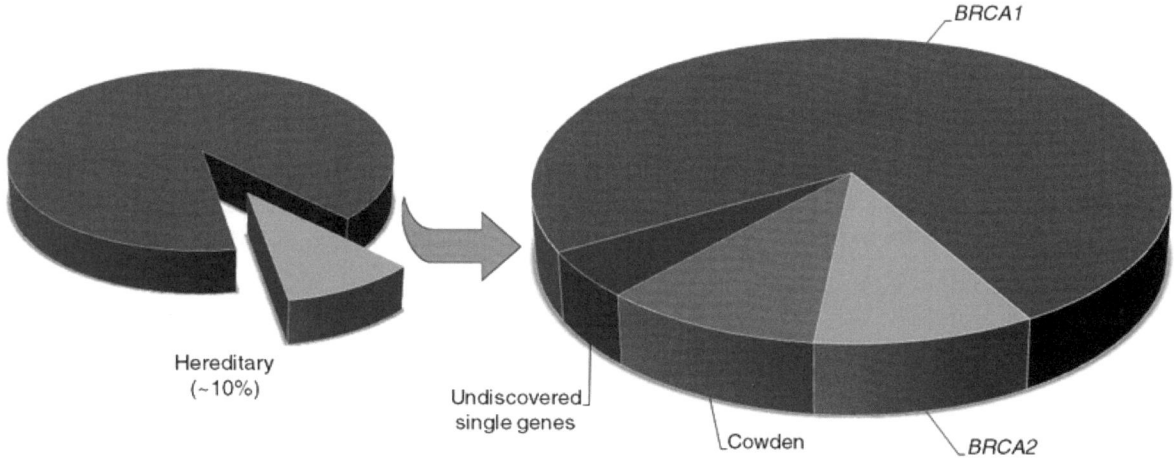

This is a typical pie chart to explain the proportions of various mutations that contribute to hereditary breast cancer.

FIGURE 4-10 RISK LADDER

Family History	Chance of *BRCA* Mutation (%)
Two relatives with breast cancer One relative with ovarian cancer	51.4
One relative with breast cancer One relative with ovarian cancer	39.2
Two relatives with breast cancer	30.1
One relative with breast cancer	15.8
None	6.8

This ladder shows the chance that a woman diagnosed at age 48 with breast cancer who has a family history of breast or ovarian cancer carries a *BRCA* mutation[a]. This is a risk ladder that can be used to help a woman to gauge the significance of her personal risk factors that contribute to breast cancer.

[a] Breast cancer diagnosed before age 50; ovarian cancer diagnosed at any age.

Note. Based on information from the BRCAPRO model.

FIGURE 4-11 USE OF STICK FIGURES

1 out of 8 women ...

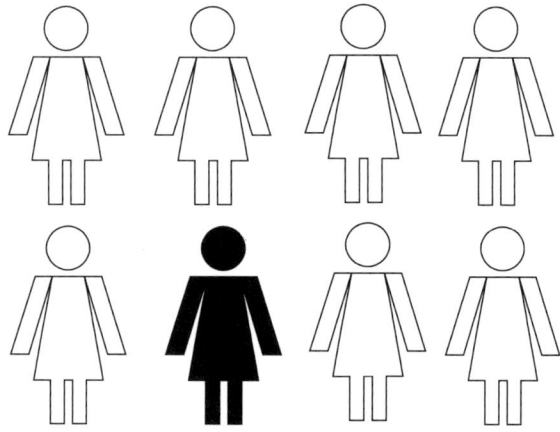

will develop breast cancer if they live to age 85.

This simple use of stick figures may be an effective means in some cases to communicate absolute risk.

FIGURE 4-12 HISTOGRAM

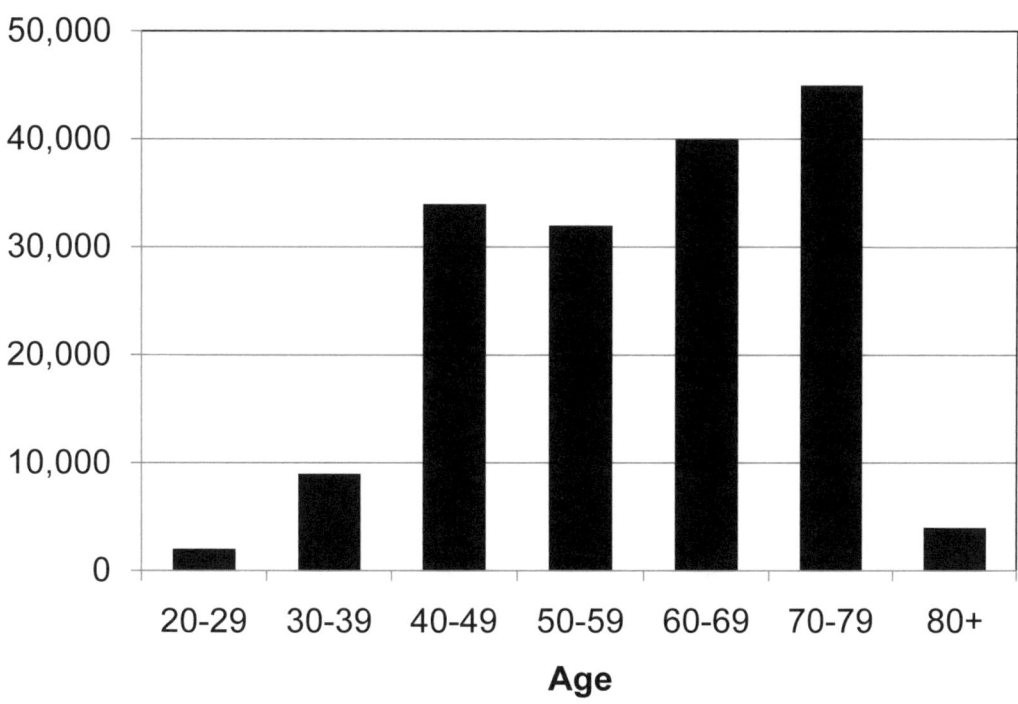

This histogram can effectively communicate breast cancer incidence rates in various age groups.

Psychosocial Issues in Risk Communication

People often have an inaccurate perception of their cancer risk even in families who are aware of their high-risk status (Hopwood, Howell, Lalloo, & Evans, 2003). Misperception of risk may influence cancer screening adherence (Pilarski, 2009). In addition, a client's anxiety can limit his or her ability to comprehend risk information. The qualitative presentation involves discussion of the meaning of the quantitative data and often touches on emotionally charged issues, such as the experience of cancer in close family members. Communication may be more effective if the healthcare professional considers psychosocial concerns that influence perception and comprehension of information. These include (Kausmeyer et al., 2006; Olsen, Dudley-Brown, & McMullen, 2006)
- Empathy (i.e., feeling with the other person and observing the world from the other's point of view)
- Other illnesses and treatments the individual and his or her family may be undergoing

- Personal control (i.e., the perception that a person can control his or her circumstances)
- Trust (i.e., accepting others without evaluating or judging them)
- Self-image and self-esteem
- Self-disclosure (i.e., any message about one's self that is communicated to others)
- Ability to navigate a complex healthcare system.

Socioeconomic and cultural differences affect beliefs about disease. Some cultures and ethnic groups have specific beliefs about cancer and what occurs during a cancer screening. Some groups are more trusting of healthcare professionals than others. These beliefs, whether accurate or not, influence perceptions of cancer risk, willingness to pursue cancer risk assessment, cancer screening, and genetic testing and are considered in risk communication.

Uncertainty also complicates risk communication. No estimate is exact and can predict exactly when or what type of disease will manifest or if a risk-management maneuver will be effective (Edwards et al., 2008). Some individuals are better able to understand and cope with the uncertainty than others. Their perception of this risk may affect choices regarding risk management (Nelson et al., 2008). No screening strategy is completely effective in detecting cancer early. The sensitivity and specificity of risk-management measures are widely variable. Furthermore, many of the risk-management strategies are not based on scientific studies of people with mutations. Often, data are extrapolated from other studies and information. This means that the certainty with which healthcare professionals can make screening recommendations may be limited at best.

Nurses also address the issue of *variable penetrance*, which is the proportion of a population that has a particular genotype or mutation that actually expresses the corresponding phenotype or cancer. In many of the genes associated with hereditary cancer, mutation penetrance is incomplete. Penetrance can change with age and a specific gene mutation and may vary considerably from family to family. Variations in penetrance can be influenced by mutation position, other genes, and factors that modify risk (e.g., diet, hormonal influences, environment). Thus, clients found to have a deleterious gene mutation live with the uncertainty of not knowing when, if at all, cancer will develop.

THE MEDIA'S ROLE IN RISK INFORMATION

Today, many sources provide health-related information to the public: radio, television news, talk shows, commercials, newspapers, magazines, and the Internet. The media often need more than numbers or complex research to make a story. A reporter usually is looking for human interest and an emotional component. Stories seem to have more of an impact if children or celebrities are involved. The subtleties of risk and technical points often are lost in these pieces of the story.

Trends have emerged regarding how the media have covered stories about cancer risk (Russell, 1999). During the 1970s and early 1980s, the focus often was on environmental carcinogens and risks. During the mid-1980s, the focus shifted to individual behaviors and lifestyle risks. With the isolation of the breast cancer susceptibility genes and the widespread use of tumor markers, such as prostate-specific antigen, the focus of news stories changed again in the 1990s. Most recently, the media have looked to stories about risk and genetic testing. Misleading coverage can result in clients requesting a specific test without sufficient background to make an informed choice or with a misunderstanding as to the benefits of the test (Lowery, Byers, Axell, Ku, & Jacobellis, 2008).

Media coverage about cancer risks in general does not address individual concerns about risk or provide sufficient detail to resolve conflicts. Many reports fail to emphasize the uncertainty involved in assessing cancer risk. Providing comprehensive, nonsensationalized information in a minute or less is difficult. Similarly, many reports fail to distinguish between absolute and relative risks. Reports about genetic testing often give little attention to the fact that such gene mutations explain only a small percentage of cases of cancer. When clients present for genetic testing, healthcare professionals should assess their source of background information regarding cancer risk and testing, determine if their perceptions are accurate, and correct misconceptions if needed.

THE LONG-TERM IMPACT OF RISK COMMUNICATION

After risk information has been communicated, the client may have difficulty remembering it. Healthcare professionals can reinforce communication about risk and recommended screening by sending clients a post-visit letter that summarizes important information. More details about counseling letters can be found in Chapter 6.

The data are unclear as to the degree to which healthcare behaviors, including adherence to cancer screening regimens, in at-risk individuals are influenced by psychological distress and whether and how much distress is a hindrance or motivator (Honda, Goodwin, & Neugut, 2005; Sweetman et al., 2006). Helping people to understand their risk accurately and options for risk reduction is still the biggest challenge in risk assessment. What enables one individual or family to understand their risk may be much different for another. For people with higher risk, more than one session may be necessary for them to accurately understand the magnitude of risk.

SUMMARY

As healthcare professionals continue to search for knowledge about minimizing risk and improving cancer treatment, genetics plays a key role. Developments in genetic testing offer a dramatic enhancement to cancer risk prediction and potentially provide a means to offer targeted risk-management strategies to those most likely to benefit from the intervention. A variety of risk models are available to predict not only the risk of developing cancer but also the risk of having a mutation in a gene associated with a specific hereditary cancer syndrome. Each model has its own inherent strengths and weaknesses. Accurate assessment is important in selecting the appropriate genetic test and most informative person to test. Communicating accurate risk information in understandable terms is a mechanism for individuals and families to understand the ramifications of genetic testing and be able to make informed decisions about their care options.

REFERENCES

Aarnio, M., Sankila, R., Pukkala, E., Salovaara, R., Aaltonen, L.A., de la Chapelle, A., et al. (1999). Cancer risk in mutation carriers of DNA-mismatch-repair genes. *International Journal of Cancer, 81*(2), 214–218.

Akobeng, A.K. (2008). Communicating the benefits and harms of treatments. *Archives of Disease in Childhood, 93*(8), 710–713.

American Society of Clinical Oncology. (2003). American Society of Clinical Oncology policy statement update: Genetic testing for cancer susceptibility. *Journal of Clinical Oncology, 21*(12), 2397–2406.

Antoniou, A.C., Pharoah, P.D., Narod, S., Risch, H.A., Eyfjord, J.E., Hopper, J.L., et al. (2005). Breast and ovarian cancer risks to carriers of the *BRCA1* 5382insC and 185delAG and *BRCA2* 6174delT mutations: A combined analysis of 22 population based studies. *Journal of Medical Genetics, 42*(7), 602–603.

Balmaña, J., Stockwell, D.H., Steyerberg, E.W., Stoffel, E.M., Deffenbaugh, A.M., Reid, J.E., et al. (2006). Prediction of *MLH1* and *MSH2* mutations in Lynch syndrome. *JAMA, 296*(12), 1469–1478.

Berry, D.A., Parmigiani, G., Sanchez, J., Schildkraut, J., & Winer, E. (1997). Probability of carrying a mutation of breast-ovarian cancer gene *BRCA1* based on family history. *Journal of the National Cancer Institute, 89*(3), 227–238.

Bradbury, A., & Olufumilayo, O.I. (2006). The case for individualized screening recommendations for breast cancer. *Journal of Clinical Oncology, 24*(21), 3328–3330.

Carey, J.M., & Burgman, M.A. (2008). Linguistic uncertainty in qualitative risk analysis and how to minimize it. *Annals of the New York Academy of Sciences, 1128*, 13–17.

Consensus Panel on Genetic/Genomic Nursing Competencies. (2009). *Essentials of genetic and genomic nursing: Competencies, curricula guidelines, and outcome indicators* (2nd ed.). Silver Spring, MD: American Nurses Association.

Constantin, C.M., Faucett, A., & Lubin, I.M. (2005). A primer on genetic testing. *Journal of Midwifery and Women's Health, 50*(3), 197–204.

Domchek, S., & Antoniou, A. (2007). Cancer risk models: Translating family history into clinical management. *Annals of Internal Medicine, 147*(7), 515–517.

Domchek, S., Eisen, A., Calzone, K., Stopfer, J., Blackwood, A., & Weber, B.L. (2003). Application of breast cancer risk prediction models in clinical practice. *Journal of Clinical Oncology, 21*(4), 593–601.

Edwards, A., Gray, J., Clarke, A., Dundon, J., Elwyn, G., Gaff, C., et al. (2008). Interventions to improve risk communication in clinical genetics: Systematic review. *Patient Education and Counseling, 71*(1), 4–25.

Fagerlin, A., Ubel, P.A., Smith, D.M., & Zikmund-Fisher, B.J. (2007). Making numbers matter: Present and future research in risk communication. *American Journal of Health Behavior, 31*(Suppl. 1), S47–S56.

Fears, T.R., Guerry, D., IV, Pfeiffer, R.M., Sagebiel, R.W., Elder, D.E., Halpern, A., et al. (2006). Identifying individuals at high risk of melanoma: A practical predictor of absolute risk. *Journal of Clinical Oncology, 24*(22), 3590–3596.

Finkel, A.M. (2008). Perceiving others' perceptions of risk: Still a task for Sisyphus. *Annals of the New York Academy of Sciences, 1128*, 121–137.

Frank, T.S., Deffenbaugh, A.M., Reid, J.E., Hulick, M., Ward, B.E., Lingenfelter, B., et al. (2002). Clinical characteristics of individuals with germ line mutations in *BRCA1* and *BRCA2*: Analysis of 10,000 individuals. *Journal of Clinical Oncology, 20*(6), 1480–1490.

Freedman, A.N., Seminara, D., Gail, M.H., Hartge, P., Colditz, G.A., Ballard-Barbash, R., et al. (2005). Cancer risk prediction models: A workshop on development, evaluation, and application. *Journal of the National Cancer Institute, 97*(10), 715–723.

Green, R.C., Green, J.S., Buehler, S.K., Robb, J.D., Daftary, D., Gallinger, S., et al. (2007). Very high incidence of familial colorectal cancer in Newfoundland: A comparison with Ontario and 13 other population-based studies. *Familial Cancer, 6*(1), 53–62.

Grimes, D.A., & Schulz, K.F. (2008). Making sense of odds and odds ratios. *Obstetrics and Gynecology, 111*(2, Pt. 1), 423–426.

Hampel, H., Frankel, W.L., Martin, E., Arnold, M., Khanduja, K., Kuebler, P., et al. (2005). Screening for the Lynch syndrome (hereditary nonpolyposis colorectal cancer). *New England Journal of Medicine, 352*(18), 1851–1860.

Honda, K., Goodwin, R.D., & Neugut, A.I. (2005). The associations between psychological distress and cancer prevention practices. *Cancer Prevention and Detection, 29*(1), 25–36.

Hopwood, P., Howell, A., Lalloo, F., & Evans, G. (2003). Do women understand the odds? Risk perceptions and recall of risk information in women with a family history of breast cancer. *Community Genetics, 6*(4), 214–223.

Hoskins, K.F., Zwaagstra, A., & Ranz, M. (2006). Validation of a tool for identifying women at high risk for hereditary breast cancer in population-based screening. *Cancer, 107*(8), 1769–1776.

Jemal, A., Siegel, R., Ward, E., Hao, Y., Xu, J., Murray, T., et al. (2008). Cancer statistics, 2008. *CA: A Cancer Journal for Clinicians, 58*(2), 71–96.

Jemal, A., Siegel, R., Ward, E., Hao, Y., Xu, J., & Thun, M. (2009). Cancer statistics, 2009. *CA: A Cancer Journal for Clinicians, 59*(4), 224–249.

Jenkins, M.A., Baglietto, L., Dowty, J.G., Van Vliet, C.M., Smith, L., Mead, L.J., et al. (2006). Cancer risks for mismatch repair gene mutation carriers: A population-based early onset case-family study. *Clinical Gastroenterology and Hepatology, 4*(4), 289–298.

John, E.M., Miron, A., Gong, G., Phipps, A.I., Felberg, A., Li, F.P., et al. (2007). Prevalence of pathogenic *BRCA1* mutation carriers in 5 U.S. racial/ethnic groups. *JAMA, 298*(24), 2869–2876.

Katki, H.A. (2007). Incorporating medical interventions into carrier probability estimation for genetic counseling. *BMC Medical Genetics, 8*, Article 13. Retrieved December 10, 2009, from http://www.biomedcentral.com/1471-2350/8/13

Kausmeyer, D.T., Lengerich, E.J., Kluhsman, B.C., Morrone, D., Harper, G.R., & Baker, M.J. (2006). A survey of patients' experiences with the cancer genetic counseling process: Recommendations for cancer genetics programs. *Journal of Genetic Counseling, 15*(6), 409–431.

Klein, W.M., & Stefanek, M.E. (2007). Cancer risk elicitation and communication: Lessons from the psychology of risk perception. *CA: A Cancer Journal for Clinicians, 57*(3), 147–167.

Kristoffersson, U. (2008). Regulatory issues for genetic testing in clinical practice. *Molecular Biotechnology, 40*(1), 113–117.

Lin, K.M., Shashidharan, M., Thorson, A.G., Ternent, C.A., Blatchford, G.J., Christensen, M.A., et al. (1998). Cumulative incidence of colorectal and extracolonic cancers in *MLH1* and *MSH2* mutation carriers of hereditary nonpolyposis colorectal cancer. *Journal of Gastrointestinal Surgery, 2*(1), 67–71.

Lindor, N.M., McMaster, M.L., Lindor, C.J., & Greene, M.H. (2008). Concise handbook of familial cancer susceptibility syndromes—second edition. *Journal of the National Cancer Institute Monographs, 2008*(38), 1–93.

Lipkus, I.M. (2007). Numeric, verbal, and visual formats of conveying health risks: Suggested best practices and future recommendations. *Medical Decision Making, 27*(5), 696–713.

Lowery, J.T., Byers, T., Axell, L., Ku, L., & Jacobellis, J. (2008). The impact of direct-to-consumer marketing of cancer genetic testing on women according to their genetic risk. *Genetics in Medicine, 10*(12), 888–894.

Lynch, H.T., Boland, C.R., Rodriguez-Bigas, M.A., Amos, C., Lynch, J.F., & Lynch, P.M. (2007). Who should be sent for genetic testing in hereditary colorectal cancer syndromes? *Journal of Clinical Oncology, 25*(23), 3524–3542.

Mantelli, M., Barile, M., & Ciotti, P. (2002). High prevalence of the G101W germ line mutation in the CDKN2A (P16(ink4a)) gene in 62 Italian malignant melanoma families. *American Journal of Medical Genetics, 107*(3), 214–221.

Matloff, E.T., Moyer, A., Shannon, K.M., Niendorf, K.B., & Col, N.F. (2006). Healthy women with a family history of breast cancer: Impact of a tailored genetic counseling intervention on risk perception, knowledge, and menopausal therapy decision making. *Journal of Women's Health, 15*(7), 843–856.

National Comprehensive Cancer Network. (2009a). *NCCN Clinical Practice Guidelines in Oncology™: Colorectal cancer screening* [v.1.2009]. Retrieved May 11, 2009, from http://www.nccn.org/professionals/physician_gls/PDF/colorectal_screening.pdf

National Comprehensive Cancer Network (2009b). *NCCN Clinical Practice Guidelines in Oncology™: Genetic/familial high-risk assessment: Breast and ovarian cancer* [v.1.2009]. Retrieved April 23, 2009, from http://www.nccn.org/professionals/physician_gls/PDF/genetics_screening.pdf

Nelson, W., Reyna, V.F., Fagerlin, A., Lipkus, I., & Peters, E. (2008). Clinical implications of numeracy: Theory and practice. *Annals of Behavioral Medicine, 35*(3), 261–274.

O'Doherty, K., & Suthers, G.K. (2007). Risky communication: Pitfalls in counseling about risk, and how to avoid them. *Journal of Genetic Counseling, 16*(4), 409–417.

Olsen, S., Dudley-Brown, S., & McMullen, P. (2006). Case for blending pedigrees, genograms and ecomaps: Nursing's contribution to the "big picture." *Nursing and Health Sciences, 4*(4), 295–308.

Oncology Nursing Society. (2006a). *Cancer predisposition genetic testing and risk assessment counseling* [Position statement]. Retrieved April 4, 2008, from http://www.ons.org/publications/positions/CancerPredisposition.shtml

Oncology Nursing Society. (2006b). *The role of the oncology nurse in cancer genetic counseling* [Position statement]. Retrieved April 4, 2008, from http://www.ons.org/publications/positions/CancerGeneticCounseling.shtml

Parmigiani, G., Berry, D., & Aguilar, O. (1998). Determining carrier probabilities for breast cancer-susceptibility genes *BRCA1* and *BRCA2*. *American Journal of Human Genetics, 62*(1), 145–158.

Parmigiani, G., Chen, S., Iversen, E.S., Friebel, T.M., Finkelstein, D.M., & Anton-Culver, H. (2007). Validity of models in predicting *BRCA1* and *BRCA2* mutations. *Annals of Internal Medicine, 147*(7), 441–450.

Pilarski, R. (2009). Risk perception among women at risk for hereditary breast and ovarian cancer. *Journal of Genetic Counseling, 18*(4), 303–312.

Potter, B.K., Avard, D., Graham, I.D., Entwistle, V.A., Caulfield, T.A., Chakraborty, P., et al. (2008). Guidance for considering ethical, legal, and social issues in health technology assessment: Application to genetic screening. *International Journal on Technology Assessment in Health Care, 24*(2), 412–422.

Ries, L.A.G., Melbert, D., Krapcho, M., Stinchcomb, D.G., Howlader, N., Horner, M.J., et al. (Eds.). (2008). *SEER cancer statistics Review, 1975–2005*. Bethesda, MD: National Cancer Institute. Retrieved April 22, 2009, from http://seer.cancer.gov/csr/1975_2005

Rimer, B.K., Briss, P.A., Zeller, P.K., Chan, E.C., & Woolf, S.H. (2004). Informed decision making: What is its role in cancer screening? *Cancer, 101*(Suppl. 5), 1214–1228.

Risch, H.A., McLaughlin, J.R., Cole, D.E.C., Rosen, B., Bradley, L., Fan, I., et al. (2006). Population *BRCA1* and *BRCA2* mutation frequencies and cancer penetrances: A kin-cohort study in Ontario, Canada. *Journal of the National Cancer Institute, 98*(23), 1694–1706.

Robson, M.E. Storm, C.D., Weitzel, J., Wollins, D.S., Offit, K., & American Society of Clinical Oncology. (2010). American Society of Clinical Oncology policy statement update: Genetic and genomic testing for cancer susceptibility. *Journal of Clinical Oncology, 28*(5), 893–901.

Russell, C. (1999). Living can be hazardous to your health: How the news media cover cancer risks. *Journal of the National Cancer Institute Monographs, 1999*(25), 167–170.

Simard, J., Dumont, M., Moisan, A.M., Gaborieau, V., Malouin, H., Durocher, F., et al. (2007). Evaluation of *BRCA1* and *BRCA2* mutation prevalence, risk prediction models and a multistep testing approach in French-Canadian families with high risk of breast and ovarian cancer. *Journal of Medical Genetics, 44*(2), 107–121.

Stigliano, V., Assisi, D., Cosimelli, M., Palmirotta, R., Giannarelli, D., Mottolese, M., et al. (2008, September 19). Survival of hereditary non-polyposis colorectal cancer patients compared with sporadic colorectal cancer patients. *Journal of Experimental and Clinical Cancer Research, 27,* Article 39. Retrieved September 21, 2009, from http://www.jeccr.com/content/27/1/39

Sweetman, J., Watson, M., Norman, A., Bunstead, Z., Hopwood, P., Melia, J., et al. (2006). Feasibility of familial PSA screening: Psychosocial issues and screening adherence. *British Journal of Cancer, 94*(4), 507–512.

Tai, Y.C., Domchek, S., Parmigiani, G., & Chen, S. (2007). Breast cancer risk among male *BRCA1* and *BRCA2* mutation carriers. *Journal of the National Cancer Institute, 99*(23), 1811–1814.

Tan, D.S., Rothermundt, C., Thomas, K., Bancroft, E., Eeles, R., Shanley, S., et al. (2008). "BRCAness" syndrome in ovarian cancer: A case-control study describing the clinical features and outcome of patients with epithelial ovarian cancer associated with *BRCA1* and *BRCA2* mutations. *Journal of Clinical Oncology, 26*(34), 5530–5536.

Trepanier, A., Ahrens, M., McKinnon, W., Peters, J., Stopfer, J., Grumet, S.C., et al. (2004). Genetic cancer risk assessment and counseling: Recommendations of the National Society of Genetic Counselors. *Journal of Genetic Counseling, 13*(2), 83–114.

Tucker, W., & Ferson, S. (2008). Strategies for risk communication: Evolution, evidence, experience. *Annals of the New York Academy of Sciences, 1128,* ix–xii.

Umar, A., Boland, C.R., Terdiman, J.P., Syngal, S., de la Chapelle, A., Rüschoff, J., et al. (2004). Revised Bethesda Guidelines for hereditary nonpolyposis colorectal cancer (Lynch syndrome) and microsatellite instability. *Journal of the National Cancer Institute, 96*(4), 261–268.

Vasen, H.F., Möslein, G., Alonso, A., Bernstein, I., Bertario, L., Blanco, I., et al. (2007). Guidelines for the clinical management of Lynch syndrome (hereditary non-polyposis cancer). *Journal of Medical Genetics, 44*(6), 353–356.

Watson, P., Ashwathnarayan, R., Lynch, H.T., & Roy, H.K. (2004). Tobacco use and increased colorectal cancer risk in patients with hereditary nonpolyposis colorectal cancer (Lynch syndrome). *Archives of Internal Medicine, 164*(22), 2429–2431.

Weitzel, J.N., Lagos, V., Blazer, K.R., Nelson, R., Ricker, C., Herzog, J., et al. (2005). Prevalence of *BRCA* mutations and founder effect in high-risk Hispanic families. *Cancer Epidemiology, Biomarkers and Prevention, 14*(7), 1666–1671.

Weitzel, J.N., Lagos, V.I., Cullinane, C.A., Gambol, P.J., Culver, J.O., Blazer, K.R., et al. (2007). Limited family structure and *BRCA* gene mutation status in single cases of breast cancer. *JAMA, 297*(23), 2587–2595.

Yoon, P.W., Scheuner, M.T., Peterson-Oehlke, K.L., Gwinn, M., Faucett, A., & Khoury, M.J. (2002). Can family history be used as a tool for public health and preventive medicine? *Genetics in Medicine, 4*(4), 304–310.

Zikmund-Fisher, B.J., Fagerlin, A., Roberts, T.R., Derry, H.A., & Ubel, P.A. (2008). Alternate methods of framing information about medication side effects: Incremental risk versus total risk of occurrence. *Journal of Health Communication, 13*(2), 107–124.

CHAPTER 5

Delivering Genetic Education and Counseling Services

Karen Greco, PhD, RN, MSN, ANP-BC, and Cathleen M. Goetsch, MSN, RN, ARNP, AOCNP®

Professional Responsibilities Domain:
- Advocate for clients' access to desired genetic and genomic services and resources, including support groups
- Advocate for the rights of all clients for autonomous, informed genetic- and genomic-related decision making and voluntary action
- Recognize when one's own attitudes and values related to genetic and genomic science may affect care provided to clients

Professional Practice Domain:
Nursing Assessment: Applying/Integrating Genetic and Genomic Knowledge
- Assess clients' knowledge, perceptions, and responses to genetic and genomic information
- Develop a plan of care that incorporates genetic and genomic assessment information

Identification
- Identify ethical, ethnic and ancestral, cultural, religious, legal, fiscal, and societal issues related to genetic and genomic information and technologies

Provision of Education, Care, and Support
- Provide clients with interpretation of selective genetic and genomic information or services
- Provide clients with credible, accurate, appropriate, and current genetic and genomic information, resources, services, and technologies specific to each client that facilitate decision making

(Consensus Panel on Genetic/Genomic Nursing Competencies, 2009)

INTRODUCTION

Genetic counseling is the process of collecting genetic information and communicating the health implications of that information to a client and his or her family in a supportive environment. Traditionally, genetic counseling is nondirective in that it presents options, not imperatives, and providers take special care to be sensitive to the emotional and psychosocial needs, culture, and healthcare beliefs of the client and his or her family or significant others. The focus is on helping the client and family to understand their potential genetic risk, options for risk reduction and risk management, and other complex issues related to genetic information so that this information may be used effectively in making health-related decisions. Genetic counseling includes interpretation of family history and other health information to assess disease risk, providing education about inheritance patterns, genetic testing, and management options, and helping clients to understand the medical, psychological, and familial implications of genetic and genomic contributions to disease and disease risk (National Society of Genetic Counselors [NSGC], 2009).

Genetic counseling as defined in the *Genetics/Genomics Nursing: Scope and Standards of Practice* (International Society of Nurses in Genetics [ISONG] & American Nurses Association, 2007, p. 56) is

> An exchange of information between genetics healthcare professionals and

clients. The genetics healthcare professional seeks to impartially and completely provide comprehensive information regarding the medical facts of, and expectations for, the course of the disorder and its expected course, mode of inheritance, recurrence risks, and diagnostic and treatment options, to promote adjustment and to support the chosen course of action.

The cancer genetic risk assessment and counseling process includes assessment, determination of risk, communication about the risk, and interpretation of cancer risk information in terminology that clients and families can understand (National Cancer Institute [NCI], 2009a). Education about the basic principles of cancer and cancer genetics and information about relevant inherited cancer risk syndromes is provided. Counseling sessions also address the availability and indication for cancer predisposition genetic testing; the risks and benefits of such testing; cancer screening and risk-reduction options depending on the test results; implications for other family members; and ethical, legal, and psychosocial issues related to cancer risk assessment and the provision of genetic information, including concerns about privacy and discrimination (Offit & Thom, 2007). Nurses who provide genetic education and counseling must understand the importance of ethical issues such as confidentiality, privacy, and informed consent. Accurate, appropriate information assists clients and family members to make informed choices.

THE ROLE OF NURSES IN GENETIC COUNSELING

Cancer genetic counseling continues to be a specialty field with a limited number of trained and experienced providers. Many oncology nurses became involved in cancer genetics through the evolution of cancer risk assessment programs where the primary focus is on identifying nonhereditary cancer risk factors, providing cancer screening recommendations, and discussing risk-reduction options for individuals at average or moderate risk for cancer. Oncology nursing practice has evolved to include cancer genetics (Greco, 2000; Mahon, 2000). Nurses are now members of multidisciplinary teams providing cancer risk education and counseling services.

As part of a multidisciplinary team, RNs are involved in case finding. Clients and families may be in need of cancer genetic services in the context of
- History taking
- Questions asked by clients or their family members
- Comments made by clients or family indicating lack of understanding
- Potential for genetic risk related to their cancer diagnosis or risk
- Information for therapeutic decision making.

Nurses are often in the situation to make these assessments and observations. Clients and family members may feel comfortable sharing concerns or questions with nurses who have more face-to-face time with them than other members of the healthcare team. Individuals with early-onset cancers, more than one cancer, and bilateral disease in paired organs, as well as families with more than three related cancers in close relatives on the same side of the family, and patterns of cancer in families that suggest known inherited cancer risk syndromes raise the suspicion of inherited cancer risk. These individuals or families are candidates for referral for consultation and education regarding potential inherited risk assessment and risk management.

Nurses providing cancer genetic risk assessment, counseling, and education have guidance from professional nursing organizations regarding training and education in cancer genetics. The Oncology Nursing Society (ONS, 2009) has advised that nurses who provide cancer risk education and counseling have advanced education in human genetics and oncology. ISONG recognizes the role of advanced practice and baccalaureate-prepared nurses in genetics. Credentialing for these nurses is offered based on training and experience in genetics (Monsen, 2005). More about the scope of cancer genetics nursing practice can be found Chapter 1, and for information about credentialing, see Chapter 14.

Providing Cancer Genetic Counseling and Education

Several program designs are available for delivering cancer genetic counseling and education services (Trepanier et al., 2004). Service delivery often is based on an institution's service approach and staffing. Establishing a genetic counseling and education program is described in Chapter 6. The provision of counseling and education is inherent in each model. Figure 5-1 describes the fundamental areas of the genetic counseling and education process.

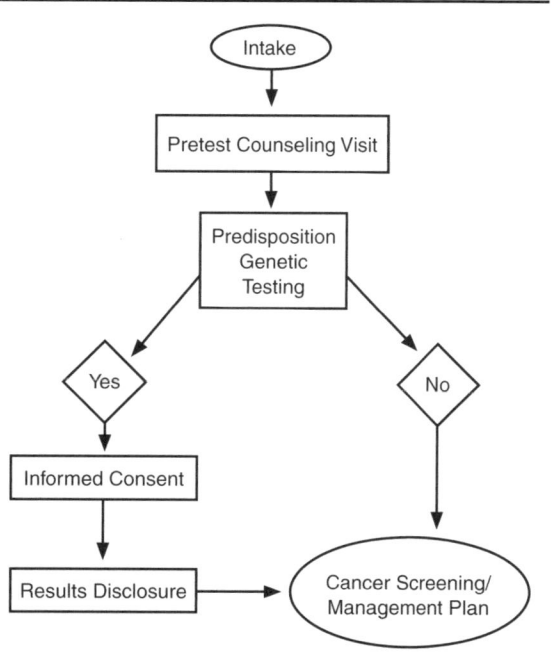

FIGURE 5-1   CANCER GENETIC COUNSELING AND EDUCATION MODEL

Genetic Counseling and Education Delivery Options

A great deal of information is conveyed in cancer risk assessment and genetic counseling visits. Many programs or clinics that provide cancer genetic services give clients information packets in preparation for an initial appointment or to those who inquire about services. The information can help clients to decide if cancer risk assessment and counseling is right for them. By having the client provide answers to initial questions and gather information before the session, the information in the completed packet can save much time during the appointment by reviewing basic information. This leaves more time during the appointment for discussion about the client's specific concerns. These packets may include
- Information on what to expect from the counseling sessions.
- The type of information and services the client can expect to receive.

- A brochure describing the program's or clinic's services.
- Other relevant educational resources related to cancer risk assessment and genetic testing (e.g., brochures, DVDs, Web sites).
- Forms for the collection of personal and family history information that will be needed for the risk assessment.

After the counseling session, providing the client with handouts that summarize and illustrate the session content or a counseling letter that reviews the information discussed is helpful. The client can refer to the materials after the session to reinforce information provided. DVDs and interactive computer programs can be a helpful way of providing genetic information. See Table 5-1 for resources related to cancer genetic counseling.

Motivation for Cancer Genetic Risk Assessment

Many factors can motivate a person to seek cancer genetic services or influence a provider to refer a client for genetic counseling regarding hereditary cancer risk or for cancer predisposition genetic testing. An unaffected person may be concerned about his or her own cancer risk because of a strong family history of cancer or because a family member has been found to carry a mutation associated with a hereditary cancer syndrome. A person diagnosed with cancer may be concerned about his or her potential risk of subsequent cancers or the potential cancer risk in offspring or other relatives. A provider may be searching for a basis for making cancer-screening and risk-reduction recommendations. In studies regarding breast or ovarian cancer, the most common reasons that clients cited for wanting predisposition testing were to learn about their children's cancer risk, to have more cancer screening tests, to take better care of themselves, to feel more reassured, and to make childbearing decisions (Staton, Kurian, Cobb, Mills, & Ford, 2007).

TABLE 5-1   Genetics Education Resources for Individuals and Families

Resource	Description	Web Site
Videos about genetics and the Human Genome Project	Titles include • Banking Our Genes • Gene Blues: Dilemmas of DNA Testing • Deadly Inheritance • The Burden of Knowledge • A Question of Genes: Inherited Risks • Patterns of Inheritance: Understanding Genetics • Heredity and Mutation	www.ornl.gov/sci/techresources/Human_Genome/education/videos.shtml
Printed materials from the National Cancer Institute	Printed educational materials that can be ordered free of charge. Examples include • Genetic Testing for Breast Cancer Risk: It's Your Choice • Understanding Gene Testing	https://cissecure.nci.nih.gov/ncipubs
Online tutorials from the National Cancer Institute	Pamphlets about cancer in both English and Spanish including topics on genetics and genomics	http://newscenter.cancer.gov/sciencebehind

Similar findings have been reported in families with hereditary colon cancer (Hadley et al., 2004, 2008).

Intake Process

During the intake process, the nurse determines what services the client and the referring healthcare provider are requesting and establishes if their expectations are realistic. Nurses who provide cancer genetic counseling and education assess the client's expectations of the process and need to be aware that the referring provider, the client, and the client's family may not have the same expectations. The provider may want to use the inherited cancer risk assessment and genetic test results to make decisions about selection and timing of cancer treatment or risk-reducing surgery. The client, however, may not be ready to deal with the psychological and family issues related to testing, sharing results, or making decisions about risk-reducing surgery. Furthermore, the time in which definitive treatment decisions are needed often is much shorter than the time needed to undergo genetic counseling and testing. The client and healthcare provider who are requesting genetic services are educated regarding what services are available, timelines, and potential outcomes. Detailed information on the intake process, including the collection of family and medical history, is presented in Chapter 3.

Counseling From a Psychosocial Perspective

During the initial counseling session, the nurse who is providing genetic counseling discusses with the client the potential psychosocial implications of receiving information about cancer risk. If predisposition genetic testing is being considered, it also is important to discuss potential emotional responses to receiving genetic test results. Clients who have been diagnosed with cancer often have psychosocial needs different from those who have not. For example, someone recently diagnosed with cancer who is referred for cancer predisposition genetic testing may be coping with multiple issues and may not be ready to undergo testing, which could lead to more psychosocial and family stressors.

Psychological distress can impede the client's ability to receive information. Psychological issues may include fear of cancer or medical procedures, past negative experiences with cancer, unresolved loss and sorrow, feelings of guilt about passing on a mutation to children, anxiety about learning test results, and concern about the effect of the results on other family members. Several studies have shown the hereditary cancer risk counseling process to be beneficial whether testing is done or not and regardless of the test results, including hereditary breast/ovarian cancer syndrome (HBOC), hereditary nonpolyposis colon cancer syndrome (Lynch syndrome), and inherited medullary thyroid cancer (Geirdal et al., 2005; Keatts & Itano, 2006; Keller et al., 2008; Low, Bower, Kwan, & Seldon, 2008; Reichelt, Heimdal, Møller, & Dahl, 2004; Watson et al., 2004). However, it is important for clients to know how to access additional support services, such as those of a psychologist, social worker, or support group. Discussing with the client the importance of support during the counseling and testing process, and offering options such as bringing a family member or friend with them to the counseling session can be very beneficial. Many of the details of this assessment can be gleaned during the rest of the history collection, including concurrent stressors and usual coping style and methods (see Figure 5-2).

FIGURE 5-2 NURSING CONSIDERATIONS REGARDING THE PSYCHOSOCIAL IMPACT OF GENETIC INFORMATION

1. Assessment of issues prior to testing may enhance receipt of information. Nursing assessment includes the assessment of
   - Current stressors
   - Past cancer experiences and unresolved grief
   - Risk perception and its related impact (e.g., anxiety, symptom monitoring)
   - Past coping strategies and psychiatric history
   - Access to social and professional supports
   - The client's understanding of how genetic information may affect him or her and the family.
2. Estimate of time to have genetic testing results available and support during the time the client and family are waiting for results
3. Assessment of immediate reaction to genetic test results. This includes
   - Identifying and validating feelings
   - Assessing the impact of the results on the client and his or her perception of their impact on family members and significant others
   - Being aware of psychosocial or ethical issues that may arise regarding third-party notification.
4. Knowing when and where to refer individuals for psychological counseling
5. Post-test counseling follow-up to assess the long-term impact of test results and to establish a plan to maintain contact for updating risk and risk management

---

ELEMENTS OF CANCER RISK ASSESSMENT, EDUCATION, AND COUNSELING

The Concept of Risk

This section will present a brief overview of issues that are typical of and unique to genetic counseling, especially pertaining to cancer risk. Determination of risk is discussed in greater detail in Chapter 4. The concept of risk is relevant to the communication of the level of risk and education regarding risk management choices including genetic testing, if appropriate.

Assessing Perception of Risk

Nurses assess the clients' perception of their own cancer risk, especially for the cancer or cancers present in their family or for their risk for recurrence of a cancer for which they have been diagnosed. How clients perceive their cancer risk often seems to depend more on their emotional responses and experiences than the actual numeric risk (Bjorvatn et al., 2007; Schneider, 2002). Genetic counseling has been shown to help women to develop more accurate views of their personal breast cancer risk and to worry less about developing breast cancer (Matloff, Moyer, Shannon, Niendorf, & Col, 2006). Similarly, individuals at risk for hereditary breast or colon cancer who received genetic counseling had lower anxiety, decreased overestimation of cancer risk, increased knowledge, and a more positive view of participating in cancer screening and risk reduction (Pieterse, Ausems, Van Dulmen, Beemer, & Bensing, 2005; van Asperen et al., 2004).

Education and Counseling About Cancer Risk

During genetic counseling, clients usually are presented with estimates of their risk for developing specific types of cancer and the likelihood that they have a genetic mutation associated with cancer risk (Trepanier et al., 2004; U.S. Preventive Services Task Force [USPSTF], 2005). Clients may think that genetic testing can provide a concrete explanation of why cancer has occurred in their families and perceive genetic testing as a diagnostic tool that will give a clear answer about whether a person will or will not develop cancer. Similarly, healthcare providers often want to use genetic information to make decisions about the treatment of cancer or precancerous conditions without understanding the uncertainties associated with genetic assessment and cancer predisposition testing. In the majority of cases, even when family and personal history are indicative of inherited cancer risk, current genetic testing may not provide definitive information. A positive cancer predisposition test does not mean a person absolutely will develop cancer; a negative cancer predisposition test does not mean a person is free from cancer risk. Communicating the uncertainty associated with genetic testing is an essential part of the genetic counseling and education process. Remember that the majority of cancer risk assessments are not likely to indicate a potential hereditary cancer syndrome. Communicating risk information to patients in a way that facilitates patient understanding and addressing the psychological issues related to the communication of cancer risk information are essential components of cancer risk assessment (Greco & Mahon, 2004).

ISSUES RELATED TO CANCER GENETIC TESTING

Indications for Testing

More than 50 hereditary cancer syndromes are described, many for which cancer susceptibility genetic testing is currently available. The second edition of the *Concise Handbook of Familial Cancer Syndromes* describes 54 syndromes, many of which have testing available (Lindor, McMaster, Lindor, & Greene, 2008). Several sets of clinical guidelines are available to assist clinicians in determining who is appropriate to undergo cancer genetic testing based on the information gathered in the cancer risk assessment. More information also is available at the GeneTests Web site and NCI's Web site (see resources in Chapter 16). Refer to Chapters 3 and 4 for an overview of this information. A few commonly used professional guidelines are presented here. The American Society of Clinical Oncology (ASCO, 2003; Robson et al., 2010) recommends that cancer genetic testing be offered when

> 1) the individual has personal or family history features suggestive of a genetic cancer susceptibility condition, 2) the test can be adequately interpreted, and 3) the results will aid in diagnosis or influence the medical or surgical management of the patient or family members at hereditary risk of cancer. (ASCO, 2003, p. 2397)

For some hereditary cancer syndromes, offering referral for hereditary cancer risk assessment and genetic testing, if appropriate, already is considered standard of practice. HBOC

(*BRCA1* and *BRCA2* genes), Lynch syndrome (*MSH2, MLH1, MLH6,* and *PMS2* genes), and familial adenomatous polyposis (FAP) (*APC* and *MYH* genes) are examples (Daly, 2005; Eng, Hample, & de la Chapell, 2000). These are the cases that oncology nurses are most likely to encounter and indicate a referral for genetic counseling and testing. Commercial testing is available for less common hereditary cancer syndromes (Greco & Mahon, 2004). For more information about the availability of genetic tests and to search a laboratory directory, visit www.genetests.org.

The National Comprehensive Cancer Network (NCCN, 2009a, 2009b) has useful algorithms for screening and managing risk for breast/ovarian and colorectal inherited risk syndromes. USPSTF (2005) referral criteria for women at risk for HBOC can be found at www.ahrq.gov/clinic/uspstf05/brcagen/brcagenrs.htm#clinical. These guidelines recommend that testing for *BRCA1* and *BRCA2* be limited to adults older than 18 years.

Not all individuals who meet criteria for medical necessity for predisposing testing will pursue testing as an option. Many reasons for refusing or avoiding testing exist. Healthcare professionals should explore these barriers with the patient and review options for managing them (see Figure 5-3).

FIGURE 5-3   BARRIERS TO CANCER GENETIC TESTING

- Lack of knowledge regarding the availability or applicability of testing
- High cost of tests
- Worries about insurance issues
- Lack of referral or request for consult by the managing healthcare provider
- Waiting for results may delay definitive cancer treatment
- Perception that confirming that risk exists somehow makes the disease occur
- Perception that confirming that risk exists somehow makes the diagnosis of disease a real possibility
- Belief that whatever happens is supposed to happen
- Fear that no risk-reduction methods exist or are effective
- Limited availability of genetic counseling resources
- Ambivalence about learning risk status
- Guilt regarding being the transmitter of harmful genetic qualities
- Social, economic, educational, racial, and ethnic factors
- Confidentiality concerns
- Fear of blood draw, screening, and other medical procedures

Note. Based on information from Brandt et al., 2008; Halbert, 2006; Rose et al., 2005; Schlich-Bakker et al., 2007.

INFORMED DECISION MAKING RELATED TO CANCER GENETIC TESTING

Deciding Whether to Undergo Testing

When deciding whether to pursue cancer predisposition testing, clients and family members have to weigh the options, risks, benefits, and limitations in light of each person's unique situation. The decision is a very personal one, and the issues are different for each individual. Not everyone who has a personal or family history that increases the risk of carrying a germ line gene mutation wants to know his or her genetic status. For some, however, the uncertainty of not knowing their genetic mutation status may cause anxiety that limits their ability to effectively proceed with screening, risk reduction, and treatment decisions. Motivations for genetic testing may include learning if offspring are at an increased risk and finding out if additional screening is needed (Esplen et al., 2007).

As has been well documented in other areas of health care, individuals from disadvantaged socioeconomic groups, from minority racial or ethnic populations, or with limited education have less access to services, are less likely to be referred for counseling or have testing, and are more likely to have increased anxiety related to implications of results (Armstrong, Micco, Carney, Stopfer, & Putt, 2005; Halbert et al., 2005; Halbert, Kessler, Stopfer, Domchek, & Wileyto, 2006; Mellon, Berry-Bobovski, Gold, Levin, & Tainsky, 2006; Nanda et al., 2005). The availability of predictive genetic testing often is dependent on ethnic background, geographical location, or ability to pay. Therefore, nurses have to consider reimbursement concerns as affecting clients' decision making about genetic testing.

Emotional Responses to Cancer Genetic Testing

Nurses can assist clients to become aware of their personal perceptions, health beliefs, psychological status, and personality characteristics that may influence their decision making and response to genetic testing, for example, considering how test results may affect the client. Individuals who undergo genetic testing may experience various reactions, such as relief, guilt, loss, or distress whether or not they are found to carry a cancer-predisposing genetic mutation. Early studies showed that women found to carry a *BRCA1* mutation had higher levels of post-test psychological distress than did women who tested negative, with the highest levels of test-related distress among mutation carriers with no personal history of cancer or cancer-related surgery (Croyle, Smith, Botkin, Baty, & Nash, 1997; Lerman et al., 1996). Later research found that women who underwent cancer-related genetic counseling had no increased anxiety and better attitudes toward screening (Braithwaite, Emery, Walter, Prevost, & Sutton, 2004; Broadstock, Michie, & Marteau, 2000). Similarly, a study of participants undergoing Lynch syndrome genetic testing found that participants affected with cancer did not have increased anxiety or distress regardless of mutation status. Unaffected carriers, however, experienced short-term increases in depression, anxiety, and cancer worry (Gritz et al., 2005). Clients have to be aware that emotional reactions are expected and most often short term.

Clients receiving cancer genetic services often have lost loved ones to cancer or may have had cancer themselves. Many families have survived multiple losses or had multiple family members diagnosed with cancer, and each of these experiences has left an emotional imprint. Nurses may be able to provide counseling and support, but all nurses have the responsibility to recognize the potential for distress and to be prepared to refer clients for appropriate support services. The words of one client, a woman whose parents were diagnosed with breast cancer and who herself had a genetic predisposition to the disease, described how her experience molded her attitude and outlook:

> The agony of watching my mother die from breast cancer is like a pencil mark [on] a piece of paper: It made an emotional imprint that can never be erased, and it caused me to view breast cancer as a disease that can never be survived. (Prouser, 2000, p. 153)

Family Issues

Genetic information is unique in that it has implications for family members as well as for the individual undergoing genetic testing. Healthcare professionals have a responsibility to inform clients prior to testing that if they test positive for a cancer-predisposing gene mutation, family members related by blood may carry the same mutation. Where appropriate, encourage the client to contact family members and recommend that they receive genetic counseling and applicable healthcare services. Questions from family members about their own cancer risk and healthcare issues will arise, especially if family members attend genetic counseling sessions with the client. Addressing these questions can be challenging. Advising a separate counseling session for the family member may best address each person's needs. Other issues, such as the testing of minors, if relevant, and the timing for the disclosure of genetic information to family members, are discussed. Some clients feel a sense of responsibility to have testing for their children. Others are concerned about confidentiality and privacy issues. Some feel guilt about having possibly passed on a mutation.

Disclosing Results to Family Members

Clients often choose which family members to tell about their test results, and some have distress with sharing their test results (Wagner et al., 2005). Clear communication with the client regarding the impact of informative test results for other family members helps to facilitate a plan prior to testing for sharing this information (Doukas, 2003). Genetic providers can assist individuals to consider the concerns of both themselves and their families using the family covenant as a helpful way to address boundaries of privacy and information sharing within the family. The family covenant helps genetic providers consider what information should be confidential and with respect to whom. Doukas recommends discussing with clients the boundaries of confidentiality, their definition of family, and how they want to share their genetic test results. Clients may be concerned that sharing their test results could be emotionally upsetting to family members or adversely affect family relationships. Discussing these issues prior to genetic testing and helping the client to develop a disclosure plan can alleviate anxiety.

In certain situations, healthcare providers have a duty to inform a family member that a potential health risk to other family members may be present. Institutions can consider policies regarding informing family members that they could be at risk for a hereditary condition or disease, if effective screening and risk-reduction measures are available, and if evidence is clear that withholding such information could result in harm to the family member (Leung, Mariman, van der Wouden, van Amergongen, & Weijer, 2000). Four states' case laws apply to "duty to warn" and identify the conflict between ethical obligations to respect the privacy of genetic information versus the potential liabilities resulting from failure to notify at-risk relatives (NCI, 2009a; Offit, Groeger, Turner, Wadsworth, & Weiser, 2004).

Disclosing or not disclosing genetic results to children has the potential for causing negative sequelae. When test results are shared without adequate preparation, potential consequences include lowered self-esteem, inability to integrate with peers, parent-child bonding issues, and stigmatization. When results are not disclosed to children, a climate of secrecy can develop or parents may act in an overprotective manner (Tercyak, Peshkin, DeMarco, Brogan, & Lerman, 2002). Parents can benefit from discussion about sharing test results with their adolescent or young adult children with preparation regarding age-appropriate information about the results. Balancing the test results with information about the available risk-reduction options fosters better adaptation for children and their future health behaviors (Bradbury et al., 2009). The child's cognitive stage and emotional maturity are considered in all aspects of the genetic testing process.

Testing Minors

In general, testing a minor for a specific hereditary disorder or syndrome is discouraged unless testing would result in a clear medical benefit to the child. For example, if someone in the family has tested positive for a mutation in the *APC* gene, associated with FAP, testing children as young as 10 years old is reasonable because if a mutation is found, annual colon screening begins at age 10–15 (NCCN, 2009a). Another example relates to multiple endocrine neoplasia type 2. When this condition is suspected, testing for a mutation in the *RET* gene is recommended because the risk of medullary thyroid cancer is very high, and prophylactic thyroidectomy often is done in childhood (Kouvaraki et al., 2005; Wiesner & Snow-Bailey, 2005). In other cases, if test results would not benefit a child, they could harm the child if they trigger stigmatization by parents, siblings, or others. Children also may be too young to understand the significance of genetic information (Dickens, Pei, & Taylor, 1996).

A review of five policy, guidelines, or position statements regarding genetic testing of children for adult-onset conditions from the United States, the United Kingdom, and Canada concluded that all the statements were in favor of genetic carrier testing when the results could provide beneficial medical interventions such as monitoring or where the use of screening would be deemed necessary or reduced. The papers cautioned against predictive testing for adult-onset conditions where the conclusions from the testing do not affect the use of resources (i.e., medical intervention). In these cases, genetic testing is best deferred until adulthood (Hogben & Boddington, 2005). The ASCO statement on genetic testing for cancer susceptibility maintains that the decision to offer childhood genetic testing should consider not only the risk of childhood malignancy but also the evidence associated with screening and risk-reduction interventions for that disorder (ASCO, 2003; Robson et al., 2010). However, researchers advocate for a reevaluation of current genetic testing practices now in preparation for future benefit (Haga & Terry, 2009).

Testing Vulnerable Populations

Genetic education, counseling, and testing involve special considerations when used in vulnerable populations. Potentially vulnerable populations include children, prisoners, traumatized and comatose patients, terminally ill patients, older people who are cognitively impaired or institutionalized, minorities, students, employees, and individuals from outside the United States (U.S. Department of Health and Human Services [DHHS] Protection of Human Subjects, 2005). The delineation of what constitutes a vulnerable population can be broadened to include multiple individuals and groups depending on their personal and social circumstances, and thus each client is assessed for vulnerability to determine when special actions are necessary to facilitate informed decision making (ISONG, 2002). This assessment guides the determination of whether another legally authorized representative needs to be involved in the counseling, informed consent, and testing process. Nurses can advocate for those vulnerable clients who need enhanced interventions to facilitate informed decisions.

PREPARING FOR GENETIC TESTING

Informed Consent

Facilitating informed consent for cancer predisposition genetic testing means providing enough information about the risks, benefits, limitations, and alternatives associated with predisposition testing for both clients and family members to enable the client to decide whether to proceed. Alternatives to genetic testing, such as DNA banking and increased screening, also are discussed. Clients are provided with sufficient information to understand the limitations of testing, the interpretation of results, and what each potential result might mean. Discussion also includes psychosocial implications and the potential for insurance risk or employment discrimination. Clients are provided with information on how their genetic information will be kept confidential and that additional testing will not be performed without informed consent. They also are made aware of their options for medical follow-up (Greco & Mahon, 2004).

The process of obtaining informed consent includes discussion of the following (Trepanier et al., 2004).

- Purpose of the test and who is the most informative person to test
- General information about the gene or genes involved in the test
- Possible test results
- Accuracy of the test
- Alternatives to genetic testing
- Process for testing (e.g., the amount of blood to be drawn)
- Cost of testing
- Risks of genetic discrimination
- Psychosocial implications of testing
- Limitations of testing
- Confidentiality of test results
- Time for results to become available and how results will be communicated
- Use of test results, including medical screening and risk-reduction measures

When cancer predisposition testing is involved, the provider documents in the medical record all components of the informed consent process that were covered. Such documentation lists the specific content discussed, including an evaluation of the client's understanding of the issues, and accompanied by appropriately signed consent forms. Include family history documentation. Record whether the client was asked about additional information needs. Include any information the client may have requested and whether he or she received it. Document that the client received a copy of the signed consent form that outlines potential risks, benefits, and limitations of genetic testing.

Economic Considerations

Many insurance companies now cover predisposition testing for cancer if criteria of medical necessity are met. Insurance eligibility criteria vary according to insurance company and policy-specific requirements of medical necessity. Cancer predisposition genetic testing can be expensive and whether the client's insurance will cover the test is a major consideration for clients who are contemplating testing. Commercial laboratories that perform the tests also may be sources of current insurance guideline information for determining individual client eligibility. Most major insurers have policy guidelines with criteria for medical necessity for cancer genetic testing available on their Web sites. These usually are reviewed and updated regularly.

Many insurance companies require preauthorization for genetic counseling and testing. This involves informing the insurance company why services are needed and including certain medical information about the cancer history of the client and his or her family. Many insurers will ask for a letter of medical necessity prior to approval. These letters are concise, include the rationale for the specific genetic test and the syndrome diagnosis, and contain only the information about the client and family history that the insurer needs to make a coverage decision. Strip pedigrees of all labels that identify family members other than the insured individual. Include or offer as an addendum information from the scientific literature regarding the justification for testing and provide references. See Shappell and Matloff (2001) and Bombard (2002) for examples of letters of medical necessity. Request the client's permission to submit this letter, as he or she may elect to self-pay and not inform the insurance company.

Discrimination and Confidentiality Concerns

Several federal laws regulate and limit the potential for discrimination based on genetic information. The most recent federal regulatory protections are provided by the Genetic Information Nondiscrimination Act (GINA) of 2008, which currently defines genetic information as genetic tests (e.g., individuals, family member, fetus, embryo), family history, and any request for, or receipt of, genetic services or participation in clinical research that includes genetic services (DHHS Office for Human Research Protections, 2009). GINA is aimed at protecting people from discrimination by health insurers and employers on the basis of genetic information (National Human Genome Research Institute [NHGRI], 2008a). The final regulation took effect May 2009 for health insurers and November 2009 for employers. For more information, see Chapter 11.

Other protective regulations besides GINA include both federal and state laws such as the Health Insurance Portability and Accountability Act (HIPAA) of 1996 (DHHS, 2006). HIPAA regulations apply only to health insurance and do not address disability, long-term care, or life insurance. State laws regulate the use of genetic information and are intended to help protect the confidentiality of genetic information and to prevent insurance and workplace discrimination and may provide additional protections beyond those provided by federal laws. A searchable database for state laws can be found on the NHGRI Web site (2008b). See Chapter 11 for more information.

Clients may be concerned about undergoing testing or releasing the results of genetic tests to their insurance companies, fearing that the result will be health insurance cancellation or an insurance rate increase. They also may believe that if the insurance company pays for a genetic test, the company will have access to the test results. If a client applies to the insurance company for genetic testing reimbursement, the insurance company will know that the client underwent genetic testing and that he or she met eligibility criteria. HIPAA permits disclosure of protected health information to a covered entity, including health insurance companies, health maintenance organizations, company health plans, and government health plans, such as Medicare, Medicaid, the military, and Veterans Administration, for the purposes of payment without the individual's authorization (Uses and Disclosures for Treatment, Payment, and Health Care Operations, 2003). If a client subsequently applies for risk-reducing surgery or screening tests based on genetic test results, the insurance company may require the client to document necessity before pay is issued for these procedures. Clients should be informed of what state and federal protections exist, the limitations of those protections, and potential insurance discrimination issues.

Performing the Test

The genetic professional ordering the test will provide the client with details about the type of sample needed and a brief description of the collection process, as well as any associated risks. Usually, the test involves either a blood sample or a swab of the inside of the cheek. The provider also will explain the approximate timetable for processing the sample and when the results are expected, as well as how the client will be notified with the outcome and if the laboratory will make contact during the waiting period. The genetic professional also will provide the client with contact information and resources if questions or concerns arise while the test is being processed.

If the client is sent to a local laboratory to have a blood specimen drawn, the clinician will explain that the laboratory may charge an additional phlebotomy fee that may or may not be covered by the insurance company. Some outside laboratories that conduct genetic testing provide testing kits with packaging materials and a postage-paid envelope for mailing the specimen to the testing facility. The client can take these materials to a local laboratory for specimen collection. This laboratory, however, may charge a processing fee for packaging and mailing the specimen.

PRETEST EDUCATION REGARDING POTENTIAL TEST RESULTS

Before an individual is tested, he or she is educated regarding potential test outcomes, including both the medical and psychological implications of potential test results. The results of predisposition genetic tests generally fall into four major categories: **true positive** or deleterious, **true negative** or negative for a known mutation in the family, uninformative, and variant of uncertain significance (see Figure 5-4).

True Positive or Deleterious Result

A true positive occurs when a mutation known to be associated with increased cancer risk or altered gene function is found. A true-positive predisposition genetic test result in an unaffected client does not necessarily mean that the client has or will get cancer. Clients may have various reactions to a positive test (Esplen et al., 2004). Clients may feel shock, disbelief, or anger, causing feelings of anxiety, depression, or hopelessness. Others may feel relieved that the explanation for their personal or familial cancers has been found.

Clients may have concerns about telling family members their test results and may worry about family reactions. If other family members also have been tested, dissimilar results may

FIGURE 5-4. TEST RESULTS

Positive or Deleterious
- It is most informative to first test a family member who has the disease.
- If that person is found to have an altered gene (positive), the specific change is referred to as a "known mutation" or deleterious.
- Other family members can then be tested to see if they also carry that specific alteration.
- A positive test result indicates that a person has inherited a known deleterious mutation and has an increased risk of developing certain cancers.
- A positive result does not indicate whether cancer will actually develop or when, only that the risk is increased.

True Negative or Negative for a Known Mutation in the Family
- If someone in a family has a known mutation, testing other family members for that specific gene alteration can provide information about their cancer risk.
- If a family member tests negative for the known mutation in that family, he or she has not inherited the susceptibility to cancer coming from that branch of the family. This test result is called a *true negative*.
- Having a true-negative test result does not mean that a person will not get cancer; it means that the person's risk of cancer is not increased because of the cancer family history in that branch of the family. However, other cancer risk factors, including a family history on the other side of the family, still influence risk.

Uninformative
- In cases where no known mutation previously has been identified in a family with a history of cancer, a negative test is not informative.
- The person may have an alteration that was not identified by the test (a false negative).
- An alteration in another gene that increases the person's cancer risk may be present, but testing was not performed on that gene and therefore is not detectable by this test.

Ambiguous or Variant of Uncertain Significance
- If the test shows a change in a gene that has not been associated with cancer in other people, that result may be interpreted as ambiguous or uncertain.
- Everyone has genetic alterations. Many do not increase the risk of disease, so sometimes whether a specific change affects a person's risk of developing cancer is unknown.
- More research is needed to determine implications of these genetic alterations and cancer risk.

Note. Based on information from National Cancer Institute, 2009b.

affect family relationships. Individuals may feel isolated from those who do not understand the feelings associated with learning one's genetic status. A parent feeling guilty about the possibility of having passed a mutation to a child is common. Additional areas of concern include worry over possible insurance or workplace discrimination, concern over potential increased healthcare costs associated with screening and risk-reduction interventions, and uncertainty about unproven risk-management options. These issues can cause additional stress on relationships with family members who may already be dealing with multiple losses.

People with inherited predisposition to cancer are concerned not only regarding their own positive results, but also about the process and effects of disclosing the information to their families (Hamilton, Bowers, & Williams, 2005). Most cancer survivors anticipate disclosing test results to relatives and physicians (Esplen et al., 2007). In a study of 16 families with Lynch syndrome, most indicated that all family members should know about the presence of a mutation in the family, with family members themselves being the preferable informants (Pentz et al., 2005).

Some individuals report that they expected to have a positive result and experience relief when they receive test results because the reason for excessive cancer in their families and early ages at onset has been found. As a result of the new information, individuals can make healthcare decisions about increased screening, chemoprevention, or risk-reducing surgery. The ability to take these potentially lifesaving actions may provide a sense of empowerment. Potentially, this ability to affect their own health course can reduce feelings of uncertainty and anxiety. A positive result also may help to solidify family relationships and increase support for those who test positive. Identifying cancer and mutation carrier risk for other family members can unify the family in a common cause.

True-Negative Result or Negative for a Known Mutation in the Family

A true-negative result occurs when a close blood relative of the client has a known cancer predisposition mutation, and the client tests negative for the same mutation. A more accurate description of cancer risk can be made because the true-negative result suggests that the client's risk is the same as that of the general population when he or she has no other family history and no other risk factors. Individuals receiving true-negative results often are relieved. Their level of anxiety and cancer worry decreases. In most cases, people who receive a true-negative result can return to the screening levels recommended for the general population unless they have other risk factors. In addition, as a result of testing, these clients have the knowledge that they have not passed the family-specific predisposition mutation to their offspring.

Some clients develop a false sense of security about cancer risk related to the negative test result. Recommended screening and risk-reduction behaviors may decrease. A true-negative result does not mean that the client will not get cancer. He or she will still have the age-related risk for specific cancers. Additionally, a client's cancer risk still may be increased by nongenetic factors such as lifestyle choices or carcinogen exposure, as well as other genes associated with increased cancer risk and genes that were not evaluated in the test. Cases are documented of women who test negative for a known *BRCA* mutation in the family and later develop breast cancer. This is known as a *phenocopy*, which means that the breast cancer in a woman without a mutation mimics the breast cancer in the same family where other women have a *BRCA* mutation. These phenocopy cases in *BRCA1* and *BRCA2* families suggest that familial factors such as environment, hormonal factors, or the effect of modifier genes may be shared (Katki, Gail, & Greene, 2007; Smith et al., 2007). These factors confer an increased cancer risk for a true-negative female. A discussion regarding continued diligence for cancer screening is warranted.

In a few cases, an individual's anxiety and cancer worry may not decrease even with a negative test result. Clients may feel insecure in relinquishing heightened cancer screening. Furthermore, because a mutation is known to be in the family, the negative result may elicit feelings of survivor guilt or alienation as a result of no longer sharing a cancer risk that is similar to that of other family members.

Uninformative or Negative Finding Without a Family-Specific Mutation Known

A negative finding without a known mutation in the family is categorized as indeterminate, uninformative, or inconclusive. This test result, also called negative in the absence of a known mutation, means that genetic predisposition to cancer is neither confirmed nor excluded. Individual or family member risk of initial or subsequent cancers cannot be accurately predicted based on this finding. This result is difficult to interpret and may result from the following.

- No known mutation has been identified in a family member with cancer. This result may be a true negative, but it cannot be confirmed without identifying a harmful mutation in an affected family member.
- If an affected family member has been tested and no mutation is detected, the cancers in the family may be the result of another inherited abnormality or a gene mutation for which testing is not available.

The indeterminate result may leave a client confused, disappointed, and uncertain about the cause of the cancers in his or her family or how to plan for screening and risk-reduction interventions. The client and the family still are considered to have an elevated cancer risk, although the exact level of risk cannot be accurately accessed. Further testing for other inherited factors may become available in the future, which may provide more clarity for the individual and family.

Ambiguous Test Result or Variant of Unknown Significance

A finding of a variant of uncertain clinical significance is a test that shows a novel DNA change or genetic variation whose association with cancer risk is unknown. Whether the finding is in an affected or unaffected family member, the results cannot be interpreted to either exclude or confirm an association with increased cancer risk.

This type of result can occur when a new DNA variation is found but not enough scientific information exists to determine if the variant is associated with an increased cancer risk. Mutations of uncertain clinical significance usually are missense mutations or splice-site mutations in an intron. These mutations may affect messenger RNA splicing. However, at the time of identification, whether the variant causes a significant functional protein change cannot be determined (Schneider, 2002).

A variant of uncertain clinical significance is difficult to explain and understand. The client and family may experience similar feelings to those previously described for individuals with negative results in the setting of a personal or family history of cancer. In some cases, testing laboratories will test other close family members free of charge in an attempt to clarify the meaning of the variant by accumulating more information about whether the variant is present in other individuals affected with disease. Informed consent for such testing is required, and the client and family are counseled that the testing will provide no additional personal health information and may provide no beneficial information for their family in the foreseeable future (ISONG, 2005). A mechanism should be established for following up with clients when further testing is requested and when a result has been reclassified.

RESULTS DISCLOSURE AND POST-TEST COUNSELING

Interpreting Test Results

Disclosing the results of the test is in part a review, because potential outcomes were discussed in the pretest counseling session. One of the most important points for the client to understand is that a positive predisposition genetic test result does not necessarily mean that the client will get cancer. Likewise, a true-negative test result does not mean the client is free from cancer risk. Whether an unaffected client will be diagnosed with cancer or whether an affected client will be diagnosed with a different cancer cannot be predicted. Cancer predisposition genetic testing is undertaken in the hope of identifying modifiable risk to reduce the chance of cancer mortality. Estimation of cancer risk is complicated by ongoing changes occurring as more research information is accumulated.

Predisposition genetic testing is used to help determine the probability that a client may be diagnosed with a certain cancer or cancers in the future, which can be used to guide medical decision making. Correctly estimating the risk of certain cancers is complicated, however, because the cancer risk estimates associated with certain mutations are changing as more information becomes available.

Settings and Methods

Genetic test results usually are disclosed in person at a clinic visit. As mentioned previously, the clinician and the client discuss how test results will be disclosed prior to testing. Clients will sometimes request to have test results disclosed by telephone, which is becoming more common. However, not everyone wants to receive phone results, so assessing an individual's preference or need for in-person genetic test result disclosure is essential (Jenkins et al., 2007). An in-person encounter also might be warranted for clients who require notification of complex results, express high anxiety, or indicate an unclear understanding of difficult concepts.

Nurses should discuss the logistics of a phone disclosure session with clients who choose to receive the information in this manner. The conversation is optimal when it takes place in a private location with minimal distractions and allocation of sufficient time for the session. Encouraging the patient to consider these issues when scheduling a phone appointment is helpful because some settings are less conducive to thoughtful interaction, discussion, and privacy. Cellular phones for results disclosure are discouraged. Providing resources and contact information for future clarification of information or support is important. Research related to results disclosure by telephone is limited; however, this model can be effective, and adverse outcomes have not been demonstrated (DeMarco et al., 2007; Jenkins et al., 2007; Shanley et al., 2007).

Family members sometimes undergo genetic testing together, especially if a cancer-predisposing mutation was found recently in a family member. In this situation, family members may request a group visit for post-test counseling results disclosure. The nurse can prepare the individual and family ahead of time to consider the family dynamics, social environment, and personal implications so that they are aware of the potential ramifications of this approach. One way to address this issue and still maintain confidentiality is to disclose test results to family members individually, and after all family members have received their results, offer them the opportunity to ask questions in a group setting. To maintain confidentiality, two waiting rooms may be necessary, one for family members awaiting results disclosure and another for those who have received their test results.

Ethical Issues

Ethical issues, such as the confidentiality of genetic test results, privacy of genetic information, and informed consent if genetic test results are to be disclosed to a third party, are addressed in counseling sessions. Clients are provided with information to understand how their genetic information will be protected and under what circumstances that information can be released (Burke, Pinsky, & Press, 2001). For a review of these issues, see Chapter 11.

Providing Psychosocial Support as Test Results Are Revealed

Genetic testing is usually a one-time event, but the results of testing can have a lasting impact, especially for people who test positive. Support groups are a typical means of helping people to deal with significant health issues. Because of the confidential nature of predisposition testing, however, gathering people together to help each other to deal with the results of predisposition testing may be infeasible. Even if confidentiality is not a concern, the number of individuals needed for a support group may be available only in large metropolitan areas. Some people have turned to the Internet as a means for finding others for support. For additional resources, visit NHGRI's patient advocacy page (www.genome.gov/27527633). People without a previous cancer diagnosis who test positive may be most in need of some type of follow-up psychological support at the time they receive genetic test results because they may not yet be receiving support services through a cancer program.

Healthcare providers have much to learn about the psychological and psychosocial follow-up needs of clients after predisposition testing. A systematic review of research assessing the impact of predictive genetic testing indicates that most do not experience adverse psychological effects after notification of positive genetic test results (Broadstock et al., 2000). However, for those individuals who had difficulty in dealing with stressful issues in the past, they may experience both short- and long-term increased distress (Gritz et al., 2005; Shiloh, Koehly, Jenkins, Martin, & Hadley, 2008). A lack of informative studies about the types of support required and counseling provided to affect emotional outcomes limits current knowledge (Broadstock et al.). Supporting the client when test results are revealed by offering the client a few minutes to sit quietly and process the information regardless of the test result can be helpful. If genetic test results are disclosed by telephone, offer the client the option to schedule an in-person appointment. All clients need a follow-up plan. During the results disclosure visit, discuss with the client a follow-up plan. Clients also should be offered a follow-up visit or telephone call. Although some clients may think that they can predict how they will respond to receiving genetic test results and what screening and risk-reduction measures they wish to follow, this can change after test results are disclosed.

Group Counseling and Alternatives to In-Person Counseling

Although in-person cancer risk counseling is the preferred method of providing the service, alternatives have been explored to overcome barriers of geography and scarcity of service providers. Some examples include video conferencing and telephone conferencing. Brown, Moglia, and Grumet (2006–2007) discussed alternative forms of providing genetic counseling and techniques for augmenting traditional face-to-face counseling such as telephone counseling. Helmes, Culver, and Bowen (2006) reported that participants counseled by phone or in person had similar outcomes resulting in decreased cancer worry and perception of risk, and the two counseling methods were equally well received. No knowledge or economic measures were included in this study. Similarly, another study (Jenkins et al.,

2007) found that no differences were reported in anxiety and general well-being measures between phone and in-person results disclosure, with both groups reporting satisfaction with services. A measured gain in knowledge persisted throughout the 12-month follow-up period, and knowledge scores were comparable for those receiving phone or in-person test results. However, greater costs in travel and time were associated with in-person results disclosure.

Telephone counseling has limitations in that body language communication cues are lost, one cannot use images to help explain concepts during the conversation, obtaining signed forms is more difficult, and sessions can be time-consuming and often are not billable. Telephone counseling is used more commonly to disclose genetic test results after an in-person visit has occurred (Jenkins et al., 2007).

A few programs now offer genetic services through telemedicine programs in conjunction with telephone counseling. Research related to telephone counseling is limited; however, this model can be effective (Helmes et al., 2006; Shanley et al., 2007). DeMarco et al.'s (2007) review of studies using telephone counseling and telemedicine as a means of expanding the scope of this service and extending its reach to individuals who might otherwise not have access to a risk assessment clinic showed equal benefits and satisfaction compared to traditional methods of delivery.

With limited availability of and increased demand for cancer-related genetic testing, original and innovative educational methods may be considered. Green et al. (2004) compared the effectiveness of a computer-based decision aid with standard genetic counseling, finding both in-person counseling and computer-based counseling to be rated highly by the participants. The interactive computer program was more effective at increasing knowledge of breast cancer genetics among women at low risk of carrying a mutation, but traditional genetic counseling was better at reducing anxiety and facilitating accurate risk perceptions. Green et al. (2005) also reported that the use of the computer-based decision aid before counseling sessions shortened the overall education time associated within the counseling session. This allowed for more time during the counseling session to focus on the individual's personal concerns and issues.

Some programs offer small-group classes, lasting an hour or two, in which an oncology nurse or genetic counselor provides basic information about the genetics of cancer, hereditary and other risk factors, and risk-reduction and surveillance options. For many people, this type of setting allows them to obtain information and ask questions in a nonthreatening environment before deciding if they want to schedule an appointment. In a randomized study of 211 Ashkenazi Jewish women comparing genetic counseling with psychosocial group counseling, both methods reduced breast cancer worry, cancer risk perception, and interest in having genetic testing (Bowen, Burke, Culver, Press, & Crystal, 2006). Additionally, no significant differences were reported in a study of 112 individuals at high risk for having a *BRCA* mutation in knowledge and psychological and satisfaction outcomes when comparing traditional individual pretest counseling to group pretest education followed by brief individual counseling (Calzone et al., 2005). The limitations of group discussion include how to best accommodate individual needs in a group setting, privacy concerns, group influence on decision making, increased frustration at not being eligible for genetic testing, increased need for follow-up, and difficulty booking group appointments (Ridge et al., 2009).

Family group counseling is another model that is sometimes used (Lynch, 2001). Genetic counseling of families can be provided to multiple family members in a group setting if this is agreeable to the family. This model is especially useful when a mutation in the family is known and multiple family members are interested in genetic counseling and genetic testing. In addition to being time efficient, the advantages of this model are that family members all receive the same information, provide support to one another, and help to clarify information for each other. When the family is large, having one family member serve as the organizer of the genetic counseling session is helpful. Usually the family member organizing the session contacts other family members who may want to participate. Each family member who wants to participate in the group counseling session is asked to contact the genetic professional in advance and indicate that he or she wants to attend. When family members are educated together, time needs to be allocated to address the questions and needs of each person. One disadvantage with family group counseling is the potential influence of family dynamics on individual decisions through family coercion. Individual attendees should be informed about this possibility.

CANCER SCREENING, RISK REDUCTION, AND FOLLOW-UP

Current screening and risk-reduction recommendations are based on estimated levels of risk. For individuals with known cancer predisposition mutations, recommendations for risk management are made with the guidance of prior studies and expert opinions (e.g., guidelines for screening and follow-up of individuals with Lynch syndrome mutations [NCCN, 2009a]). For example, evidence supports enhanced breast cancer screening with magnetic resonance imaging in addition to mammogram, and prophylactic mastectomy and oophorectomy as cancer risk-reduction interventions in women with HBOC (Dowdy, Stefanek, & Hartmann, 2004; Olopade & Artioli, 2004; Pavelka, Li, & Karlan, 2007; Rebbeck et al., 2004; Saslow et al., 2007).

NCCN is an excellent source for evidence-based cancer screening guidelines, including algorithms for screening and cancer risk management of high-risk individuals and those with hereditary risk. Another excellent source for current cancer screening guidelines is the National Guideline Clearinghouse (NGC), which is a searchable database of evidence-based clinical practice guidelines. NGC is an initiative of DHHS's Agency for Healthcare Research and Quality. Components of a cancer screening and risk-reduction plan can be found in Figure 5-5. These plans usually include the combination of enhanced screening, chemoprevention, and risk-reducing surgery.

Genetic information generally is released to the primary healthcare provider and to the referring healthcare provider with the client's specific written consent because it is considered necessary for continuity of care, as specifically

FIGURE 5-5 COMPONENTS OF A CANCER SCREENING AND RISK-REDUCTION PLAN

- Recommended interventions and frequency of suggested cancer screening tests
- Recommended frequency of examinations by a healthcare provider
- Potential risks and benefits of potential risk-reduction interventions such as chemoprevention and prophylactic surgery
- Information about lifestyle, dietary, and environmental factors known to increase cancer risk
- Any follow-up recommendations regarding additional clinic visits or referrals to outside programs or healthcare providers

Note. From "Cancer Genetics Nursing Practice: Impact of the Double Helix," by K. Greco, 2000, *Oncology Nursing Forum, 27*(Suppl. 9), pp. 29–33. Copyright 2000 by Oncology Nursing Society. Adapted with permission.

addressed in the HIPAA statutes. If the client asks not to release cancer predisposition test results to a healthcare provider, the need for information exchange to ensure appropriate care is discussed. Optimally, genetic nurses discuss with clients prior to testing whether they intend to release the genetic test results to their healthcare providers and the potential implications of their decision.

SUMMARY

Genetic information regarding cancer predisposition has implications for the entire family, not just the client. The predictive nature of genetic test results may alter individuals' concept of their health, even if they have no history of cancer or evidence of disease. The knowledge that one has a cancer-predisposing mutation can be life changing and have long-term consequences for clients and their families. Health decisions are based on this information, and family relationships can be affected. Cancer predisposition DNA testing does not provide definitive answers but can aid in risk-management decision making. Clients may fear discrimination, so they should be provided with information about the protections available to them. Individuals and families seeking and receiving information about inherited risk should be provided with both recommendations for proceeding onward with health-maintenance activities and support for their unique psychosocial challenges.

Oncology nurses have a pivotal role in caring for clients who have cancer risk–related genetic syndromes. They offer clients and their families information about pertinent research studies. Additionally, nurses are needed to conduct research studies to learn more about the long-term healthcare needs of people with a genetic risk for cancer. Oncology nurses who provide genetic counseling and education have additional training giving them the knowledge and skills to address the complex issues involved in providing genetic education, counseling, predisposition genetic testing, and cancer risk management.

REFERENCES

American Society of Clinical Oncology. (2003). American Society of Clinical Oncology policy statement update: Genetic testing for cancer susceptibility. *Journal of Clinical Oncology, 21*(12), 2397–2406.

Armstrong, K., Micco, E., Carney, A., Stopfer, J., & Putt, M. (2005). Racial differences in the use of *BRCA1/2* testing among women with a family history of breast or ovarian cancer. *JAMA, 293*(14), 1729–1736.

Bjorvatn, C., Eide, G.E., Hanestad, B.R., Øyen, N., Havik, O.E., Carlsson, A., et al. (2007). Risk perception, worry, and satisfaction related to genetic counseling for hereditary cancer. *Journal of Genetic Counseling, 16*(2), 211–212.

Bombard, A. (2002). Insurance justification letters [Letter to the editor]. *Journal of Genetic Counseling, 11*(1), 75.

Bowen, D.J., Burke, W., Culver, J.O., Press, N., & Crystal, S. (2006). Effects of counseling Ashkenazi Jewish women about breast cancer risk. *Cultural Diversity and Ethnic Minority Psychology, 12*(1), 45–56.

Bradbury, A.R., Patrick-Miller, L., Pawlowski, K., Ibe, C.N., Cummings, S.A., Hlubocky, F., et al. (2009). Learning of your parent's *BRCA* mutation during adolescence or early adulthood: A study of offspring experiences. *Psycho-Oncology, 18*(2), 200–208.

Braithwaite, D., Emery, J., Walter, F., Prevost, T., & Sutton, T. (2004). Psychological impact of genetic counseling for familial cancer: A systematic review and meta-analysis. *Journal of the National Cancer Institute, 96*(2), 122–133.

Brandt, R., Ali, Z., Sabel, A., McHugh, T., & Gilman, P. (2008). Cancer genetics evaluation: Barriers to and improvements for referral. *Genetic Testing, 12*(1), 9–12.

Broadstock, M., Michie, S., & Marteau, T. (2000). Psychological consequences of predictive genetic testing: A systematic review. *European Journal of Human Genetics, 8*(10), 731–738.

Brown, K.L., Moglia, D.M., & Grumet, S. (2006–2007). Genetic counseling for breast cancer risk: General concepts, challenging themes and future directions. *Breast Disease, 27,* 69–96.

Burke, W., Pinsky, L.E., & Press, N.A. (2001). Categorizing genetics tests to identify their ethical, legal, and social implications. *American Journal of Medical Genetics, 106*(3), 233–240.

Calzone, K.A., Prindiville, S.A., Jourkiv, O., Jenkins, J., DeCarvalho, M., Wallerstedt, D.B., et al. (2005). Randomized comparison of group versus individual genetic education and counseling for familial breast and/or ovarian cancer. *Journal of Clinical Oncology, 23*(15), 3455–3464.

Consensus Panel on Genetic/Genomic Nursing Competencies. (2009). *Essentials of genetic and genomic nursing: Competencies, curricula guidelines, and outcome indicators* (2nd ed.). Silver Spring, MD: American Nurses Association.

Croyle, R., Smith, K., Botkin, J., Baty, B., & Nash, J. (1997). Psychological responses to *BRCA1* mutation testing: Preliminary findings. *Health Psychology, 16*(1), 63–72.

Daly, P.A. (2005). Genetic counseling in breast and colorectal cancer. *Annals of Oncology, 16*(Suppl. 2), ii163–ii169.

DeMarco, T.A., Smith, K.L., Nusbaum, R.H., Peshkin, B.N., Schwartz, M.D., & Isaacs, C. (2007). Practical aspects of delivering hereditary cancer risk counseling. *Seminars in Oncology, 34*(5), 369–378.

Dickens, B., Pei, N., & Taylor, K. (1996). Legal and ethical issues in genetic testing and counseling for susceptibility to breast, ovarian, and colon cancer. *Canadian Medical Association Journal, 154*(6), 813–818.

Doukas, D. (2003). Genetics providers and the family covenant: Connecting individuals with their families. *Genetic Testing, 7*(4), 315–321.

Dowdy, S.C., Stefanek, M., & Hartmann, L.C. (2004). Surgical risk reduction: Prophylactic salpingo-oophorectomy and prophylactic mastectomy. *American Journal of Obstetrics and Gynecology, 191*(4), 1113–1123.

Eng, C., Hample, H., & de la Chapell, A. (2000). Genetic testing for cancer predisposition. *Annual Review of Medicine, 52,* 371–400.

Esplen, M.J., Hunter, J., Leszcz, M., Warner, E., Narod, S., Metcalfe, K., et al. (2004). A multicenter study of supportive-expressive group therapy for women with *BRCA1/BRCA2* mutations. *Cancer, 101*(10), 2327–2340.

Esplen, M.J., Madlensky, L., Aronson, M., Rothenmund, H., Gallinger, S., Butler, K., et al. (2007). Colorectal cancer survivors undergoing genetic testing for hereditary non-polyposis colorectal cancer: Motivational factors and psychosocial functioning. *Clinical Genetics, 72*(5), 394–401.

Geirdal, A.Ø., Reichelt, J.G., Dahl, A.A., Heimda, L.K., Maehle, L., Stormorken, A., et al. (2005). Psychological distress in women at risk of hereditary breast/ovarian or HNPCC cancers in the absence of demonstrated mutations. *Familial Cancer, 4*(2), 121–126.

Greco, K. (2000). Cancer genetics nursing practice: Impact of the double helix. *Oncology Nursing Forum, 27*(Suppl. 9), 29–36.

Greco, K.E., & Mahon, S. (2004). Common hereditary cancer syndromes. *Seminars in Oncology Nursing, 20*(3), 164–177.

Green, M.J., Peterson, S.K., Baker, M.W., Friedman, L.C., Harper, G.R., Rubinstein, W.S., et al. (2005). Use of an education computer program before genetic counseling for breast cancer susceptibility: Effects on duration and content of counseling sessions. *Genetics in Medicine, 7*(4), 221–229.

Green, M.J., Peterson, S.K., Baker, M.W., Harper, G.R., Friedman, L.C., Rubinstein, W.S., et al. (2004). Effect of a computer-based decision aid on knowledge, perceptions, and intentions about genetic testing for breast cancer susceptibility: A randomized controlled trial. *JAMA, 28*(4), 442–452.

Gritz, E.R., Peterson, S.K., Vernon, S.W., Marani, S.K., Baile, W.F., Watts, B.G., et al. (2005). Psychological impact of genetic testing for hereditary nonpolyposis colorectal cancer. *Journal of Clinical Oncology, 23*(9), 1902–1910.

Hadley, D., Jenkins, J., Dimond, E., DeCarvalho, M., Kirsch, I., & Palmer, C. (2004). Colon cancer screening practices following genetic counseling and testing for hereditary non-polyposis colorectal cancer (HNPCC). *Journal of Clinical Oncology, 22*(1), 40–44.

Hadley, D., Jenkins, J., Steinberg, S., Liewehr, D., Moller, S., Martin, J., et al. (2008). Perceptions of cancer risks and predictors of colon and endometrial cancer screening in women undergoing genetic testing for Lynch syndrome. *Journal of Clinical Oncology, 26*(6), 948–954.

Haga, S., & Terry, S. (2009). Ensuring the safe use of genomic medicine in children. *Clinical Pediatrics, 48*(7), 703–708. Retrieved May 25, 2009, from http://cpj.sagepub.com/cgi/rapidpdf/0009922809335736v1

Halbert, C.H. (2006). Genetic counseling and testing for breast cancer risk in African Americans. *Leonard Davis Institute of Health Economics (LDI) Issue Brief, 12*(1), 1–4.

Halbert, C.H., Brewster, K., Collier, A., Smith, C., Kessler, L., Weathers, B., et al. (2005). Recruiting African American women to participate in hereditary breast cancer research. *Journal of Clinical Oncology, 23*(31), 7967–7973.

Halbert, C.H., Kessler, L., Stopfer, J.E., Domchek, S., & Wileyto, E.P. (2006). Low rates of acceptance of *BRCA1* and *BRCA2* test results among African American women at increased risk for hereditary breast-ovarian cancer. *Genetic Medicine, 8*(9), 576–582.

Hamilton, R.J., Bowers, B.J., & Williams, J.K. (2005). Disclosing genetic test results to family members. *Journal of Nursing Scholarship, 37*(1), 18–24.

Helmes, A.W., Culver, J.O., & Bowen, D.J. (2006). Results of a randomized study of telephone versus in-person breast cancer risk counseling. *Patient Education and Counseling, 64*(1–3), 96–103.

Hogben, S., & Boddington, P. (2005). Policy recommendations for carrier testing and predictive testing in childhood: A distinction that makes a real difference. *Journal of Genetic Counseling, 14*(4), 271–281.

International Society of Nurses in Genetics. (2002). *Position statement: Genetic counseling for vulnerable populations: The role of nursing*. Retrieved May 25, 2009, from http://www.isong.org/about/ps_vulnerable.cfm

International Society of Nurses in Genetics. (2005). *Position statement: Informed decision-making and consent: The role of nursing*. Retrieved May 25, 2009, from http://www.isong.org/about/ps_consent.cfm

International Society of Nurses in Genetics & American Nurses Association. (2007). *Genetics/genomics nursing: Scope and standards of practice*. Washington, DC: American Nurses Association.

Jenkins, J., Calzone, K., Dimond, E., Liewehr, D., Steinberg, S., Jourkiv, O., et al. (2007). Randomized comparison of phone versus in-person *BRCA1/2* predisposition genetic test result disclosure counseling. *Genetics in Medicine, 9*(8), 487–495.

Katki, H.A., Gail, M.H., & Greene, M.H. (2007). Breast-cancer risk in *BRCA*-mutation-negative women from *BRCA*-mutation-positive families. *Lancet Oncology, 8*(12), 1042–1043.

Keatts, E.L., & Itano, J. (2006). Medullary thyroid cancer and the impact of genetic testing. *Clinical Journal of Oncology Nursing, 10*(5), 571–575.

Keller, M., Jost, R., Haunstetter, C.M., Sattel, H., Schroeter, C., Bertsch, U., et al. (2008). Psychosocial outcome following genetic risk counseling for familial colorectal cancer: A comparison of affected patients and family members. *Clinical Genetics, 74*(5), 414–424.

Kouvaraki, M., Shapiro, S., Perrier, N., Cote, G., Gagel, R., Hoff, A., et al. (2005). *RET* proto-oncogene: A review and update of genotype-phenotype correlations in hereditary medullary thyroid cancer and associated endocrine tumors. *Thyroid, 15*(6), 531–544.

Lerman, C., Narod, S., Schulman, K., Hughes, C., Gomez-Caminero, A., Bonney, G., et al. (1996). *BRCA1* testing in families with hereditary breast-ovarian cancer: A prospective study of patient decision making and outcomes. *JAMA, 275*(24), 1885–1892.

Leung, W.C., Mariman, E.C., van der Wouden, J.C., van Amergongen, H., & Weijer, C. (2000). Results of genetic testing: When confidentiality conflicts with a duty to warn relatives. *BMJ, 321*(7274), 1464–1466.

Lindor, N.M., McMaster, M.L., Lindor, C.J., & Greene, M.H. (2008). Concise handbook of familial cancer susceptibility syndromes—second edition. *Journal of the National Cancer Institute Monographs, 2008*(38), 1–93.

Low, C.A., Bower, J.E., Kwan, L., & Seldon, J. (2008). Benefit finding in response to *BRCA1/2* testing. *Annals of Behavioral Medicine, 35*(1), 61–69.

Lynch, H.T. (2001). Family information service and hereditary cancer. *Cancer, 91*(4), 625–628.

Mahon, S.M. (2000). The role of the nurse in developing cancer screening programs. *Oncology Nursing Forum, 27*(Suppl. 9), 19–27.

Matloff, E.T., Moyer, A., Shannon, K.M., Niendorf, K.B., & Col, N.F. (2006). Healthy women with a family history of breast cancer: Impact of a tailored genetic counseling intervention on risk perception, knowledge, and menopausal therapy decision making. *Journal of Women's Health, 15*(7), 843–856.

Mellon, S., Berry-Bobovski, L., Gold, R., Levin, N., & Tainsky, M.A. (2006). Communication and decision making about seeking inherited cancer risk information: Findings from female survivor-relative focus groups. *Psycho-Oncology, 15*(3), 193–208.

Monsen, R.B. (Ed.). (2005). *Genetics nursing portfolios: A new model for credentialing*. Silver Spring, MD: American Nurses Association.

Nanda, R., Schumm, L.P., Cummings, S., Fackenthal, J.D., Sveen, L., Ademuyiwa, F., et al. (2005). Genetic testing in an ethnically diverse cohort of high-risk women: A comparative analysis of *BRCA1* and *BRCA2* mutations in American families of European and African ancestry. *JAMA, 294*(15), 1925–1933.

National Cancer Institute. (2009a). *Cancer genetics risk assessment and counseling (PDQ®)*. Retrieved May 19, 2009, from http://www.cancer.gov/cancertopics/pdq/genetics/risk-assessment-and-counseling/healthprofessional

National Cancer Institute. (2009b). *Genetic testing for BRCA1 and BRCA2: It's your choice*. Retrieved May 19, 2009, from http://www.cancer.gov/cancertopics/factsheet/Risk/BRCA

National Comprehensive Cancer Network. (2009a). *NCCN Clinical Practice Guidelines in Oncology™: Colorectal cancer screening* [v.1.2009]. Retrieved June 3, 2009, from http://www.nccn.org/professionals/physician_gls/f_guidelines.asp

National Comprehensive Cancer Network. (2009b). *NCCN Clinical Practice Guidelines in Oncology™: Genetic/familial high risk assessment: Breast and ovarian*. Retrieved June 3, 2009, from http://www.nccn.org/professionals/physician_gls/PDF/genetics_screening.pdf

National Human Genome Research Institute. (2008a). *Genetic Information Nondiscrimination Act of 2008*. Retrieved May 25, 2009, from http://www.genome.gov/10002328

National Human Genome Research Institute. (2008b). *NHGRI Policy and Legislation Database*. Retrieved May 25, 2009, from http://www.genome.gov/PolicyEthics/LegDatabase/pubsearch.cfm

National Society of Genetic Counselors. (2009). *Genetic counseling as a profession*. Retrieved May 19, 2009, from http://www.nsgc.org/consumer/definition.cfm

Offit, K., Groeger, E., Turner, S., Wadsworth, E., & Weiser, M. (2004). The "duty to warn" a patient's family members about hereditary disease risks. *JAMA, 292*(12), 1469–1473.

Offit, K., & Thom, P. (2007). Ethical and legal aspects of cancer genetic testing. *Seminars in Oncology, 34*(5), 435–443.

Olopade, O., & Artioli, G. (2004). Efficacy of risk-reducing salpingo-oophorectomy in women in *BRCA-1* and *BRCA-2* mutations. *Breast Journal, 10*(Suppl. 1), S5–S9.

Oncology Nursing Society. (2009, March). *Cancer predisposition genetic testing and risk assessment counseling.* Retrieved May 25, 2009, from http://www.ons.org/publications/positions/CancerPredisposition.shtml

Pavelka, J.C., Li, A.J., & Karlan, B.Y. (2007). Hereditary ovarian cancer-assessing risk and prevention strategies. *Obstetrics and Gynecology Clinics of North America, 34*(4), 651–665.

Pentz, R.D., Peterson, S.K., Watts, B., Vernon, S.W., Lynch, P.M., Koehly, L.M., et al. (2005). Hereditary nonpolyposis colorectal cancer family members' perceptions about the duty to inform and health professionals' role in disseminating genetic information. *Genetic Testing, 9*(3), 261–268.

Pieterse, A.H., Ausems, M.G., Van Dulmen, A.M., Beemer, F.A., & Bensing, J.M. (2005). Initial cancer genetic counseling consultation: Change in counselees' cognitions and anxiety and association with addressing their needs and preferences. *American Journal of Medical Genetics Part A, 137*(1), 27–35.

Prouser, N. (2000). Case report: Genetic susceptibility testing for breast and ovarian cancer—a client's perspective. *Journal of Genetic Counseling, 9*(2), 153–159.

Rebbeck, T.R., Friebel, T., Lynch, H.T., Neuhausen, S.L., van't Veer, L., Garber, J.E., et al. (2004). Bilateral prophylactic mastectomy reduces breast cancer risk in *BRCA1* and *BRCA2* mutation carriers: The PROSE Study Group. *Journal of Clinical Oncology, 22*(6), 1055–1062.

Reichelt, J.G., Heimdal, K., Møller, P., & Dahl, A.A. (2004). *BRCA1* testing with definitive results: A prospective study of psychological distress in a large clinic-based sample. *Familial Cancer, 3*(1), 21–28.

Ridge, Y., Panabaker, K., McCullum, M., Portigal-Todd, C., Scott, J., & McGillivray, B. (2009). Evaluation of group genetic counseling for hereditary breast and ovarian cancer. *Journal of Genetic Counseling, 18*(1), 87–100.

Robson, M.E. Storm, C.D., Weitzel, J., Wollins, D.S., Offit, K., & American Society of Clinical Oncology. (2010). American Society of Clinical Oncology policy statement update: Genetic and genomic testing for cancer susceptibility. *Journal of Clinical Oncology, 28*(5), 893–901.

Rose, A.L., Peters, N., Shea, J.A., & Armstrong, K. (2005). Attitudes and misconceptions about predictive genetic testing for cancer risk. *Community Genetics, 8*(3), 145–151.

Saslow, D., Boetes, C., Burke, W., Harms, S., Leach, M.O., Lehman, C.D., et al. (2007). American Cancer Society guidelines for breast screening with MRI as an adjunct to mammography. *CA: A Cancer Journal for Clinicians, 57*(2), 75–89.

Schlich-Bakker, K.J., ten Kroode, H.F., Wárlám-Rodenhuis, C.C., van den Bout, J., & Ausems, M.G. (2007). Barriers to participating in genetic counseling and *BRCA* testing during primary treatment for breast cancer. *Genetic Medicine, 9*(11), 766–777.

Schneider, K. (2002). *Counseling about cancer: Strategies for genetic counseling* (2nd ed.). New York: Wiley-Liss.

Shappell, H., & Matloff, E. (2001). Writing effective insurance justification letters for cancer genetic testing: A streamlined approach. *Journal of Genetic Counseling, 10*(3), 331–341.

Shanley, S., Myhill, K., Doherty, R., Ardern-Jones, A., Hall, S., Vince, C., et al. (2007). Delivery of cancer genetics services: The Royal Marsden telephone clinic model. *Familial Cancer, 6*(2), 213–219.

Shiloh, S., Koehly, L., Jenkins, J., Martin, J., & Hadley, D. (2008). Monitoring coping style moderates emotional reactions to genetic testing for hereditary nonpolyposis colorectal cancer: A longitudinal study. *Psycho-Oncology, 17*(8), 746–755.

Smith, A., Moran, A., Boyd, M.C., Bulman, M., Shenton, A., Smith, L., et al. (2007). Phenocopies in *BRCA1* and *BRCA2* families: Evidence for modifier genes and implications for screening. *Journal of Medical Genetics, 44*(1), 10–15.

Staton, A.D., Kurian, A.W., Cobb, K., Mills, M.A., & Ford, J.M. (2007). Cancer risk reduction and reproductive concerns in female *BRCA1/2* mutation carriers. *Familial Cancer, 7*(2), 179–186.

Tercyak, K., Peshkin, B., DeMarco, T., Brogan, B., & Lerman, C. (2002). Parent-child factors and their effect on communicating *BRCA1/2* test results to children. *Patient Education and Counseling, 47*(2), 145–153.

Trepanier, A., Ahrens, M., McKinnon, W., Peters, J., Stopfer, J., Grumet, S., et al. (2004). Genetic cancer risk assessment and counseling: Recommendations of the National Society of Genetic Counselors. *Journal of Genetic Counseling, 13*(2), 83–114.

U.S. Department of Health and Human Services Protection of Human Subjects, 45 C.F.R. § 46 (2005). Retrieved June 17, 2009, from http://www.hhs.gov/ohrp/documents/OHRPRegulations.pdf

U.S. Department of Health and Human Services. (2006). *Does the HIPAA privacy rule protect genetic information?* Retrieved October 18, 2008, from http://www.hhs.gov/hipaafaq/about/354.html

U.S. Department of Health and Human Services Office for Human Research Protections. (2009, March). *Guidance on the Genetic Information Nondiscrimination Act: Implications for investigators and institutional review boards.* Retrieved June 17, 2009, from http://www.hhs.gov/ohrp/humansubjects/guidance/gina.html

Uses and Disclosures for Treatment, Payment, and Health Care Operations, 45 C.F.R. § 164.506 (2003). Retrieved September 29, 2009, from http://www.hhs.gov/ocr/privacy/hipaa/understanding/coveredentities/sharingfortpo.pdf

U.S. Preventive Services Task Force. (2005). Genetic risk assessment and *BRCA* mutation testing for breast and ovarian cancer susceptibility. *Annals of Internal Medicine, 143*(5), 355–361.

van Asperen, C.J., Jonker, M.A., Jacobi, C.E., van Diemen-Homan, J.E., Bakker, E., Breuning, M.H., et al. (2004). Risk estimation for healthy women from breast cancer families: New insights and new strategies. *Cancer Epidemiology, Biomarkers and Prevention, 13*(1), 87–93.

Wagner, A., van Kessel, I., Kriege, M.G., Tops, C.M., Wijnen, J.T., Vasen, H.F., et al. (2005). Long-term follow-up of HNPCC gene mutation carriers: Compliance with screening and satisfaction with counseling and screening procedures. *Familial Cancer, 4*(4), 295–300.

Watson, M., Foster, C., Eeles, R., Eccles, D., Ashley, S., Davidson, R., et al. (2004). Psychosocial impact of breast/ovarian (*BRCA1/2*) cancer-predictive genetic testing in a UK multi-centre clinical cohort. *British Journal of Cancer, 91*(10), 1787–1794.

Wiesner, G.L., & Snow-Bailey, K. (2005, March 7). *Multiple endocrine neoplasia type 2*. Retrieved May 25, 2009, from http://www.ncbi.nlm.nih.gov/bookshelf/br.fcgi?book=gene&part=men2

CHAPTER 6
Establishment of a Cancer Genetic Risk Assessment Program

Bridget LeGrazie, MSN, RN, APNc, AOCN®, APNG, and Agnes Masny, MSN, MPH, BS, RN, CRNP

Professional Practice Domain:
Identification
- Identify clients who may benefit from specific genetic and genomic information and services based on assessment data
- Identify credible, accurate, appropriate, and current genetic and genomic information, resources, services, and technologies specific to given clients

Provision of Education, Care, and Support
- Collaborate with healthcare providers in providing genetic and genomic health care
- Collaborate with insurance providers and payers to facilitate reimbursement for genetic and genomic healthcare services

(Consensus Panel on Genetic/Genomic Nursing Competencies, 2009)

INTRODUCTION

The demand for cancer genetic risk assessment services in the community is on the rise and nurses play a key role in both the development and provision of these services. Ten to fifteen percent of people with cancer are estimated to have an underlying inherited predisposition to the disease. Asking about a family history of cancer or making a referral for cancer risk counseling has become recommended practice for oncology healthcare providers. The American Society of Clinical Oncology (ASCO) issued a statement indicating that clinical oncologists have the responsibility to ascertain the families at risk for inherited forms of cancer (ASCO, 2003; Robson et al., 2010; Zon et al., 2009). This translates into a greater need for cancer risk assessment services to accommodate these referrals. Until recently, National Cancer Institute (NCI)-designated cancer centers and other academic centers have been on the forefront of offering these services. A survey of NCI-designated cancer centers found that 82% provide cancer risk assessment services (Epplein, Koon, Ramsey, & Potter, 2005). Furthermore, the American College of Surgeons (ACS) Commission on Cancer stated in its cancer program standards that genetic testing and counseling is a supportive service that is offered either on site or by referral (ACS, 2009).

As cancer risk assessment enters mainstream oncologic practice, an increasing number of administrators consider offering cancer genetic risk assessment programs (CGRAPs) in their institutions or in their private practices independently or in collaboration with an academic research program (Daly, Stearman, Masny, Sein, & Mazzoni, 2005; MacDonald et al., 2006). When choosing to deliver services as complex as risk assessment, genetic counseling, and testing, providers consider the time and expertise necessary for competent service delivery (Mac-

Donald et al.; Sein, Mazzoni, Masny, & Stearman, 2004; Stopfer, 2000). Research will continue to identify genetic variants that modify risk and genomic markers to screen for early cancer and improve tailored risk-reduction strategies. Future cancer risk assessment programs most likely will become a key component of a cancer center's oncology service line. These programs will offer a wide range of cancer risk assessment for both inherited and sporadic types of cancers with genetic and genomic testing for cancer predisposition, in some instances for cancer treatment decisions, as well as a variety of risk reduction, behavioral, and surgical interventions aimed at decreasing cancer rates. Currently, most cancer risk assessment programs focus on the known factors contributing to cancer risk with genetic risk assessment for hereditary predisposition. Therefore, this chapter will address the main components of a CGRAP and points to consider when deciding whether to start a program.

NEEDS ASSESSMENT AND PLANNING

Needs Assessment

The first thing to consider before starting a CGRAP is whether to initiate a program or to refer clients to an existing program in the area. CGRAPs currently operate in many cities and towns across the United States. Consult NCI's Web site for the searchable *Cancer Genetics Services Directory* (http://cancernet.nci.nih.gov/search/geneticsservices) or the National Society of Genetic Counselors Web site for a list of genetic counselors by specialty (www.nsgc.org/resourcelink.cfm). These lists will help to determine whether CGRAP services are accessible to clients in your geographic area.

Regardless of whether programs are readily available in the area, consider performing a needs assessment. A CGRAP needs assessment identifies and evaluates existing community resources, availability of skilled providers, gaps in current services or unmet needs of high-risk individuals, and strategies for program planning and quality assurance. A needs assessment also raises awareness of the potential development of the service and may stimulate interest in the program. See Figure 6-1 for considerations that need preliminary evaluation prior to establishing a CGRAP.

Strategic Planning Committee

At the institutional level, it may be helpful to establish a strategic planning committee to garner administrative support for the program. Forming a multidisciplinary strategic planning committee to sort out program feasibility, risks versus benefits, mission and goals, timelines, and overall vision for the CGRAP is helpful in this endeavor (MacDonald et al., 2006; Snyder et al., 2003). A strategic planning committee can provide institutional input on the following.
- Determine administrative commitment: Does the administration see the value of a CGRAP? Is administrative financial support available for a CGRAP?
- Indentify medical staff support. Having a physician champion interested in cancer prevention and control serves as a driving force for program development and bridges communication with the administrative, medical, and nursing staff.
- Explore types of CGRAP programs, such as those with a research component or collaboration versus traditional clinical service.

FIGURE 6-1 NEEDS ASSESSMENT: CONSIDERATIONS FOR INITIATING A CANCER GENETIC RISK ASSESSMENT PROGRAM

- Are cancer genetic risk assessment programs available within the community?
- Are existing data (e.g., tumor board or hospital screening data) available to assess potential service needs?
- To determine the number of potential clients for the program, obtain the number of cancer clients served by the cancer center from the institution's cancer registry. From that number, 5%–10% will be affected by hereditary predisposition syndromes (Daly et al., 2005), thus providing an estimate of potential clients of such genetic services.
- What community input has been gathered?
  - Sampling community representatives about starting a program
  - Establishing community interest
  - Survey approach or community forum to identify priority needs for risk assessment services
- What financial support will be given to start and sustain the program?
- Are administrative and clinical interest and support available?
- Will the program be integrated into existing clinic structures or a stand-alone risk assessment program?
- What type of multidisciplinary team will be employed to deliver service?
- What clinical and interdepartmental staff will plan the clinic's vision, mission, goals, and implementation?

Note. Based on information from Daly et al., 2005; National Cancer Institute, 2008.

- Determine the clinical partnerships or consultations needed to operate a CGRAP such as staff from pathology, surgery, gastroenterology, and gynecology from within the institution or the community.
- Establish institutional policies and procedures for the CGRAP such as referral, intake, pre-appointment screening and evaluation, counseling processes, and procedures for communicating with referring primary care providers or specialists providing follow-up.
- Plan for operational issues such as resources, billing mechanisms, staffing needs, information management, space, equipment, and mechanisms to ensure confidentiality and security of personal health information including genetic data.
- Establish capital and operating budgets. Identify revenue or funding sources, knowing that a CGRAP may not be a direct revenue generating program in its first years of operation.
- Develop goals for quality assurance that are in accordance with the institution's quality assurance policies.
- Develop a marketing plan to inform the public about the services and to communicate with community physicians, other healthcare providers, and those within the hospital where the program is being established. Prepare a brochure or other informational materials about the CGRAP and involve the media or plan events that provide visibility for the program.
- The strategic plan provides the opportunity for administrative and clinical staff to determine an effective infrastructure for the CGRAP and day-to-day operational needs. See Table 6-1 for further considerations for strategic planning.

Development of a Multidisciplinary Team

A primary consideration for CGRAP planning is identifying staff who will provide the services. The disciplines that comprise the CGRAP represent the varied skills needed to ensure

TABLE 6-1. Strategic Planning Considerations

Planning Dimension	Purpose	Considerations
Programmatic Development		
Strategic plan Establish mission, goals, and objectives Develop program timeline Marketing	Provides up-front administrative and clinical backing Helps to identify program need and specific cancer types; best fit for this type of clinic (e.g., a high-risk breast program in a breast center versus a gastrointestinal [GI] risk assessment program in a GI clinic)	Requires up-front time commitment and lead time for establishment of a program. Established goals and procedures provide a standardized approach for client care and cancer risk counseling.
Administrative Aspects		
Staffing requirements Training Facility infrastructure Capital equipment needs Information management Billing system and establishment of fee schedule HIPAA and institutional review board (IRB) compliance	Clearly identifies costs involved Helps to identify appropriate staff needed to establish multidisciplinary team Establishes institutional mechanisms for confidentiality and client protections Identifies lines of responsibility and accountability (e.g., MD in charge)	Program costs must be weighed against client and community outcomes. May identify that a phase-in period of training is necessary. Few IRBs have sufficient genetics background to assess appropriateness of genetic protocols. Successful programs require administrative and medical staff support.
Clinical Policies and Procedures		
Client identification Intake/eligibility assessment Education Risk assessment Informed consent Genetic counseling and testing Genetic test results disclosure Follow-up and surveillance	Intake procedures to expand family history in order to identify high-risk individuals Establishes mechanisms for client recruitment and triage of appropriate high-risk individuals Establishes counseling procedures, number of visits, and estimated time spent with proband Establishes mechanisms for obtaining informed consent prior to testing research versus clinical testing Develops institutional policy on medical management recommendations for high-risk populations	Multiple mechanisms for referral for both community and in-house are available (e.g., computerized, face-to-face, telephone). Computerized genetic education versus face-to-face strategies involve different level of staffing (e.g., computerized program can be viewed prior to counseling requiring only administrative support). Informed consent in a research setting versus a clinical service requires regulatory oversight. Mechanisms for ongoing review of literature and clinical updates are necessary.
Quality Assurance		
Ongoing program evaluation/audit	Identifies outcome indicators to track progress of program, identifies programmatic issues, and provides opportunity for remediation of problems	Mechanisms for audit may include input from administrative and program staff as well as outside reviewer to assess clinical utility of new technologies in high-risk populations.

Note. Adapted with permission from Agnes Masny, Familial Cancer Risk Assessment Program, Fox Chase Cancer Center, Philadelphia, PA.

that risk assessment, education, counseling, and medical management are delivered to meet the needs of the client medically and psychosocially. A multidisciplinary team approach is a way to provide clients with the most comprehensive cancer risk assessment, which also offers a complement of specific expertise, support, and consultation for the entire team. The team's staff can be drawn from the institution or by contractual or consultative arrangements with other CGRAPs and clinical or academic groups. Programs have reported staffing to include a geneticist or oncologist specially trained in genetics, a genetic counselor, and an oncology nurse specially trained in genetics; some also include a psychologist and a social worker (Daly et al., 2005). Some programs also may include specialists such as gastroenterologists, endocrinologists, dermatologists, surgeons, gynecologic oncologists, or others as needed to address the needs of clients with different cancer syndromes. According to a survey of NCI-designated cancer centers, 28% of programs had an RN as part of their risk assessment staff and 13% included a nurse practitioner (Epplein et al., 2005). Most of the programs staffed a genetic counselor (96%) followed by a medical geneticist or medical oncologist (61%); other specialties were gynecologic oncologists and health educators (Epplein et al.). See Figure 6-2 for multidisciplinary provider considerations.

Careful consideration of professional requirements for the team in terms of certification and credentialing, education (oncology and genetics), and licensure is suggested. ASCO's 2003, 2009, and 2010 policy statements recommend training for health professionals who provide cancer genetic assessment and risk-reduction counseling (ASCO, 2003; Robson et al., 2010; Zon et al., 2009). Other practice and educational considerations for nurses are presented in Chapters 1 and 13.

Financial Considerations

Most oncology services prepare an operating budget that shows a projected net income compared to operating expenses prior to launching a new ser-

FIGURE 6-2 MULTIDISCIPLINARY PROVIDER CONSIDERATIONS FOR TEAM MEMBERS, CONSULTATIVE STAFF, AND SPECIALISTS

Team members for cancer genetic risk assessment program (CGRAP)
- Medical/surgical/gynecologic oncologists[1]
- Gastroenterologist or gynecologist[1]
- Clinical geneticists[1]
- Nurse/nurse practitioner
- Genetic counselor
- Program coordinator (i.e., someone who oversees administrative and operational issues of the CGRAP)
- Health educator
- Support staff (e.g., intake coordinator, scheduler, billing specialist, information specialist, data manager)

Consultative members to the team (may be institutional staff, consultants to program)
- Psychologist or social worker
- Pathologist—to help to verify pathology reports or establish procedures for specific tumor testing (e.g., microsatellite instability or immunohistochemistry testing for colon tumors)
- Research or academic affiliates—contacts with experts in cancer genetics to assist with opinion for cancer syndrome/testing options or recommendations for genetic research studies and medical management issues

Referral specialists for further workup, medical management, or risk-reducing interventions
- Genetic specialist for evaluation of other genetic conditions
- Gynecologic oncologist/surgeon/plastic surgeon for risk-reducing surgery
- Dermatologist/urologist/gastroenterologist/gynecologist for screening as needed

[1]Practice setting for CGRAP may determine type of medical staff. This listing does not imply that all the medical professionals listed are part of the team.

Note. Based on information from Epplein et al., 2005.

vice. A revenue impact study has been suggested as a way to determine program expenses and projected revenues for the CGRAP (Ho, 2004). This type of financial planning assesses the operating costs for all expected budgetary items compared to projected revenues. The needs assessment data can help to project the number of expected clients for the CGRAP. Information from insurers or established fee for service per expected client gives potential revenues. The projected income is then compared to expenses. Examples of expense items are
- Salaries and benefits for professional and support staff based on expected time and effort in the CGRAP. Time and effort includes both direct and indirect service. (Initial training expenses and in-service updates are incorporated into salary support calculations.)
- Facility expenses such as offices, telephone, copiers and computers, mailings, medical records, and secure storage
- Client education and counseling resources such as software program for taking family histories, educational materials
- Marketing materials such as brochures or media advertisement about the program.

Reimbursement for CGRAP services often is insufficient to balance expenses. An ASCO survey showed that lack of reimbursement was one of the main barriers to establishing risk assessment services in oncology practice (Ganz et al., 2006). However, CGRAPs have shown downstream indirect revenue, such as those generated for medical management when clients are referred back to the institution for screening and other risk-reduction strategies such as prophylactic surgery or the care rendered to clients who develop cancer and are treated at the same institution (Ho, 2004). Some institutions consider CGRAPs loss leaders. Because CGRAPs offer cutting-edge genetic and genomic services, institutional funds or donors may be seeking to support novel services. Revenue sources beyond service reimbursement can be explored. Examples of projected revenues are
- Institutional revenues such as grants, endowments, or foundation funding (These sources may be temporary or for program startup.)
- Institutional support for salaries and equipment
- Reimbursement for CGRAP services (e.g., fee-for-service, insurance reimbursement)
- Projected downstream revenues.

Reimbursement

CGRAPs vary in their billing strategies, including charging a fee for service, billing insurers, or offering the service at no cost (Zon et al., 2006). Fee for service may be itemized per visit (see the Visit Designs section later in this chapter) or have a packaged fee that covers multiple visits. To determine the fee for service, calculate fees associated with the projected expenses. These fees include but are not limited to salaries for staff providing cancer risk assessment, education, counseling, phlebotomy services, test or tissue sample packaging fees, time taken for documentation and acquisition of medical records, and pathology for the client and family members. The fees are then compared to other established CGRAPs as well as a third-party payer's fees for the same or similar services. The institution's fee for service is set according to a percentage set by the third party (e.g., Medicare, Medicaid, managed care insurers) (National Society of Genetic Counselors, 2008).

Administrators who are establishing the program should consider the pros and cons of fee-for-service billing. Some advantages are having immediate payment, saving time related to the billing process, decreasing the cost of staff who prepare and process billing, and having a payment mechanism for those clients who do not want their insurer involved or whose insurance plan does not cover genetic education and counseling services. The disadvantages are potentially limiting the number of clients because of the limited ability to pay an out-of-pocket cost and losing clients to another institution that accepts insurance payment. A sliding fee scale based on the client's ability to pay or establishing a fund for hardship cases may be explored.

Three categories of service are considered for billing and reimbursement: (a) the cost of the genetic test, (b) cancer risk education and counseling, and (c) evaluation and management services.

Cost of Genetic Testing

Commercial and research laboratories provide testing for the majority of familial cancer syndromes. Listings of commercial and research laboratories can be found on the National Center for Biotechnology Information's GeneTests Web site (www.geneclinics.org). The site provides peer-reviewed information on genetic tests, clinical manifestations, and management (see Table 6-2).

Payment for the genetic test often requires preauthorization with the client's insurer and determination of coverage amount. Establishing this billing process for genetic testing is important prior to ordering tests, because clients need notification about potential costs or copayments and the options for payment.

TABLE 6-2   Resources for Establishing a Billing Process

Resource	Contact Information
GeneTests is a peer-reviewed Web site funded by a contract with the National Institutes of Health. The site provides genetic testing information and laboratories offering testing.	www.genetests.org Link to "Gene Reviews," then search for the cancer syndrome or cancer type, then chose "testing" for listing of commercial and research laboratories offering testing.
ICD Online resource for ICD-9 codes or manuals	www.cdc.gov/nchs/icd.htm
Current Procedural Terminology (CPT): Online resources for CPT codes	https://catalog.ama-assn.org/Catalog/cpt/cpt_search.jsp
The National Plan and Provider Enumeration System: Site to apply for a National Provider Identifier (NPI)	https://nppes.cms.hhs.gov Phone: 800-465-3203 or TYY 800-629-2326
HIPAA Health Care Provider Taxonomy Code Set: Site to obtain needed code for an NPI application	www.wpc-edi.com/content/view/793/1
Evaluation and Management Services Guide: Provides CPT code information for evaluation and management services	www.cms.hhs.gov/MLNProducts/downloads/eval_mgmt_serv_guide.pdf
National Society of Genetic Counselors (NSGC) Billing and Reimbursement Toolkit (accessible by NSGC members)	www.nsgc.org

Some laboratories assist with obtaining insurance authorization and payment of the genetic tests. Contact with the specific laboratory will help to determine authorization support services and billing policies. Some laboratories prefer institutional billing; this means that an institution or practice has an established account with the laboratory. With institutional billing, the laboratory doing the testing directly charges the institution ordering the test. The billing and reimbursement for the testing is then sought by the ordering facility. Institutions that do not have the capability of providing specialized tests may have to consider institutional billing. For example, colon tumor testing for microsatellite instability (MSI) and immunohistochemistry (IHC) may entail sending the tissue for analysis to another facility. Payment coverage for the MSI and IHC testing needs to be arranged prior to sending the sample. Involving the billing department therefore is helpful in establishing institutional billing.

Billing and Reimbursement for Cancer Risk Education and Counseling Services

Several steps are needed to establish a formal payment policy for cancer risk assessment and counseling services. See Figure 6-3 for the suggested steps to establish billing procedures. Billing policies need to be established for each third-party insurer along with coding designations for the services provided. The billing department in the institution or practice can help to determine coverage for the scope of services offered and by what healthcare provider. Contacting the institution's contracted payers, insurers, and Medicare carrier can help to determine if a formal reimbursement policy exists or can be negotiated for these services. Currently, institutions may have to advocate independently for reimbursement with third parties. The third-party insurers may require dialogue and education from the administrators or healthcare providers on the multidisciplinary team regarding the complexity and the benefits of cancer risk assessment and counseling in order to establish a formal policy for payment.

As noted earlier in this chapter, poor reimbursement for education and counseling has been a barrier to implementing CGRAPs. A survey of 15 national medical plans and three Medicare carrier medical directors examined the policies for billing and reimbursement of cancer prevention counseling services (Zon et al., 2006). The study showed that many insurers cover different components of a risk assessment service for high-risk individuals but often do not have preventive counseling coverage policies in place. However, an ASCO initiative is

FIGURE 6-3 SUGGESTED STEPS TO ESTABLISH CANCER GENETIC RISK ASSESSMENT PROGRAM (CGRAP) BILLING PROCEDURES

1. Determine what billing process the institution will use (i.e., fee for service, billing insurance, or combination or both).
2. Obtain information from institution's third-party payers regarding reimbursement policy for cancer risk assessment services. May need to advocate for reimbursement of CGRAP services.
3. Determine appropriate Common Procedural Terminology and International Classification of Diseases codes for billing with the help of personnel who are experienced in coding and billing.
4. Apply for a National Provider Identifier (NPI) number with appropriate Health Care Provider Taxonomy code.
5. Consider a pilot period for billing. Establish a time period to bill and evaluate third-party payers' level of reimbursement. The institution may need to renegotiate formal billing policy for CGRAP services.
6. Consider credentialing in a nursing specialty. Some third-party payers and insurance carriers require credentialing in order to reimburse the nursing service.

under way to improve reimbursement with third-party payers for preventive counseling services (Zon et al., 2009).

Cancer risk counseling services billed to an insurer will need to have procedural and diagnosis coding designations. The coding designations are the Current Procedural Terminology (CPT) codes and the *International Classification of Diseases* (ICD) (see Figure 6-4 for procedural and diagnostic codes). Because the coding rules can be complex and are revised regularly, establishing service codes with staff trained in billing and coding (i.e., staff from the billing or coding department) is advisable.

In order to receive reimbursement, nurses providing genetic cancer risk education and counseling must have a National Provider Identifier (NPI) number. The Centers for Medicare and Medicaid Services (CMS) adopted the NPI system in 2006 in response to the 1996 Health Insurance Portability and Accountability Act (HIPAA), which mandated the adoption of a uniform unique health provider identifier for all healthcare providers, not just Medicare providers, for use in standard electronic transactions (CMS, 2005, 2009). However, having an NPI number does not guarantee reimbursement by Medicare for genetic education and counseling services. Although the NPI number was adopted for Medicare and Medicaid, almost all insurance plans and payers request it. Because healthcare providers who conduct standard transactions as adopted under HIPAA are covered healthcare providers, they need an NPI number to bill for standard transactions.

Nurses can apply individually for an NPI number online (see Table 6-2). Some institutions apply for individual provider numbers, whereas others apply for group provider numbers. Therefore, nurses should check first with their institution about applying for an NPI number. The application for an NPI number asks for a provider code. HIPAA established a standard set of codes for electronic billing transactions called *healthcare provider taxonomy codes* (see Table 6-2 for the taxonomy code set). Nurses have several categories of codes such as registered nurse,

FIGURE 6-4 PROCEDURAL AND DIAGNOSTIC CODING

What is a CPT code?
CPT is an acronym for Current Procedural Terminology. The purpose of the coding system is to provide uniform language that accurately describes medical, surgical, and diagnostic services.

A CPT code is a five-digit numeric code that is used to describe medical, surgical, radiology, laboratory, anesthesiology, and evaluation/management services of physicians, hospitals, and other healthcare providers. CPT codes are published by the American Medical Association and revised on a regular schedule. CPT is a registered trademark of the American Medical Association.

What is an ICD code?
International Classification of Diseases (ICD) coding system is used to code signs, symptoms, injuries, diseases, and conditions. The ICD is maintained jointly by the National Center for Health Statistics (NCHS) and the Centers for Medicare and Medicaid Services (CMS).

Are both the ICD code and CPT code needed for billing?
Yes, both codes are needed because of the relationship between the ICD (diagnosis) code and the CPT (procedure or service rendered) code. The diagnosis that is coded (ICD) supports the medical necessity of the procedure or service (CPT).

What are evaluation and management codes?
Evaluation and management (E/M) codes refer specifically to services provided by physicians, nurse practitioners, clinical nurse specialists, and physician assistants for history and physical examinations, consultations, and medical decision making. The CPT guidelines apply to the reporting of E/M services because the CPT code justifies the level of the service billed.

Note. Information for this figure was compiled from the resources listed in Table 6-2.

nurse practitioner, and clinical nurse specialist. A nurse certified as a genetic counselor may apply for an NPI number using either a genetic counseling or nursing code. Nurses credentialed by the Genetic Nursing Credentialing Commission or trained with a specialty in genetics can apply using a nursing code appropriate for their level of training. The institution's billing or coding department can help to determine the most appropriate code.

Billing for Evaluation and Management Services

Evaluation and management (E/M) services refer to clinical visits or consultations provided by physicians, nurse practitioners, clinical nurse specialists, and physician assistants for history and physical examinations, consultations, and medical decision making. The CPT guidelines apply to the reporting of E/M services because the CPT code defines the level of the service provided and therefore what is billed. The level of service is the amount of face-to-face time spent with a client and the complexity of the medical decision making. Documentation is required for the amount of time spent in education and counseling as it relates to the medical decision (see Table 6-2).

INSTITUTIONAL POLICY CONSIDERATIONS

Procedures and Policies

Developing written CGRAP procedures and policies is helpful. Policies and procedures ensure a standardized approach to clients and their needs. For example, policies and procedures can cover such things as what information is collected and when, the process and minimum standards for risk education and counseling, and how genetic test results will be given and by whom. A privacy policy can cover where genetic information is stored and how genetic information is shared. These policies provide safeguards for staff, consistency in care delivery, and a mechanism for staff when confronted with requests for exceptions. Most institutions also require a practice protocol for their medical and nursing staff members who provide clinical services. Guidelines such as those from the National Comprehensive Cancer Network (NCCN) can be utilized for practice protocols (NCCN, 2009).

Client Identification

Clients can come to a CGRAP from a variety of sources; therefore, policies or strategies for identification of clients within an institution or community should be developed. Establishment of guidelines of what constitutes a high-risk client can be developed based on existing evidence and guidelines such as the NCCN guidelines. In-house and community physicians (e.g., oncologists, gynecologists, gastroenterologists, primary care providers, surgeons) and nurses are in a position to identify those clients needing a referral. Education for these providers or having referral forms highlighting the "red flags" of familial cancers are examples of identification strategies. Some institutions have all individuals complete a family history form at the time of mammography or colonoscopy to identify high-risk clients (Lee et al., 2005; Nathanson, Zisman, Julian, McCaffrey, & Rubin, 2008). Ohio State University studied the use of kiosks where all new and established clients input their family history.

They found this method to be helpful in identifying individuals who needed a referral to their CGRAP (Sweet, Bradley, & Westman, 2002). Routinely collecting a family history is a practice decision that also requires a procedure to determine who will review the family history to decide which clients or families need further evaluation.

Another strategy that can be used to identify clients is to develop clinical or pathologic criteria to identify clients who are having surgery or other treatments and who would also benefit from risk assessment. ASCO recommended that practitioners recognize indications for genetic testing (ASCO, 2003; Robson et al., 2010). For example, 25% of multifocal medullary thyroid cancer is because of germ line mutations in the *RET* oncogene with a 4% rate of de novo mutations (Lindor, McMaster, Lindor, & Greene, 2008). The American College of Obstetricians and Gynecologists (ACOG) has recommended genetic risk assessment for any patient with high-grade serous ovarian cancer, primary peritoneal cancer, or fallopian tube cancer (Lu et al., 2009). Tumor expression profiles conducted for targeted therapy selection also may identify individuals with hereditary cancer risk. MSI testing of colon tumors is used to predict treatment response to adjuvant chemotherapy (Bertagnolli et al., 2009); yet, MSI results have implications for further evaluation for Lynch syndrome (Hampel et al., 2008). These client identification strategies carry with them considerations for how an institution or practice will establish policies to identify high-risk clients, communicate with other departments about these policies, and provide client education and informed consent when surgical or pathologic results may give genetic information that affects the client and his or her family.

Referral policies need to be developed once criteria are established to identify high-risk individuals or information about the CGRAP program is made known to the public. Some examples of referral considerations include

- Will the CGRAP accept self-referrals, or do clients need to have a referral from a healthcare provider?
- Will the referred clients have to meet any personal or family history criteria for program entry?
- What mechanism of communication will be established with the referring provider?
- What process will be established for in-house referrals? Will in-house staff provide referral information to the client, or will the in-house staff directly contact the CGRAP about the referral?

Selection of Genetic Test and Laboratory

A family history that exhibits a hereditary pattern of cancer may fit a number of cancer syndromes with different genes responsible for different syndromes. For example, nonmedullary thyroid cancer and early-onset breast and uterine cancers may cluster in a family. These cancers are suggestive of different cancer syndromes (see Chapter 3). The selection of the most likely cancer syndrome, a differential list of cancer syndromes, and which gene to test first are decisions that often are complex and need to be considered by the multidisciplinary team. Having procedures for how family histories are evaluated, similar to tumor board reviews, will help with the selection of the most likely cancer syndrome and the respective gene or genes to test. Some institutions have regular multidisciplinary pedigree evaluation meetings regarding the selection of cancer syndromes and gene-testing strategies. As previously mentioned, a CGRAP that has a specific disease focus, such as breast cancer, needs policies and procedures for how cancer risk assessment, testing, and referral will be provided for other cancer syndromes that are identified.

Most clinical laboratories follow the Clinical Laboratory Improvement Act (CLIA) regulations that monitor personnel qualifications, laboratory quality assurance standards, documentation, and validation of laboratory tests (Hudson et al., 2006). However, a CLIA specialty for genetic testing is not offered, and CLIA was not designed to assess the clinical validity of laboratory tests. Clinical validity measures the association of a test result with a disorder. For example, finding a *MEN* mutation in a patient correlates with a diagnosed medullary thyroid cancer. If genetic predisposition testing is performed, clinical validity measures the accuracy of predicting a future clinical outcome based on prevalence and penetrance data (Secretary's Advisory Committee on Genetics, Health, and Society, 2008). Although a genetic test may be available, the CGRAP needs a policy or process for evidence-based review and guidelines for when to use a commercially or research-based genetic test. Many existing CGRAPs have periodic journal clubs or evidence-based reviews to evaluate new data or guidelines. Professional organizations such as the U.S. Preventive Services Task Force (2005) have provided an evidence-based review and recommendations for the use of *BRCA* testing. The Centers for Disease Control and Prevention supports an online resource for reviews of new genetic and genomic technologies called Evaluation of Genomic Applications in Practice and Prevention (2009). If research genetic testing is conducted, a policy for providing test results also is needed. Some research laboratories give the ordering provider research test results with the recommendation that the test result be repeated and verified in a CLIA-approved laboratory.

When selecting a laboratory to do genetic testing, it is important for the CGRAP team to know what method of genetic testing the laboratory uses to detect mutations, such as **polymerase chain reaction**, microarray, or immunoassay of proteins, along with what is being measured in the sample (e.g., a genetic sequence or a protein). Having information about the genetic test's corresponding sensitivity and specificity, how test results are given and interpreted, and if laboratory personnel are available for questions also are essential in choosing a genetic testing laboratory. Different laboratories may have varied procedures for blood sample collection, storage, and shipping. Policies and procedures for both the selection of gene tests and laboratories need to be established as part of a program's operational plan and reviewed regularly to incorporate new data, guidelines, or recommendations, as well as for quality assurance.

Direct-to-Consumer Marketing

Genetic testing companies are marketing directly to the community as well as healthcare providers. A policy should be written on how the CGRAP will collaborate with other community providers who may be ordering genetic testing. The policy can address how to accept referrals for clients already tested who may not understand their results or who request post-test counseling. Collaboration with healthcare providers who order genetic testing may make them aware of the CGRAP services and encourage their interest in referring clients. The CGRAP can become familiar with the state's policies on direct-to-consumer marketing and create institutional policies in accordance with state guidance. To check the institution's state policy, visit the Genetics and Public Policy Center (2007) online. This site provides a listing of direct-to-consumer marketing testing statutes and regulations by state.

Information Management and Confidentiality

Genetic information is considered medical information. As CGRAPs become part of clinical services, institutions are including the cancer risk assessment and genetic testing information as part of the client's medical record. Established HIPAA policies regulating protected information (CMS, 2005) applies to all information collected in a CGRAP. Because family history information applies to other family members besides the client, confidentiality issues related to demographics and identifiers of family members need to be addressed. Tracking a client's personal and family cancer history, test results, long-term screening follow-up, clinical course, and clinical trial involvement (if applicable) requires a relational database and someone who can both understand and manage the data that are captured. Genetic databases are available commercially or can be developed by the CGRAP using computerized programs. Collecting and tracking data of CGRAP clients, such as cancer screening visits, risk-reducing surgeries, or chemoprevention use, may serve to track institutional revenues related to the services provided.

CHOOSING A TYPE OF CANCER GENETIC RISK ASSESSMENT PROGRAM

Scope of Services

In defining what type of program to create, providers can consider the NCCN practice guidelines for the components of genetics cancer risk assessment as a guide to the scope of services that are feasible for the institution to offer. The NCCN guidelines give criteria for whom to refer for breast and ovarian cancer and gastrointestinal cancer risk assessment. In addition, the guidelines recommend assessment of the client's genetic testing knowledge; a detailed family, medical, and surgical history; and a focused physical examination when necessary to evaluate other physical findings associated with familial cancer syndromes. In view of these guidelines, determining a program's scope of services addresses how the institution will provide the cancer genetic risk assessment components, specifically identification and referral for individuals needing cancer genetic risk assessment, collection of family and medical history, education and counseling for genetic testing, physical examination, and clinical follow-up. Programs providing clinical follow-up typically include cancer screening, risk-reduction measures with chemoprevention or surgery, follow-up of client and family medical history, and behavioral and emotional concerns related to high-risk or mutation carrier status.

CGRAPs may have a narrow or broad disease focus in their approach. If a program will focus on one specific hereditary cancer syndrome, such as breast and ovarian cancer, a policy needs to define how to identify, manage, or refer clients with other suspected hereditary cancer syndromes. Programs with a comprehensive risk assessment approach provide services for all suspected familial cancer syndromes.

Long-term client follow-up is another component of some CGRAPs that may include tracking compliance to screening recommendations, providing updates about genetic tests, or risk-reduction strategies. Some comprehensive cancer centers provide follow-up and screening as part of research and longitudinal studies (Epplein et al., 2005). A distinct needs assessment would need to be undertaken for CGRAP programs considering a specialized high-risk follow-up clinic. Establishing a follow-up clinical service would require a similar planning process to evaluate service and screening availability and gaps in the community, as well as staffing and financial support.

Cancer Genetic Risk Program Designs

Several different types of cancer risk assessment and counseling program designs are available. Examples that will be explored in detail within this chapter include
- Identifying and referring high-risk clients to an existing CGRAP in the community
- Establishing a CGRAP within the institution or practice
- Establishing a CGRAP with a research collaboration.

Identifying and Referring Clients to an Existing Cancer Genetic Risk Assessment Program

After conducting the community needs assessment previously discussed in this chapter, referral of clients to an established CGRAP is an option. This approach would involve performing a cancer risk assessment to determine those clients at risk for cancer and cancer syndromes and then referring them to another established program. Another option is to collaborate with an existing program and offer the ability to provide services on-site at the CGRAP's facility. Some existing CGRAPs share staff across institutions. A referral approach may be beneficial if the estimated volume of high-risk clients is low or if administrative and financial support is lacking. A possible limitation of the "identify and refer" design is that the referring institution could lose revenue if services for screening, risk reduction, and management of cancer are provided another healthcare provider outside your CGRAP.

Establishing a Cancer Genetic Risk Assessment Program Within the Institution or Practice

A CGRAP within an institution or office practice can provide on-site comprehensive care by staff employed by the institution so that all care is provided "in-house." The benefit of this design is the established mechanisms for referral and the dedicated staff who are receiving ongoing cancer genetics–specific in-services and training. Other benefits to having a dedicated CGRAP in an institution or office is the opportunity for revenue by keeping the clients' clinical management within the institution, not losing clients to competing organizations, and achieving recognition in the community for providing "high-tech" or "state-of-the-art" care.

Limitations of the stand-alone design are that reimbursement for education and counseling may not support a self-sustaining CGRAP. Therefore, the CGRAP may need institutional support and mechanisms to track revenues. Another limitation is where clients will be referred for medical follow-up. Epplein et al. (2005) noted that 38% of comprehensive cancer centers provide clinical follow-up. A stand-alone program without a clinical evaluation and follow-up program may lack the capacity to provide ongoing follow-up and reevaluation, recommended screening and medical management, and risk-reduction options for clients. For example, a program may perform a thorough family history assessment and genetic testing but not provide clinical screening. The client then relies on his or her oncologist or private medical doctor for the clinical follow-up. Procedures for communicating medical management recommendations need to be established to prevent fragmented care.

Establishing a Cancer Genetic Risk Assessment Program With Research Collaboration

Several CGRAPs offer a combination of risk assessment with a research component or collaboration. Some programs conduct independent clinical and molecular research related to high-risk populations and are part of academic centers or comprehensive cancer centers. Other CGRAPs collaborate with academic centers to implement research or refer clients to research studies. Research programs may offer clinical, behavioral, or molecular studies performed in the context of a protocol approved by an institutional review board (IRB). Still other programs are a combination of the two, in which a clinical program operates as a billable service or fee-for-service in conjunction with a research program offering participation in a research study either during or after the clinical service. Issues of informed consent or informed decision making are essential to either approach. Whether or not a CGRAP is strictly a clinical service or has a research component or collaboration, benefits and limitations should be considered.

Benefits of a clinical program include that most clients are tested through a commercial laboratory; the service is provided in the community near the client; and test results may be returned more quickly than if the testing was done through a research mechanism. Benefits of a research-based program include potential access to newer genetic testing technologies, as well as screening or chemopreventive strategies undergoing study. Research-based programs offer increased client protection because of the scrutiny of the IRB prior to client accrual and greater assurance of understanding with the use of informed consents. Collaboration with an academic or research program may offer access to cancer genetic experts or consultation regarding additional genetic testing that may be available only through research studies. One of the limitations of research-based programs is that the client may not receive results. The biggest barriers to the development of a genetics program in the community are (a) lack of qualified staff, (b) maintaining current knowledge, (c) funding, (d) education of staff, and (e) referral sources. The relationship with an academic institution can address many of these barriers.

Some authors suggest that community CGRAPs develop a relationship with an academic risk program (Daly et al., 2005; MacDonald et al., 2006). Once a gene mutation is identified, the client may pursue clinical trials or enter into a family registry with prospective follow-up or screening. Follow-up studies for clients with non-informative results are being conducted to help to identify other cancer susceptibility genes, modifier genes, or newer genetic technology to increase the sensitivity of testing. Research on carriers of deleterious mutations include the penetrance of specific mutation loci, phenotypic disease characteristics associated with specific mutations, and the effectiveness of current clinical management and screening. An example of the benefit of collaborative research is a study about the benefits of bilateral salpingo-oophorectomy based on whether the woman was a *BRCA1* or *BRCA2* mutation carrier (Kauff et al., 2008). Eleven collaborating cancer centers worked 10 years to accrue 1,000 *BRCA* mutation carriers after oophorectomy. Research collaborations are helping to validate clinical benefits of risk-reduction measures and to elucidate genotype-phenotype correlations for individuals with inherited susceptibility.

WHAT A CANCER GENETIC RISK ASSESSMENT PROGRAM LOOKS LIKE

How Clients Discover the Cancer Genetic Risk Assessment Program

The marketing strategy influences the CGRAP's visibility and how individuals find services. Marketing is an ongoing component of the CGRAP that initially increases awareness of a program, continues to make the program visible, and chronicles its success in the community. Many people who have a family history may seek out the services of a CGRAP. Ways that clients search for services include searching the Internet, asking their primary healthcare provider or specialist, calling a comprehensive cancer center to ask about a program near them, or reading a newspaper story or seeing a report on television about a hereditary cancer that raised their personal suspicion. The CGRAP should be visible on the institution's Web site, brochures should be available in physician offices and around the hospital, and media coverage of the CGRAP should be utilized to help clients searching for services.

Primary healthcare providers are often the first to field questions about familial cancer risk (Daly et al., 2005). Although increasing numbers of primary care providers are taking cancer family histories, many do not have adequate information or do not feel competent in performing a cancer risk assessment (Sabatino, McCarthy, Phillips, & Burns, 2007; Tyler & Snyder, 2006). Primary care providers conducting risk assessment have had low rates of referral for further risk assessment or genetic evaluation (Burke et al., 2009). To address the educational need of local healthcare providers, the CGRAP team can

- Offer educational programs (e.g., grand rounds, clinical conferences based on a significant case, in-services, tumor boards, office visits, departmental meetings)
- Publish articles in staff and hospital newsletters that are distributed to community providers
- Volunteer to speak about cancer genetics at professional meetings
- Provide program brochures for physician offices.

Intake

Intake is information that is collected from the potential client by phone prior to the initial visit to determine the client's eligibility for the program and so that the nurse and counselor can prepare for the counseling session. A list of frequently asked questions for the intake staff to refer to will minimize the number of calls transferred to other team members, minimize time spent on the phone, and increase caller satisfaction. Consider the following to streamline the referrals into the CGRAP.

- Who will handle the calls? Have clients register and be triaged through a centralized number with a specific intake coordinator or institutional call center.
- What information is collected at intake? Each CGRAP will decide what information is needed for the client's chart, such as insurance information, demographics, and who referred the client.
- Perform an initial assessment of the client's interest and perception of risk. In many cases, a client's perceptions have been shaped by living in a family in which multiple cancer diagnoses and deaths have occurred (Berliner & Fay, 2007).
- Discuss what the CGRAP has to offer and the CRGAP process and associated costs.

The process used to collect family or medical history may include

- Phone intake—If family history is collected via telephone, additional staffing may be needed. If additional staff is not available, this may mean meeting the client's immediate need for information and deferring history taking until the initial visit with the nurse.
- Online family history tool—The U.S. Surgeon General's Family Health Portrait is a free, online tool (Feero, Bigley, Brinner, & Family Health History Multi-Stakeholder Workgroup of the American Health Information Community, 2008).
- Mailed family history tool—In many cases, initial contact is made by telephone, with program materials and family medical history forms mailed to the client prior to the initial visit.

Visit Designs

ASCO has recommended that education and counseling are required parts of the cancer risk assessment and precede genetic testing and disclosure of results (ASCO, 2003; Robson et al., 2010. The components covered in each visit will depend upon the client's learning style or availability. This variability in clients will call for the nurse or counselor to have flexibility in the number of visits required for each client. The cancer risk assessment and counseling process may require one or more sessions and generally includes

- Detailed, multifaceted assessment of the client's medical and family history
- Determination of the risk of cancer or indication for genetic testing based on evidence of an inherited cancer syndrome
- Education and counseling specific to risks and eligibility for genetic testing
- Pretest counseling, including risks, benefits, and limitations, as well as obtaining informed consent for testing if applicable
- Disclosure of genetic test results if applicable
- Establishment of a cancer risk management plan and clinical follow-up.

The risk assessment process can be done over two or three visits (Epplein et al., 2005). Table 6-3 shows how cancer risk education and counseling can be provided in a two- or three-visit design. An initial risk assessment visit may last two hours if assessment, education, risk communication, and counseling are completed consecutively, whereas a results disclosure session generally may be completed in 30–60 minutes.

Options for education include in-person education, group education followed by brief individual sessions, or the use of an interactive computer program, Web site, or telephone education prior to the first visit. Current research shows that clients find education helpful and suggest enhanced educational techniques, such as newsletters and videotapes or DVDs (Kausmeyer et al., 2006). Clients have benefited from receiving information prior to their first visit (Collins, Halliday, Warren, & Williamson, 2000).

Telemedicine or phone result disclosure may be an option for clients who cannot travel to the CGRAP because of distance or health barriers (Jenkins et al., 2007). More research is needed in the area of telemedicine or telephone genetic test result disclosure; however, other non-genetic results currently are delivered by phone, for example, HIV or cancer diagnosis results.

Client Follow-Up

Each CGRAP may choose a different strategy for client follow-up, depending on the program procedures, such as

- Sending a follow-up letter to the client and client's referring physicians or healthcare providers
- Telephone follow-up
- Communicating to clients as new genetic information is discovered.

Sending a follow-up letter that summarizes the risk assessment visit or disclosure visit, along with a customized cancer risk management plan, to the client and the referring healthcare provider is standard practice. The recommended care can then be provided by the CGRAP's follow-up clinic if one is established, the client's healthcare provider, a specialist in the area, or a high-risk clinic at an academic institution. Such a letter serves as a reminder for the client and as legal documentation of the information and recommendations

TABLE 6-3   Components of Cancer Risk Education and Counseling by a Two- or Three-Visit Design

Activity	Two-Visit Design		Three-Visit Design		
	1st Visit	2nd Visit	1st Visit	2nd Visit	3rd Visit
Collection of risk information	Prior to or at 1st visit		Prior to or in between 1st and 2nd visits		
Cancer risk education	Prior to 1st visit via multimedia education if available or at 1st visit		At first visit		
Personal, medical, and family history and psychosocial assessment	Prior to or at 1st visit		In between 1st and 2nd visits		
Estimation of cancer risk and mutation carrier probability	Prior to 1st visit or at 1st visit		In between 1st and 2nd visits		
Communication of risk information	At 1st visit			At 2nd visit	
Pretest counseling	At 1st visit			At 2nd visit	
Blood draw	At 1st visit or appointment for blood draw after 1st visit			At 2nd visit or appointment for blood draw after 2nd visit	
Disclosure counseling		At 2nd visit			At 3rd visit
Cancer risk-reduction, screening, medical management plan	At 1st visit if client not pursuing testing	At 2nd visit after test results or make clinical appointment		At 2nd visit if client not pursuing testing	At 3rd visit after test results or make clinical appointment
Physical examination at any visit	Optional	Optional		Optional	Optional

given. Consider which team members will sign the follow-up letters ahead of time. Generally, the nurse counselor prepares and signs the letter; however, other members of the multidisciplinary team also may sign it. Also, consider what the CGRAP intuitional policies are regarding the client giving permission to release information to their healthcare providers.

Telephone follow-up is used to assess how the client is coping with the information and to ascertain the extent to which the client intends to comply with recommendations, including medical management and family dissemination if indicated. Consider the development of an institutional policy for follow-up and notification of family members at risk. Primarily, the CGRAP staff counsels the client to notify family members about their risk of being carriers or their risk for cancer. Documentation of the recommendation may protect the clinician of "failure to notify" other family members (ASCO, 2003; Schneider et al., 2006). Having printed materials for clients to share with their family members about the types of genetic test results, the meaning of these results for family members, and contact information is helpful. A follow-up telephone call can determine if the client has followed through with family notification. If a client's family members are interested in being tested and live far away, the follow-up call provides an opportunity for staff to provide referral resources where the client's relatives can obtain genetic counseling closer to home.

Another facet of long-term follow-up is a policy for recontacting clients. Genetic test results finding a variant of uncertain significance (VUS) must have a mechanism in place for recontacting clients. In most instances, the laboratory notifies the ordering provider if the VUS has been reclassified as a deleterious mutation or a benign polymorphism. The responsibility lies with CGRAP staff to notify the client about the reclassification. Other genetic and genomic discoveries may have an impact on participating clients or family health care, such as new genes and new testing technologies. The institutional policy regarding recontacting clients needs to be included in the overall CGRAP plan. If the institution does not have the resources to recontact clients with new developments, a statement can be added to the genetic test consent forms or client and referring physician letters indicating that the client is responsible for staying in touch with the CGRAP annually for new developments. Clients referred to an academic institution where they can enroll in research studies may have ongoing communication via newsletters or education programs. These strategies also can be used in clinical programs through a newsletter or electronic mailing lists.

QUALITY ASSURANCE

Quality assurance plans are a systematic approach to monitoring, assessing, and improving the quality of care. Many institutions providing cancer care have established measures based on the Institute of Medicine's (2001) framework to assess quality care for effectiveness, accessibility, and availability, as well as patient satisfaction with the care experience, use of services, cost of care, and informed health choice. This framework has been designed to ensure that cancer care would increase the likelihood of desired health outcomes and be consistent with current evidence. This approach facilitates comparison of health outcomes with national outcomes, adherence to best practice models, and current professional knowledge and skills based on training and adherence to clinical standards and guidelines.

Little data exist on quality assurance measures for cancer genetic risk assessment and counseling. Some CGRAP measures studied have used chart audits to find appropriate referrals for cancer risk assessment (Washburn et al., 2005) and program audits of staff competencies, documentation, and regulatory issues (Sein et al., 2004). Although several studies have been conducted on approaches to education and counseling (Collins et al., 2000; Wang, Gonzalez, Milliron, Strecher, & Merajver, 2005), a systematic review of trials evaluating interventions for familial breast cancer risk assessment found that the evidence on how best to deliver cancer genetic risk assessment services is insufficient (Sivell, Iredale, Gray, & Coles, 2007). Although further research will establish evidence on best practices, staff performance, and the impact of CGRAPs on health outcomes, this does not preclude the establishment of quality assurance plans.

Possible quality assurance plans may include the evaluation of clinical standards, staff performance, and client satisfaction via program evaluation or clinical audits. Patient satisfaction and health outcomes can be collected through follow-up questionnaires. Staff performance measures in cancer risk assessment can be written into job descriptions and annual evaluations. Other measures based on standard quality assurance plans can include the following.

- Clinical outcomes
  - Adherence to guidelines for education and counseling, medical management, and HIPAA regulations
  - Adherence to institutional policies for the CGRAP
  - Outcomes (e.g., number of clients counseled, number referred for further genetic or medical consultation)
- Staff performance
  - Compliance with ASCO recommendations for training
  - Staff supervision measures
  - Nursing adherence to *Scope and Standards of Practice and Essentials of Genetic and Genomic Nursing: Competencies, Curricula Guideline, and Outcome Indicators*
  - Staff evaluation
  - Number of consultations with experts
- Blood specimens
  - Measures to ensure that blood samples are correctly labeled, test request forms are accurate, and results are matched with the right sample
  - A double-check of labeling is reasonable, using both a colleague and the client to validate that what is written on the blood tube and test request form is accurate
- Client satisfaction (questionnaires or interviews)
  - Determines satisfaction with overall program, process, and client outcome
  - Assesses client communication with physician, nurse or genetic counselor, and other program staff. Was information clear? Were questions answered? Were recommendations given; if so, were the recommendations clear and services accessible?
  - Evaluates if client was treated with respect
  - Assesses if facility/space offered privacy
  - Would the client refer someone to the institution's CGRAP?
  - Is a mechanism for reporting adverse events available?
  - Are cancer events and stage of diagnosis documented (early diagnosis may show program impact)?
  - How were client complaints handled?

SUMMARY

Cancer genetic and genomic information is and will continue to be a necessary component of the delivery of appropriate risk reduction and diagnostic and prescribed care regimens recommended to individuals at risk for or being treated for cancer. Planning for the establishment of a CGRAP is a time-intensive endeavor that requires a multitude of resources and collaborative efforts that extend within and outside an institution or office. A competently staffed, well-developed CGRAP provides a valuable benefit to the community, clients, their families, and healthcare providers who grapple with the molecular complexities of inherited cancer syndromes and are concerned about communication and management of individual cancer risk.

The importance of continued research in the area of CGRAPs cannot be overstated. A gap in knowledge exists regarding optimal visit designs, mechanisms to ensure clients follow through with a referral to a CGRAP, and quality assurance measures. These gaps in knowledge will not close without continued research on the high-risk population now being served by emerging CGRAPs in communities across the country. Nurses hold a critical role in the delivery of CGRAP services and are positioned to facilitate continued collaboration with research centers and professional organizations to help close the knowledge gap.

REFERENCES

American College of Surgeons. (2009). Community outreach. In *Commission on cancer: Cancer program standards* (Rev. ed., pp. 69–74). Chicago: Author.

American Society of Clinical Oncology. (2003). American Society of Clinical Oncology policy statement update: Genetic testing for cancer susceptibility. *Journal of Clinical Oncology, 21*(12), 2397–2406.

Berliner, J.L., & Fay, A.M. (2007). Risk assessment and genetic counseling for hereditary breast and ovarian cancer: Recommendations of the National Society of Genetic Counselors. *Journal of Genetic Counseling, 16*(3), 241–260.

Bertagnolli, M.M., Niedzwiecki, D., Compton, C.C., Hahn, H.P., Hall, M., Damas, B., et al. (2009). Microsatellite instability predicts improved response to adjuvant therapy with irinotecan, fluorouracil, and leucovorin in stage III colon cancer: Cancer and Leukemia Group B Protocol 89803. *Journal of Clinical Oncology, 27*(11), 1814–1821.

Burke, W., Culver, J., Pinsky, L., Hall, S., Reynolds, S.E., Yasui, Y., et al. (2009). Genetic assessment of breast cancer risk in primary care practice. *American Journal of Medical Genetics Part A, 149A*(3), 349–356.

Centers for Medicare and Medicaid Services. (2005). *Health insurance portability and accountability act of 1996.* Retrieved May 22, 2009, from http://www.cms.hhs.gov/HIPAAGenInfo/Downloads/HIPAALaw.pdf

Centers for Medicare and Medicaid Services. (2009). *National provider identifier standards.* Retrieved April 30, 2009, from http://www.cms.hhs.gov/NationalProvIdentstand

Collins, V., Halliday, J., Warren, R., & Williamson, R. (2000). Assessment of education and counseling offered by a familial colorectal cancer clinic. *Clinical Genetics, 57*(1), 48–55.

Consensus Panel on Genetic/Genomic Nursing Competencies. (2009). *Essentials of genetic and genomic nursing: Competencies, curricula guidelines, and outcome indicators* (2nd ed.). Silver Spring, MD: American Nurses Association.

Daly, M.B., Stearman, B., Masny, A., Sein, E., & Mazzoni, S. (2005). How to establish a high-risk cancer genetics clinic: Limitations and successes. *Current Oncology Reports, 7*(6), 469–474.

Epplein, M., Koon, K.P., Ramsey, S.D., & Potter, J.D. (2005). Genetic services for familial cancer patients: A follow-up survey of National Cancer Institute Cancer Centers. *Journal of Clinical Oncology, 23*(21), 4713–4718.

Evaluation of Genomic Applications in Practice and Prevention. (2009, May). *EGAPP reviews.* Retrieved May 25, 2009, from http://www.egappreviews.org

Feero, W.G., Bigley, M.B., Brinner, K.M., & Family Health History Multi-Stakeholder Workgroup of the American Health Information Community. (2008). New standards and enhanced utility for family health history information in the electronic health record: An update from the American Health Information Community's Family Health History Multi-Stakeholder Workgroup. *Journal of the American Medical Informatics Association, 15*(6), 723–728.

Ganz, P.A., Kwan, L., Somerfield, M.R., Alberts, D., Garber, J.E., Offit, K., et al. (2006). The role of prevention in oncology practice: Results from a 2004 survey of American Society of Clinical Oncology members. *Journal of Clinical Oncology, 24*(18), 2948–2957.

Genetics and Public Policy Center. (2007). *Survey of direct-to-consumer testing statutes and regulations.* Retrieved April 19, 2009, from http://www.dnapolicy.org/resources/DTCStateLawChart.pdf

Hampel, H., Frankel, W.L., Martin, E., Arnold, M., Khanduja, K., Kuebler, P., et al. (2008). Feasibility of screening for Lynch syndrome among patients with colorectal cancer. *Journal of Clinical Oncology, 26*(35), 5783–5788.

Ho, C. (2004). How to develop and implement a cancer genetics risk assessment program: Clinical and economic considerations. *Oncology Issues, 19*(6), 22–26.

Hudson, K.L., Murphy, J.A., Kaufman, D.J., Javitt, G.H., Katsanis, S.H., & Scott, J. (2006). Oversight of U.S. genetic testing laboratories. *Nature Biotechnology, 24*(9), 1083–1090.

Institute of Medicine. (2001). *Crossing the quality chasm: A new health system for the 21st century.* Retrieved June 6, 2009, from http://www.iom.edu/Object.File/Master/27/184/Chasm-8pager.pdf

Jenkins, J., Calzone, K.A., Dimond, E., Liewehr, D.J., Steinberg, S.M., Jourkiv, O., et al. (2007). Randomized comparison of phone verses in-person BRCA1/2 predisposition genetic test result disclosure counseling. *Genetics in Medicine, 9*(8), 487–495.

Kauff, N.D., Domchek, S.M., Friebel, T.M., Robson, M.E., Lee, J., Garber, J.E., et al. (2008). Risk-reducing salpingo-oophorectomy for the prevention of BRCA1- and BRCA2-associated breast and gynecologic cancer: A multicenter, prospective study. *Journal of Clinical Oncology, 26*(8), 1331–1337.

Kausmeyer, D.T., Lengerich, E.J., Kluhsman, B.C., Morrone, D., Harper, G.R., & Baker, M.J. (2006). A survey of patient's experiences with the cancer genetic counseling process: Recommendations for cancer genetics programs. *Journal of Genetic Counseling, 15*(6), 409–431.

Lee, R., Beattie, M., Crawford, B., Mak, J., Stewart, N., Komaromy, M., et al. (2005). Recruitment, genetic counseling, and BRCA testing for underserved women at a public hospital. *Genetic Testing, 9*(4), 306–312.

Lu, K., Kauff, N., Powell, C.B., Chen, L.M., Cass, I., Lancaster, L., et al. (2009). Hereditary breast and ovarian cancer syndrome. *Gynecologic Oncology, 113*(1), 6–11.

Lindor, N.M., McMaster, M.L., Lindor, C.J., & Greene, M.H. (2008). Concise handbook of familial cancer susceptibility syndromes (2nd ed.). *Journal of the National Cancer Institute Monographs, 2008*(38), 1–93.

MacDonald, D.J., Sand, S., Kass, F., Blazer, K.R., Congleton, J., Craig, J., et al. (2006). The power of partnership: Extending comprehensive cancer center expertise in clinical cancer genetics to community breast cancer centers. *Seminars in Breast Disease, 9*(1), 39–47.

Nathanson, J.W., Zisman, T.L., Julian, C., McCaffrey, S., & Rubin, D.T. (2008). Identification of patients at increased risk for colorectal cancer in an open access endoscopy center. *Journal of Clinical Gastroenterology, 42*(9), 1025–1031.

National Cancer Institute. (2008). *Making health communication programs work.* Retrieved November 23, 2009, from http://www.cancer.gov/pinkbook

National Comprehensive Cancer Network. (2009). *Guidelines for detection, prevention, and risk reduction.* Retrieved April 12, 2009, from http://www.nccn.org/professionals/physician_gls/f_guidelines.asp

National Society of Genetic Counselors. (2008). *Billing and reimbursement toolkit: Billing for genetic counselors.* Retrieved April 11, 2009, from http://www.nsgc.org/members_only/tools/br_index.cfm

Robson, M.E., Storm, C.D., Weitzel, J., Wollins, D.S., Offit, K., & American Society of Clinical Oncology. (2010). American Society of Clinical Oncology policy statement update: Genetic and genomic testing for cancer susceptibility. *Journal of Clinical Oncology, 28*(5), 893–901.

Sabatino, S.A., McCarthy, E.P., Phillips, R.S., & Burns, R.B. (2007). Breast cancer risk assessment and management in primary care: Provider attitudes, practices, and barriers. *Cancer Detection and Prevention, 31*(5), 375–383.

Schneider, K.A., Chittenden, A.B., Branda, K.J., Keenan, M.A., Joffe, S., Patenaude, A.F., et al. (2006). Ethical issues in cancer genetics: 1) Whose information is it? *Journal of Genetic Counseling, 15*(6), 491–503.

Secretary's Advisory Committee on Genetics, Health, and Society. (2008). *U.S. system of oversight of genetic testing: A response to the charge of the secretary of health and human services.* Retrieved May 26, 2009, from http://oba.od.nih.gov/oba/SACGHS/reports/SACGHS_oversight_report.pdf

Sein, E., Mazzoni, S., Masny, A., & Stearman, B. (2004). Process evaluation of community-based cancer risk assessment programs. *Oncology Issues, 19*(6), 32–36.

Sivell, S., Iredale, R., Gray, J., & Coles, B. (2007). Cancer genetic risk assessment for individuals at risk of familial breast cancer. *Cochrane Database of Systematic Reviews* 2007, Issue 2. Art. No.: CD003721. DOI: 10.1002/14651858.CD003721.pub2.

Snyder, L.A., Soballe, D.B., Lahl, L.L., Nehrebecky, M.E., Soballe, P.W., & Klein, P.M. (2003). Development of the breast cancer education and risk assessment program. *Oncology Nursing Forum, 30*(5), 803–808.

Stopfer, J.E. (2000). Genetic counseling and clinical cancer genetics services. *Seminars in Surgical Oncology, 18*(4), 347–357.

Sweet, K.M., Bradley, T.L., & Westman, J.A. (2002). Identification and referral of families at high risk for cancer susceptibility. *Journal of Clinical Oncology, 20*(2), 528–537.

Tyler, C.V., Jr., & Snyder, C.W. (2006). Cancer risk assessment: Examining the family physician's role. *Journal of the American Board of Family Medicine, 19*(5), 468–477.

U.S. Preventive Services Task Force. (2005). Genetic risk assessment and BRCA mutation testing for breast and ovarian cancer susceptibility: Recommendation statement. *Annals of Internal Medicine, 143*(5), 355–361.

Wang, C., Gonzalez, R., Milliron, K.J., Strecher, V.J., & Merajver, S.D. (2005). Genetic counseling for BRCA1/2: A randomized controlled trial of two strategies to facilitate the education and counseling process. *American Journal of Medical Genetics Part A, 134A*(1), 66–73.

Washburn, N.J., Sommer, V.K., Spencer, S.E., Simmons, S.K., Adkins, B.W., Rogers, M.R., et al. (2005). Outpatient genetic risk assessment in women with breast cancer: One center's experience. *Clinical Journal of Oncology Nursing, 9*(1), 49–53.

Zon, R., Towle, E., Ndoping, M., Levinson, J., Colbert, A., & Williams, C. (2006). Reimbursement for preventive counseling services. *Journal of Oncology Practice, 2*(5), 214–218.

Zon, R.T., Goss, E., Vogel, V.G., Chlebowski, R.T., Jatoi, I., Robson, M.E., et al. (2009). American Society of Clinical Oncology position statement: The role of the oncologist in cancer prevention and risk assessment. *Journal of Clinical Oncology, 27*(6), 986–993.

CHAPTER 7

Genome-Wide Association Studies and Cancer

Lucia A. Hindorff, PhD, MPH, and Teri A. Manolio, MD, PhD

Professional Responsibilities Domain:
- Incorporate genetic and genomic technologies and information into registered nurse practice

(Consensus Panel on Genetic/Genomic Nursing Competencies, 2009)

INTRODUCTION

The completion of the human genome sequence and human haplotype maps of the most common form of genetic variation, the single nucleotide polymorphism (SNP), have led to a dramatic transformation in research into the genetics of common and **complex diseases** such as cancer (Altshuler et al., 2005; Frazer et al., 2007; Manolio, Brooks, & Collins, 2008). An estimated 10 million "common" SNPs or single-letter differences occur among individuals in the spelling of the 3 billion nucleotides that compose the human genome. SNPs that are located very close together on a chromosome tend to be inherited as a group or "haplotype block" so that one does not need to measure all 10 million SNPs, but only a subset of them to capture much of a person's genetic variation. Determining the frequencies and patterns of inheritance across SNPs was the goal of the International HapMap Consortium (International HapMap Project, 2003), which facilitated the development of cost-effective genotyping technologies that assay hundreds of thousands of SNPs across the genome in **genome-wide association** (GWA) studies. The National Institutes of Health Office of Extramural Research (n.d.) defines a GWA study as "any study of genetic variation across the entire human genome that is designed to identify genetic associations with observable traits (such as blood pressure or weight), or the presence or absence of a disease or condition." Implicit in this definition is that sufficient numbers of SNPs are genotyped to capture the vast majority of common variation (i.e., variant alleles [alternate forms of a gene or chromosomal locus that differ in DNA sequence] with a frequency of at least 5% in a population) throughout the entire genome. The goal is to identify common SNPs that may be associated with common diseases. Such studies typically involve hundreds of thousands of SNPs and are not limited to known genes or regulatory regions. Instead, they use hundreds of thousands of SNPs to assess genetic variation genome-wide in an almost "agnostic" fashion (Carlson, 2006), not hypothesis driven or limited. The current generation of genetic association studies relies on the **common disease, common variant hypothesis**, which suggests that genetic influences on many common diseases will be at least partly attributable to a limited number of allelic variants (one or a few at each major disease locus) that are present in more than 1%–5% of the population (Carlson; Collins, Guyer, & Charkravarti, 1997; Reich & Lander, 2001). A well-known example of a common SNP that has been related to disease is the variation in apolipoprotein E associated with risk of Alzheimer disease (Poirier et al., 1995).

The first association study commonly considered to be truly genome-wide was published in March 2005 (Klein et al., 2005), and by August 2008, more than 170 such studies had identified more than 300 genetic variants associated with more than 60 complex diseases and traits (Hindorff, Junkins, & Manolio, 2008; Manolio et al., 2008). In cancer alone, 15 SNPs associated with prostate cancer, eight SNPs associated with breast cancer, six SNPs associated with colorectal cancer, and two SNPs associated with lung cancer have been identified in 18 studies, most within 2007 and 2008 (see Table 7-1). Media reports publicizing associations between genetic variants and disease occur on a near-daily basis, yet these new findings, exciting as they may be, are generally some ways off from clinical application. Despite this, private companies (e.g., 23andme [www.23andme.com], deCODEme [www.decodeme.com], Navigenics [www.navigenics.com]) are beginning to market targeted genetic testing for specific diseases directly to consumers, as well as full research-grade genome-wide scans involving hundreds of thousands of SNPs.

What are health practitioners to make of this onslaught of information? How does it differ from that generated by studies of candidate genes such as *BRCA1* or Mendelian disorders such as hereditary nonpolyposis colorectal cancer? How does one explain these new findings to patients, or advise on whether to get tested for the "next new gene for disease X"? The goal of this chapter is to enable the reader to read and understand a GWA study sufficiently to apply its findings to practice where appropriate, and to explain it to patients when asked.

First, fundamental concepts of genetic epidemiology are introduced by tracing the progression of genetic association studies from **linkage** findings to candidate genes to GWA studies (see Figure 7-1). Next, examples of GWA studies in cancer are highlighted to illustrate more detailed methods and complexities in interpreting results. Opportunities for clinical application of GWA findings are then discussed, accompanied by criteria to help evaluate when a study will be clinically useful. Finally, several online resources for further information and enrichment are described.

THE ROAD TO GENOME-WIDE SCANS

As in any epidemiologic study, an association between a genetic variant and an outcome can be inferred by studying groups of individuals distinguished by whether or not they have the outcome of interest. Genetic epidemiology has the advantage that the risk factors of interest (the genetic variants) are passed from parents to children and are shared among closely related individuals. For this reason, early genetic epidemiology studies focused on families, often families with many affected relatives, making it more likely that a genetic basis for disease would be found. The presence or absence of a family history of a serious disease like cancer can be obtained readily from a patient, although accuracy may be a factor (Guttmacher, Collins, & Carmona, 2004).

Strong familial clustering of disease often, but not always, suggests a genetic basis. This is how variants in genes associated with very high risk of cancer in certain families were identified,

TABLE 7-1 Genome-Wide Association Results in Prostate, Breast, Colorectal, and Lung Cancer

Strongest SNP-Risk Allele	Genomic Region	Genes in or Near Region	Risk Allele Frequency	Odds Ratio [95% Confidence Interval]	P-value	Author
Prostate Cancer						
rs16901979-A	8q24.21	Intergenic	0.03	1.79 [1.53–2.11]	1×10^{-12}	Gudmundsson, Sulem, Manolescu, et al., 2007
rs6983267-G	8q24.21	Intergenic	0.50	1.26 [1.13–1.41]	9×10^{-13}	Yeager et al., 2007
rs4430796-A	17q12	TCF2	0.49	1.22 [1.15–1.30]	1×10^{-11}	Gudmundsson, Sulem, Steinthorsdottir, et al., 2007
rs1859962-G	17q24.3	gene-poor region	0.46	1.20 [1.14–1.27]	3×10^{-10}	
rs5945572-A	Xp11.22	GSPT2, MAGED1, NUDT10, NUDT11, LOC340602	0.35	1.23 [1.16–1.30]	4×10^{-13}	Gudmundsson et al., 2008
rs721048-A	2p15	EHBP1	0.19	1.15 [1.10–1.21]	8×10^{-9}	
rs10993994-T	10q11.23	MSMB	0.40	1.25 [1.17–1.34]	9×10^{-29}	Eeles et al., 2008
rs2735839-G	19q13.33	KLK3	0.85	1.20 [1.10–1.33]	2×10^{-18}	
rs7931342-G	11q13.2	Intergenic	0.51	1.19 [1.11–1.27]	2×10^{-12}	
rs9364554-T	6q25.3	NR	0.29	1.17 [1.08–1.26]	6×10^{-10}	
rs6465657-C	7q21.3	LMTK2	0.46	1.12 [1.05–1.20]	1×10^{-9}	
rs10993994-T	10q11.23	MSMB	0.40	1.16 [1.04–1.29]	7×10^{-13}	Thomas et al., 2008
rs4962416-C	10q26.13	CTBP2	0.27	1.17 [1.05–1.30]	2×10^{-7}	
rs10896449-G	11q13.2	Intergenic	0.52	1.10 [0.98–1.23]	2×10^{-8}	
Breast Cancer						
rs2981582-G	10q26.13	FGFR2	0.38	1.26 [1.23–1.30]	2×10^{-76}	Easton et al., 2007
rs3803662-C	16q12.1	TNCR9/ LOC643714	0.25	1.20 [1.16–1.24]	1×10^{-36}	
rs889312-A	5q11.2	MAP3K1	0.28	1.13 [1.10–1.16]	7×10^{-20}	
rs13281615-T	8q24.21	Intergenic	0.40	1.08 [1.05–1.11]	5×10^{-12}	
rs3817198-T	11p15.5	LSP1	0.30	1.07 [1.04–1.11]	3×10^{-9}	
rs1219648-G	10q26.13	FGFR2	0.40	1.20 [1.07–1.42]	1×10^{-10}	Hunter et al., 2007
rs13387042-A	2q35	Intergenic	0.50	1.20 [1.14–1.26]	1×10^{-13}	Stacey et al., 2007
rs3803662-T	16q12.1	Near TNRC9	0.27	1.28 [1.21–1.35]	6×10^{-19}	

(Continued on next page)

TABLE 7-1 Genome-Wide Association Results in Prostate, Breast, Colorectal, and Lung Cancer *(Continued)*

Strongest SNP-Risk Allele	Genomic Region	Genes in or Near Region	Risk Allele Frequency	Odds Ratio [95% Confidence Interval]	P-value	Author
rs2180341-G	6q22.33	ECHDC1, RNF146	0.21	1.41 [1.25–1.59]	3×10^{-8}	Gold et al., 2008
Colorectal Cancer						
rs6983267-G	8q24.21	Intergenic	0.49	1.27 [1.16–1.39]	1×10^{-14}	Tomlinson et al., 2007
rs10505477-A	8q24.21	ORF DQ515897	0.50	1.17 [1.12–1.23]	3×10^{-11}	Zanke et al., 2007
rs4939827-T	18q21.1	SMAD7	0.52	1.16 [1.09–1.27]	1×10^{-12}	Broderick et al., 2007
rs3802842-C	11q23.1	Intergenic	0.43	1.11 [1.08–1.15]	6×10^{-10}	Tenesa et al., 2008
rs16892766-C	8q23.3	EIF3H	0.07	1.27 [1.20–1.34]	3×10^{-18}	Tomlinson et al., 2007
rs10795668-G	10p14	Intergenic	0.67	1.12 [1.10–1.16]	3×10^{-13}	
Lung Cancer						
rs8034191-C	15q25.1	CHRNA5, CHRNA3, CHRNB4, IREB2, PSMA4, LOC123688	0.34	1.30 [1.23–1.37]	5×10^{-20}	Hung et al., 2008
rs8034191-G	15q25.1	LOC123688 CHRNA3, CHRNA5, PSMA4	NR	1.30 [1.15–1.47]	3×10^{-18}	Amos et al., 2008

NR—not reported; SNP—single nucleotide polymorphism

Only studies published through April 2008 with at least one association significant at 9.9×10^{-7} or less are shown, regardless of number of SNPs tested. Odds ratios range from 1.08 to 2.10. Gene regions corresponding to SNPs were identified from the UCSC Genome Browser. Named genes refer to either the most plausible candidate gene(s) within the associated region or the gene nearest the (currently known) most associated SNP in a region, with the associated region being determined by the linkage disequilibrium structure.

Note. From "A HapMap Harvest of Insights Into the Genetics of Common Disease," by T.A. Manolio, L.D. Brooks, and F.S. Collins, 2008, *Journal of Clinical Investigation, 118*(5), p. 1597. Copyright 2008 by American Society of Clinical Investigation. Adapted with permission.

such as the *TP53* gene in Li-Fraumeni syndrome (Malkin, 1994), *APC* in familial adenomatous polyposis (Bodmer, 2006), or *Rb* in retinoblastoma (DiCiommo, Gallie, & Bremner, 2000). Family studies initially were used to assess *heritability*, or familial clustering, of disease, as was typically done in studies of twins. Such studies were used to identify stronger similarities in disease characteristics between monozygotic twins (sharing all of their genetic content) than between dizygotic twins (sharing on average half of their genetic content), implying a genetic basis for the disease (Khoury, Beaty, & Cohen, 1993). Examination of inheritance patterns within nuclear families or multigenerational pedigrees suggested genetic transmission in **dominant**, **recessive**, or X-linked fashion and were important in identifying genes related to sickle-cell disease, cystic fibrosis, and familial hypercholesterolemia (Khoury et al.). Linkage studies involving at first sibling pairs and then large pedigrees were important predecessors to GWA studies.

The idea of genotyping anonymous markers (genetic variants of known location that serve as signposts to a specific region of association on a particular chromosome) originated in linkage studies where family members were genotyped for hundreds of such markers typically spaced about 10 million base pairs apart. Evidence that markers and disease traits were inherited together, or linked, was important evidence for a genetic basis for disease, particularly if the causative gene could be identified within the chromosomal region that showed evidence of linkage. These regions often contained dozens or hundreds of genes, so this preliminary evidence needed to be narrowed by **fine-mapping**, or adding many more markers within the linkage region to identify the specific genetic difference (with luck, even the specific nucleotide base change) producing the strongest linkage signal.

Family studies have the distinct advantage of controlling for ethnicity or ancestry differences between people with and without the disease, a situation often referred to as **population stratification**. This is important because even subtle differences in ancestry between cases and controls can confound results by demonstrating associations with variants unrelated to disease but differing because the ancestral origin of the individuals is different (Cardon & Abecasis, 2003). Conditions much more common in one ethnic group compared to another, such as diabetes in Pima Indians compared to people of European ancestry, will appear to be associated with all the thousands of alleles that differ in frequency between the

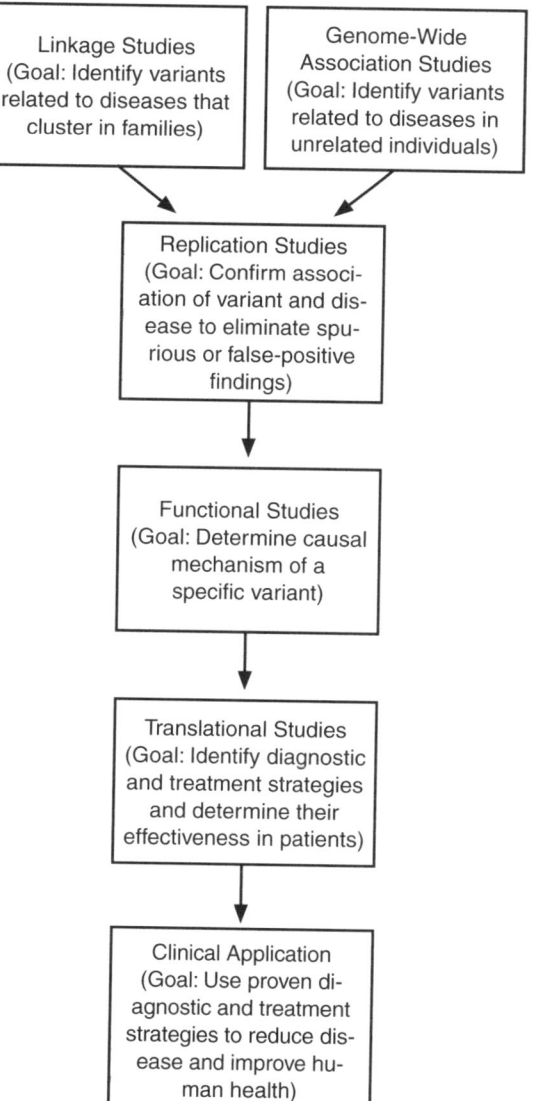

FIGURE 7-1 FLOW OF GENETIC STUDIES POTENTIALLY LEADING TO CLINICAL APPLICATION

Pima and other groups, even if those alleles have nothing to do with diabetes risk (Knowler, Williams, Pettitt, & Steinberg, 1988). In addition, an extended family displaying strong patterns of inheritance, especially for early-onset disease, often yields a strong genetic signal that might otherwise be indistinguishable from smaller signals, because of common environmental factors that families often share. Variants found in this way are often of large effect but may be relatively rare outside of that specific family or ethnic group, such as the *TP53* mutation in cancer-prone families (Malkin, 1994), or may appear to have different effects in people without strong family histories of disease, such as the *BRCA1* mutation in breast cancer (Struewing et al., 1997). The generalizability or relevance on a population-wide basis of variants identified within heavily affected families has appeared to be limited. In addition, extended families or even parent-offspring trios or sibling pairs often are more difficult to recruit into studies than unrelated individuals and, for many outcomes, require much larger sample sizes (Cordell & Clayton, 2005; Risch & Merikangas, 1996). Additionally, family studies may be less successful in identifying causal genes for outcomes with multiple contributing genes (Hirschhorn & Daly, 2005).

For these reasons, and because high-throughput genotyping technologies (platforms assaying hundreds of thousands of SNPs for less than $500 per sample) have evolved to the point that the smaller lengths of chromosomes shared between less closely related or unrelated individuals can be assayed reliably, studies of complex diseases are shifting away from linkage studies in families and toward association studies of unrelated individuals. Often these are case-control studies in which individuals with the outcome of interest (cases) are recruited along with individuals representing the population from which the cases arose but who do not have the disease (controls). This study design affords the advantage of identifying a large number of cases up front, compared to a cohort design in which a population-based sample of initially healthy individuals is followed prospectively for the outcome, but only a small proportion of the sample ultimately will develop the disease. The advantages presented by case-control studies in terms of ease and cost (large numbers of cases often are readily identifiable through specialty clinics or medical records) must be balanced against the often-selected nature of the cases who must survive the disease long enough to come to medical attention, be diagnosed, and entered into studies (Collins, 2004). Case-control studies also are prone to many other biases, such as recall bias in reporting exposures among cases compared to controls, and these biases can be more difficult to control than cohort studies, though careful attention to study design and minimization of bias is needed in both approaches (Manolio, Bailey-Wilson, & Collins, 2006).

The form of genetic variation most often assayed in the current generation of genetic association studies is the SNP, a single-letter difference in the spelling of the DNA. The two (typically, but rarely three or more) alternative forms, or alleles, and the precise chromosomal location of SNPs throughout the genome have been catalogued in databases such as dbSNP (www.ncbi.nlm.nih.gov/projects/SNP) and the University of California, Santa Cruz Genome Browser (http://genome.ucsc.edu/cgi-bin/hgGateway). Early genetic association studies typically genotyped single SNPs in candidate genes, or genes that were known or strongly suspected to be involved in the disease process. Because genotyping was so expensive, early studies often focused on SNPs in known functional regions of the genes, such as the protein coding regions (exons) or regulatory regions (promoters). Demonstration of an association between a variant and an observed disease or trait (phenotype) was regarded commonly as the definitive step in confirming biologically driven genetic hypotheses that were identified from laboratory or clinical findings. As technology developed, it became possible to perform multiple genotyping reactions simultaneously on a single individual (Hirschhorn & Daly, 2005). Studies naturally expanded to examining multiple SNPs within a gene, as well as one or a few SNPs within multiple candidate genes.

As information about genetic variation accumulated, several points became apparent. The strength of many genetic associations often was relatively modest, with less than a twofold difference in disease risk associated with carrying a particular allele. A typical association study, however, was only large enough to detect very strong associations or associations with very common alleles, and many associations were missed (Chanock et al., 2007; Ioannidis, Trikalinos, Ntzani, & Contopoulos-Ioannidis, 2003; Todd, 2006). Associations were likely to be missed because it simply was not possible to survey the majority of common genetic variations in a comprehensive manner. Also, data emerging from the **International HapMap Project** on patterns of **linkage disequilibrium**, a tendency for nearby SNPs on a chromosome to be inherited together, enabled researchers to be more successful in choosing SNPs that were proxies for many other nearby SNPs (**tagSNPs**), thus maximizing the information content within a minimal set of genotyped SNPs.

Robust associations in these early studies did not always correspond to expected genes or functional regions of genes, and studies naturally broadened to encompass larger sweeps of the genome. The HapMap and other genomic resources utilized linkage disequilibrium information to assemble a minimum subset of common SNPs necessary to survey significant portions of the genome. As genotyping platforms providing thousands and then hundreds of thousands of genotypes became commercially available, the prospect of conducting a genome-wide survey of genetic variation that was not dependent on prespecifying the correct genes became a reality.

Without a need to focus on candidate genes, researchers were able to design association studies that were not driven by an as-yet-imperfect knowledge of genome structure or function, but could theoretically encompass nearly all common genetic variation (Collins et al., 1997). The underlying hypothesis of this research thus progressed from SNPs in candidate genes being associated with disease to common variations across the genome being associated with common disease. An important caveat to GWA studies is that even a small error rate (e.g., 1% or less) applied across the very large number of statistical tests performed can yield an unwieldy number of **false-positive** results, as well as many **nominally significant** findings likely as a result of chance alone.

Because a goal of GWA studies is to identify genomic regions that include functional variants, so that disease etiology can be understood and potential treatments developed, careful attention must be given to the study design to help to distinguish true from false-positive results. The cost of genotyping hundreds of thousands or millions of SNPs to assay the majority of genomic variation in an individual is substantial and must be weighed against the need for larger sample sizes to detect smaller effects or rarer alleles (Ioannidis et al., 2003). The most common design is a multistage design, where intensive genome-wide genotyping is performed in an initial set of participants, and only the most promising associations judged by strict statistical criteria as being highly unlikely to be caused by chance are further investigated in one or more replication populations.

In summary, genome-wide scans evolved from studies of many dozens or even hundreds of families using a few hundred genetic markers to studies of many thousands of unrelated individuals using hundreds of thousands of markers, permitting interrogation of disease associations across the genome at an unprecedented level of precision. Care must be taken in genome-wide research to ensure associations are replicated in multiple studies to reduce the risk of false-positive findings or spurious associations. These studies have identified more than 300 variants associated with more than 60 diseases and traits, many of which are not located in any known genes and carry relatively low increased risk of disease. See Figure 7-2 for additional information on GWA studies.

FIGURE 7-2 GENOME-WIDE ASSOCIATION STUDY FACTS

What is a genome-wide association study?
A genome-wide association study is an approach that involves rapidly scanning hundreds of thousands of markers across the complete sets of DNA, or genomes, of many people to find genetic variations associated with a particular disease. Once new genetic associations are identified, researchers can use the information to develop better strategies to detect, treat, and prevent the disease. Such studies are particularly useful in finding genetic variations that contribute to common, complex diseases, such as asthma, cancer, diabetes, heart disease, and mental illnesses.

How are genome-wide association studies conducted?
To carry out a genome-wide association study, researchers use two groups of participants: people with the disease being studied and similar people without the disease. Researchers obtain DNA from each participant, usually by drawing a blood sample or by rubbing a cotton swab along the inside of the mouth to harvest cells.

Each person's complete set of DNA, or genome, is then purified from the blood or cells, placed on tiny chips and scanned on automated laboratory machines. The machines quickly survey each participant's genome for strategically selected markers of genetic variation, which are called single nucleotide polymorphisms, or SNPs.

If certain genetic variations are found to be significantly more frequent in people with the disease compared to people without disease, the variations are said to be "associated" with the disease. The associated genetic variations can serve as powerful pointers to the region of the human genome where the disease-causing problem may reside.

However, the associated variants themselves may not directly cause the disease. They may just be "tagging along" with the actual causal variants. For this reason, researchers often need to take additional steps, such as sequencing DNA base pairs in that particular region of the genome, to identify the exact genetic change involved in the disease.

What are the major types of genetic variation?
Variations—inter-individual differences at the level of DNA; one or more base pairs has undergone a change; the change could be at random or caused by an environmental factor such as radiation or a virus
- SNPs are the most common, occurring about once every 300 bases
- Copy number variations—Some DNA repeats itself (e.g., AAGAAGAAGAAG), and a variation in the number of repeats can occur.

How will genome-wide association studies benefit human health?
The impact on medical care from genome-wide association studies could potentially be substantial. Such research is laying the groundwork for the era of personalized medicine, in which the current one-size-fits-all approach to medical care will give way to more customized strategies. The information may enable health professionals to tailor prevention programs to each person's unique genetic makeup. In addition, if a patient does become ill, the information can be used to select the treatments most likely to be effective and least likely to cause adverse reactions in that particular patient.

Note. From *Genome-Wide Association Studies* and *Talking Glossary of Genetic Terms*, by National Institutes of Health National Human Genome Research Institute, 2009. Retrieved October 6, 2009, from http://www.genome.gov/20019523#1 and http://www.genome.gov/Glossary.

ANATOMY OF A GENOME-WIDE ASSOCIATION STUDY

By April 2008, results from several GWA studies in prostate, breast, colorectal, and lung cancer had been reported (see Table 7-1). Typically, these studies included patients under clinical care, often at tertiary care medical centers, and compared the patients to disease-free individuals selected from a variety of settings. Reports from these studies typically provide the **reference SNP (rs) number** as identified from the human genome sequence database and the specific allele associated with increased risk, as well as the genomic region in which it occurs and any nearby genes. This information sometimes differs between reports for the same SNP, as in rs803419 for lung cancer, because different investigators use slightly different versions of genomic databases or define association regions somewhat differently, but these differences are typically minor (Hung et al., 2008; Thorgeirsson et al., 2008). GWA reports also usually include estimates of **allele frequency**, **odds ratios**, and **p values**. Associations were replicated robustly for genes such as *TCF2*, *FGFR2*, *LSP1*, and *SMAD7* and for chromosomal regions without known genes, such as the 8q24 locus. Several reports included successful replication in populations with diverse ancestral backgrounds, increasing the confidence and generalizability of the findings (Gudmundsson, Sulem, Manolescu, et al., 2007). In addition, because populations of recent African ancestry have greater diversity and shorter stretches of linkage disequilibrium (International HapMap Consortium, 2003), demonstrating an association in these populations often permits the researcher to narrow the region to fewer SNPs or genes that tend to be inherited together in these populations.

Because a substantial proportion of GWA study associations were located in genes previously unsuspected to be related to cancer or in regions entirely outside of known genes, the hypothesis-free, "agnostic" approach may be more successful than candidate gene approaches in identifying new genetic variants important to cancer etiology. Intriguingly, one of these hits in the chromosome 8q24 region was independently identified in multiple studies of prostate, breast, and colorectal cancer (Easton et al., 2007; Gudmundsson, Sulem, Manolescu, et al., 2007; Tomlinson et al., 2007; Yeager et al., 2007; Zanke et al., 2007). Extensive additional research is needed to determine the functional significance of SNPs demonstrated to be associated with disease, both inside and outside of known candidate genes.

As noted previously, GWA studies generally feature a multistage sampling design, because performing genome-wide genotyping on all participants in both the initial and replication samples, who may number in the tens of thousands, is not cost-effective and often not necessary. For example, Zanke et al. (2007) conducted an initial study of nearly 100,000 SNPs in a population of 1,226 prostate cancer cases and 1,239 controls (see Figure 7-3). From this stage 1 or initial GWA "discovery" study, three successive replication studies were undertaken to determine which smaller subset of SNPs were replicated in each population. Variations on this basic design are common. Studies may enrich the initial case-control sample for familial cases of disease to help identify stronger associations (Easton et al., 2007; Tomlinson et al., 2007; Zanke et al., 2007). Including replication populations of a different ancestral background can help to assess whether study findings are generalizable across diverse populations (see Table 7-2). In this example, the rs16901979-A allele on chromosome 8 had an allele frequency of about 2%–4% in the four European ancestry populations studied (Iceland, Spain, Netherlands, Chicago) and fairly similar odds ratios except for a stronger risk in the Chicago sample. The African American sample, however, had a much higher frequency of this allele (greater than 40%) and a somewhat lower odds ratio, but confidence intervals on the odds ratios across groups overlapped widely. The higher allele frequency may be important in interpreting the higher incidence and more severe course of prostate cancer in African Americans (Jones & Wenzel, 2005).

Unfortunately, most GWA studies thus far have been conducted in populations of European ancestry, though this is changing (Manolio et al., 2007). It is worth noting that to date, no consensus has been established on the ideal relative sizes of the initial and replication populations, nor on the proportion of SNPs to carry forward (Hoover, 2007; Skol, Scott, Abecasis, & Boehnke, 2007), but in general, larger initial sample sizes are more likely to detect less common variants or variants of smaller effect. Conversely, large effect sizes in small studies are more likely to be overestimates or even spurious associations, so more credence should be placed in a large odds ratio (greater than 2) derived from a large study than a small one.

In summary, GWA studies provide key information on SNPs associated with disease including the reference SNP number, the risk allele and its frequency, the associated odds ratio and p-value, and nearby genes that might be implicated in the disease association. Most studies to date have been conducted in European ancestry populations.

IDENTIFYING PROMISING GENOMIC REGIONS

GWA genotyping is performed on commercial platforms or genotyping arrays, typically assaying 100,000 SNPs or more. The SNPs selected for these platforms tend to be common in frequency; those with allele frequencies of 5%

FIGURE 7-3   MULTISTAGE SAMPLING DESIGN FOR COLORECTAL CANCER STUDY

Stage 1: Ontario Familial Colorectal Cancer Registry
Purpose: Comprehensively survey common variation throughout the genome, without regard to function

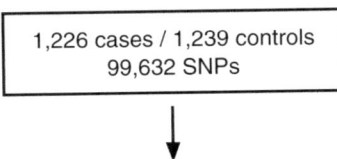

1,226 cases / 1,239 controls
99,632 SNPs

Stage 2: Seattle and Newfoundland case-control studies
Purpose: Replication of top SNPs from Stage 1

1,139 cases / 1,055 controls
1,143 SNPs

Stage 3: Scotland case-control study of early onset disease
Purpose: Replication of top SNPs from Stage 2

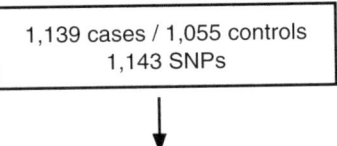

975 cases / 1,002 controls
76 SNPs

Stage 4: Scotland case-control study of early onset disease
Purpose: Replication of top SNPs from Stage 3

1,910 cases / 1,985 controls
9 SNPs

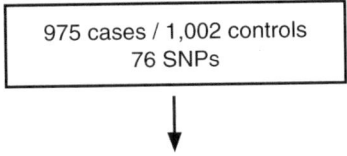

SNP—single nucleotide polymorphism

The experimental stage 1 and three sequential validation stages (2–4) are illustrated, with the number of successfully genotyped affected individuals and controls and the number of analyzed markers.

Note. From "Genome-Wide Association Scan Identifies a Colorectal Cancer Susceptibility Locus on Chromosome 8q24," by B.W. Zanke, C.M. Greenwood, J. Rangrej, R. Kustra, A. Tenesa, S.M. Farrington, et al., 2007, *Nature Genetics, 39*(8), p. 990. Copyright 2007 by Nature Publishing Group. Reprinted with permission.

TABLE 7-2 Association of rs16901979-A on Chromosome 8q24 With Prostate Cancer in Iceland, Spain, the Netherlands, and the United States

Study Population	Frequency		Odds Ratio (95% Confidence Interval)	P-value
	Affected Individuals	Controls		
European Ancestry				
Iceland	0.07	0.04	1.80 (1.47–2.20)	9.9×10^{-9}
Spain	0.07	0.04	1.71 (1.17–2.49)	5.2×10^{-3}
The Netherlands	0.03	0.02	1.58 (0.96–2.58)	0.07
Chicago	0.05	0.02	2.43 (1.32–4.50)	4.6×10^{-3}
All European	NR	0.03	1.79 (1.53–2.11)	1.1×10^{-12}
African-American Ancestry				
Baltimore	0.50	0.43	1.34 (1.09–1.64)	4.9×10^{-3}

NR—not reported

Note. From "Genome-Wide Association Study Identifies a Second Prostate Cancer Susceptibility Variant at 8q24," by J. Gudmundsson, P. Sulem, A. Manolescu, L.T. Amundadottir, D. Gudbjartsson, A. Helgason, et al., 2007, *Nature Genetics, 39*(5), p. 633. Copyright 2007 by Nature Publishing Group. Adapted with permission.

or less or in chromosomal regions not captured by the HapMap, such as centromeres and telomeres, are not well represented (Manolio et al., 2008). The number of SNPs on the platform directly correlates with the proportion of common variation tagged by the genotyped SNPs within each platform, though cross-platform comparisons are not always consistent. The Affymetrix® 500,000 platform, for example, provided similar genomic coverage to the Illumina® 317,000 platform because of differences in the approaches used to select the SNPs (Frazer et al., 2007). Affymetrix and Illumina are two companies that produced the genotyping platforms used in the majority of GWA studies to date. Genotyping platforms of 500,000–1 million SNPs have been estimated to capture 67%–89% of common SNP variation in populations of European and Asian ancestry and 46%–66% of variation in populations of recent African ancestry (Frazer et al.). Higher density platforms now also include probes for **copy number variants** that are not well tagged by SNPs. Copy number variants that feature stretches of genomic sequence that are deleted or duplicated in varying numbers have gained increasing attention because of their apparent high frequency and potential effect on gene expression (McCarroll & Altshuler, 2007). Most variations in the human genome can now be studied by genotyping a carefully selected few hundred thousand to one million genetic variants, a small proportion of the 10 million or so common variants that are thought to exist (Manolio et al., 2008).

Assessing the quality of both the individual samples to be genotyped and the individual SNPs to be assayed is crucial to ensuring the validity of a GWA study. Because SNPs are chosen for replication in a second-stage study primarily based on statistical evidence of associations (typically p-values), errors in association statistics can lead either to false-positive SNPs being carried forward to subsequent stages that should not have been, or to false-negative SNPs that should have been carried forward but were not. It is critical that investigators in GWA studies minimize genotyping errors and clearly describe their efforts to do so, as an error rate of even 0.1% among one million separate assays can lead to 1,000 false associations. Missing genotype data also can be very problematic, as they can bias results and lead to incorrect conclusions if data are not missing at random (and they rarely are).

Criteria for genotyping quality and for reporting quality control measures have been published and should include checks for sample quality and identity even prior to initiating genotyping (Chanock et al., 2007). Rare variants with **minor allele frequencies** of 1% or less in a given set of samples, even if they were more frequent in the reference samples used to develop the genotyping platform, can be very difficult to genotype reliably and often are excluded from data analysis. Other checks should ensure

- High concordance between duplicate samples
- High SNP "call rate," or proportion of samples for which an SNP can be measured (typically greater than 95%)
- Low rate of deviations from **Hardy-Weinberg equilibrium**, which typically indicates genotyping error
- Low rate of **Mendelian errors** of allelic transmission, which can be detected only if family members are included.

Once the initial stage of genotyping is complete, investigators perform tests of association between each SNP and the outcome. These association tests typically take one of two forms: (a) comparisons of allele or genotype frequencies in cases and controls using chi-square or Fisher exact tests, or (b) comparisons of levels of a continuous trait in people with and without a specific allele using t-tests or across three genotype classes (those with two copies of the minor allele or "minor allele homozygote," those with one copy of the minor allele or "heterozygote," and those with no copies of the minor allele, or "major allele homozygote") using analysis of variance (Burton, Tobin, & Hopper, 2005). For binary outcomes when participants either have the outcome or not (such as the presence or absence of prostate cancer), **relative risks** or odds ratios are estimated by dividing a measure of disease incidence or prevalence in one genotype group by the incidence in another genotype group. For continuous outcomes or measures spanning a range of possible values (such as height or cholesterol level), the results often are reported as an X-unit difference in the trait when comparing one genotype group to another, but continuous outcomes are not common in cancer studies.

Calculation of these SNP versus outcome associations involves fairly straightforward analyses that are familiar to those with an epidemiology or biostatistics background, but the challenge in this context is that they are repeated hundreds of thousands of times within a single study. Each SNP is then ranked by the significance of its association with the outcome (typically by smallest to largest p-value), and a prespecified number of "interesting" SNPs. Typically, SNPs with the smallest p-values are carried forward for genotyping in second- and third-stage replication populations.

To date, the criteria for selecting SNPs to carry forward to subsequent stages have not been agreed upon completely. Many investigators focus entirely on choosing SNPs with the smallest p-values and may carry a very large number forward into the second stage, whereas others may rely on prior knowledge, imperfect as it is, of potential gene function to carry forward specific SNPs. For example, at a cutoff of p = 0.05, out of every 100 SNPs tested, 5 would be declared statistically significant by chance alone. With the current generation of genotyping platforms that assay hundreds of thousands of SNPs, setting significance thresholds at this level will yield a large number of SNPs to be carried forward, perhaps more than the investigator can afford, and including many that are not likely to be associated with the disease at all. The advantage of carrying forward large numbers of SNPs is that it minimizes false negatives or SNPs that did not reach high significance in the initial sample, but this practice may do so subsequently when the initial and replication populations are combined. This is illustrated by the prostate cancer study of Thomas et al. (2008), in which two of the newly identified SNPs that were most significant in the combined replication phases ranked 24,233 and 24,407 in significance of the 27,000 carried over into the second stage.

Ultimately, researchers wish to distinguish the small number of true-positive signals from the large number of false-positive signals, but this may not be possible in the initial stages of a GWA study. To minimize the possibility of false-positive results, p-value thresholds have been adjusted to as low as 10^{-7} or 10^{-8}, but researchers commonly acknowledge that this is a conservative threshold likely to yield **false-negative** findings (missed associations) as well as false-positive ones (spurious associations). Another approach is to incorporate information about each SNP's hypothesized function to quantify the chance that a result is a false positive (Zanke et al., 2007). Using this approach, only the SNPs with the lowest probability of being a false-positive result based on available biologic information are carried forward. Another possible option is to rank the associations in terms of their population risk based on high prevalence, strong effect, or susceptibility to modification and to follow up the SNPs with the most potential for public health impact, though this approach is uncommon.

A typical table of results from a GWA study includes allele frequencies, relative risk estimates (usually expressed as odds ratios), and p-values for an "interesting" SNP at each stage of the study, as shown in Table 7-1. Visual representations of the massive amounts of resulting association data include genome-wide plots showing all associations across the genome from the "p" end of chromosome 1 to the "q" end of chromosome 22 or the X and Y chromosomes (see Figure 7-4). Association statistics often are shown as the $-\log_{10}$ of the p-value, so that p = 0.01 would be plotted as "2" on the y-axis and p = 10^{-7} as "7." A more focused view of an associated region is given in a locus plot showing the specific region of association, the SNPs tested, and the linkage disequilibrium relationships between them (see Figure 7-5). Genes or messenger RNA (mRNA) transcripts in the region often are indicated as well, which can help to suggest SNPs that may be playing a true causative role in the disease.

Journal editors generally require one or more replication samples even for publication of an initial study (Freimer & Sabatti, 2007; Todd, 2006), with subsequent papers then attempting to replicate or extend the findings to other populations or related phenotypes to strengthen the evidence for an etiologic role of the variant. If the associations are judged to be similar among the various stages, a pooled estimate combining all studies is appropriate and yields a more stable result because of the larger sample size (Zeggini et al., 2008).

In summary, GWA genotyping identifies genomic regions associated with disease and likely to contain a causal genetic variant. Stringent quality control standards are needed to avoid spurious findings or missing important associations. Analyses testing for these associa-

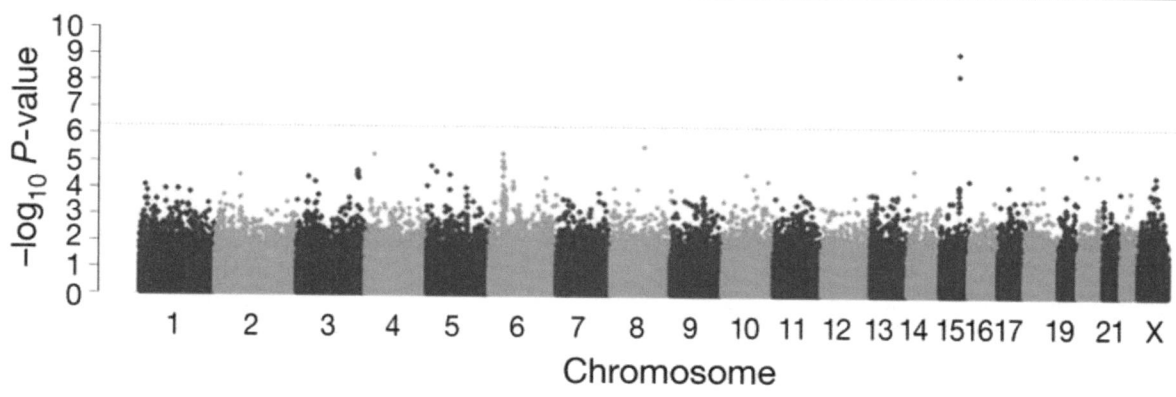

FIGURE 7-4. GENOME-WIDE PLOT OF ASSOCIATIONS OF 310,000 SINGLE NUCLEOTIDE POLYMORPHISMS WITH LUNG CANCER

This figure displays the distribution of $-\log_{10}$ p-values for the association between a SNP and lung cancer across the 22 autosomes and chromosome X. Each association is designated as a single point; the gray line indicates the 5×10^{-7} threshold of statistical significance. Two SNPs on chromosome 15 exceed this threshold.

Note. From "A Susceptibility Locus for Lung Cancer Maps to Nicotinic Acetylcholine Receptor Subunit Genes on 15q25," by R.J. Hung, J.D. McKay, V. Gaborieau, P. Boffetta, M. Hashibe, D. Zaridze et al., 2008, *Nature, 452*(7187), p. 634. Copyright 2008 by Nature Publishing Group. Reprinted with permission.

tions are relatively straightforward and generally are conducted one SNP at a time, though aggregating the findings across hundreds of thousands of SNPs is complicated by the potential for false-positive findings. This is typically addressed by testing the most strongly associated SNPs in a second or third replication study.

REPLICATION IN INDEPENDENT STUDIES

Replication of the findings from an initial GWA publication in subsequent independent populations is essential to establish the overall credibility of a genetic association. The strong emphasis placed on replication in GWA studies is in part because of the legacy of candidate gene studies where the literature contains many examples of initial reports of genetic associations that were not convincingly replicated (Hirschhorn, Lohmueller, Byrne, & Hirschhorn, 2002; Lohmueller, Pearce, Pike, Lander, & Hirschhorn, 2003; Manolio, Boerwinkle, O'Donnell, & Wilson, 2004). In a seminal review of this problem, Hirschhorn et al. showed that only 6 candidate gene associations of 600 were significant in 75% or more of reported publications. Statistical criteria for replication initially tended to vary across genetic association studies, but consensus criteria for replication in GWA studies have been published (Chanock et al., 2007). Ideally, replication should be demonstrated in populations with similar if not identical phenotype (disease or trait) definitions and similar distributions of other factors related to disease. Replication studies also should use the same genetic model (e.g., dominant, recessive, X-linked) and should be of similar magnitude and

FIGURE 7-5 LOCUS PLOT OF THE 8Q24 REGION AND COLORECTAL CANCER

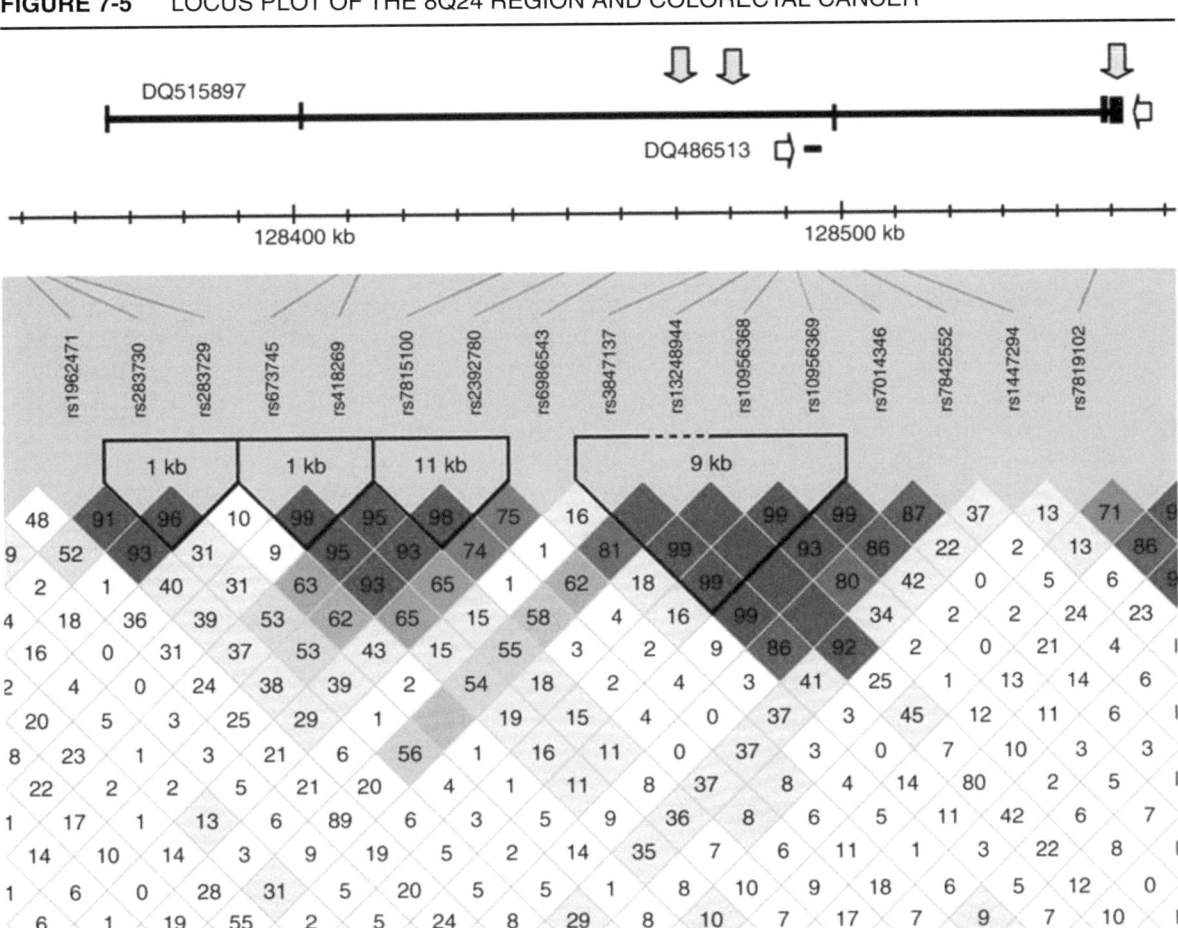

The top two lines denote the location of single nucleotide polymorphism (SNP) rs10505477 associated with colorectal cancer and nearby SNPs within the 8q24 region. The vertical lines denote boundaries of the mRNA transcripts DQ515897 and DQ486513. The shaded portion displays linkage disequilibrium (LD) information for pairs of nearby SNPs from stage 1. Darker squares correspond to comparisons with higher LD. SNPs rs10505477 and rs6983267, found within the indicated region of LD, are associated with the colon cancer phenotype.

Note. From "Genome-Wide Association Scan Identifies a Colorectal Cancer Susceptibility Locus on Chromosome 8q24," by B.W. Zanke, C.M. Greenwood, J. Rangrej, R. Kustra, A. Tenesa, S.M. Farrington, et al., 2007, *Nature Genetics, 39*(8), p. 992. Copyright 2007 by Nature Publishing Group. Reprinted with permission.

direction as the initial study. In addition, replication should be performed in studies large enough to distinguish the proposed effect from no effect, accounting for the fact that initial studies often overestimate the magnitude of an effect, and subsequent studies should be adequately powered to detect smaller effects. Most studies adopt a strict threshold for statistical significance in the initial stage (e.g., $p < 10^{-7}$) but may relax that threshold somewhat for follow-up studies because the number of hypotheses tested is lower when fewer SNPs are assayed. The precise choice of statistical thresholds probably is less important than the specification of replication criteria before the data are analyzed to preserve the unbiased nature of the GWA study.

As noted repeatedly throughout this chapter, replication in independent study samples is essential for identifying a robust association between a genetic variant and disease.

FINE MAPPING AND BEYOND: HINTS AT BIOLOGIC FUNCTION

Once an association is reliably identified, either in the initial study or in subsequent replication studies, more research must be conducted to identify the true causal SNP because SNPs on genotyping platforms are selected primarily for tagging the largest number of neighboring SNPs and not for biologic function. This process of "checking out the neighborhood" around an associated SNP (Witte, 2007) often is referred to as fine mapping in which all known SNPs in the region of the tagged SNP showing the association are tested for strength and consistency of their associations with the trait. Patterns of linkage disequilibrium or associations among SNPs also can provide clues to nearby SNPs or genes to investigate further. If two SNPs nearly always are inherited together, for example, and one is a functional SNP that changes the amino acid sequence of the resulting protein while its nearby tag SNP is assayed by the platform, this may be good evidence that the functional SNP plays a role in disease etiology.

Because genotyping platforms are limited to common SNPs, rarer variants not on the platform may be missed and actually may be causing the observed association signal. Sequencing of regions surrounding the associated SNP, which involves determining the precise genetic sequence, nucleotide by nucleotide, in a small sample of participants, can identify rare SNPs that might be tremendously important in disease causation (Cohen, Boerwinkle, Mosley, & Hobbs, 2006). Functional studies in cells, tissues, or animal models also strengthen the evidence for a particular SNP as playing a causal role in disease.

CHALLENGES FOR GENOME-WIDE ASSOCIATION STUDIES: PRESENT AND FUTURE

Some important statistical and biologic limitations of GWA studies also must be recognized. The strict statistical threshold used to identify promising SNPs for replication may exclude true causal regions that do not meet the cutoff if the causal variants are represented poorly by the SNPs on the platform, have small effects, or are rare in frequency. Nearly all replication attempts focus on replicating positive signals from previous studies. However, the problem of false negatives, or potentially missing a valid association, is also a major limitation of many GWA follow-up studies. Replication must be carried out in a thoughtful and systematic manner (Chanock et al., 2007). However, even when replication is carefully attempted, two studies may come to different conclusions for valid reasons (Lohmueller et al., 2003). For example, as noted previously, the association is often strongest in the initial study and weakens as additional studies are performed, which is a phenomenon termed the **winner's curse** (Lohmueller et al.). Subsequent studies that assume a similar effect size as the initial study actually may have included too few subjects to detect smaller associations and thus may fail to replicate the initial association. Other possible sources of inconsistency are population stratification, as noted previously, or **interaction** (inconsistency or modification of associations) because of other genetic or nongenetic factors (Lai et al., 2006).

Biologic considerations also may factor into the success of the GWA approach in identifying functional variants of clinical or public health significance. Early GWA studies quickly identified diseases for which associations were easily discovered and replicated (for example, Crohn disease and macular degeneration), raising the possibility that some diseases may be more amenable than others to the GWA approach. Initial results may reflect the "low-hanging fruit" of genetic associations—such as those having a large effect or high minor allele frequencies.

Diseases complicated by **genetic heterogeneity** (different genes or variants that cause disease in different ancestral groups) or by genes that depend on the presence of another genetic variant or environmental factor for the expression of a disease state will be more difficult to study. For many complex diseases such as cancer, genetic variants that have been identified in GWA studies and convincingly replicated are associated with small effects (that is, relative risks or odds ratios of less than 1.5).

Are such effects too small to be meaningful? In some cases, perhaps not. Small effects may reflect the imprecision in choosing a genetic variant for genotyping that imperfectly tags the true causal variant, which actually may demonstrate a larger effect. Or, they may represent a mixture of at-risk individuals, most at little to no risk, but some at high risk. More importantly, they may provide clues to biologic pathways or therapeutic targets for which drugs can be developed that may help everyone, even if they do not carry the causal variant (Manolio et al., 2008). Finally, even small relative risks may have a public health impact if the baseline risk in the general population is very high and the genetic variant is common. One of the greatest challenges to the success of GWA studies will be diseases caused by rare variants for which the common disease/common variant hypothesis does not hold (Collins et al., 1997; Manolio et al., 2008).

CLINICAL IMPLICATIONS AND FUTURE DIRECTIONS

Although GWA studies are reported prominently in scientific journals and in other media, the current generation of data is far from ready to be integrated into clinical care (Pearson & Manolio, 2008). As discussed previously, many SNPs identified from such studies have unknown function. Additionally, unlike many Mendelian disorders, SNPs from GWA studies in complex diseases do not predict unequivocally who will develop disease and who will remain free of it; rather, people who have a particular genotype have a greater risk of developing disease compared to people who do not.

The distinction between disease prediction and disease susceptibility is worth noting because for many common variants, a substantial number of individuals who do not have the at-risk genotype may develop disease anyway because of environmental or other factors. Indeed, for common diseases such as hypertension or diabetes, environmental or lifestyle factors may play such a strong role relative to genetics that many individuals with the genotype will develop disease for reasons that probably are unrelated to genotype (Cooper, 2003). Individuals who carry the genotype may not develop disease if other important factors are not present; this concept is perhaps more intuitive considering that an SNP with a frequency of 40% does not have high predictive power if the outcome only occurs in a few percent of the population. Although exceptions exist, most SNPs identified from GWA studies in cancer exhibit modest associations (odds ratios well below 2, see Table 7-1). A positive family history, which is often simpler to obtain, typically carries a three- to fourfold increased risk and is extremely useful in identifying people to target for more intensive screening (Guttmacher et al., 2004; Yoon et al., 2002). Given that the variants found to date explain such a small proportion of the familial clustering of cancer, one might conclude that either very many more variants are to be found or that the identified variants interact with environmental factors that also are shared by family members.

Identifying subgroups of individuals in whom SNP outcome associations differ according to the presence or absence of other SNPs or environmental factors might be more clinically useful. An important limitation to the SNPs on current genome-wide platforms is the focus on common genetic variation. If the true underlying biology of some cancers depends on rare variants that differ among affected individuals, GWA studies are unlikely to have the large numbers of participants necessary to detect these associations.

Although very few (arguably no) SNPs identified by GWA studies currently are ready for clinical application, health practitioners would still benefit from learning how to interpret a GWA study and from thinking critically about the steps necessary for integration of such SNPs into clinical care. With the increasing emphasis placed on the very large population sizes necessary to identify robust findings, interest has generated in recruiting participants from large hospitals or health organizations, where electronic medical records serve as a rich and largely untapped data resource. Patients are becoming more aware of population genetic research, either through media reports or direct marketing of personal genomic services, and are likely to rely on their primary care providers for informed decision making. Genetic variants influencing response to pharmacologic treatment or other interventions are already beginning to be identified, and genetic testing in this context may serve an important role in risk stratification or tailored therapies (Maitland, Vasisht, & Ratain, 2006; Workman, 2001). At the very least, the revolution in GWA studies is helping to shape the discussion and policy around personalized medicine. Treating each patient with the right treatment at the right time is a central goal of clinical care, whether it ultimately relies on genetic information or not.

What sort of criteria would help advance a GWA study finding toward the clinic? First, the study must be scientifically sound. Results should generalize beyond the initial population and demonstrate consistency across important subgroups such as those defined by age, sex, or race. Interested readers of scientific literature may consider published advice on important questions to ask when reading a GWA study (Hattersley & McCarthy, 2005; Pearson & Manolio, 2008) (see Figure 7-6). An additional factor to consider is the strength and significance of the association. Ideally, SNPs should demonstrate an appreciable relative risk (e.g., size of the odds ratio or relative risk) as well as the public health significance (e.g., absolute risk or **population attributable risk**). Finally, genetic information will have perhaps the greatest healthcare impact when it can be used to allocate healthcare resources to individuals who would receive a specific and unique benefit not offered to the population at large.

SUMMARY

GWA studies use high-throughput genotyping technologies to assay hundreds of thousands of SNPs and relate them to cancer and cancer-related traits. In cancer alone, more than 30 SNPs and a dozen genes have been associated with breast, prostate, colorectal, and lung cancer. Many of these genes were not previously suspected of playing a role in cancer, and some of the strongest SNP associations are in genomic regions containing no genes at all.

GWA studies represent a powerful new tool for identifying genetic variants related to cancer, but they have important limitations, including their potential for false-positive and false-negative results and for biases related to the selection of study subjects and genotyping errors. Their primary use for the foreseeable future likely will be the investigation of biologic pathways of disease causation and normal health and development. Clinical application of these findings will require firm evidence that testing for them adds information to known risk factors (e.g., age, smoking, family history for cancer), that effective interventions are available, that improved outcomes justify the associated costs, and that obtaining this information does not have serious adverse consequences for individuals and their families. Although GWA findings are clearly many steps removed from actual clinical use at present, specific applications of these findings in prevention and treatment now are actively being pursued.

FIGURE 7-6 TEN BASIC QUESTIONS TO ASK ABOUT A GENOME-WIDE ASSOCIATION STUDY

1. Are the cases defined clearly and reliably so that they can be compared with patients typically seen in clinical practice?
2. Are case and control participants demonstrated to be comparable to each other on important characteristics that might also be related to genetic variation and to the disease?
3. Was the study of sufficient size to detect modest odds ratios or relative risks (1.3–1.5)?
4. Was the genotyping platform of sufficient density to capture a large proportion of the variation in the population studied?
5. Were appropriate quality control measures applied to genotyping assays, including visual inspection of cluster plots and replication on an independent genotyping platform?
6. Did the study reliably detect associations with previously reported and replicated variants (known positives)?
7. Were stringent corrections applied for the many thousands of statistical tests performed in defining the p-value for significant associations?
8. Were the results replicated in independent population samples?
9. Were the replication samples comparable in geographic origin and phenotype definition, and if not, did the differences extend the applicability of the findings?
10. Was evidence provided for a functional role for the gene polymorphism identified?

Note. From "How to Interpret a Genome-Wide Association Study," by T.A. Pearson and T.A. Manolio, 2008, *JAMA, 299*(11), p. 1342. Copyright 2008 by American Medical Association. Reprinted with permission.

RESOURCES

GWA study literature accumulates at a rapid pace and readers may wish to consult the following resources, adapted from a catalog of Internet resources for clinicians (Uhlmann & Guttmacher, 2008) for updated information. Also included are several resources that address general principles of evaluating GWA studies that are broadly applicable.

For Healthcare Providers or Researchers

- Office of Population Genomics, National Human Genome Research Institute, National Institutes of Health (www.genome.gov/19518660): This office promotes multidisciplinary research in epidemiology and genomics by applying genomic technologies to existing population and clinical studies and developing new population resources for investiga-

tion of genetic and environmental contributions to complex diseases. Includes an up-to-date catalog of novel SNPs identified from published GWA studies.
- Office of Public Health Genomics, Centers for Disease Control and Prevention (www.cdc.gov/genomics): This office promotes the integration of genomics into public health research, policy, and practice in order to improve the lives and health of all people. Includes a curated database of GWA studies as part of the HuGENet knowledge base.
- Department of Energy Genome Glossary (www.ornl.gov/sci/techresources/Human_Genome/glossary): An excellent, comprehensive glossary of genetic terms from the Department of Energy Human Genome Program.
- GeneTests (www.genetests.org): A publicly funded medical genetics information resource developed for physicians, other healthcare providers, and researchers. Includes expert-authored disease reviews and a directory of genetic testing laboratories.
- Cancer Genetics Services Directory (www.cancer.gov/search/genetics_services): This directory lists professionals who provide services related to cancer genetics such as cancer risk assessment, genetic counseling, genetic susceptibility testing, and others.
- Genetic and Rare Diseases Information Center (http://rarediseases.info.nih.gov): This office coordinates research and information on rare diseases at the National Institutes of Health and for the rare diseases community.
- OMIM® (Online Mendelian Inheritance in Man, www.ncbi.nlm.nih.gov/sites/entrez?db=OMIM): This database is a catalog of human genes and genetic disorders authored and edited by Dr. Victor A. McKusick and his colleagues at Johns Hopkins and elsewhere, developed for the Internet by the National Center for Biotechnology Information.
- Centers for Disease Control and Prevention (www.cdc.gov/genomics/famhistory/famhist.htm): An excellent compilation of resources and tools for understanding and promoting the use of family history information for the improvement of health.
- American Medical Association Physician Resources (www.ama-assn.org/ama/pub/category/2380.html): A series of family history tools that can aid the health provider in collecting family history information for prenatal, pediatric, and adult patients.
- National Society of Genetic Counselors (www.nsgc.org/consumer/familytree/index.cfm): An instructive resource for learning how to record a family history.
- National Guideline Clearinghouse (www.guideline.gov): A public resource for evidence-based clinical practice guidelines (search for "genetics" and name of condition).
- National Coalition for Health Professional Education in Genetics (www.nchpeg.org): A coalition of health professional organizations whose purpose is to promote health professional education and access to information about advances in human genetics. Includes core competencies and core genetic principles important for all healthcare professionals.
- International Society of Nurses in Genetics (www.isong.org): An organization whose goals include enabling a forum for education and support for nurses providing genetic health care, promoting the integration of the nursing process into the delivery of genetic healthcare services, and advancing nursing research in human genetics. Includes a comprehensive list of nursing-specific resources for research, practice, and education.

For Patients or Consumers
- Genetics Home Reference (www.ghr.nlm.nih.gov): A consumer-friendly resource providing information about the effects of genetic variations on human health. Includes infor-

mation on specific genes and diseases, as well as concepts and tools for understanding human genetics.

- U.S. Surgeon General's Family History Initiative (https://familyhistory.hhs.gov): The starting point for accessing My Family Health Portrait, an easy-to-use tool that allows users to create a personalized and computerized family health history report.
- National Center for Biotechnology Information Genes and Disease (www.ncbi.nlm.nih.gov/books/bv.fcgi?rid=gnd): This resource is a collection of articles that discuss genes and the diseases that they cause, organized by parts of the body that they affect.
- Genetic Alliance (family history tools and resources for consumers) (www.geneticalliance.org/tools): A series of dynamic resources that emphasize expanded access to quality vetted information, including family history resources, and a guide for patients and professionals.

REFERENCES

Altshuler, D., Brooks, L.D., Chakravarti, A., Collins, F.S., Daly, M.J., & Donnelly, P. (2005). A haplotype map of the human genome. *Nature, 437*(7063), 1299–1320.

Amos, C.I., Wu, X., Broderick, P., Gorlov, I.P., Gu, J., Eisen, T., et al. (2008). Genome-wide association scan of tag SNPs identifies a susceptibility locus for lung cancer at 15q25.1. *Nature Genetics, 40*(5), 616–622.

Bodmer, W.F. (2006). Cancer genetics: Colorectal cancer as a model. *Journal of Human Genetics, 51*(5), 391–396.

Broderick, P., Carvajal-Carmona, L., Pittman, A.M., Webb, E., Howarth, K., Rowan, A., et al. (2007). A genome-wide association study shows that common alleles of SMAD7 influence colorectal cancer risk. *Nature Genetics, 39*(11), 1315–1317.

Burton, P.R., Tobin, M.D., & Hopper, J.L. (2005). Key concepts in genetic epidemiology. *Lancet, 366*(9489), 941–951.

Cardon, L.R., & Abecasis, G.R. (2003). Using haplotype blocks to map human complex trait loci. *Trends in Genetics, 19*(3), 135–140.

Carlson, C.S. (2006). Agnosticism and equity in genome-wide association studies. *Nature Genetics, 38*(6), 605–606.

Chanock, S.J., Manolio, T., Boehnke, M., Boerwinkle, E., Hunter, D.J., Thomas, G., et al. (2007). Replicating genotype-phenotype associations. *Nature, 447*(7145), 655–660.

Cohen, J.C., Boerwinkle, E., Mosley, T.H., Jr., & Hobbs, H.H. (2006). Sequence variations in PCSK9, low LDL, and protection against coronary heart disease. *New England Journal of Medicine, 354*(12), 1264–1272.

Collins, F.S. (2004). The case for a U.S. prospective cohort study of genes and environment. *Nature, 429*(6990), 475–477.

Collins, F.S., Guyer, M.S., & Charkravarti, A. (1997). Variations on a theme: Cataloging human DNA sequence variation. *Science, 278*(5343), 1580–1581.

Consensus Panel on Genetic/Genomic Nursing Competencies. (2009). *Essentials of genetic and genomic nursing: Competencies, curricula guidelines, and outcome indicators* (2nd ed.). Silver Spring, MD: American Nurses Association.

Cooper, R.S. (2003). Gene-environment interactions and the etiology of common complex disease. *Annals of Internal Medicine, 139*(5, Pt. 2), 437–440.

Cordell, H.J., & Clayton, D.G. (2005). Genetic association studies. *Lancet, 366*(9491), 1121–1131.

DiCiommo, D., Gallie, B.L., & Bremner, R. (2000). Retinoblastoma: The disease, gene, and protein provide critical leads to understand cancer. *Seminars in Cancer Biology, 10*(4), 255–269.

Easton, D.F., Pooley, K.A., Dunning, A.M., Pharoah, P.D., Thompson, D., Ballinger, D.G., et al. (2007). Genome-wide association study identifies novel breast cancer susceptibility loci. *Nature, 447*(7148), 1087–1093.

Eeles, R.A., Kote-Jarai, Z., Giles, G.G., Olama, A.A., Guy, M., Jugurnauth, S.K., et al. (2008). Multiple newly identified loci associated with prostate cancer susceptibility. *Nature Genetics, 40*(3), 316–321.

Frazer, K.A., Ballinger, D.G., Cox, D.R., Hinds, D.A., Stuve, L.L., Gibbs, R.A., et al. (2007). A second generation human haplotype map of over 3.1 million SNPs. *Nature, 449*(7164), 851–861.

Freimer, N.B., & Sabatti, C. (2007). Human genetics: Variants in common diseases. *Nature, 445*(7130), 828–830.

Gold, B., Kirchhoff, T., Stefanov, S., Lautenberger, J., Viale, A., Garber, J., et al. (2008). Genome-wide association study provides evidence for a breast cancer risk locus at 6q22.33. *Proceedings of the National Academy of Sciences, 105*(11), 4340–4345.

Gudmundsson, J., Sulem, P., Manolescu, A., Amundadottir, L.T., Gudbjartsson, D., Helgason, A., et al. (2007). Genome-wide association study identifies a second prostate cancer susceptibility variant at 8q24. *Nature Genetics, 39*(5), 631–637.

Gudmundsson, J., Sulem, P., Rafnar, T., Bergthorsson, J.T., Manolescu, A., Gudbjartsson, D., et al. (2008). Common sequence variants on 2p15 and Xp11.22 confer susceptibility to prostate cancer. *Nature Genetics, 40*(3), 281–283.

Gudmundsson, J., Sulem, P., Steinthorsdottir, V., Bergthorsson, J.T., Thorleifsson, G., Manolescu, A., et al. (2007). Two variants on chromosome 17 confer prostate cancer risk, and the one in *TCF2* protects against type 2 diabetes. *Nature Genetics, 39*(8), 977–983.

Guttmacher, A.E., Collins, F.S., & Carmona, R.H. (2004). The family history—more important than ever. *New England Journal of Medicine, 351*(22), 2333–2336.

Hattersley, A.T., & McCarthy, M.I. (2005). What makes a good genetic association study? *Lancet, 366*(9493), 1315–1323.

Hindorff, L.A., Junkins, H.A., & Manolio, T.A. (2008). *A catalog of published genome-wide association studies.* Retrieved August 23, 2008, from http://www.genome.gov/gwastudies

Hirschhorn, J.N., & Daly, M.J. (2005). Genome-wide association studies for common diseases and complex traits. *Nature Reviews: Genetics, 6*(2), 95–108.

Hirschhorn, J.N., Lohmueller, K., Byrne, E., & Hirschhorn, K. (2002). A comprehensive review of genetic association studies. *Genetics in Medicine, 4*(2), 45–61.

Hoover, R.N. (2007). The evolution of epidemiologic research: From cottage industry to "big" science. *Epidemiology, 18*(1), 13–17.

Hung, R.J., McKay, J.D., Gaborieau, V., Boffetta, P., Hashibe, M., Zaridze, D., et al. (2008). A susceptibility locus for lung cancer maps to nicotinic acetylcholine receptor subunit genes on 15q25. *Nature, 452*(7187), 633–637.

Hunter, D.J., Kraft, P., Jacobs, K.B., Cox, D.G., Yeager, M., Hankinson, S.E., et al. (2007). A genome-wide association study identifies alleles in *FGFR2* associated with risk of sporadic postmenopausal breast cancer. *Nature Genetics, 39*(7), 870–874.

International HapMap Consortium. (2003). The International HapMap Project. *Nature, 426*(6968), 789–796.

Ioannidis, J.P., Trikalinos, T.A., Ntzani, E.E., & Contopoulos-Ioannidis, D.G. (2003). Genetic associations in large versus small studies: An empirical assessment. *Lancet, 361*(9357), 567–571.

Jones, R.A., & Wenzel, J. (2005). Prostate cancer among African-American males: Understanding the current issues. *Journal of National Black Nurses' Association, 16*(1), 55–62.

Khoury, M.J., Beaty, T.H., & Cohen, B.H. (1993). *Fundamentals of genetic epidemiology.* New York: Oxford University Press.

Klein, R.J., Zeiss, C., Chew, E.Y., Tsai, J.Y., Sackler, R.S., Haynes, C., et al. (2005). Complement factor H polymorphism in age-related macular degeneration. *Science, 308*(5720), 385–389.

Knowler, W.C., Williams, R.C., Pettitt, D.J., & Steinberg, A.G. (1988). Gm3;5,13,14 and type 2 diabetes mellitus: An association in American Indians with genetic admixture. *American Journal of Human Genetics, 43*(4), 520–526.

Lai, C.Q., Corella, D., Demissie, S., Cupples, L.A., Adiconis, X., Zhu, Y., et al. (2006). Dietary intake of n-6 fatty acids modulates effect of apolipoprotein A5 gene on plasma fasting triglycerides, remnant lipoprotein concentrations, and lipoprotein particle size: The Framingham Heart Study. *Circulation, 113*(17), 2062–2070.

Lohmueller, K.E., Pearce, C.L., Pike, M., Lander, E.S., & Hirschhorn, J.N. (2003). Meta-analysis of genetic association studies supports a contribution of common variants to susceptibility to common disease. *Nature Genetics, 33*(2), 177–182.

Maitland, M.L., Vasisht, K., & Ratain, M.J. (2006). *TPMT, UGT1A1*, and *DPYD*: Genotyping to ensure safer cancer therapy? *Trends in Pharmacological Sciences, 27*(8), 432–437.

Malkin, D. (1994). Germ line *p53* mutations and heritable cancer. *Annual Review of Genetics, 28*, 443–465.

Manolio, T.A., Bailey-Wilson, J.E., & Collins, F.S. (2006). Genes, environment and the value of prospective cohort studies. *Nature Reviews Genetics, 7*(10), 812–820.

Manolio, T.A., Boerwinkle, E., O'Donnell, C.J., & Wilson, A.F. (2004). Genetics of ultrasonographic carotid atherosclerosis. *Arteriosclerosis, Thrombosis, and Vascular Biology, 24*(9), 1567–1577.

Manolio, T.A., Brooks, L.D., & Collins, F.S. (2008). A HapMap harvest of insights into the genetics of common disease. *Journal of Clinical Investigation, 118*(5), 1590–1605.

Manolio, T.A., Rodriguez, L.L., Brooks, L., Abecasis, G., Ballinger, D., Daly, M., et al. (2007). New models of collaboration in genome-wide association studies: The Genetic Association Information Network. *Nature Genetics, 39*(9), 1045–1051.

McCarroll, S.A., & Altshuler, D.M. (2007). Copy-number variation and association studies of human disease. *Nature Genetics, 39*(Suppl. 7), S37–S42.

National Institutes of Health Office of Extramural Research. (n.d.). *Genome-wide association studies (GWAS).* Retrieved October 5, 2009, from http://grants.nih.gov/grants/gwas

Pearson, T.A., & Manolio, T.A. (2008). How to interpret a genome-wide association study. *JAMA, 299*(11), 1335–1344.

Poirier, J., Delisle, M.C., Quirion, R., Aubert, I., Farlow, M., Lahiri, D., et al. (1995). Apolipoprotein E4 allele as a predictor of cholinergic deficits and treatment outcome in Alzheimer disease. *Proceedings of the National Academy of Sciences, 92*(26), 12260–12264.

Reich, D.E., & Lander, E.S. (2001). On the allelic spectrum of human disease. *Trends in Genetics, 17*(9), 502–510.

Risch, N., & Merikangas, K. (1996). The future of genetic studies of complex human diseases. *Science, 273*(5281), 1516–1517.

Skol, A.D., Scott, L.J., Abecasis, G.R., & Boehnke, M. (2007). Optimal designs for two-stage genome-wide association studies. *Genetic Epidemiology, 31*(7), 776–788.

Stacey, S.N., Manolescu, A., Sulem, P., Rafnar, T., Gudmundsson, J., Gudjonsson, S.A., et al. (2007). Common variants on chromosomes 2q35 and 16q12 confer susceptibility to estrogen receptor-positive breast cancer. *Nature Genetics, 39*(7), 865–869.

Struewing, J.P., Hartge, P., Wacholder, S., Baker, S.M., Berlin, M., McAdams, M., et al. (1997). The risk of cancer associated with specific mutations of *BRCA1* and *BRCA2* among Ashkenazi Jews. *New England Journal of Medicine, 336*(20), 1401–1408.

Tenesa, A., Farrington, S.M., Prendergast, J.G., Porteous, M.E., Walker, M., Haq, N., et al. (2008). Genome-wide association scan identifies a colorectal cancer susceptibility locus on 11q23 and replicates risk loci at 8q24 and 18q21. *Nature Genetics, 40*(5), 631–637.

Thomas, G., Jacobs, K.B., Yeager, M., Kraft, P., Wacholder, S., Orr, N., et al. (2008). Multiple loci identified in a genome-wide association study of prostate cancer. *Nature Genetics, 40*(3), 310–315.

Thorgeirsson, T.E., Geller, F., Sulem, P., Rafnar, T., Wiste, A., Magnusson, K.P., et al. (2008). A variant associated with nicotine dependence, lung cancer and peripheral arterial disease. *Nature, 452*(7187), 638–642.

Todd, J.A. (2006). Statistical false positive or true disease pathway? *Nature Genetics, 38*(7), 731–733.

Tomlinson, I., Webb, E., Carvajal-Carmona, L., Broderick, P., Kemp, Z., Spain, S., et al. (2007). A genome-wide association scan of tag SNPs identifies a susceptibility variant for colorectal cancer at 8q24.21. *Nature Genetics, 39*(8), 984–988.

Uhlmann, W.R., & Guttmacher, A.E. (2008). Key Internet genetics resources for the clinician. *JAMA, 299*(11), 1356–1358.

Witte, J.S. (2007). Multiple prostate cancer risk variants on 8q24. *Nature Genetics, 39*(5), 579–580.

Workman, P. (2001). New drug targets for genomic cancer therapy: Successes, limitations, opportunities and future challenges. *Current Cancer Drug Targets, 1*(1), 33–47.

Yeager, M., Orr, N., Hayes, R.B., Jacobs, K.B., Kraft, P., Wacholder, S., et al. (2007). Genome-wide association study of prostate cancer identifies a second risk locus at 8q24. *Nature Genetics, 39*(5), 645–649.

Yoon, P.W., Scheuner, M.T., Peterson-Oehlke, K.L., Gwinn, M., Faucett, A., & Khoury, M.J. (2002). Can family history be used as a tool for public health and preventive medicine? *Genetics in Medicine, 4*(4), 304–310.

Zanke, B.W., Greenwood, C.M., Rangrej, J., Kustra, R., Tenesa, A., Farrington, S.M., et al. (2007). Genome-wide association scan identifies a colorectal cancer susceptibility locus on chromosome 8q24. *Nature Genetics, 39*(8), 989–994.

Zeggini, E., Scott, L.J., Saxena, R., Voight, B.F., Marchini, J.L., Hu, T., et al. (2008). Meta-analysis of genome-wide association data and large-scale replication identifies additional susceptibility loci for type 2 diabetes. *Nature Genetics, 40*(5), 638–645.

SECTION III

Genomics and Cancer Care

CHAPTER 8   TUMOR PROFILING

CHAPTER 9   PHARMACOGENOMICS

CHAPTER 10 TARGETED THERAPIES

CHAPTER 8
Tumor Profiling

Cathleen M. Goetsch, MSN, RN, ARNP, AOCNP®

Professional Practice Domain:
Nursing Assessment: Applying/Integrating Genetic and Genomic Knowledge
- Demonstrate an understanding of the relationship of genetics and genomics to health, prevention, screening, diagnostics, prognostics, selection of treatment, and monitoring of treatment effectiveness

Identification
- Identify clients who may benefit from specific genetic and genomic information and services based on assessment data

Provision of Education, Care, and Support
- Perform interventions and treatments appropriate to clients' genetic and genomic healthcare needs
- Use genetic and genomic–based interventions and information to improve clients' outcomes

(Consensus Panel on Genetic/Genomic Nursing Competencies, 2009)

INTRODUCTION

The terms *gene profiling, molecular profiling, molecular signature, gene signature tumor profiling,* and *tumor profiling* often are used interchangeably. The National Cancer Institute (NCI, n.d.) online *Dictionary of Cancer Terms* defines a genetic profile as "information about specific genes, including variations and gene expression, in an individual or in a certain type of tissue." Tumor profiling techniques are used to determine the differences between how genes are expressed in normal versus cancerous tissue. These differences, in which genes are turned on or off, can be recognized as a tumor-specific molecular profile or genetic signature. Recognizing such differences may help to diagnose a disease, establish prognosis, or predict an individual's response to various treatments. Oncology nurses play a vital role in teaching clients about these new technologies. Advanced practice oncology nurses may be in the position to identify who might need such testing and order appropriate testing. Making clients aware of ongoing studies and assisting them in accessing research opportunities is another key nursing responsibility in improving clients' outcomes.

THE NEED FOR TUMOR PROFILING

In the pregenomic age, cancer treatment decisions were made based on patient and provider tolerance of potential toxicity versus potential benefit (Coates & Simes, 1992; Duric et al., 2005; Simes & Coates, 2001). Traditionally, cancer treatments have been designed and studied for safety and efficacy by looking at the aggregate response of groups of individuals with cancer that arose from the same tissue (e.g., colon cancer). Experience and research had shown that no treatment could be effective in all cases, but no methods existed to identify when benefit would occur in an individual case.

The need to better identify individual tumor and patient differences was recognized. Tumor-specific factors that might distinguish patient prognosis and response to treatments were sought. Describing tumors by cell appearance, amount of differentiation, differential staining, and proliferative potential were among the early efforts for modern tumor profiling.

Some of the earliest and most effective advances in tumor profiling occurred in breast cancer, including the discovery of estrogen and progesterone receptors and more recently the ability to identify *HER2* gene overexpression. Attempts to clarify risk versus benefit of treatments in a given patient situation, using such tumor-specific factors, led to the development of various decision aids. As an example, various models and tools exist to assist patients in making decisions in the selection of treatment for breast and colon cancer (e.g., National Comprehensive Cancer Network [NCCN] algorithms, St. Gallen guidelines, the statistical model Adjuvant! Online—see Table 8-1 for Web addresses).

In the genomic era, the hope for better recognition of who needs treatment, what kind, and how much has begun to be attainable. Identifying tumor-specific factors that affect disease prognosis and designing treatments to target such factors has begun already. Rapid progress in molecular technology and genomic understanding is a legacy of the **Human Genome Project**. Advancing the understanding of molecular and genetic profiles of specific cancer cells remains a major initiative of NCI.

The Cancer Genome Anatomy Project (CGAP) is one aspect of NCI's integrated genomics focus (http://cgap.nci.nih.gov). CGAP was created with the goal of supporting research to discover gene expression profiles that distinguish cancer cells from normal cells. However, to understand where we are now requires going back and reflecting on how we got here. This chapter will present the historical background of tumor profiling, current status of knowledge, and practice related to molecular profiling, ongoing research, and future directions.

TABLE 8-1 Web Sites Using the TNM System for Prognosis Prediction and Treatment Decision Making

Web Site	Address
Adjuvant! Online	www.adjuvantonline.com/index.jsp
National Comprehensive Cancer Network	www.nccn.org
St. Gallen International Consensus Conference	http://annonc.oxfordjournals.org/cgi/reprint/18/7/1133

BEGINNINGS OF TUMOR PROFILING

The TNM System

In an effort to base cancer treatment on a scientific foundation, tumor factors that affect prognosis were examined. Historically, these factors were clinical-pathologic features of tumors: primary tumor size (T), histologic grade, lymph node involvement (N), and spread to distant sites (M). The TNM system of grading tumor severity, initially proposed in 1953 and first published in 1959, is accepted internationally as an indicator of patient prognosis (Gospodarowicz et al., 2004). In the genomic era, molecular factors, both genomic and proteomic of the tumor and the patient, combined with traditional tumor information truly characterize cancer prognosis (Burke, 2004). However, the questions that concern oncology healthcare providers remain the same:

> 1) Does this individual patient need any therapy (i.e., is the natural history of the disease sufficiently poor to warrant therapy)? 2) If this patient has a poor prognosis without therapy, which therapy, combination of therapies, or succession of therapies will provide the highest probability of survival and the best quality of life? . . . 3) What toxic effects and side effects will this patient experience with a particular therapy, and are there any measures that can be taken to mitigate or eliminate these therapeutic harms? (Burke, 2004, p. 1409)

Estrogen Receptor Status

One of the first successes at recognizing molecular-level tumor factors that affected patient outcomes looked at the presence or absence and number of specific cell receptors and proteins. Estrogen receptors (ERs) in breast cancer are a classic example (Jensen & Jordan, 2003). Jensen and Jacobson proposed the presence of the receptors in 1962, and Toft and Gorski (1966) first isolated ERs in rat tissue. In 1971, this knowledge was used to show that effective response to hormone ablative surgery (the standard of care for adjuvant breast cancer treatment in the first 70 years of the 20th century) was related to the presence of ERs (ER positive) on the tumor cells (Jensen, Block, Smith, Kyser, & DeSombre, 1971). During the early 1970s, studies of women with advanced breast cancer who were ER positive showed response to an antiestrogen compound (Ward, 1973). Presentations at the NCI 1974 Breast Cancer Task Force Workshop established the utility of the ER assay in predicting response to tamoxifen (Jensen & Jordan). With recognition of the importance of ER status, tamoxifen became the first molecular-targeted cancer therapy. Unfortunately, it was only applicable for about 60%–70% of breast cancer cases.

HER2 Oncogene Overexpression

As effectiveness of chemotherapy for breast cancer improved with implementation of treatment strategies validated in clinical trials, a portion of breast cancers (20%–30%) seemed more aggressive and chemoresistant. Initially described in 1985 by King, Kraus, and Aaronson, research at the molecular level led to results that linked *ERBB2* gene (also known as *HER2*, a homolog for the *neu* mouse oncogene) overexpression to the neoplastic growth of mammary tumor cells (Kraus, Popescu, Amsbaugh, & King, 1987). Previous evidence supported the supposition that overexpression of such genes could precede gene amplification in the development of multidrug resistance (Roninson et al., 1986). Soon after, the overexpression HER2 protein in breast cancer tissue was shown to be a negative prognostic factor for stage at diagnosis, risk of recurrence or progression, and death (Klijn, Berns, Bontenbal, & Foekens, 1993; Klijn, Berns, & Foekens, 1993; Seshadri, Matthews, Dobrovic, & Horsfall, 1989; Slamon et al., 1987). In short order, the *ERBB2*

(*HER2/neu*) gene was sequenced (Tal et al., 1987) and located at 17q12-q21.32 (Popescu, King, & Kraus, 1989). (For discussion of the implications of *HER2* overexpression on treatment, see Chapter 10.)

ADVANCES IN TUMOR PROFILING: MOLECULAR PROFILING

The Human Genome Project spurred major advances in technology that provided tools for assessing tumor characteristics at the genomic level. As these tools became available, tumor profiling efforts began in earnest. Molecular genetic characteristics of tumors could now be identified. The next step was to look for combinations of various genetic factors in tumors that could be distinguished as a predictive signature or profile.

The methods of performing gene profiling are known by many names. Also called gene signature profiling or microarray analysis, this is a technique of simultaneously measuring gene activity. Determining which genes are active or switched on allows tumor subgroups to be identified. The information found is then studied for its applicability in predicting treatment response and risk of relapse in individual tumors (NCI, n.d.).

Gene Profiling Techniques

Although each cell in a human's tissue initially contains all the same genetic information, only a limited number of genes are active or switched on at any one time. The active genes vary from tissue to tissue and form a unique gene expression profile, or a molecular signature. The molecular signature of cancer cells is different from that of normal cells and may vary among individuals having the same type of cancer. These somatic (acquired) changes result in altered production and function of the gene products (proteins), and the differences can be measured using either DNA or protein analysis.

DNA Microarrays

Microarray analysis is a method of examining how multiple genes interact and are regulated. Using this method, thousands of gene sequences can be examined on an area the size of a regular microscope slide. Molecular signature identification begins with collecting and preparing the tissue of interest. Active genes are identified because they are making messenger RNA (mRNA) as an initial step in protein synthesis, whereas inactive genes, which are not switched on, are not (see Figures 8-1 and 8-2). (See Chapter 2 for a review of the DNA to RNA to protein process.) Each unique protein is templated from mRNA that is specific for it alone, and the mRNA can be separated from the rest of the cellular material by chemical means.

The mRNA molecules are collected and used to make multiple copies of single-stranded complementary DNA (cDNA) using the real-time polymerase chain reaction (RT-PCR) technique (University of Utah Genetic Science Learning Center, 2008). The cDNA is then used to build a microarray platform containing multiple copies of a gene of interest (see Figure 8-3). Using fluorescent tagged bases (adenine = A, thymine = T, cytosine = C, and guanine = G), cDNA probes (short lengths of cDNA) made from a tissue of interest can then be hybridized (i.e., reformed into a double-stranded DNA molecule) on a DNA microarray slide that may hold hundreds or thousands of areas, each containing a different gene (functional DNA

FIGURE 8-1 HOW DOES DNA MICROARRAY TECHNOLOGY WORK?

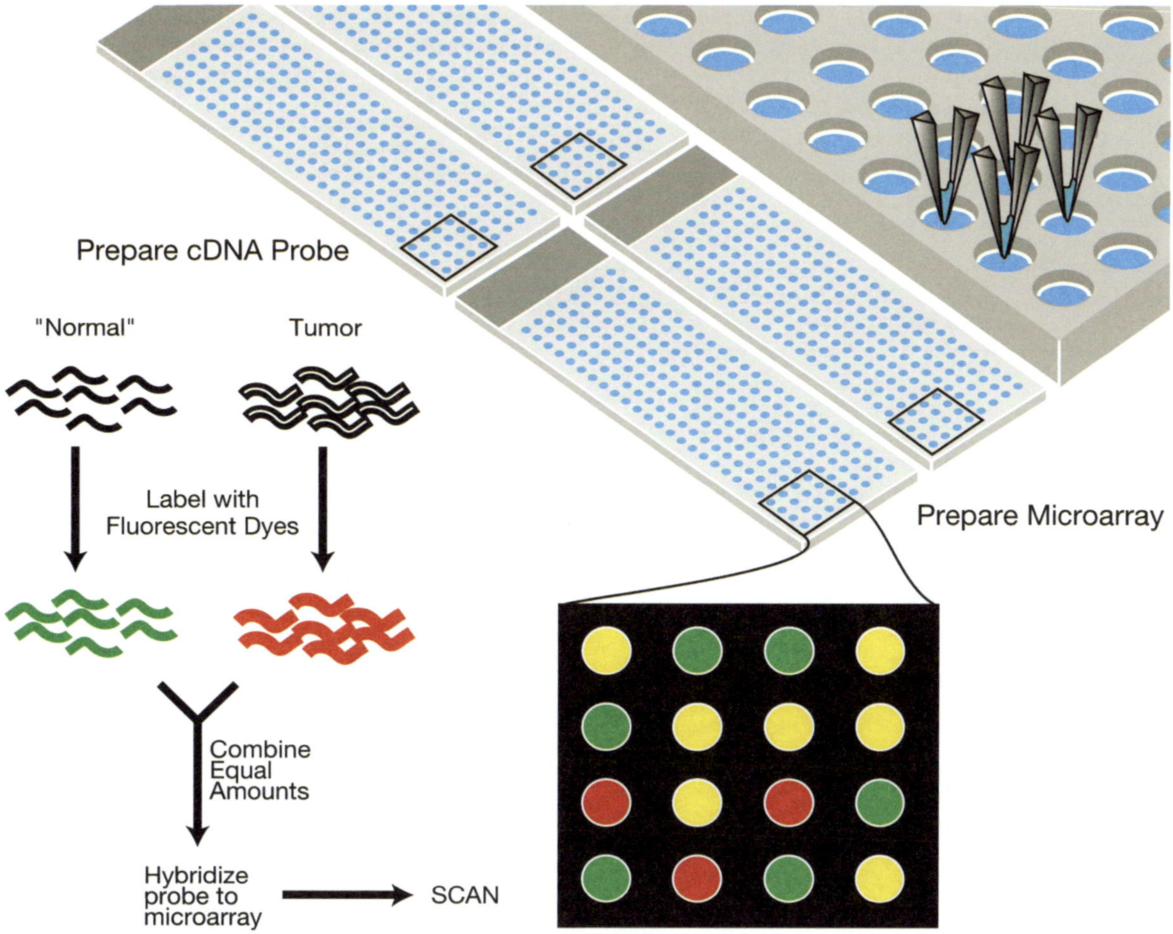

mRNA is obtained from tumor and nearby normal tissue. Fluorescent tags are applied to create "probes." The probes are exposed to microarray where attachment to complementary DNA occurs (hybridization). Electronic scanning detects which genes are active (switched on) by recording the amount of fluorescent color emitted. Highly active genes will appear brighter. Differences between the normal and the cancerous tissues can be seen.

Green spots represent genes switched on in a cancer cell. Red spots mean genes switched on in the normal cell. Yellow spots are caused by mixing red and green fluorescence, and represent genes whose expression is roughly the same in both cell types, and black spots, or absence of fluorescence, represent genes not being expressed in either cell type.

Note. Figure courtesy of the National Human Genome Research Institute. Retrieved December 22, 2009, from http://www.genome.gov/10000533.

sequence). If a cDNA sample of interest (the probe) has a sequence that is complementary to the DNA on a given spot, the probe will hybridize or bond to the spot (see Figure 8-4). This hybridization is detectable by its fluorescence because of the tags placed during the formation of the cDNA probes (see Figure 8-5).

FIGURE 8-2.   DNA MICROARRAY

A technique used to assess expression of multiple genes at one time by fixing DNA to a glass slide, attaching labeled fluorescent probes to complementary DNA strands, and then measuring the brightness of each fluorescent dot.

Note. Based on information from University of Utah Genetic Science Learning Center, 2008.

FIGURE 8-3.   cDNA MICROARRAY PLATFORM WITH MULTIPLE AREAS OF SINGLE GENE CONCENTRATION

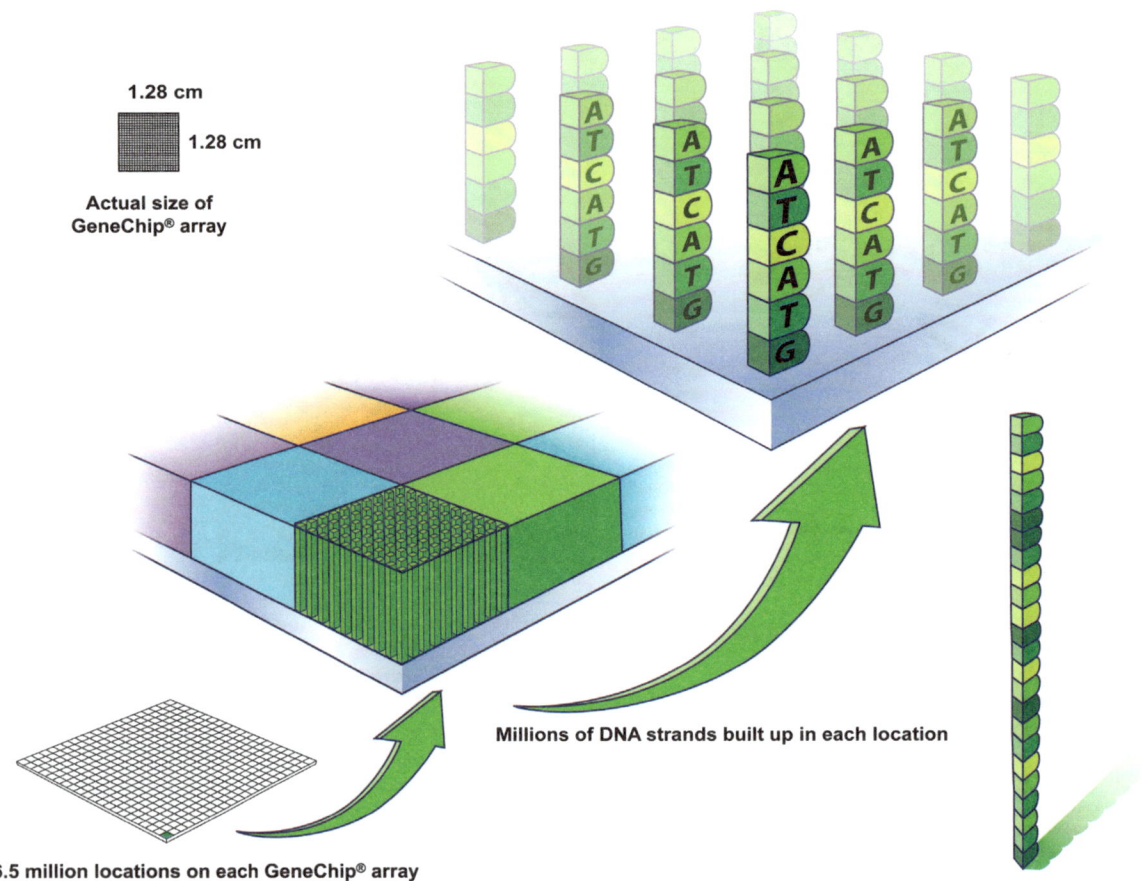

Each spot on the array contains millions of copies of cDNA. The chip contains multiple areas with different single genes in each area.

Note. Image courtesy of Affimetrix. Used with permission.

FIGURE 8-4 HYBRIDIZATION OF SAMPLES (MESSENGER RNA WITH FLUORESCENT TAG BINDS TO COMPLEMENTARY DNA)

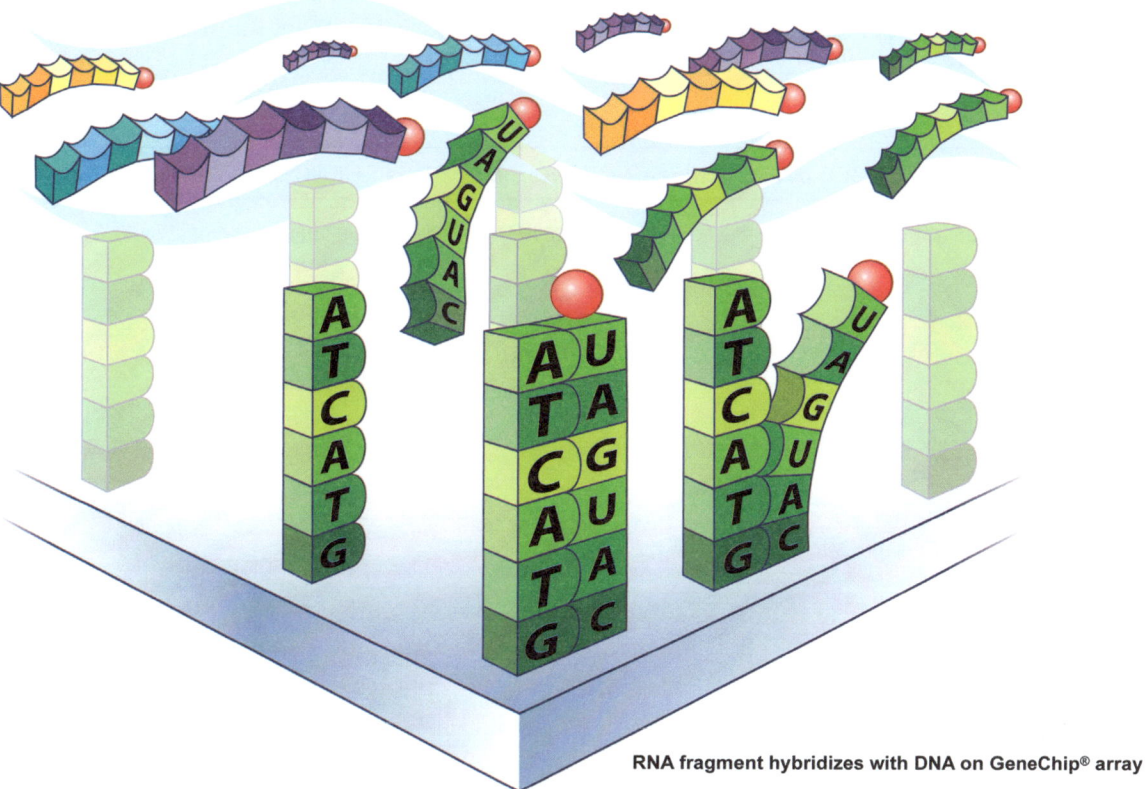

When a fluorescent tagged mRNA molecule finds a cDNA that shares the same gene of origin, hybridization occurs, as complementary base pairs combine.

Note. Image courtesy of Affimetrix. Used with permission.

Thus, each spot on a DNA microarray is an independent assay for the presence of a different cDNA sequence. Excess DNA is at each assay spot so that more than one sample probe can hybridize to it at once without competition (Buhler, 2002). This allows tissue samples tagged with different colors to be compared for activity in the same genes (see Figure 8-1). Although this procedure can be done by hand, a mechanized process is faster and more accurate. Computers are essential in collecting, analyzing, and managing the data.

The ability to perform DNA microarray analysis to pinpoint unique molecular signatures was a major leap forward in the quest to further cancer research at the genomic level. The use of reverse transcriptase polymerase chain reaction was a key tool in the process. Its utility in a clinical setting, however, initially was limited by its need for fresh or fresh-frozen tissue for mRNA extraction. The capability to use archived tissue to obtain the same information was a major breakthrough (Esteva et al., 2005). One method being used to minimize cellular damage in order to ensure accurate DNA and protein patterns are preserved in cancer and normal cells is laser capture microdissection (Fuller, Palmer-Toy, Erlander, & Sgroi, 2003). This technology will continue to develop and expand as illustrated by the availability of digital gene expression profiling, which increases the speed, input, and output of the analysis (Blow, 2009).

FIGURE 8-5   DIFFERENCES IN FLUORESCENCE INDICATING DIFFERENCES IN GENE EXPRESSION

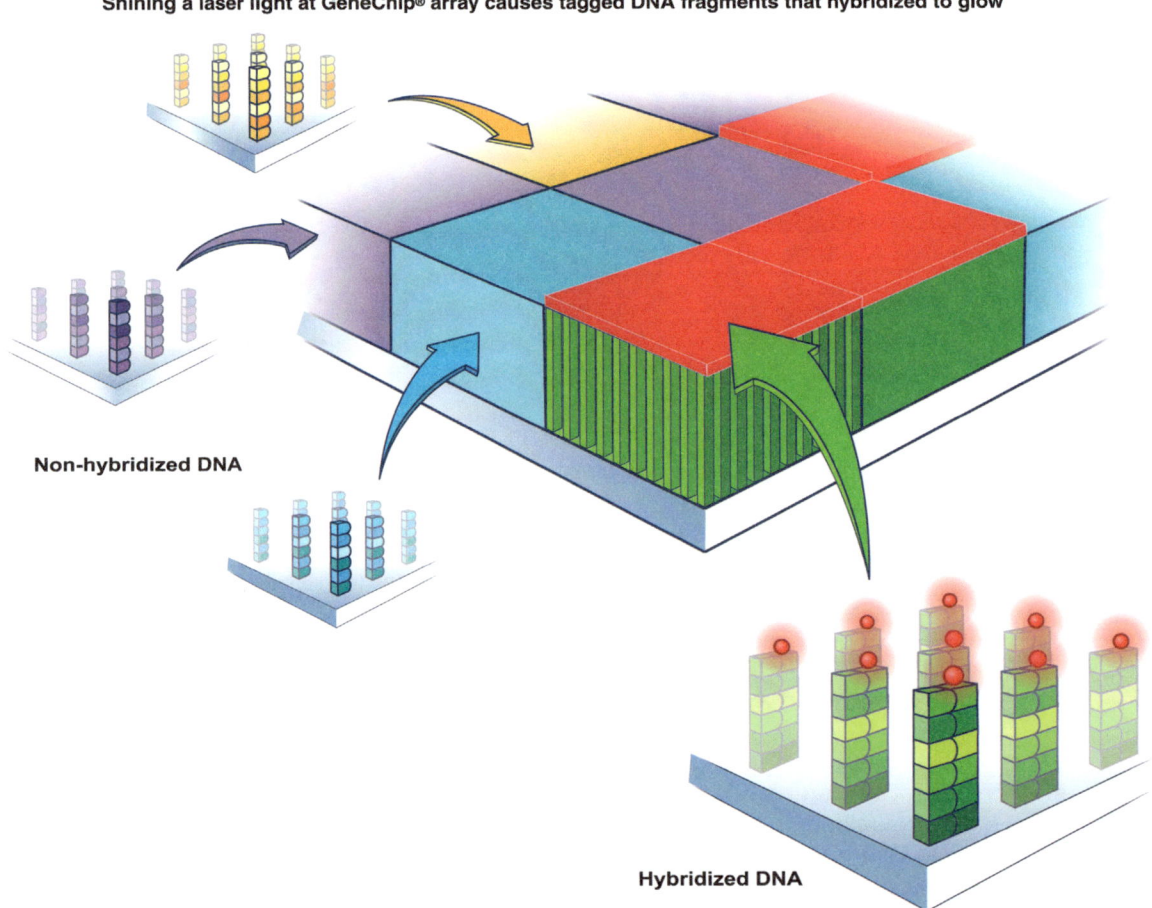

The fluorescent dye attached to the mRNA allows the presence and amount of binding that occurred to be detected when activated by laser light. The intensity of the fluorescence detected is representative of an activated gene from the tissue of interest, tumor versus normal.

Note. Image courtesy of Affimetrix. Used with permission.

Laser-Capture Microdissection

This technique employs a low-energy laser beam and special transfer film to harvest only the desired cell or cells out of formalin-fixed, paraffin-embedded (FFPE) tissue sections. The harvested cells can be used to extract mRNA and proceed as described previously to make cDNA for use with DNA microarrays. Alternatively, proteins present in the selected cells can be used to map the protein pattern. Another advantage to laser capture microdissection technique is the ability to capture separate sets of cells from normal, precancerous, cancerous, and other tissue of interest, all from the same patient's biopsy sample.

Real-Time Polymerase Chain Reaction

One of the limitations of RT-PCR is its qualitative nature. By finding a way to quantify the process as it progresses, the amount of gene activity in the original tissue can be assessed. Several commercial products are available that incorporate this technology. Oncotype DX® (Genomic Health, Inc.) tumor expression profile for breast cancer, discussed later in this chapter, is an example. An explanation of the RT-PCR process is available from Davidson College (www.bio.davidson.edu/Courses/Molbio/MolStudents/spring2003/Pierce/realtimepcr.htm).

Clinical Use of Gene Signature Tumor Profiling

Although powerful, microarray technology has limitations. It can show differences between gene expressions, but it cannot verify whether a gene is switched on or off. If a gene is switched on, this method cannot determine if a functional protein is being formed; protein profiling or protein expression analysis can be used for this purpose. Furthermore, this technology can only identify variation; it does not fix the problem detected. Potential uses for this technology include identification of cancer-specific gene expression, markers for metastasis, subtypes of cancers, new molecular targets for drug development, and variation in drug metabolism.

Gene expression profiling is most advanced in breast cancer, with landmark initial work reported in 2000 of multigene signature assays as a gauge of prognosis and to predict response to therapy (Perou et al., 2000; Sørlie et al., 2001). Several gene signature assays (also known as gene profile arrays or molecular profiles) for breast cancer exist. Some are already in use in clinical practice and are reviewed later in this chapter. Discussion of work in other cancer types will follow.

Gene-Expression Signature Technology in Breast Cancer

Oncotype DX

One of the first microarray technology tools to have wide clinical use in cancer care is Oncotype DX. This is an RT-PCR–based gene expression profiling test that quantifies the risk of distant recurrence in patients with node-negative, ER-positive breast cancer based on their individual tumor signature. One of the qualities of the test that adds to its clinical utility is the ability to run the assay on FFPE, archived tissue.

The Oncotype DX assay was developed using stored FFPE tissue samples from previous large clinical trials of ER-positive, node-negative breast cancers treated with or without tamoxifen or with tamoxifen and with or without chemotherapy. These tumors were used to identify genes of interest that eventually were narrowed to a 21-gene assay. Genes in the assay reflected proliferation rate, invasive potential, ER activity factors, *HER2* expression, other genes with cancer-related activity, and five reference genes. Using the assay, an algorithm that correlated clinical outcome with gene expression was developed. Initial analysis showed this gene profile could be used to generate a score that correlated with the risk of breast cancer recurrence (Paik et al., 2004).

Using a scale of 1–100, point values were assigned categories: high (greater than or equal to 31), intermediate (18–30), and low (less than 18) risk of recurrence within 10 years. The recurrence score expressed recurrence risk as a point on a continuous risk curve. Tumors with low recurrence score profiles were associated with low risk of recurrence within 10 years, whereas tumors with high recurrence scores showed the highest rate of 10-year recurrence (see Figure 8-6).

Recurrence prediction using recurrence scores has similarities but also significant differences to the recurrence estimates made using the Adjuvant! Online algorithm, which is based on the TNM system. Paik (2007) compared the correlation between the recurrence score and the Adjuvant! Online estimates for recurrence and found patient outcomes related more closely to the recurrence score than to the Adjuvant! Online prediction.

Benefits of adjuvant treatment also were shown to differ by recurrence score category. In a retrospective analysis, women with tumors that had a low to intermediate recurrence score were most likely to benefit from tamoxifen therapy and less likely to have added benefit from chemotherapy. Women with ER-positive, node-negative tumors that showed a high recurrence score benefited more from combined chemotherapy and tamoxifen than from tamoxifen alone (Paik et al., 2006). Recognition of the importance of this tool is reflected in the recent changes in the NCCN guidelines for breast cancer treatment and the most recent American Society of Clinical Oncology (ASCO) clinical guidelines for tumor marker use in breast cancer treatment (Harris et al., 2007; NCCN, 2009). The 2007 ASCO guidelines noted that level I and level II evidence (see Figure 8-7) supports the use of Oncotype DX to guide selection of tamoxifen alone or tamoxifen plus adjuvant chemotherapy in early-stage ER-positive, *HER2* non-overexpressing breast cancers.

In newly diagnosed patients with node-negative, ER-positive breast cancer, the Oncotype DX assay can be used to predict the risk of recurrence in patients treated with tamoxifen. Oncotype DX may be used to identify patients who are predicted to obtain the most therapeutic benefit from adjuvant tamoxifen and may not require adjuvant chemotherapy. In addition, patients with high recurrence scores appear to achieve more benefit from adjuvant chemotherapy than from tamoxifen (Evaluation of Genomic Applications in Practice and Prevention Working Group, 2009; Harris et al., 2007).

Although NCCN is more conservative, the guidelines recommend that evaluation with Oncotype DX be considered in making adjuvant therapy decisions for women with breast cancer with the following characteristics: (a) ductal, lobular, mixed ductal and lobular, or metaplastic histology; (b) tumor pathologic grades pT1–pT3 with pN0–pN1mic (less than or equal to 2 mm axillary metastasis) and M0; and (c) tumor size is 0.6–1 cm grade 2 or 3 or unfavorable features (angiolymphatic invasion, high nuclear grade, or high histologic grade), or tumors larger than 1 cm (NCCN, 2009). In each of these guidelines, the recommendations for treatment are based on the recurrence score, with low recurrence scores (greater than 18) indicating endocrine therapy only, intermediate recurrence scores (18–30) in-

FIGURE 8-6 RATE OF DISTANT RECURRENCE AS A CONTINUOUS FUNCTION OF THE RECURRENCE SCORE

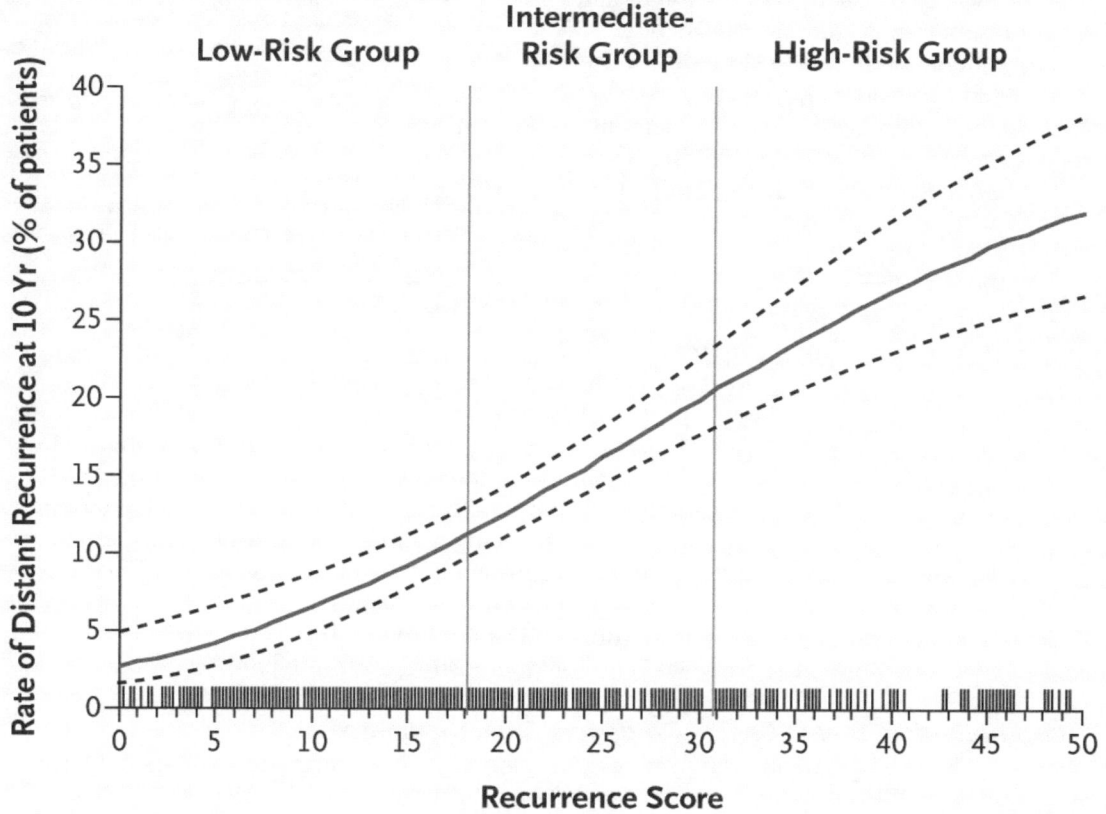

The continuous function was generated with use of a piecewise log-hazard ratio model 28. The dashed curves indicate the 95% confidence interval. The rug plot on top of the x-axis shows the recurrence score for individual patients in the study.

The x-axis shows the recurrence score for individual breast cancer patients, demonstrating use of tumor gene profiling could predict risk of recurrence.

Note. From "A Multigene Assay to Predict Recurrence of Tamoxifen-Treated, Node-Negative Breast Cancer," by S. Paik, S. Shak, G. Tang, C. Kim, J. Baker, M. Cronin, et al., 2004, *New England Journal of Medicine, 351*(27), p. 2824. Copyright 2004 by Massachusetts Medical Society. Reprinted with permission.

dicating chemotherapy considered in addition to endocrine therapy, and high recurrence scores (greater than 30) bringing a recommendation for both adjuvant endocrine therapy and chemotherapy.

The consensus opinion in the European community is more reserved. At the 2007 St. Gallen Conference on treatment for early breast cancer, an assessment of the technology was made by a panel of experts. The group found that not enough quality and quantity of evidence was available to recommend the use of the available gene profiling to guide treatment selection (Goldhirsch et al., 2007).

Despite this controversy, another indication of the mainstream United States' acceptance of the use of Oncotype DX is the availability of insurance coverage. Medicare and many private insurers cover the testing. Also, reimbursement assistance is available through the Genomic Access Program of Genomic Health, Inc.

MammaPrint

MammaPrint™ (Agendia, Inc.) is a 70-gene expression profiling test that is based on work from the Netherlands Cancer Institute (van de Vijver et al., 2002; van't Veer et al., 2002). It has been shown to have prognostic relevance in patients with untreated breast cancer who are younger than age 61 with node-negative tumors less than 5 cm in size (Bueno-de-Mesquita et al., 2007; Espinosa et al., 2005). This test received clearance from the U.S. Food and Drug Administration in mid-2007 for marketing in the United States for these indications. When compared with recurrence risk using Adjuvant! Online, the 70-gene profile provided independent prognostic information (Buyse et al., 2006). The downside for clinical utility is the requirement for fresh or fresh-frozen tumor tissue for analysis, something that is not readily available in standard practice in the United States, and the clinical benefit of the assay has yet to be demonstrated (Simon, 2006).

Rotterdam Breast Cancer Prognosis Gene Signature

This 76-gene profile was developed using tumors from untreated women of all ages stratified for ER status. This profile was reported to discriminate between those who had high versus low risk to develop distant metastases within five years. What distinguishes this assay from MammaPrint and Oncotype DX is the inclusion of ER-negative tumors, with strong prognostic association seen in subgroups of premenopausal women and in those with small (10–20 mm) tumors (Wang et al., 2005). Foekens, Atkins, Zhang, Sweep, and Harbeck (2006) published a validation study that confirmed the 76-gene signature assessment had a strong correlation to prognosis for ER-positive breast cancer smaller than 2 cm in size, independent of menopause status. Prognostic scores were compared to both the St. Gallen criteria and the Adjuvant! Online estimate, with an almost 40% reduction in the number of women who would have had chemotherapy treatment recommended (Desmedt et al., 2007; Wang et al., 2005).

Invasiveness Gene Signature

The 186-gene invasiveness gene signature (IGS) was evaluated for its association with overall survival and metastasis-free survival in patients with breast cancer or other types of cancer (Liu et al., 2007). Women with high-risk early breast cancer were sorted using the IGS into good and poor prognostic categories. For those with good prognosis by IGS, the 10-year rate of metastasis-free survival was 81%; however, those with a poor

---

FIGURE 8-7 RANKING LEVELS OF EVIDENCE

- Level I: Evidence obtained from at least one properly designated randomized controlled trial
- Level II-1: Evidence obtained from well-designed controlled trials without randomization
- Level II-2: Evidence obtained from well-designed cohort or case-control analytic study, preferably from more than one center or research group
- Level II-3: Evidence obtained from multiple time series with or without the intervention
- Level III: Opinions of respected authorities based on clinical experience, descriptive studies, or reports of expert committees

Note. Based on information from Harris et al., 2007.

prognosis had only a 57% metastasis-free survival rate. Other tumors for which the IGS showed prognostic correlation included prostate cancer, lung cancer, and medulloblastoma.

Combining and Refining Gene Profiles

As observed by Henry and Hayes (2007), the clinical utility and reproducibility of all of these methods are still being studied. One of the confounders in evaluating the significance and validity of the gene signature work to date has been the lack of overlap of genes used in the various gene signature profiles. Hu et al. (2006) examined the various different profiles looking for a unifying theory with a more novel method. Using publicly available breast cancer gene expression data sets, they combined the different genes from five breast tumor molecular assays and derived a new 1,300-gene profile. With the new gene set, they were able to group tumors into four subtypes. Described in prior research (Sørlie, Perou, et al., 2006; Sørlie et al., 2001; Sørlie, Wang, et al., 2006), each tumor subtype had a distinct gene expression profile that correlated with patient outcomes. Designated LumA, LumB, Basal-like, and *HER2*+/ER–, the LumA tumor type had the best prognosis, whereas the *HER2*+/ER–, Basal-like, and LumB groups had significantly worse clinical outcomes. With the new gene profile, better predictability of recurrence-free survival ($p = 0.01$), overall survival ($p = 0.009$), and disease-specific survival ($p = 0.04$) was obtained compared to standard TNM predictions (Hu et al.).

Quality of the Evidence Supporting Current Assays

Using head-to-head comparison on the same set of samples, Fan et al. (2006) performed analysis with several of the cancer gene signature assays available at the time (intrinsic subtypes, 70-gene profile, wound response, recurrence score, and the two-gene ratio) and compared them to the Rotterdam 76-gene signature. They found good agreement with four of the five assay methods in ability to predict significant differences in relapse-free and overall survival with the low- and high-recurrence risk stratification (the exception was the two-gene ratio method).

Another review of the evidence supporting the technology utilized in clinical practice comes from the Agency for Healthcare Research and Quality (Marchionni et al., 2008). Strong retrospective evidence showed that the Oncotype DX gene expression assay added clinically meaningful information beyond standard prognostic indices for predicting distant spread and chemotherapy benefit, which offer clear treatment implications. In contrast, although the MammaPrint gene expression assay showed the ability to separate tumors into risk categories, it was not clear that the MammaPrint assay added clinical utility to current methods. Using another set of tumors, Haibe-Kains et al. (2008) found three of the breast cancer signature profiles—the 70-gene, the 76-gene, and the gene expression grade index signatures—had similar ability to predict distant metastatic disease–free survival and improved the current non–genomic-based methods of predicting survival.

Predicting Chemotherapy Response

Looking at women undergoing neoadjuvant therapy for breast cancer provides an opportunity to correlate the gene signature results with tumor response to chemotherapy; however, results to date have been mixed. Sørlie, Perou, et al. (2006) found little correlation between gene profile results and response to two different chemotherapy types. In contrast, Bonnefoi et al. (2007) reported good correlation between signature and response when therapy was chosen using the signature information.

Clinical Trials

Both the MammaPrint and the Oncotype DX are being evaluated in prospective randomized trials to confirm validity and to show utility, as well as to better understand the middle ground in the prognostic scoring. TAILORx (Trial Assigning IndividuaLized Options for Treatment [Rx], is examining whether the Oncotype DX 21-gene signature is effective in assigning patients to the most appropriate and effective therapy (NCI, 2006). To date, the results from using the Oncotype DX recurrence score have been most accurate in the lowest and the highest risk categories. For the purposes of the trial, the intermediate recurrence score group (11–25) was assigned randomly to either hormonal therapy only or hormonal therapy and chemotherapy. Women with low recurrence score received hormonal therapy only, and those with high recurrence score tumors received chemotherapy and hormonal therapy. The aim of the study is that the intermediate group randomization will result in more information to direct treatment decisions in an area of current uncertainty.

The MammaPrint 70-gene profile is being used as a stratification tool in a large European study (European Organisation for Research and Treatment of Cancer, 2007). MINDACT (Microarray In Node-negative Disease may Avoid ChemoTherapy) is a prospective randomized study comparing the gene signature assay with the common clinical-pathologic criteria (TNM staging) and looking for accuracy in selecting whether patients need adjuvant chemotherapy in node-negative breast cancer (Mook, van't Veer, Rutgers, Piccart-Gebhart, & Cardoso, 2007). This study compares the usual recommendations for chemotherapy (Goldhirsch et al., 2007) to whether the participant's tumor has a high or low risk of recurrence. More information about the study is available at the NCI Clinical Trials Web site (http://clinicaltrials.gov/ct2/show/NCT00433589?term=MINDACT&rank=1).

Both of these trials will answer important different but related clinical questions. However, it will take years for the results to be available. Meanwhile, the clinical use of gene signature methodology proceeds despite limited evidence to guide decision making by healthcare providers.

CURRENT WORK

Researchers also are developing studies that seek metastasis signatures of solid tumors. Current work focuses on choosing and developing cancer therapeutics that will ensure the appropriate person is treated in the most effective way, and that those not likely to benefit from treatment are spared its side effects. Although breast cancer studies have led the way, researchers are studying many other cancer types.

Microarrays have been developed for use in assessing ovarian, head and neck, prostate, colon, cervical, and pancreatic cancer cancers (Iorio et al., 2007; Schlecht et al., 2007; Setlur et al., 2007; Wang et al., 2004; Zhai et al., 2007; Zhao et al., 2007). Progression markers for melanoma have been found using molecular profiling (Bertucci et al., 2007). In January 2008, two groups reported progress on the use of molecular markers in predicting prognosis and choosing therapy for lung cancer (Azzoli, Park, Pao, Zakowski, & Kris, 2008;

Yu et al., 2008). The ability of microarray analysis to predict response to radiotherapy also has been examined (Ogawa, Murayama, & Mori, 2007; Rimkus et al., 2008). Hoshida et al. (2008) studied the feasibility of genome-wide expression profiling of tissues from patients with hepatocellular carcinoma. They demonstrated a reproducible gene-expression signature that correlated with survival and were able to do so using FFPE tissues. The application of microarray in this context to better inform therapeutic decision making currently is being investigated.

Work in lymphoma also has begun (see Figure 8-8). Studies using molecular profiling have been done for Burkitt lymphoma (Dave et al., 2006), diffuse large B-cell lymphoma (Lenz et al., 2008), and follicular lymphoma (Schwaenen et al., 2008). Candidate genes have been identified that correlate with inferior survival in follicular lymphoma, and gene

FIGURE 8-8 DNA MICROARRAY ANALYSIS OF BURKITT LYMPHOMA AND DIFFUSE LARGE B-CELL LYMPHOMA

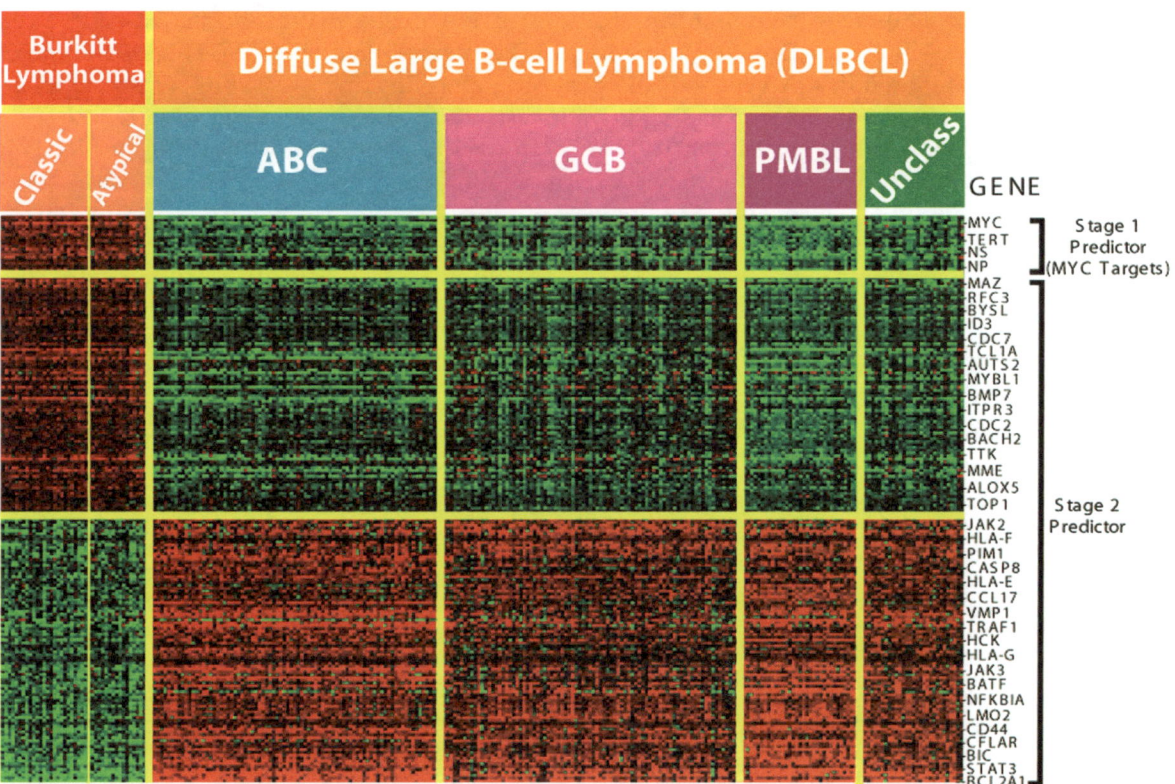

Colors indicate levels of gene expression. Green indicates genes that are overexpressed in normal cells compared to lymphoma cells. Red indicates genes that are overexpressed in lymphoma cells compared to normal cells.

Note. From "Molecular Diagnosis of Burkitt's Lymphoma," by S.S. Dave, K. Fu, G.W. Wright, L.T. Lam, P. Kluin, E.J. Boerma, et al., 2006, New England Journal of Medicine, 354(23), p. 2435. Figure courtesy of the National Cancer Institute.

signatures may assist in diagnosis of Burkitt lymphoma. Horlings et al. (2008) reported success in using tumor profiling assays to aid in diagnosing adenocarcinoma tumor type in patients with unknown primary at the time of disease discovery. This capability is expected to result in better patient outcomes, as the most effective treatment can be given if the tumor type is known.

FAST FORWARD INTO THE FUTURE

As new knowledge and technology arrive at an avalanche pace, the U.S. National Institutes of Health have made extensive efforts to coordinate advances in genomics. Attempts to facilitate research and information distribution have been the main areas of focus. Several programs pertinent to cancer genomics have been launched as a part of those efforts. NCI's Office of Cancer Genomics (n.d.) aims "to enhance understanding of the molecular mechanisms of cancer, with the ultimate goal of improving the prevention, early detection, diagnosis, and treatment of cancer."

An important aspect of U.S. government efforts to support the genomics revolution is the Evaluation of Genomic Applications in Practice and Prevention (EGAPP) project. The Centers for Disease Control and Prevention Office of Public Health Genomics (2007) initiated this project with the goal of establishing and evaluating a systematic, evidence-based process for assessing genetic tests and other applications of genomic technology, especially in transition from research to clinical and public health practice. This project was created in response to concerns about the current status of genetic testing implementation and oversight. Not the least of the concerns was the need to have evidence to support the efficacy and cost-effectiveness of tests before they are marketed. Analytic validity, the ability to measure the expression of mRNA by breast cancer tumor cells, clinical validity, the ability of the test to accurately and reliably identify or predict the recurrence, and clinical utility, the balance of benefit to harm, were all considered when the EGAPP group decided the available evidence was insufficient to warrant a recommendation for or against use of tumor profiling as it existed at the time of publication (EGAPP Working Group, 2009). Ongoing evaluation by groups such as EGAPP and NCCN will need to continue, with recommendations and standards being revised frequently to keep up with the rapid advances in the technology. Efforts to evaluate and compare new assays are challenged by the (a) imprecise definitions of what constitutes normal expression in different assays, (b) difficulty in comparing assay techniques with dissimilar methods of showing validity, and (c) the heterogeneity of both normal and tumor tissues being assayed (King & Sinha, 2001).

COORDINATION OF EFFORTS

Molecular, Biochemical, and Genomic

As part of the technologic advances spurred by the Human Genome Project, a flurry of studies of specific molecular factors and their impact on cancer ensued. The director of NCI called for a coordination of research efforts to identify multiple molecular tumor characteristics by making archived tumor samples available for researchers. The Program for the Assessment of Clinical Cancer Tests made grants available, with archived tissue from prior NCI-sponsored clinical trials as a source of large numbers of tissue samples made available for study. Strategic Partnering to Evaluate Cancer Signatures provided awards for programs to work on breast cancer, prostate cancer, lung cancer, lymphoma, sarcoma, and leukemia.

NCI CGAP began in 1996 and studies the molecular changes at the genomic level that occur as a normal cellular DNA undergoes transformation to a cancerous DNA. NCI's Initiative for Chemical Genetics (NCI ICG) public access laboratory was established in 2002 with the goal of accelerating the development of new cancer strategies and therapies, focusing on small molecules. The strategy is to unite synthetic chemistry and cancer biology (Tolliday et al., 2006). Through the use of molecular probes, activation or inactivation of targeted protein functions can be used to promote antitumor activity and discover new therapeutic approaches for cancer. Data derived from the NCI ICG are deposited into the ChemBank Web site (http://chembank.broad.harvard.edu) and become available to the research community at-large within one year. Information is available at www.broadinstitute.org/science/programs/chemical-biology/initiative-chemical-genetics.

Bioinformatics and Biotechnical Information

Since 1997, NCI's Center for Bioinformatics (NCICB) has launched a major effort to integrate molecular and clinical cancer-related information within a unified biomedical informatics framework and, in 2007, published the NCI Thesaurus to assist in that endeavor. The thesaurus provides accurate, comprehensive, shared terminology that includes topics such as cancers, drugs, therapies, anatomy, genes, pathways, cellular and subcellular processes, proteins, and research results to date (Sioutos et al., 2007). It also models how these things relate to each other and how bioinformatics can assist in the advancement of knowledge in these areas. NCICB helps to increase the rate of scientific discovery by facilitating translational research by building tools and resources that enable information sharing along the continuum from the research laboratory to clinical utility. More information about NCICB is available at http://ncicb.nci.nih.gov.

The National Center for Biotechnology Information (NCBI) is another information coordination resource. It provides molecular biology information, creates public databases, conducts research in computational biology, develops software tools for analyzing genome data, and disseminates biomedical information. The goal is better understanding of molecular processes affecting human health and disease. NCBI can be accessed at www.ncbi.nlm.nih.gov.

The Cancer Genome Atlas is a collaboration between the National Human Genome Research Institute and NCI aimed at elucidating the molecular basis of cancer by identifying the full complement of genomic changes associated with a given cancer. This effort will test the feasibility of a large-scale systematic approach to identify genetic alterations in human cancers. Initial efforts will be aimed at three tumor types (brain, lung, and ovarian cancers). Expression profiles and genomic changes associated with each cancer sample will be analyzed. This will be followed by the sequencing of genes with altered function in the specific tumor types. Data collected through this project are likely to provide insights into functional aspects of gene regulation and its role in cancer biology in these three cancers. The hope is that identifying new genes and chromosomal regions of interest will serve to improve cancer outcomes. Additionally, a comprehensive, publicly available database will be created. Advanced technology platforms will play key roles in the genomic analysis, and open access to current technology-based data management and analysis by the scientific community will be an essential component of success. Thus far, this research network has published results on glioblastoma (Cancer Genome Atlas Research Network, 2008). The Cancer Genome Atlas Web site can be accessed at http://cancergenome.nih.gov.

SUMMARY

Initial efforts at tumor profiling to guide cancer treatment decisions involved pathologic descriptions of cancer cell appearance along with tumor size and spread. Identification of molecular markers (e.g., ER positivity and *HER2* overexpression) that were associated with breast cancer prognosis and disease recurrence led to development of targeted treatments (e.g., tamoxifen, aromatase inhibitors, trastuzumab, lapatinib). Advances in tumor profiling were spurred by the technologic progress that occurred during the sequencing of the human genome. Multigene tumor profiles have been found in many tumor types. The use of these profiles in clinical care to guide choices of treatment has begun despite the preliminary nature of the data to support their use. The pace of these advances has been dizzying, making the healthcare professional's task of keeping current a daunting one (see Table 8-2 for resources). Patients often have questions regarding the applicability of genomic technology to their own care (O'Neill et al., 2007). Professional oncology care providers are challenged not only to maintain their own knowledge base, but also to act as resources of accurate information for their patients and colleagues, as well as to encourage patients to participate in research that will advance future care.

TABLE 8-2   Information and Education Resources for Molecular Genomics Technology

Web Site	Address
National Cancer Institute (NCI) Center for Bioinformatics	http://ncicb.nci.nih.gov
NCI's Initiative for Chemical Genetics	www.broad.mit.edu/node/757
NCI's Understanding Cancer Series: Cancer Genome Project	www.cancer.gov/cancertopics/understandingcancer/CGAP
NCI's Understanding Cancer Series: Molecular Diagnostics	www.cancer.gov/cancertopics/understandingcancer/moleculardiagnostics
National Center for Biotechnology Information (NCBI)	www.ncbi.nlm.nih.gov
A Science Primer (NCBI)	www.ncbi.nlm.nih.gov/About/primer/index.html
University of Utah Genetic Science Learning Center	http://learn.genetics.utah.edu

REFERENCES

Azzoli, C.G., Park, B.J., Pao, W., Zakowski, M., & Kris, M.G. (2008). Molecularly tailored adjuvant chemotherapy for resected non-small cell lung cancer: A time for excitement and equipoise. *Journal of Thoracic Oncology, 3*(1), 84–93.

Bertucci, F., Pages, C., Finetti, P., Rochaix, P., Lamant, L., Devilard, E., et al. (2007). Gene expression profiling of human melanoma cell lines with distinct metastatic potential identifies new progression markers. *Anticancer Research, 27*(5A), 3441–3449.

Blow, N. (2009). Transcriptomics: The digital generation. *Nature, 458*(7235), 239–242.

Bonnefoi, H., Potti, A., Delorenzi, M., Mauriac, L., Campone, M., Tubiana-Hulin, M., et al. (2007). Validation of gene signatures that predict the response of breast cancer to neoadjuvant chemotherapy: A substudy of the EORTC 10994/BIG 00-01 clinical trial. *Lancet Oncology, 8*(12), 1071–1078.

Bueno-de-Mesquita, J.M., van Harten, W.H., Retelm, V.P., van't Veer, L.J., van Dam, F.S., Karsenberg, K., et al. (2007). Use of 70-gene signature to predict prognosis of patients with node-negative breast cancer: A prospective community-based feasibility study (RASTER). *Lancet Oncology, 8*(12), 1079–1087.

Buhler, J. (2002). *Anatomy of a comparative gene expression study.* Retrieved January 7, 2008, from http://www.cs.wustl.edu/~jbuhler/research/array/

Burke, H.B. (2004). Outcome prediction and the future of the TNM staging system. *Journal of the National Cancer Institute, 96*(19), 1408–1409.

Buyse, M., Loi, S., van't Veer, L., Viale, G., Delorenzi, M., Glas, A.M., et al. (2006). Validation and clinical utility of a 70-gene prognostic signature for women with node-negative breast cancer. *Journal of the National Cancer Institute, 98*(17), 1183–1192.

Cancer Genome Atlas Research Network. (2008). Comprehensive genomic characterization defines human glioblastoma genes and core pathways. *Nature, 455*(7216), 1061–1068.

Centers for Disease Control and Prevention Office of Public Health Genomics. (2007, December). *Genetic testing.* Retrieved October 6, 2009, from http://www.cdc.gov/genomics/gtesting/index.htm

Coates, A.S., & Simes, R.K. (1992). Patient assessment of adjuvant treatment in operable breast cancer. In D.J. Williams (Ed.), *Introducing new treatments for cancer: Practical, ethical, and legal problems* (pp. 447–458). New York: Wiley.

Consensus Panel on Genetic/Genomic Nursing Competencies. (2009). *Essentials of genetic and genomic nursing: Competencies, curricula guidelines, and outcome indicators* (2nd ed.). Silver Spring, MD: American Nurses Association.

Dave, S.S., Fu, K., Wright, G.W., Lam, L.T., Kluin, P., Boerma, E., et al. (2006). Molecular diagnosis of Burkitt's lymphoma. *New England Journal of Medicine, 354*(23), 2431–2442.

Desmedt, C., Piette, F., Loi, S., Wang, Y., Lallemand, F., Haibe-Kains, B., et al. (2007). Strong time dependence of the 76-gene prognostic signature for node-negative breast cancer patients in the TRANSBIG multicenter independent validation series. *Clinical Cancer Research, 13*(11), 3207–3214.

Duric, V.M., Stockler, M.R., Heritier, S., Boyle, F., Beith, J., Sullivan, A., et al. (2005). Patients' preferences for adjuvant chemotherapy in early breast cancer: What makes AC and CMF worthwhile now? *Annals of Oncology, 16*(11), 1786–1794.

Espinosa, E., Fresno-Vara, J.A., Redondo, A., Sanchez, J.J., Hardisson, D., Zamora, P., et al. (2005). Breast cancer prognosis determined by gene expression profiling: A quantitative reverse transcriptase polymerase chain reaction study. *Journal of Clinical Oncology, 23*(29), 7278–7285.

Esteva, F.J., Sahin, A.A., Cristofanill, M., Coombes, K., Lee, S.J., Baker, J., et al. (2005). Prognostic role of a multigene reverse transcriptase-PCR assay in patients with node-negative breast cancer not receiving adjuvant systemic therapy. *Clinical Cancer Research, 11*(9), 3315–3319.

European Organisation for Research and Treatment of Cancer. (2007). *EORTC Trial 10041 (BIG 3-04)—MINDACT.* Retrieved January 13, 2008, from http://www.eortc.be/services/unit/mindact/MINDACT_websiteii.asp

Evaluation of Genomic Applications in Practice and Prevention Working Group. (2009). Recommendations from the EGAPP Working Group: Can tumor gene expression profiling improve outcomes in patients with breast cancer? *Genetics in Medicine, 11*(1), 66–73.

Fan, C., Oh, D.S., Wessels, L., Weigelt, B., Nuyten, D.S., Nobel, A.B., et al. (2006). Concordance among gene-expression-based predictors for breast cancer. *New England Journal of Medicine, 355*(6), 560–569.

Foekens, J.A., Atkins, D., Zhang, Y., Sweep, F.C., & Harbeck, N. (2006). Multicenter validation of a gene expression–based prognostic signature in lymph node–negative primary breast cancer. *Journal of Clinical Oncology, 24*(11), 1665–1671.

Fuller, A.P., Palmer-Toy, D., Erlander, M.G., & Sgroi, D.C. (2003). Laser capture microdissection and advanced molecular analysis of human breast cancer. *Journal of Mammary Gland Biology and Neoplasia, 8*(3), 335–345.

Goldhirsch, A., Wood, W.C., Gelber, R.D., Coates, A.S., Thürlimann, B., & Senn, H.J. (2007). Opinion on use of molecular profiling for breast cancer treatment choice. Progress and promise (Highlights of the Tenth Saint Gallen conference, Switzerland: International expert consensus on the primary therapy of early breast cancer). *Annals of Oncology, 18*(7), 1133–1144.

Gospodarowicz, M.K., Miller, D., Groome, P.A., Greene, F.L., Logan, P.A., & Sobin, L.H. (2004). The process for continuous improvement of the TNM classification. *Cancer 100*(1), 1–5.

Haibe-Kains, B., Desmedt, C., Piette, F., Buyse, M., Cardoso, F., Van't Veer, L., et al. (2008). Comparison of prognostic gene expression signatures for breast cancer. *BMC Genomics, 9*, 394.

Harris, L., Fritsche, H., Mennel, R., Norton, L., Ravdin, P., Taube, S., et al. (2007). American Society of Clinical Oncology 2007 update of recommendations for the use of tumor markers in breast cancer. *Journal of Clinical Oncology, 25*(33), 5287–5312.

Henry, N.L., & Hayes, D.F. (2007). Use of gene-expression profiling to recommend adjuvant chemotherapy for breast cancer. *Oncology, 21*(11), 1301–1311.

Horlings, H.M., van Laar, R.K., Kerst, J.M., Helgason, H.H., Wesseling, J., van der Hoeven, J.J., et al. (2008). Gene expression profiling to identify the histogenetic origin of metastatic adenocarcinomas of unknown primary. *Journal of Clinical Oncology, 26*(27), 4435–4441.

Hoshida, Y., Villanueva, A., Kobayashi, M., Peix, J., Chiang, D.Y., Camargo, A., et al. (2008). Gene expression in fixed tissues and outcome in hepatocellular carcinoma. *New England Journal of Medicine, 359*(19), 1995–2004. Retrieved October 20, 2008, from http://content.nejm.org/cgi/content/full/NEJMoa0804525v1#F2

Hu, Z., Fan, C., Oh, D.S., Marron, J.S., He, X., Qaqish, B.F., et al. (2006). The molecular portraits of breast tumors are conserved across microarray platforms. *BMC Genomics, 7*, 96.

Iorio, M.V., Visone, R., Di Leva, G., Donati, V., Petrocca, F., Casalini, P., et al. (2007). MicroRNA signatures in human ovarian cancer. *Cancer Research, 67*(18), 8699–8707.

Jensen, E.V., Block, G.E., Smith, S., Kyser, K., & DeSombre, E.R. (1971). Estrogen receptors and breast cancer response to adrenalectomy. *Journal of the National Cancer Institute Monographs, 1971*(34), 55–70.

Jensen, E.V., & Jacobson, H.I. (1962). Basic guides to the mechanism of estrogen action. *Recent Progress in Hormonal Research, 18*, 387–414.

Jensen, E.V., & Jordan, V.C. (2003). The estrogen receptor: A model for molecular medicine. *Clinical Cancer Research, 9*(6), 1980–1989.

King, C.R., Kraus, M.H., & Aaronson, S.A. (1985). Amplification of a novel v-erbB-related gene in a human mammary carcinoma. *Science, 229*(4717), 974–976.

King, H.C., & Sinha, A.A. (2001). Gene expression profile analysis by DNA microarrays: Promise and pitfalls. *JAMA, 286*(18), 2280–2288.

Klijn, J.G., Berns, E.M., Bontenbal, M., & Foekens, J.A. (1993). Cell biological factors associated with the response of breast cancer to systemic treatment. *Cancer Treatment Reviews, 19*(Suppl. B), 45–63.

Klijn, J.G., Berns, E.M., & Foekens, J.A. (1993). Prognostic factors and response to therapy in breast cancer. *Cancer Surveys, 18*, 165–198.

Kraus, M.H., Popescu, N.C., Amsbaugh, S.C., & King, C.R. (1987). Overexpression of the EGF receptor-related protooncogene erbB-2 in human mammary tumor cell lines by different molecular mechanisms. *European Molecular Biology Organization Journal, 6*(3), 605–610.

Lenz, G., Wright, G.W., Emre, N.C., Kohlhammer, H., Dave, S.S., Davis, R.E., et al. (2008). Molecular subtypes of diffuse large B-cell lymphoma arise by distinct genetic pathways. *Proceedings of the National Academy of Sciences, 105*(36), 13520–13525.

Liu, R., Wang, X., Chen, G.Y., Dalerba, P., Gurney, A., Hoey, T., et al. (2007). The prognostic role of a gene signature from tumorigenic breast-cancer cells. *New England Journal of Medicine, 356*(3), 217–226.

Marchionni, L., Wilson, R.F., Marinopoulos, S.S., Wolff, A.C., Parmigiani, G., Bass, E.B., et al. (2008, January). Impact of gene expression profiling tests on breast cancer outcomes. *Evidence Report/Technology Assessment No. 160* [AHRQ Publication No. 08-E002]. Rockville, MD: Agency for Healthcare Research and Quality. Retrieved October 25, 2008, from http://www.ahrq.gov/clinic/tp/brcgenetp.htm

Mook, S., van't Veer, L.J., Rutgers, E.J., Piccart-Gebhart, M.J., & Cardoso, F. (2007). Individualization of therapy using MammaPrint: From development to the MINDACT trial. *Cancer Genomics and Proteomics, 4*(3), 147–155.

National Cancer Institute. (2006, March). *Clinical Trials: PDQ®: Phase III randomized study of adjuvant combination chemotherapy and hormonal therapy versus adjuvant hormonal therapy alone in women with previously resected axillary node-negative breast cancer with various levels of risk for recurrence (TAILORx Trial).* Retrieved January 13, 2008, from http://www.cancer.gov/clinicaltrials/ECOG-PACCT-1

National Cancer Institute. (n.d.). *Dictionary of cancer terms: Genetic profile.* Retrieved October 20, 2008, from http://www.cancer.gov/dictionary/?searchTxt=genetic+profile&btnGo.x=0&btnGo.y=0&sgroup=Starts+with&lang=

National Cancer Institute Office of Cancer Genomics. (n.d.). *Mission and goals.* Retrieved October 8, 2009, from http://ocg.cancer.gov/overview

National Comprehensive Cancer Network. (2009). *NCCN Clinical Practice Guidelines in Oncology™: Breast cancer* [v.1.2010]. Retrieved November 16, 2009, from http://www.nccn.org/professionals/physician_gls/PDF/breast.pdf

O'Neill, S.C., Brewer, N.T., Lillie, S.E., Morrill, E.F., Dees, E.C., Carey, L.A., et al. (2007). Women's interest in gene expression analysis for breast cancer recurrence risk. *Journal of Clinical Oncology, 25*(29), 4628–4634.

Ogawa, K., Murayama, S., & Mori, M. (2007). Predicting the tumor response to radiotherapy using microarray analysis. *Oncology Reports, 18*(5), 1243–1248.

Paik, S. (2007). Development and clinical utility of a 21-gene recurrence score prognostic assay in patients with early breast cancer treated with tamoxifen. *Oncologist, 12*(6), 631–635.

Paik, S., Shak, S., Tang, G., Kim, C., Baker, J., Cronin, M., et al. (2004). A multigene assay to predict recurrence of tamoxifen-treated, node-negative breast cancer. *New England Journal of Medicine, 351*(27), 2817–2826.

Paik, S., Tang, G., Shak, S., Kim, C., Baker, J., Kim, W., et al. (2006). Gene expression and benefit of chemotherapy in women with node-negative, estrogen receptor-positive breast cancer. *Journal of Clinical Oncology, 24*(23), 3726–3734.

Perou, C.M., Sørlie, T., Eisen, M.B., van de Rijn, M., Jeffrey, S.S., Rees, C.A., et al. (2000). Molecular portraits of human breast tumours. *Nature, 406*(6797), 747–752.

Popescu, N.C., King, C.R., & Kraus, M.H. (1989). Localization of the human erbB-2 gene on normal and rearranged chromosomes 17 to bands q12-21.32. *Genomics, 4*(3), 362–366.

Rimkus, C., Friederichs, J., Boulesteix, A.L., Theisen, J., Mages, J., Becker, K., et al. (2008). Microarray-based prediction of tumor response to neoadjuvant radiochemotherapy of patients with locally advanced rectal cancer. *Clinical Gastroenterology and Hepatology, 6*(1), 53–61.

Roninson, I.B., Chin, J.E., Choi, K.G., Gros, P., Housman, D.E., Fojo, A., et al. (1986). Isolation of human mdr DNA sequences amplified in multidrug-resistant KB carcinoma cells. *Proceedings of the National Academy of Sciences, 83*(12), 4538–4542.

Schlecht, N.F., Burk, R.D., Adrien, L., Dunne, A., Kawachi, N., Sarta, C., et al. (2007). Gene expression profiles in HPV-infected head and neck cancer. *Journal of Pathology, 213*(3), 283–293.

Schwaenen, C., Viardot, A., Berger, H., Barth, T.F., Bentink, S., Döhner, H., et al. (2008). Microarray-based genomic profiling reveals novel genomic aberrations in follicular lymphoma which associate with patient survival and gene expression status. *Genes, Chromosomes and Cancer, 48*(1), 39–54. Retrieved October 20, 2008, from http://www3.interscience.wiley.com/journal/121427561/abstract

Seshadri, R., Matthews, C., Dobrovic, A., & Horsfall, D.J. (1989). The significance of oncogene amplification in primary breast cancer. *International Journal of Cancer, 43*(2), 270–272.

Setlur, S.R., Royce, T.E., Sbonerk, A., Mosquera, J.M., Demichelis, F., Hofer, M.D., et al. (2007). Integrative microarray analysis of pathways dysregulated in metastatic prostate cancer. *Cancer Research, 67*(21), 1296–1303.

Simes, R.J., & Coates, A.S. (2001). Patient preferences for adjuvant chemotherapy of early breast cancer: How much benefit is needed? *Journal of the National Cancer Institute Monographs, 2001*(30), 146–152.

Simon, R. (2006). Development and evaluation of therapeutically relevant predictive classifiers using gene expression profiling. *Journal of the National Cancer Institute, 98*(17), 1169–1171.

Sioutos, N., de Coronado, S., Haber, M.W., Hartel, F.W., Shaiu, W.L., & Wright, L.W. (2007). NCI Thesaurus: A semantic model integrating cancer-related clinical and molecular information. *Journal of Biomedical Informatics, 40*(1), 30–43.

Slamon, D.J., Clark, G.M., Wong, S.G., Levin, W.J., Ullrich, A., & McGuire, W.L. (1987). Human breast cancer: Correlation of relapse and survival with amplification of the HER-2/neu oncogene. *Science, 235*(4785), 177–182.

Sørlie, T., Perou, C.M., Fan, C., Geisler, S., Aas, T., Nobel, A., et al. (2006). Gene expression profiles do not consistently predict the clinical treatment response in locally advanced breast cancer. *Molecular Cancer Therapy, 5*(11), 2914–2918.

Sørlie, T., Perou, C.M., Tibshirani, R., Aas, T., Geisler, S., Johnsen, H., et al. (2001). Gene expression patterns of breast carcinomas distinguish tumor subclasses with clinical implications. *Proceedings of the National Academy of Sciences, 98*(19), 10869–10874.

Sørlie, T., Wang, Y., Xiao, C., Johnsen, H., Naume, B., Samaha, R.R., et al. (2006). Distinct molecular mechanisms underlying clinically relevant subtypes of breast cancer: Gene expression analyses across three different platforms. *BMC Genomics, 7*, 127.

Tal, M., King, C.R., Kraus, M.H., Ullrich, A., Schlessinger, J., Givol, D., et al. (1987). Human HER2 (neu) promoter: Evidence for multiple mechanisms for transcriptional initiation. *Molecular and Cellular Biology, 7*(7), 2597–2601.

Toft, D., & Gorski, J. (1966). A receptor molecule for estrogens: Isolation from the rat uterus and preliminary characterization. *Proceedings of the National Academy of Sciences, 55*(6), 1574–1581.

Tolliday, N., Clemons, P.A., Ferraiolo, P., Koehler, A.N., Lewis, T.A., Li, X., et al. (2006). Small molecules, big players: The National Cancer Institute's initiative for chemical genetics. *Cancer Research, 66*(18), 8935–8942.

University of Utah Genetic Science Learning Center. (2008). *Profiling technique: Microarray analysis.* Retrieved January 10, 2008, from http://learn.genetics.utah.edu/units/pharma/phmicroarray/

van de Vijver, M.J., He, Y.D., van't Veer, L.J., Dai, H., Hart, A.A., Voskuil, D.W., et al. (2002). A gene-expression signature as a predictor of survival in breast cancer. *New England Journal of Medicine, 347*(25), 1999–2009.

van't Veer, L.J., Dai, H., van de Vijver, M.J., He, Y.D., Hart, A.A., Mao, M., et al. (2002). Gene expression profiling predicts clinical outcome of breast cancer. *Nature, 415*(6871), 530–536.

Wang, Y., Jatkoe, T., Zhang, Y., Mutch, M.G., Talantov, D., Jiang, J., et al. (2004). Gene expression profiles and molecular markers to predict recurrence of Dukes' B colon cancer. *Journal of Clinical Oncology, 22*(9), 1564–1571.

Wang, Y., Klijn, J.G., Zhang, Y., Sieuwerts, A.M., Look, M.P., Yang, F., et al. (2005). Gene-expression profiles to predict distant metastasis of lymph node–negative primary breast cancer. *Lancet, 365*(9460), 671–679.

Ward, H.W. (1973). Anti-oestrogen therapy for breast cancer: A trial of tamoxifen at two dose levels. *BMJ, 1*(5844), 13–14.

Yu, S.L., Chen, H.Y., Chang, G.C., Chen, C.Y., Chen, H.W., Singh, S., et al. (2008). MicroRNA signature predicts survival and relapse in lung cancer. *Cancer Cell, 13*(1), 48–57.

Zhai, Y., Kuick, R., Nan, B., Ota, I., Weiss, S.J., Trimble, C.L., et al. (2007). Gene expression analysis of preinvasive and invasive cervical squamous cell carcinomas identifies HOXC10 as a key mediator of invasion. *Cancer Research, 67*(21), 10163–10172.

Zhao, Y.P., Chen, G., Feng, B., Zhang, T.P., Ma, E.L., & Wu, Y.D. (2007). Microarray analysis of gene expression profile of multidrug resistance in pancreatic cancer. *Chinese Medical Journal, 120*(20), 1743–1752.

CHAPTER 9

Pharmacogenomics

Julia Eggert, PhD, APRN-BC, GNP, AOCN®, and Linda Howe, PhD, RN, CNS, CNE

Professional Practice Domain:
Nursing Assessment: Applying/Integrating Genetic and Genomic Knowledge
- Demonstrate an understanding of the relationship of genetics and genomics to health, prevention, screening, diagnostics, prognostics, selection of treatment, and monitoring of treatment effectiveness

Provision of Education, Care, and Support
- Use genetic- and genomic-based interventions and information to improve clients' outcomes
- Evaluate the impact and effectiveness of genetic and genomic technology, information, interventions, and treatments on clients' outcomes

(Consensus Panel on Genetic/Genomic Nursing Competencies, 2009)

INTRODUCTION

Pharmacogenetics evolved from a combination of the disciplines of pharmacology and genetics. With the sequencing of the human genome, an improved understanding of how genetics affects responses to drugs led to the term *pharmacogenomics*. Geneticists were the first to identify the possibility of inherited tendencies causing multiple individuals to react differently to the same drugs. This exciting new knowledge is encouraging nurses to understand the role genetics may play in the selection of appropriate drug agents for patients and to observe for possible adverse responses that are genetically based. Following early genetic discoveries, today's ever-widening knowledge base of pharmacogenomics is changing the landscape of nursing practice. This chapter will examine the history of pharmacogenetics and pharmacogenomics, current discoveries, and implications for nursing practice in today's oncologic treatment and regimens.

HISTORY

In 1931, Sir Archibald Garrod of England, a physiologist, first suggested a relationship between individual reactions to drugs, environmental pollutants, and chemicals (Kalow, 2004). Nearly two decades later, J.B.S. Haldane concurred after studying biochemical reactions and forecasting idiosyncratic reactions to drugs. Though the Haldane and Garrod publications were compelling, they were hardly more than educated guesses. True pharmacogenetics actually started in the 1950s following several scientific discoveries that heralded the recognition of the new science (Kalow, 2004; Roden et al., 2006). Early discoveries included the genetic alteration that lengthens the paralysis from succinylcholine from minutes to hours; this was discovered when patients received this drug during electroshock therapy in the early 1950s. In 1953, the antitubercular drug isoniazid reportedly caused neuropathies in some patients. First thought to be a vitamin B_6 interaction, it was later confirmed through genetic research that these adverse reactions were caused by an alteration in an enzyme that degraded the drug, thus the patients had a toxic reaction from the accumulation of the drug (Kalow, 2004).

In the 1970s, several studies identified that multiple drugs caused metabolic differences among individuals, evidenced by changes in the speed of metabolism. The causative factor is now known as one of the family of enzymes, cytochrome P450 (CYP450), responsible for the metabolism of approximately 20% of drugs: CYP2D6. A decrease in efficiency of this enzyme results in the accumulation of some drugs, whereas a decrease in response can cause the lack of drug conversion to an active form. Antidepressants are a common example of drugs with accumulation potential, which could potentiate side effects, cause adverse reactions, or reach toxic levels. A decrease in response causing lack of drug conversion is exemplified by the inability of codeine to be converted to morphine, resulting in the lack of pain relief (Kalow, 2004; Roden et al., 2006).

These discoveries and publication of such research stimulated further research studies of CYP enzymes (Kalow, 2004). Today, PubMed has almost 3,100 references to the actions of CYP2D6 in humans and more than 110 single nucleotide polymorphisms (SNPs) associated with this variation in individual metabolism noted in the National Center for Biotechnology Information (NCBI) Entrez SNP database regarding differences in drug metabolism (NCBI, n.d.). A SNP is a variation in DNA sequence occurring when a single nucleotide (A, T, C, or G) DNA sequence differs between members of a population. A clarifying example is that of a cake recipe. The DNA code directs how to make a cake. Changing an ingredient could create a strawberry cake, a chocolate cake, or a pineapple upside-down cake. Replacing one single ingredient changes the flavor of the cake. Replacing one nucleotide with another changes the "flavor" of the individual. On rare occasions, an ingredient change can cause a cookie instead of a cake. This could be compared to a mutation. Once again, it is a single ingredient change, but as a rare occurrence, it is labeled as a mutation. The incorporation of multiple SNPs into each DNA blueprint creates the uniqueness of individuals.

PHARMACOGENETICS AND PHARMACOGENOMICS

The completion of the gene sequencing portion of the Human Genome Project resulted in focusing research to learn more about how genetics affects the development of diseases and responses to drug therapies. Sequencing of the human genome revealed that 99.9% of genetic material is identical between individuals. In other words, all of the physical and molecular differences that make each person unique occur because of variations in 0.1% of the DNA. In this small percentage, variations can include nucleotide repeats, insertions, deletions, and SNPs causing changes in amino acid sequence in gene products (proteins), RNA splicing, and gene transcription (Carroll, 2006; Lee, Lockhart, Kim, & Rothenberg, 2005). Some of the variations in the nucleotide (A, T, C, and G) sequences have been found to be responsible for alterations in drug responsiveness among individuals. Other variations are found to be responsible for interactions between the drugs and metabolic enzymes, receptor mutations, or disease pathways. With the completion of the Human Genome Project, SNPs are now known to be associated with what previously was termed *idiosyncratic reactions*, or an unusual response to a drug (Pepper, 2004). Being cognizant of common medications and diseases or syndromes that may be affected by these nucleotide variations is an evolving role for nurses of all specialties, including oncology.

Pharmacogenetics, the study of the role of genetics on therapeutic responses, has been investigated for years, whereas *pharmacogenomics* is the study of genetic variants ranging through an entire genome, and the resultant variances in drug effects is a relatively new area of research (Roden et al., 2006). The Human Genome Project was the major impetus in moving research from pharmacogenetics to pharmacogenomics. The processes currently being investigated include *pharmacokinetics*, how the drug is absorbed, metabolized, distributed, and excreted, and *pharmacodynamics*, the interaction of the drug and target cells that produces drug effects. Recent developments in pharmacogenomics provide the basis for the interest in individualized chemoprevention and treatment based on genetic and molecular makeup.

Pharmacokinetics

Pharmacokinetics is the study of the absorption, distribution, metabolism, and excretion of drugs from the body. Absorption is simply the movement of the drug into the vascular system for distribution into the cells. Metabolism or biotransformation is an enzyme-mediated process that alters the structure of the drug, such as transforming a drug to its active form. Excretion is the removal of the drug and the resulting metabolites from the body. This entire process determines the concentration of the drug at the receptor sites for targeted cells. SNPs can alter the rate of metabolism through the CYP450 enzyme system, resulting in changes of drug conveyance into and out of the cell with molecules such as the p-glycoprotein transporter and differences in drug effects at targeted receptor sites (Evans & McCleod, 2003; Lee et al., 2005) (see Figure 9-1).

Metabolism, or biotransformation of drugs, has two phases (Sarlis & Gourgiotis, 2005). Phase one oxidation processes are the result of CYP microsomal enzymes, which cause inactivation of the drug or the production of an active compound (e.g., codeine conversion to morphine via the CYP2D6 enzyme). Phase two is conjugation, where the drug (substrate) or its metabolite is combined with other chemicals through enzymes that catalyze compounds.

CYP450 is not a single enzyme but a group of more than 40 enzyme families that are hemoproteins similar to hemoglobin. Three of these families, CYP1, CYP2, and CYP3, are known to be important in the metabolism of drugs, whereas the others metabolize various endogenous substances such as lipids, steroids, and hormones, and some metabolize environmental toxins. Each of the three drug-metabolizing families is composed of multiple members that metabolize specific drugs (Evans & McCleod, 2003; Lee et al., 2005).

A specific nomenclature was designed to identify individual enzymes of the CYP system. This nomenclature is based on CYP, designating human cytochrome. The CYP abbreviation is followed by a numeral designating the family (CYP1), next a capital letter to designate the subfamily (CYP1A), and then a second numeral designating the gene that encodes for a single enzyme (CYP1A1) (Pepper, 2004; Roden et al., 2006). Because all of the human cytochromes use this same nomenclature, the family and subfamily are easy

FIGURE 9-1   FACTORS CONTRIBUTING TO DRUG RESPONSE

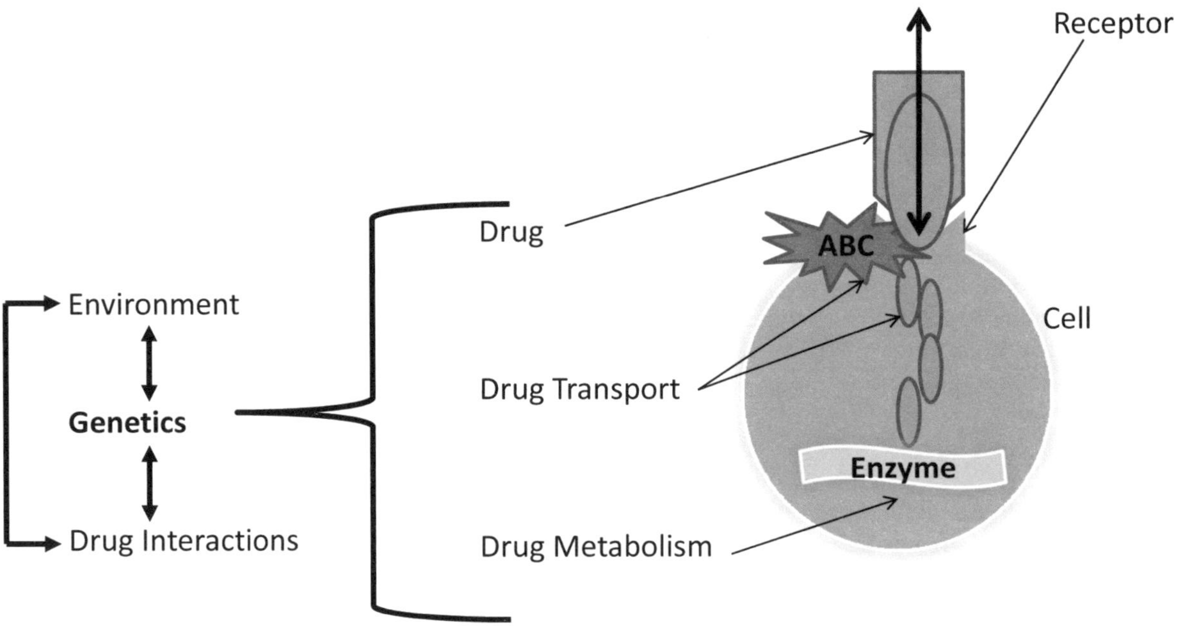

Based on information from Lee et al., 2005.

Note. From "Pharmacogenomics" (p. 142), by J. Eggert in J. Eggert (Ed.), *Cancer Basics*, 2010, Pittsburgh, PA: Oncology Nursing Society. Copyright 2010 by Oncology Nursing Society. Reprinted with permission.

to identify and remain consistent for easy communication among professionals and within the literature.

In the CYP3 family, the CYP3A subfamily performs more than 50% of the known first phase in drug metabolism (Roden et al., 2006). The predominant CYP subfamily enzyme is CYP3A4. Substrates for this enzyme are endogenous (i.e., substances produced in the body, such as steroids, fatty acids, and retinoic acids) and exogenous (i.e., substances from outside the body including drugs, chemicals, and plant products). The CYP3A4 enzyme is associated with many drug-drug and drug-food interactions. In addition to functioning in the liver, CYP3A4 also is located in intestinal mucosa where grapefruit juice may inhibit it, limiting deactivation of certain drugs, thus increasing the bioavailability of certain drugs and elevation of blood levels to possible toxic levels. One example of a drug affected by CYP3A4 is oral methotrexate (Roden et al.).

Some chemical substances increase the activity of a CYP enzyme system, called induction, and others can decrease the activity, called inhibition. If a chemical is seen as increasing the activity of the enzyme, and possibly deactivating more of the drug, then the chemical most likely has been responsible for induction. However, if the chemical prevents or inhibits the enzyme activity, the drug may not be metabolized, and blood levels of the drug may rise. Simply stated, induction and inhibition have an inverse effect on drug levels (see Figure 9-2).

Induction and inhibition actions usually are associated with drug interactions with foods (such as grapefruit juice, charbroiled foods, and cruciferous vegetables), environmental pollutants (such as cigarette smoke), and other drugs (Pepper, 2004). Some of the major substrates for enzymes of the CYP systems with important clinical implications for oncology are listed in Table 9-1.

Drug metabolism rates also affect the rate of renal excretion of the drug, inactivation of the drug, increased therapeutic action of the drug, activation of drugs called prodrugs, and the resulting increased or decreased toxicity. However, SNPs also can alter anticipated therapy results by modifying the drug target, drug uptake or activation pathways, or drug metabolism pathways (Roukos, Murray, & Briasoulis, 2007). Numerous gene variants affect drug metabolism. For example, more than 65 alleles (a variation in the gene, for example, blue versus the wild-type brown eye color) for CYP2D6 have been identified, many having mutations affecting drug metabolism (Sim, 2008).

It is important to remember that the body does not rely on just one set of genes for metabolism. In addition to the numerous CYP genes, numerous genes for enzymes facilitate metabolism outside the CYP family. Genetic changes also may affect drug transport, metabolism, and target. The environment and drug-drug interactions also can affect the variation in an individual's response to a drug (see Figure 9-1).

FIGURE 9-2 INVERSE RELATIONSHIP OF INHIBITION VERSUS INDUCTION OF DRUG ACTIVITY

Inhibition
- Drug prevents or decreases activity of the enzyme
- Drug not degraded or deactivated
- Increased toxicities
- More drug available for effect

Induction
- Drug increases enzyme activity
- More drug deactivated
- Fewer or no toxicities
- Less drug available

Pharmacodynamics

Pharmacodynamics is the study of the physiologic and biochemical effects on the body, the mechanisms on drug actions, and the relationship between drug concentration and

TABLE 9-1 Some Common Oncology-Related Substrates for Drug-Metabolizing Enzymes of Select p450 (CYP) Family Members

Drug-Metabolizing Enzyme	Drug
CYP1A2	Acetaminophen, caffeine, flutamide, methadone, naproxen, theophylline, warfarin
CYP2C19	Phenytoin, warfarin
CYP2D6	Codeine, dextromethorphan, haloperidol, morphine, ondansetron, oxycodone, paroxetine, venlafaxine, tamoxifen
CYP3A4-7	Acetaminophen, antiarrhythmics, codeine, cortisol, cyclophosphamide, doxorubicin, flutamide, hydrocortisone, macrolide antibiotics, morphine, ondansetron, paclitaxel, phenytoin, tamoxifen, trazodone, vinblastine, vincristine

Note. Based on information from Flockhart, 2009; Sarlis & Gourgiotis, 2005.

drug effect. Drug effect is caused largely by interaction with receptors on cells of target organs. This effect involves interaction with cellular proteins, many of which can have genetic variants. Human drug receptors are classified as cell surface receptors and nuclear receptors. Cell surface receptors are proteins embedded in the cell surface. These play a role in most drug effects. Nuclear receptors, contained in the cell nucleus, react to substances, which include glucocorticoids, vitamin D, hormones, and aldosterone (Kalow, 2004). Mutations in receptors can result in the receptor not binding with the drug or binding too much. Genetic variants of the targeted receptor protein can reduce drug efficacy. SNPs in drug uptake or activation of surface receptors could be responsible when the patient does not respond to the drug administered because an alteration in uptake would prevent the drug from reaching the target cell receptors, and a mutation in activation would prevent the drug from being activated and having any effect (Roukos et al., 2007).

Research from the Human Genome Project has identified some of the specific genes responsible for the production of the isoenzymes, enzymes that do the same work but differ in origination, in the CYP enzyme system. The genetic locations for some of the CYP isoenzymes have been identified on chromosomes 4, 10, 19, and 22 (Online Mendelian Inheritance in Man [OMIM], n.d.-a). Pharmacogenomics is taken into account when prescribing known cytochrome substrates. A thorough understanding of family history also is critical to determining familial drug response differences. Identified familial differences in response to a drug such as a life-threatening adverse reaction could be a polymorphism, which is passed from generation to generation. Noting this unusual occurrence could lead to altered prescriptions. Increasingly, prescriptions may be based upon genotypes found by carefully discussing the family history for unusual or different reactions to drugs.

Knowledge of genetic-based differences in a patient's drug pharmacodynamics and pharmacokinetics is used in some venues and will be used widely in the near future to individualize drug therapy. More positive patient outcomes will result, because individualized drug therapy would improve efficacy and minimize the risk of toxicity.

Effects on Metabolism

For each major drug metabolizing and elimination pathway, usually a secondary pathway can carry out these processes in the event that the original pathway is nonfunctioning. The most dramatic negative responses to drug therapy occur when the reduced ability of the primary pathway is combined with the absence of the secondary pathway. A single gene that encodes drug-metabolizing enzymes contributes to aberrant responses to substrate drugs, affecting primary pathways. Primary and secondary pathways are affected by the loss of function determined by several alleles. Individuals with homozygous mutations (the same mutation on both alleles) resulting in loss of function were the first observed to have responses widely varying from those expected (Roden et al., 2006). The "normal" individual is identified as an extensive/effective metabolizer (often written as EM) and therefore has the normal capacity for drug metabolism. Homozygous status is designated as "MM," meaning an individual has two functioning copies of the specific gene producing the enzyme for metabolism. Using "mm" to designate a homozygous mutation, these individuals are labeled as poor metabolizers. They both activate drugs and clear them. This can lead to lesser or no response if the medication is a prodrug, which requires metabolism for the drug to become active. In addition, poor metabolizers will have problems with side effects and toxicities when administered drugs that are active in their administered form. In a heterozygous individual (two different alleles), "Mm" describes an intermediate metabolizer. They will have genes for both normal and reduced metabolic activity of drugs. Finally, the ultrametabolizer can have multiple copies causing enhanced enzyme activity resulting in accelerated clearance. These individuals will have drug activity below the level of an effective dose (see Figure 9-3).

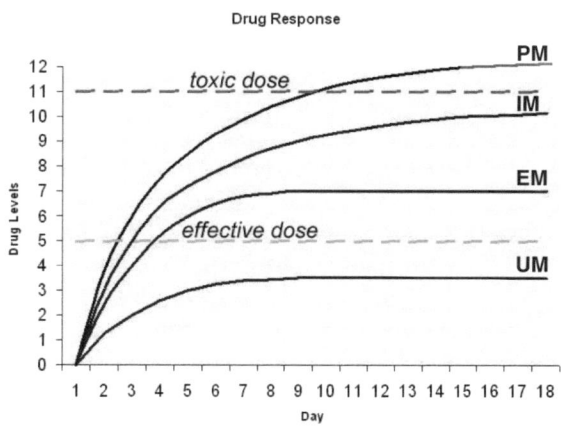

FIGURE 9-3 RELATIONSHIP OF DRUG-METABOLIZING STATUS AND EFFECTIVE DRUG DOSING

PM—poor metabolizer; IM—intermediate metabolizer; EM—effective metabolizer; UM—ultrametabolizer

Note. From *Pharmacogenetic Testing—Web Seminar: Pharmacogenetics in the Practice of Medicine,* by Genelex Corporation, n.d. Retrieved August 24, 2009, from http://www.healthanddna.com/healthcare-professional/pharmacogenetics.html. Copyright Genelex Corporation. Reprinted with permission.

Pharmacogenomics in Oncology

Oncology healthcare professionals consistently have noted interindividual differences in tumor response and tissue toxicity to chemotherapy drugs or regimens. Many of these differences are explained by age, sex, diet, and drug-drug interactions. Research results are now showing that inherited variations of genes responsible for drug disposition (metabolism and transport), and drug targets also are contributing to the variability observed in the clinical outcomes of cancer therapies (Wooin, Lockhart, Kim, & Rothenberg, 2005).

Resistance to chemotherapy agents is a major problem for patients being treated for malignancies. Molecular research and clinical trials have led to improved understanding of the biology of human cancers, how chemotherapy affects the cellular machinery of cancer, and the impact of an individual's molecular differences on his or her response to drugs (Cheng & Evans, 2005).

Known examples of pharmacogenomics can be applied to the oncology clinical setting. Of note are the enzyme systems with similar metabolic activity as described for the CYP family. These include specific SNPs in drug-metabolizing enzymes (thiopurine methyltransferase [TPMT], UDP-glucuronosyltransferase 1A1 [UGT1A1], dihydropyrimidine dehydrogenase [DPD]), drug transporters (multidrug resistance 1 [MDR1]), and drug target enzymes (thymidylate synthase and tyrosine kinase) affecting clinical outcomes for medications such as 5-fluorouracil (5-FU) and irinotecan (Wooin et al., 2005). As nurses become more knowledgeable regarding the influence of pharmacogenomics on the patient outcomes, the quality of care and quality of life for the patient will be enhanced. Several examples of where knowledge of pharmacogenomics makes a difference are described next.

POLYMORPHISMS IN DRUG-METABOLIZING ENZYMES

Thiopurine Methyltransferase and 6-Mercaptopurine

The TPMT enzyme provides the catalyst to cause 6-mercaptopurine (6-MP) to form inactive metabolites, preventing the formation of nucleotides necessary for DNA and RNA synthesis (Wooin et al., 2005). Three alleles, *TPMT*2, TPMT*3A,* and *TPMT*3C*, account for 95% of the enzyme deficiency (Lee et al., 2005). Approximately 1 in 300 individuals inherits the autosomal recessive phenotype of the TPMT enzyme causing low activity. The heterozygous phenotype (6%–11% of the population) has an intermediate activity, and the wild type (89%–94%) has high activity. Low levels of enzyme activity cause changes in the bioavailability and toxicity with 6-MP treatment so that people with this polymorphism who are treated with standard doses of 6-MP can experience a decrease in the rate of metabolism allowing prolonged levels of chemotherapeutic drug in circulation and leading to a risk of severe hematologic toxicities (Engen, Marsh, Van Booven, & McLeod, 2006; OMIM, n.d.-c). These toxicities can cause a need for hospitalization, platelet transfusions, and missed weeks of chemotherapy. Dosing with 6-MP is considered carefully with dose reductions up to 91% in the homozygous recessive phenotype and 50% in the heterozygotes. Children with acute lymphocytic leukemia who have received these dose reductions have equivalent overall survival compared to children receiving the full standard dose (Arber et al., 2003).

Commonly, 6-MP is used to treat acute lymphocytic leukemia in children, with dose intensity leading to event-free survival (Wooin et al., 2005). TPMT testing of red blood cells is now clinically available to ensure dose optimization prior to initiation of 6-MP treatment. Nurses can encourage testing to ensure optimal dosing and ultimately safe treatment of patients. Because blood transfusions can affect accurate results, parents of these young patients need to be carefully questioned regarding the length of time since the last transfusion (Evans, 2003; Lee et al., 2005). Finally, assessments targeting liver and bone marrow toxicities will promote early detection.

UDP-Glucuronosyltransferase 1A1 and Irinotecan

The enzyme UGT1A1 is responsible for linking substances to glucuronic acid in the liver enabling them to be detoxified or inactivated. The wild-type *UGT1A1* has six TATA repeats in the promoter region of the gene that directs transcription, whereas the variant (*UGT1A1*28*) has seven. These polymorphisms in the promoter region of the variant *UGT1A1*28* are associated with toxicity in patients receiving irinotecan therapy. Like other agents, irinotecan requires conversion to an active metabolite, in this case SN-38, which has a stronger inhibitory effect on topoisomerase I. The UGT1A1 enzyme promotes the activation of SN-38 and the catalytic action for bilirubin. Individuals who are homozygous for the seven TATA repeat alleles have reduced metabolism of SN-38 causing increased neutropenia plus hyperbilirubinemia. Those who are heterozygous for the seven repeat (6/7 versus 7/7) have more toxicities but not at the level of homozygous patients. Simply, individuals with homozygous and heterozygous variations in the *UGT1A1* gene have increased toxicities.

Revised dosing of irinotecan is considered for patients who are homozygous for the *UGT1A1*28* 7/7 genotype. One study found that Asians have a 70% incidence rate of the wild-type *UGT1A1* genotype, whereas Caucasians and Africans have less than a 40% rate. The heterozygous *UGT1A1* for the 6/7 genotype is found more commonly in Caucasians and less in African and Asian ethnic groups. Patients who are homozygous for the 7/7 variance are more commonly African, followed in frequency by Caucasians and Asians (Grabinski, 2007; Pangilinan, Khan, & Zalupski, 2008) (see Figure 9-4). The package insert for irinotecan recommends genotyping and that the clinical assay is available. Nurses can encourage testing for the *UGT1A1* variant. In addition, assessing for grade 4 neutropenia and hyperbilirubinemia, especially in patients who are older than 65, would be helpful. Monitoring the high-risk African population is another important intervention (see Table 9-2).

FIGURE 9-4   COMPARISON OF WILD-TYPE (TYPICAL) GENE VERSUS POLYMORPHIC VARIANT GENE RESULTING IN TOXIC EFFECT WITH IRINOTECAN

Efficient Metabolizer
Wild type *UGT1A1* gene → production of UGT1A1 enzyme + irinotecan (I) → conversion of I to active metabolite (SN-38) → normal conversion of metabolite → increased effect on cancer and bilirubin levels within normal limits.

Poor Metabolizer
Variant UGT1A1*28 (extra TATA, heterozygous or homozygous) → altered production of UGT1A1 enzyme + irinotecan (I) → altered conversion of I to active metabolite (SN-38) → significant neutropenia + hyperbilirubinemia

Note. Based on information from Wooin et al., 2005.

TABLE 9-2   Dosing Considerations for Irinotecan

Characteristics	Recommendations
Homozygous for UGT1A1*28 allele	Consider decrease of one dosing level as single and combined agent. Consider use of colony-stimulating factors. Consider use of an alternate agent to irinotecan.
Hyperbilirubinemia syndromes Patient older than 65 years Prior pelvic/abdominal irradiation Elevated baseline bilirubin level Baseline performance status of 2	Carefully review patient history for risk factors. Monitor bilirubin level as treatment progresses and compare to baseline. Monitor change in performance status.

Note. Based on information from Grabinski, 2007; Pangilinan et al., 2008.

Dihydropyrimidine Dehydrogenase and Fluorouracil

The metabolism of 5-FU is complex, with approximately 5% converted to cytotoxic agents responsible for antitumor activity and the remainder degrading into inactive metabolites excreted in the bile and urine (Mattison et al., 2006). The enzyme responsible for catalyzing the rate-limiting step of 5-FU breakdown is DPD. Alterations of the activity of DPD are associated with the adverse effects to 5-FU. DPD deficiency has been associated with several polymorphisms in the *DPYD* gene, with a guanidine to adenine (G→A) point mutation in *DPYD*2A* being one of the most common (Lee et al., 2005). The splice-site mutation (change in DNA sequence from G to A) in the gene *DPYD*2A* leads to a truncated mRNA and a defective protein with diminished enzymatic activity that is unable to deactivate 5-FU. This allows an accumulation of chemotherapy metabolites resulting in excessive toxicity and sometimes lethal consequences. Though the occurrence rates are rare for both the heterozygous (less than 3%) and homozygous (less than 1%) mutations of the gene variant, both changes result in diminished DPD enzyme activity (Mattison et al.).

No clinical practice recommendations exist because no genotyping assay is available. However, an oral uracil breath test, not routinely used in practice, has the capability of discriminating between wild-type and DPD-deficient individuals (Mattison et al., 2006).

Methylenetetrahydrofolate Reductase and Methotrexate

The methylenetetrahydrofolate reductase (MTHFR) enzyme is important in the regulation of folate metabolism, critical for DNA repair and protein synthesis (Toffoli et al., 2003). The *677C→T* polymorphism in the gene is common worldwide with the highest incidence in Caucasians (approximately 30%) and lowest in Africans (approximately 7%) (OMIM, n.d.-b). The conversion in nucleotide is associated with a change in amino acids, reducing the functionality of the enzyme, leading to hyperhomocysteinemia. This is a problem also associated with methotrexate treatments. Individuals with the *677T* polymorphisms, especially homozygotes, would be at highest risk for hyperhomocysteinemia toxicity, and careful monitoring for this toxicity when receiving methotrexate treatment is suggested (Toffoli et al.). Patients with hyperhomocysteinemia are at higher risk for blood clots and strokes. The nursing role would include monitoring for and educating about these cardiovascular problems, especially in the Caucasian population. Though African Americans are typically at higher risk for developing these conditions, the Caucasian group more commonly exhibits the *677T* polymorphism.

POLYMORPHISMS IN DRUG TRANSPORTERS

P-glycoprotein (PGP) is one example of a family of transporting proteins able to move a variety of molecules across the cellular membrane. These include hydrophobic drugs such as hormones, carcinogens, and the chemotherapeutic agents doxorubicin and paclitaxel. Because of its transporting characteristic, PGP can be found in a variety of normal tissues, including hepatocytes, proximal tubules of the kidney, the brush border of the small intestine, the colon, adrenal glands, and capillary endothelium of the brain and testes.

PGP is encoded by the *MDR1* gene and is overexpressed in multidrug resistant cancers. It also varies in expression between individuals and ethnic groups, with the *MDR1* gene variants correlated with commonly prescribed drugs such as digoxin and fexofenadine (Kummar, Gutierrez, Doroshow, & Murgo, 2006). Because these variants are more common in African Americans, this ethnic group needs to be carefully monitored for signs of drug resistance and progressive disease.

POLYMORPHISMS IN DRUG TARGETS

Changes in genes that metabolize medication promote the need to modify drug doses to minimize side effects and maximize dosing effects. Drug targets are a new area of pharmacogenomic concentration for the use of genetic technology. This section will describe target sites for treatment based on genetic variation and prognostic indicators.

Epidermal Growth Factor Receptor Inhibitors

Monoclonal Antibodies

The epidermal growth factor receptor (EGFR) family, also known as ERBB or HER, consists of four receptor tyrosine kinases: EGFR, HER2/neu, ERBB3, and ERBB4. Overamplification of these protein receptors is responsible for initiating the pathways that stimulate cell cycle progression, motility, adhesion, invasion, and angiogenesis, as well as hinder apoptosis, causing the development of cancer (Joshi & Kucherlapati, 2006; Yong, Innocenti, & Ratain, 2006).

Cetuximab is an example of a monoclonal antibody used to target EGFR. It has a high affinity for EGFR and complexes with the cell surface receptor preventing EGFR from binding with it, thus preventing internalization and stimulation of cell proliferation. Polymorphisms in EGFR have been studied to determine their predictability for clinical response in patients with metastatic colorectal cancer. One polymorphism is associated with overexpression of the EGFR protein and is believed to result from increased EGFR translation. It has been observed that patients with less cytosine adenine (CA) dinucleotide repeats in a polymorphic region of the *EGFR* gene are associated with more transcription of EGFR protein and are predictive of metastatic colorectal cancer. Fewer CA repeats were correlated especially with better clinical response to oxaliplatin therapy (Ngyuen, Tran, Lipkin, & Fruehauf, 2006).

Vascular endothelial growth factor (VEGF) is a protein secreted by oxygen-starved tissue to promote the formation of blood vessels, or angiogenesis. Cancer cells have the capability of causing hypoxia, thereby promoting angiogenesis. More than 30 SNPs have been identified in the gene for VEGF. Overexpression of VEGF is found with many tumor types. Bevacizumab is a monoclonal antibody used in combination with 5-FU for the treatment of metastatic colorectal carcinoma. It prevents VEGF from binding to its receptors by competing for those target sites. This causes increased detectable serum levels of VEGF, suggesting diminished availability to tumors. It also implies a mechanism to study for detection of a treatment response (Ngyuen et al., 2006).

Small-Molecule Inhibitors

Two examples of the small-molecule EGFR tyrosine kinase inhibitors are gefitinib and erlotinib. They work by blocking *EGFR* signal transduction (Joshi & Kucherlapati, 2006; Yong et al., 2006). Research results from several non-small cell lung cancer studies using either gefitinib or erlotinib found that tumors with somatic activating mutations (within nonsexual cells) in certain genes increase the activation of EGFR. It was calculated that 80.8% of the treatment responders had somatic mutations, whereas only 8.2% of the responders had germ line (in the ovary or sperm) mutations (Joshi & Kucherlapati). Other studies with small numbers found a correlation of these mutations with progressive disease or a small percentage of response. The "best responders" are identified as having an adenocarcinoma with bronchoalveolar histology, high EGFR expression with mutation (deletion of exon *19 > L858R*), never-smoked status, female sex, and Asian ethnicity (Joshi & Kucherlapati). An acneform rash is a common skin toxicity in patients experiencing a more favorable outcome and absent in patients with resistance (Grabinski, 2007; Yong et al.).

Several academic and commercial laboratories offer investigational use of diagnostic tests to predict patient response to EGFR-tyrosine kinase inhibitors. However, their validity is a concern because of formalin use during tumor processing and the uncertainty regarding which biomarker is best used to determine patient benefit. Pharmacogenomic testing of the *EGFR* mutation focuses on somatic mutations within the tumor, whereas most studies look for germ line polymorphisms (Grabinski, 2007; Joshi & Kucherlapati, 2006).

Chemoprevention

Cancer risk reduction always has included early detection of asymptomatic disease. As more genes, gene products, and their receptors are identified, the practice of cancer risk reduction is merging with treatment. This is enabling clinical practice to move from "the tip of the iceberg" into the deeper molecular and nuclear areas of the cell to target early at risk changes in structures. One of the best examples is the transition of tamoxifen from being only used to treat breast cancer into the realm of risk reduction because of its ability to target the estrogen nuclear receptor.

The progress in risk reduction also is evidenced by the advancement of the National Cancer Institute Cancer Prevention Program's inclusion of national cooperative groups in clinical and translation risk-reduction studies and formalization of risk-reduction science. With the predicted "aging of America," cancer risk reduction is needed more than ever. Studies have shown that carcinogenesis, atherogenesis, neurodegeneration, and other diseases of aging have molecular changes in common. The research is suggesting that a single multitargeted regimen may be used to reduce the risk of or delay a spectrum of these diseases (Lippman & Hong, 2002; Nguyen et al., 2006).

Ethnic Influences and Effects of Admixtures

The study of pharmacogenomics focuses on hereditary factors and drug response. Genetic alterations exist within various ethnic groups. CYP450 enzyme system mutations differ in various ethnic groups, possibly explaining the differences in drug responses. For instance, a percentage of population of a particular group may lack one of the isoenzymes of the CYP450 system, which forces them to utilize other metabolism pathways. The evidence shows that 7% of the Caucasian population and up to 10% of the African American population do not convert codeine to morphine because they have a defective CYP2D6 enzyme (Paice, 2007). This defect causes them to have similar pain relief from Tylenol® (McNeil-PPC, Inc.) #3 as from plain Tylenol. In addition, in the United States about half of the population is identified as *slow acetylators*. This loss of activity in CYP2D6 also results in drug accumulation and increased side effects with certain antitumor drugs. This was supported by Yan et al. (2005), who discovered 58% lower plasma levels of tamoxifen, an antiestrogen agent, in subjects who concomitantly were taking CYP2D6 inhibitors and carried a homozygous wild-type genotype than in those who did not need other antitumor drugs. These individuals are more prone to develop certain adverse reactions with drugs that are metabolized by acetylation (Pepper, 2004; Troup, Martin, McMillan, & Horton, 2005). At least 26 of 42 drug-metabolizing enzymes differ between ethnic groups (Kalow, 2001, 2004). For example, among Caucasian populations (i.e., American Caucasian, British, Polish, Swiss, Danish, German, Swedish, Spanish, Turkish, or Croatian ancestry), 1.5% (Croatian)–10% (Swiss) have CYP2D6 polymorphisms that categorize them as poor metabolizers (Bernard, Neville, Nguyen, & Flockhart, 2006). Poor metabolizers among people of African descent can range as little as 0% for Nigerians to as much as 19% of South Africans. Poor metabolizers who are Asian range from 0% (Japanese) to as much as 4.8% (Indian). Hispanics range from 2.2% among Panamanians to 6.6% among Colombians (Bernard et al.). CYP2D6 polymorphisms also can cause increased or diminished metabolism. Approximately 1%–2% of Caucasians and 51% of Asians are in this category. Significant populations of ultrametabolizers include approximately 10% of people of Spanish descent, 21% of Saudi Arabians, and 29% of Ethiopians (Bernard et al.). Additional information on drugs and ethnic variation can be found at PharmGKB, a central repository of pharmacogenetic and pharmacogenomic research, at www.pharmgkb.org.

Originally, research was centered on ethnic and race determinants for drug therapy. In the United States, however, genetic admixture (genetic variation that occurs within a single ethnic or racial group because of mixing of different populations over many generations) has occurred for centuries and is now affecting the outcomes of future research of pharmacogenetics and pharmacogenomics. The average African American in the United States has 20%–25% European ancestry, resulting in a mosaic of gene inheritance (Suarez-Kurtz & Pena, 2006). Hispanics have an even wider variation, depending on region of ancestral origin (e.g., Mexico, Puerto Rico, Central America, South America) and residence in the United States. The percentage of people with African ancestry varies widely from 1.3% of those from Mexico to 29.1% of those from Puerto Rico, and European ancestry from 4.2% of those from Mexico to 62.7% of Hispanics living in Colorado. Thirty-eight known polymorphisms result from insertions and deletions that affect drug response. Two-thirds of these polymorphisms have shown a difference between Caucasians and African Americans. However, the differences vary based on the amount of European admixture present in the African American group. Sub-Saharan Africans have a wider variation from Caucasians than African Americans. Variant alleles normally found in Europeans and not in Africans are detected in higher levels in African Americans, and conversely, lower levels in Caucasians, further indicating genomic differences based on genetic admixtures. These admixtures may confound some research, requiring consideration for individual pharmacogenetics instead of population-based pharmacogenomics for drug prescription (Suarez-Kurtz & Pena).

Disease-Related Variants

Many diseases introduce additional variants that affect therapy. Such variants are present in common diseases such as asthma, cardiac disease, and cancer. According to Roden et al. (2006, p. 754), "Disease-associated genetic variants may be inherited or arise later: such somatic cell mutations often are found in cancer, where they may arise as a consequence of the disease and may contribute to drug response." For example, two EGFR inhibitors, gefitinib and erlotinib, have widely varying responses in patients with lung cancer; some have significant tumor reduction where somatic mutations occur in the cancer cells in the tyrosine kinase domain of the receptor. Although not routinely used in practice, a screening test is now available to test for these individuals (Roden et al.). Many diseases have genetic links that must be considered when prescribing pharmacotherapy. The following section identifies some malignancies with gene or gene products that alter responses to drug therapy in the patient with cancer.

Acute Myeloid Leukemia-M3

Before the 1990s, those individuals with an *M3* variant of acute myeloid leukemia had a very poor prognosis, with only about 20% of people with this disease experiencing long-term survival (Arber et al., 2003). In the late 1970s, translocation (movement of pieces of chromosome from one chromosome to another) of the long arms of chromosomes 15 and 17 was identified. The retinoic acid receptor-alpha (RAR-α) was identified in 1990 as the specific molecular lesion producing the translocation. This led to the current regimen of an induction course of tretinoin followed by daunorubicin and cytarabine. Testing of an aspirate blood smear is used to identify the *M3* and *M3* variant characteristics. Today, 80% of individuals with an *M3* variant can anticipate long-term survival (Arber et al.).

Chronic Myeloid Leukemia

The Philadelphia chromosome (known as Ph) and its association with chronic myeloid leukemia (CML) have been well known since the discovery in 1960. When the BCR-ABL protein was identified as a tyrosine kinase, the monoclonal antibody imatinib was rapidly developed to target its cellular receptor. Imatinib is now a common treatment for patients in chronic phase CML who have not responded to interferon. Currently, other treatments have been developed based on the identification of a mutation of the *BCR-ABL* gene (Baranska et al., 2008; Druker et al., 1996). In addition, worldwide standardization of molecular monitoring for *BCR-ABL* status is being reviewed (Ross & Hughes, 2008).

TECHNOLOGIC ADVANCES APPLICABLE TO PHARMACOGENOMICS

Researchers are making progress toward cataloging the genetic variations found within the human genome. These variations could be useful in determining a patient's response to a drug. For this to happen, an individual's DNA must be sequenced to determine the presence of specific SNPs. The process of DNA sequencing is lengthy and expensive. This prevents widespread use of variant identification as a diagnostic tool for the prescription of medication. DNA microarrays (called DNA chips) show promise in making a more rapid determination of variant identification that would be affordable. This technology includes placing designated genes in rows on a microscope slide. For example, a single microarray can screen for 100,000 SNPs in less than 24 hours. In 2005, the U.S. Food and Drug Administration approved a diagnostic test for genotyping two important drug-metabolizing enzymes (CYP450 2D6 and 2C19). This assay predicts the metabolic phenotype as a poor, intermediate, extensive, or ultrarapid metabolizer (Roche Diagnostics, n.d.). As this technology advances, it potentially could be used in a healthcare provider's office prior to drug prescription, enabling personalized drug therapy. Microarray technology and expression analysis or mutation and polymorphism analysis could be used to guide drug development, drug response, and therapy development (Yang, Adelstein, & Kassis, 2009).

In the future, personalized polymorphic screenings would benefit the patient, the drug company, and the prescriber. Pharmaceutical companies could exclude drug development targeting alleles with potentially harmful or ineffective metabolism and focus on drugs with the potential for a higher efficacy level based on predicted metabolic phenotypes and population incidence. This also would have potential economic benefits because clinical trials could focus on people with specific SNPs, allowing smaller accrual numbers and less cost. Ultimately, the cost of developing drugs drops, and rapid market place availability is enhanced. The prescriber would have more confidence in the outcomes, and the patient would feel more confident in the medication individually prescribed based on disease, ethnicity, and genotype. For now, healthcare providers must be knowledgeable about the CYP450 system and be aware of the possibility of individual reactions to drugs based on that 0.1% of their DNA (Cheng & Evans, 2005). For nurses, this implies the need for increased awareness that adverse reactions can be more than a troubling problem. It could mean certain patients are receiving too high or too low a dose of their medication. Asking questions about the possibilities of testing for polymorphisms is becoming an important new role in nursing.

SUMMARY

In the world of pharmacogenomics, the future is now. Current research reveals that a significant variation among different ethnic groups and results of haplotype evaluation are providing better correlation with phenotypes than the individual polymorphisms alone. Chemoprevention is converging with cancer treatment. A major remaining deficit is that information about the human genome is based on only about one-quarter of the approximately 30,000 genes. Many of these anonymous genes will be targeted for the development of drugs designed for genetic variations (Frigal, Dracopoli, & Trent, 2005). Individuals providing care to the public need to have at least a basic understanding of pharmacogenetics and pharmacogenomics and how they relate to common oncology medications in order to educate and advocate for their patients and families. Also, implications for the public's health are in regard to reducing drug-associated morbidities and mortalities because of adverse events that could be avoided when using pharmacogenetic and genomic information. This would have therapeutic, quality-of-life, and economic secondary outcomes (van Delden, Bolt, Kalis, Derijks, & Leufkens, 2004).

REFERENCES

Arber, D.A., Stein, A.S., Carter, N.H., Ikle, D., Forman, S.J., & Slovak, M.L. (2003). Prognostic impact of acute myeloid leukemia classification. Importance of detection of recurring cytogenetic abnormalities and multilineage dysplasia on survival. *American Journal of Clinical Pathology, 119*(5), 672–680.

Baranska, M., Lewandowski, K., Gniot, M., Iwola, M., Lewandowska, M., & Komarnicki, M. (2008). Dasatinib treatment can overcome imatinib and nilotinib resistance in CML patient carrying F359I mutation of BCR-ABL oncogene. *Journal of Applied Genetics, 49*(2), 201–203.

Bernard, S., Neville, K., Nguyen, A., & Flockart, D. (2006). Interethnic differences in genetic polymorphisms of CYP2D6 in the U.S. population: Clincial implications. *Oncologist, 11*(2), 126–135.

Carroll, S.B. (2006). *The making of the fittest: DNA and the ultimate forensic record of evolution*. New York: Norton.

Cheng, Q., & Evans, W. (2005). Cancer pharmacogenomics may require both qualitative and quantitative approaches. *Cell Cycle, 4*(11), 1506–1509.

Consensus Panel on Genetic/Genomic Nursing Competencies. (2009). *Essentials of genetic and genomic nursing: Competencies, curricula guidelines, and outcome indicators* (2nd ed.). Silver Spring, MD: American Nurses Association.

Druker, B., Tamura, S., Buchdunger, E., Ohno, S., Segal, G., Fanning, S., et al. (1996). Effects of a selective inhibitor of the Abl tyrosine kinase on the growth of Bcr-Abl positive cells. *Nature Medicine, 2*(5), 561–566.

Engen, R., Marsh, S., Van Booven, D., & McLeod, H. (2006). Ethnic differences in pharmacogenetically relevant genes. *Current Drug Targets, 7*(12), 1641–1648.

Evans, W.E. (2003). Pharmacogenomics: Marshalling the human genome to individualize drug therapy. *Gut, 52*(Suppl. II), ii10–ii18. Retrieved April 26, 2008, from http://www.pubmedcentral.nih.gov/picrender.fcgi?artid=1867751&blobtype=pdf

Evans, W.E., & McCleod, H.L. (2003). Pharmacogenomics—Drug disposition, drug targets, and side effects. *New England Journal of Medicine, 348*(6), 538–549.

Flockhart, D.A. (2009). *Indiana University School of Medicine Division of Pharmacology P450 drug interaction table*. Retrieved November 29, 2009, from http://medicine.iupui.edu/clinpharm/ddis/table.asp

Frigal, E., Dracopoli, N., & Trent, M. (2005). Oncogenomics 2005 meeting report: Dissecting cancer through genome research. *Cancer Research, 65*(19), 8587–8590.

Grabinski, J. (2007). Pharmacogenomics of anticancer agents: Implications for clinical pharmacy practice. *Journal of Pharmacy Practice, 20*(3), 246–251.

Joshi, V., & Kucherlapati, R. (2006). Lung cancer genetics and pharmacogenomics. *Cytogenetic and Genome Research, 115*(3–4), 298–302.

Kalow, W. (2001). Interethnic differences in drug response. In W. Kalow, U. Meyer, & R. Tyndale (Eds.), *Pharmacogenomics* (pp. 109–134). New York: Marcel Dekker.

Kalow, W. (2004). *Pharmacogenomics: Applications to patient care*. Kansas City, MO: American College of Clinical Pharmacy.

Kummar, S., Gutierrez, M., Doroshow, J., & Murgo, A. (2006). Drug development in oncology: Classical cytotoxics and molecularly targeted agents. *British Journal of Clinical Pharmacology, 62*(1), 15–26.

Lee, W., Lockhart, C., Kim, R., & Rothenberg, M. (2005). Cancer pharmacogenomics: Powerful tools in cancer chemotherapy and drug development. *Oncologist, 10*(2), 104–111. Retrieved April 3, 2008, from http://www.TheOncologist.com/egi/content/full/10/2/104

Lippman, S.M., & Hong, W.K. (2002). Cancer prevention science and practice. *Cancer Research, 62*(18), 5119–5125.

Mattison, L., Fourie, J., Hirao, Y., Koga, T., Desmond, R., King, J., et al. (2006). The uracil breath test in the assessment of dihydropyrimidine dehydrogenase activity: Pharmacokinetic relationship between expired 13CO_2 and plasma [2-13C] dihydrouracil. *Clinical Cancer Research, 12*(2), 549–555.

National Center for Biotechnology Information. (n.d.). *CYP2D6*. Retrieved April 8, 2008, from http://www.ncbi.nlm.nih.gov/sites/entrez?db=snp&cmd=search&term=cyp2d6.

Nguyen, H., Tran, A., Lipkin, S., & Fruehauf, J.P. (2006). Pharmacogenomics of colorectal cancer prevention and treatment. *Cancer Investigation, 24*(6), 630–639.

Online Mendelian Inheritance in Man. (n.d.-a). *CYP*. Retrieved April 28, 2008, from http://www.ncbi.nlm.nih.gov/Omim/getmap.cgi?chromosome=cyp&start=-2

Online Mendelian Inheritance in Man. (n.d.-b). *Methylenetetrahydrofolate reductase (MTHFR)*. Retrieved April 26, 2008, from http://www.ncbi.nlm.nih.gov/entrez/dispomim.cgi?id=607093

Online Mendelian Inheritance in Man. (n.d.-c). *Thiopurine S-methyltransferase*. Retrieved March 9, 2008, from http://www.ncbi.nlm.nih.gov/entrez/dispomim.cgi?id=187680

Paice, J. (2007). Pharmacokinetics, pharmacodynamics, and pharmacogenomics of opioids. *Pain Management Nursing, 8*(3, Suppl. 1), S2–S5.

Pangilinan, J., Khan, G., & Zalupski, M. (2008). Irinotecan pharmacogenetics: An overview for the community oncologist. *Community Oncology, 5*(2), 99–103.

Pepper, G.A. (2004). Pharmacokinetics and pharmacodynamics. In E.Q. Youngkin, K.J. Sawin, J.F. Kissinger, & D.S. Israel (Eds.), *Pharmacotherapeutics: A primary care clinical guide* (2nd ed., pp. 50–78). Stamford, CT: Appleton and Lange.

Roche Diagnostics. (n.d.). *AmpliChip: Breakthrough in individualized treatment*. Retrieved March 8, 2008, from http://www.amplichip.us

Roden, D.M., Altman, R.B., Benowitz, N.L., Flockhart, D.A., Giacomini, K.M., & Johnson, J.A. (2006). Pharmacogenomics: Challenges and opportunities. *Annals of Internal Medicine, 145*(10), 749–757.

Ross, D., & Hughes, T. (2008). Current and emerging tests for the laboratory monitoring of chronic myeloid leukaemia and related disorders. *Pathology, 40*(3), 2331–2346.

Roukos, D., Murray, S., & Briasoulis, E. (2007). Molecular genetic tools shape a roadmap towards a more accurate prognostic prediction and personalized management of cancer. *Cancer Biology and Therapy, 6*(3), 8–12.

Sarlis, N., & Gourgiotis, L. (2005). Hormonal effects on drug metabolism through the CYP system: Perspectives on their potential significance in the era of pharmacogenomics. *Current Drug Targets—Immune, Endocrine, and Metabolic Disorders, 5*(4), 439–448.

Sim, S. (2008). *CYP2D6 nomenclature*. Retrieved April 27, 2008, from http://www.cypalleles.ki.se/cyp2d6.htm

Suarez-Kurtz, G., & Pena, S. (2006). Pharmacogenomics in the Americas: The impact of genetic admixture. *Current Drug Targets, 7*(12), 1649–1658.

Toffoli, G., Russo, A., Innocenti, F., Carona, G., Tumolo, S., Sartor, F., et al. (2003). Effect of methylenetetrahydrofolate reductase 677→T polymorphism on toxicity and homocysteine plasma level after chronic methotrexate treatment of ovarian cancer patients. *International Journal of Cancer, 103*(30), 294–299.

Troup, C., Martin, B., McMillan, C., & Horton, R. (2005). Simulated pharmacogenomics exercises for the cybertory virtual molecular biology laboratory. *IEEE Computational Systems Bioinformatics Conference Workshops. Bioengineering Conference Northeast Proceedings* (pp. 124–125). New York: IEEE.

van Delden, J., Bolt, I., Kalis, A., Derijks, J., & Leufkens, H. (2004). Tailor-made pharmacotherapy: Future developments and ethical challenges in the field of pharmacogenomics. *Bioethics, 18*(4), 303–321.

Wooin, L., Lockhart, A., Kim, R., & Rothenberg, M. (2005). Cancer pharmacogenomics: Powerful tools in cancer chemotherapy and drug development. *Oncologist, 10*(2), 104–111.

Yan, J., Desta, Z., Stearns, V., Ward, B., Ho., H., Lee, K., et al. (2005). CYP2D6 genotype, antidepressant use, and tamoxifen metabolism during adjuvant breast cancer treatment. *Journal of the National Cancer Institute, 97*(1), 30–39.

Yang, Y., Adelstein, S., & Kassis, A. (2009). Target discovery from data mining approaches. *Drug Discovery Today, 14*(3–4), 147–154.

Yong, W.P., Innocenti, F., & Ratain, M.J. (2006). The role of pharmacogenetics in cancer therapeutics. *British Journal of Clinical Pharmacology, 62*(1), 35–46.

CHAPTER 10

Targeted Therapies

Michele E. Gaguski, MSN, RN, AOCN®, CHPN, APN-C, and Susan D. Bruce, MSN, RN, OCN®

Professional Practice Domain:
Nursing Assessment: Applying/Integrating Genetic and Genomic Knowledge
- Demonstrate an understanding of the relationship of genetics and genomics to health, prevention, screening, diagnostics, prognostics, selection of treatment, and monitoring of treatment effectiveness

Provision of Education, Care, and Support
- Use genetic- and genomic-based interventions and information to improve clients' outcomes

(Consensus Panel on Genetic/Genomic Nursing Competencies, 2009)

INTRODUCTION

Cancer treatment in the 21st century is moving molecular biology from inside the laboratory to the front lines of therapy options for oncology professionals with the advent of targeted therapies. In cancer care, selection of treatment is not just based upon the staging of tumors but also takes into account the microenvironment of each cell that may range from the type of protein expressed to growth factors that signal the cells to grow. Such factors influenced by or products of the cell's communication system cause each tumor to become a unique entity and are potential targets for treatment.

Since the late 1990s, oncology healthcare professionals have seen the exponential growth of treatment options with advances in molecular research and technology. These milestones have led the way to new approaches for diagnosing, monitoring, and treating people diagnosed with cancer. Research findings from the Cancer Genome Anatomy Project (http://cgap.nci.nih.gov) and the Cancer Molecular Analysis Project (http://cmap.nci.nih.gov) began to link together the intricate workings of the tumor cell and its cell signaling and control mechanisms. As a result, cancer treatment is no longer a one-size-fits-all mentality, but utilizes personalized medicine targeted approaches, right down to the cellular workings of each individual's tumor cell. The regulation of the cell cycle, cell activation and inactivation, cell signaling, and cell growth is the basis for understanding current and future targets for drug therapies.

RATIONALE FOR TARGETED THERAPIES

Targeted therapy refers to the utilization of agents that target cancer cell–specific abnormalities and characteristics such as signaling pathways and tumor-specific genetic profiles (Hait & Hambley, 2009). For more information on tumor profiling, see Chapter 8. Mounting evidence suggests that cancer can be viewed as a "signaling disease." In cancer cells, the signaling process is defective. Targeted therapies affect cancer growth by influencing the defective communication pathways in the cancer cell. Focusing on the signal transduction pathways specific to a given cancer leaves healthy cells alone; therefore, many targeted therapies have a lower toxicity profile when compared to nontargeted traditional anticancer therapies (Hait & Hambley). Because targeted therapies aim to target only aberrant signals in malignant cells or malfunctioning gene expression, they lack many of the side effects associated with common chemotherapy. This lower toxicity profile provides the opportunity to sustain treatment throughout the projected therapy time and limits serious side effects that would warrant dose delays, reductions, and discontinuation.

Finding the right target is based on tumor biology and the molecular workings of the cell such as signaling pathways, enzyme activity, cell membrane receptors, and regulatory growth controls (Hait & Hambley, 2009). Tumor growth and progression is contingent on cell membrane receptors that control intracellular signal transduction pathways, which in turn regulates cellular behavior, including proliferation, apoptosis, angiogenesis, adhesion, and motility (Gemmill & Idell, 2003). These pathways provide a rich environment for selecting targets upon which to design cancer therapies.

HISTORY OF TARGETED THERAPY

The use of targeted therapies to treat cancer is by no means new. Hormonal manipulations to treat cancer are an early example of targeted therapy. For example, observations that bilateral salpingo-oophorectomy resulted in breast cancer regression stimulated research in the early 1900s exploring the biologic basis for this finding (Jordan, 2009). The discovery of breast cell estrogen receptors led the identification of selective estrogen receptor modulators (SERMs), which act by competing with estradiol for receptor binding and, as a result, block the action of estrogen in breast tissue while not significantly affecting the beneficial estrogen effects on the bone and heart (see Figure 10-1) (Jordan; Sengupta & Jordan, 2008). The efficacy of one such SERM, tamoxifen citrate, is well documented and has been a treatment option for estrogen receptor–positive breast cancer for more than 30 years (Jordan).

Signal Transduction-Cell Signaling Pathways

All cells regulate their function, growth, differentiation, and life span via an intricate network of biochemical and molecular messengers that are collectively referred to as "cell signaling" (Gale, 2003). Cell signaling is the complex communication system based on a network of interacting molecular signals. These signals govern basic cellular activities and coordinate cell function. The ability of cells to communicate within their microenvironment provides the foundation for normal tissue homeostasis and growth. If genetic mutations occur, the communication network could malfunction. The accumulation of errors in cell information processing is responsible for the disruption of cell function, regulatory control of cell growth, and ultimately development of cancer. Finding where the communication or signal disruption occurs forms the underpinning for targeted therapies. Targeted agents designed to address specific aspects of the cell signal may be unique to a given

FIGURE 10-1. HORMONAL TARGETED THERAPIES

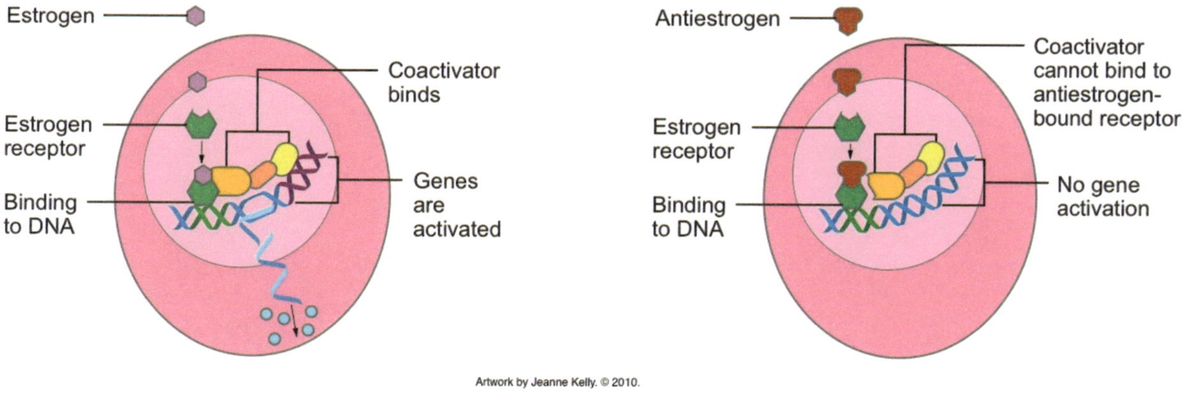

Note. From *Understanding Cancer and Related Topics: Understanding Estrogen Receptors, Tamoxifen, and Raloxifene,* by L. Kliensmith, D. Kerrigan, J. Kelley, and B. Hollen, 2006. Retrieved May 26, 2009, from http://www.cancer.gov/cancertopics/understandingcancer/estrogenreceptors/Slide13. Artwork orginally created for the National Cancer Institute. Reprinted with permission of the artist, Jeanne Kelly. Copyright 2010.

malignancy, given the complex network of signals where errors can occur (Hait & Hambley, 2009). A list of terminology specific to the signaling pathways that will be reviewed is summarized in Figure 10-2.

Signal transduction refers to the pathways in which a chemical signal is transmitted from outside the cell (extracellular) exterior to the interior (intracellular) to initiate and regulate cellular functions, including cell proliferation, apoptosis, cell motility, and angiogenesis (Battiato & Wheeler, 2005) (see Figure 10-3). These pathways are activated through ligand binding (see Figure 10-4). A ligand is any type of molecule that binds to receptors on the membrane surface of the cell or within the cell that is receiving the signal (Battiato & Wheeler). Many different types of ligands exist, including hormones and growth factors.

Receptors (represented in yellow in Figure 10-4) are proteins that can be either inside or on the cell surface. The li-

FIGURE 10-2. SIGNAL TRANSDUCTION TERMINOLOGY

Cell signaling—Network of biochemical and molecular messengers involved in the communication of cells

Dimerization—The reaction of the receptor by the ligand when two monomers (identical molecules) are paired having little structural change

Growth factor receptors—A substance made by the body that functions to regulate cell division and cell survival

Heterodimerization—The pairing of two different (hetero) receptors

Homodimerization—The pairing of two of the same (homo) receptors

Ligands—Molecular messengers, such as growth factors, that bind and activate receptors on the surface of the cell

Ligand binding—The process by which the ligand attaches itself to a specific receptor on the cell surface and activates the receptor, initiating the signaling pathway

Monomer—Single receptor in an inactive state, joins with other monomers to create polymers, which build proteins

Phosphorylation—The addition of a phosphate group to a protein molecule, which activates the cell signaling pathway

Receptors—A cell membrane protein on the inside or outside of a cell that selectively binds to a specific drug, hormone, or chemical mediators to alter cell function

Signal—Chemical language of cells

Note. Based on information from Remer, 2009; Wujcik, 2006.

FIGURE 10-3   SIGNAL TRANSDUCTION

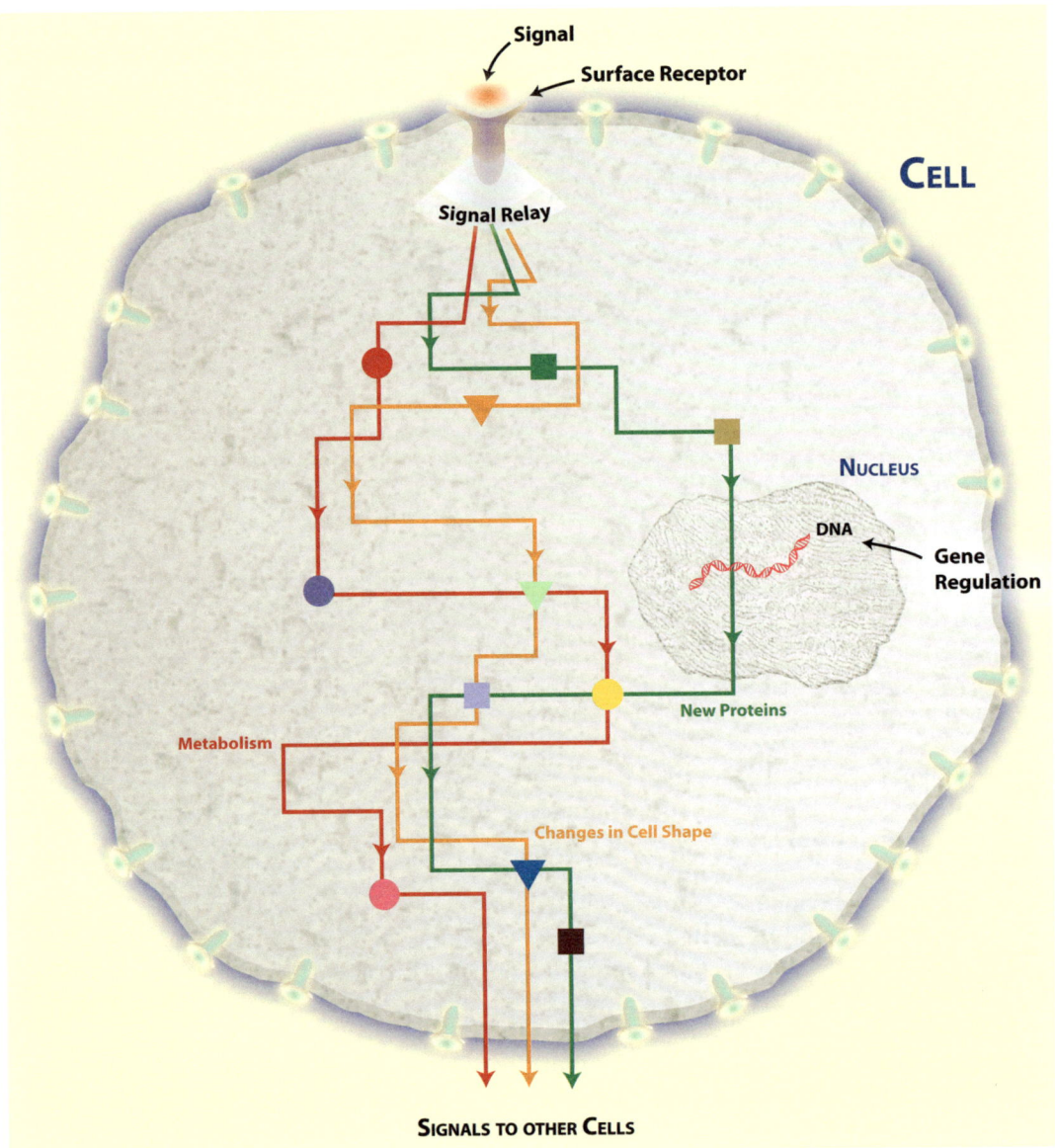

Signal transduction is the process by which a signal is carried from outside the cell to the nucleus. Signaling is initiated by a soluble ligand, such as a growth factor, hormone, antibody, or external drug, which through its binding causes the activation of cell surface receptors. This activation produces phosphorylation of the internal portion of the receptor, which in turn activates downstream signaling intermediates. In this way, the signal eventually reaches the nucleus, where it modulates a particular cellular process.

Note. From *Biological Pathways,* by National Human Genome Research Institute, 2009. Retrieved November 9, 2009, from http://www.genome.gov/images/illustrations/Biological_Pathways.pdf.

gand selectively attaches itself to the receptor, which then activates the receptor and initiates the cellular signaling pathway. This attachment of the ligand to the receptor is called ligand binding (see Figure 10-4). A cell produces a limited number of receptors based on its function, which restricts its responses to only those it needs. The binding prompts dimerization (the joining of two receptors). A dimer is a chemical or biologic entity consisting of two subunits called monomers. Homodimers are two monomers of the same type. Heterodimers are two different receptors that are able to bind together. When the receptors bind to an extracellular signaling molecule (a ligand), they become activated and generate a cascade of intracellular signals that alter the behavior of the cell. The intracellular receptor and signaling ligand need to enter the cell in order to activate them. These signaling molecules must be small, sticky, and adherent (hydrophobic) to be able to diffuse the plasma membrane (Battiato & Wheeler, 2005).

When the signal is received, activation of the signaling pathway occurs (represented in pale yellow in Figure 10-4). This is done chemically using phosphates in a process called phosphorylation, which occurs as soon as dimerization and ligand-binding take place, resulting in the cell signaling activation. Phosphorylation is the addition of a phosphate group to a protein molecule and is reversible by the removal of that phosphate group. Last, the

FIGURE 10-4 LIGAND BINDING

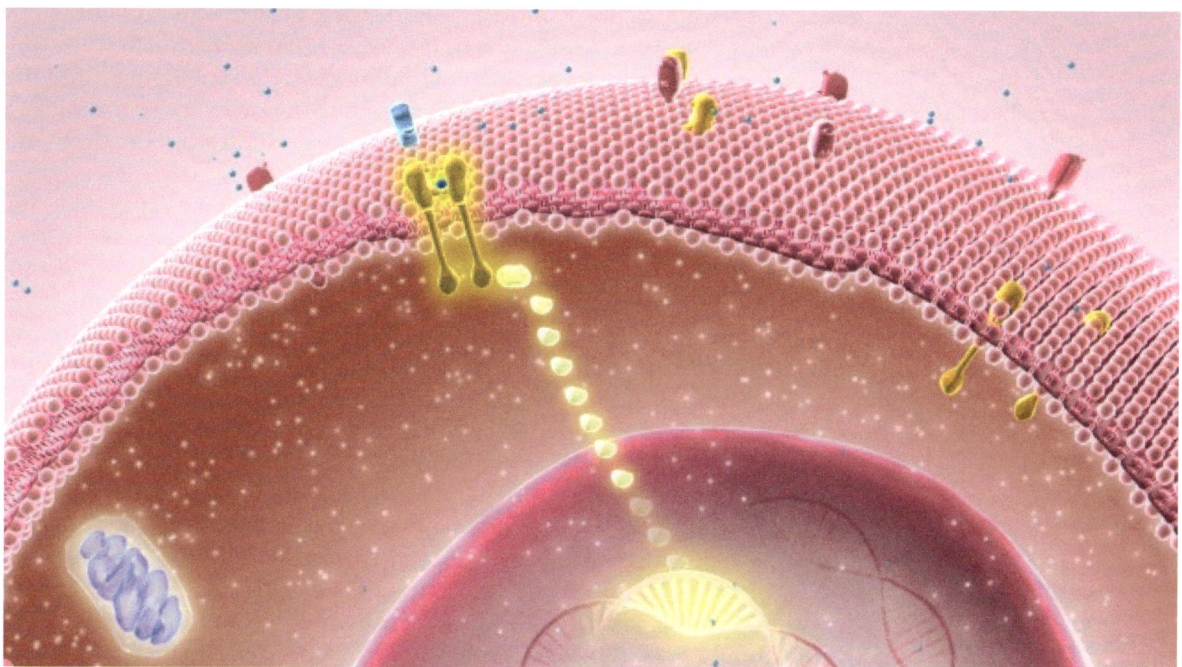

The binding of a ligand to a receptor initiates a signaling cascade that ends in the nucleus, where it stimulates cell growth, metastasis, angiogenesis, and apoptosis (cell death).

Note. From *Advances in Targeted Therapies Tutorial,* by National Cancer Institute, n.d. Retrieved December 4, 2009, from http://www.cancer.gov/cancertopics/understandingcancer/targetedtherapies/htmlcourse/page3.

output layer lies in the intracellular region that contains tyrosine kinase, which is activated through phosphorylation following dimerization. The phosphorylation of proteins is a cellular regulatory mechanism and is critical to regulating cell signaling. Signal transduction pathways are regulated to some degree by the process of protein phosphorylation. Determination of a protein's phosphorylating state is important in identifying the "on/off" state of the signaling transduction pathways. Protein phosphorylation and dephosphorylation are complex biochemical processes, which result from a cellular response to a specific stimulus. This activation leads to downstream signaling that controls the various cell activities, including cell proliferation, apoptosis, cell motility, and angiogenesis (Battiato & Wheeler, 2005; Wujcik, 2006).

Signaling molecules inside the cell participate in the transmission of the internal signal, which is a process called the intracellular signaling cascade. This mechanism occurs through the interface of one protein with another in the pathway, much like a lock and key. This provides the means by which a signal outside the cell can be transmitted to the inside of a cell and influence cell behavior (see Figure 10-3). In summary, the cell signaling pathway consists of the signal, a receptor, and the intracellular signaling cascade.

Gene Mutations and Signal Transduction

Genetic alterations can disrupt this signaling process deregulating normal cell growth, division, and programmed cell death (apoptosis). Proto-oncogenes (precursors of oncogenes or cancer genes) are normal genes that are involved in the growth and division of the cell. These proto-oncogenes code for the proteins that send a signal to the nucleus to stimulate cell division. They are part of the intracellular signaling cascade (see Figure 10-3) described previously. As the cascade progresses, one protein activates one or more proteins in the cell until the transcription factors in the nucleus activate the genes for cell division (Annenberg Media, n.d.).

Oncogenes (cancer genes) are mutated versions of the proto-oncogenes that code for these signaling molecules. Oncogenes activate the signaling cascade continuously. This facilitates the increased production of factors that stimulate cell growth. Mutations in proto-oncogenes can occur in several ways: through viruses that insert their DNA in or near the proto-oncogene; by a chromosome translocation, which refers to a break in a chromosome resulting in a chromosome section attaching itself to another chromosome resulting in a genetic rearrangement; or by an increase in the number of copies of the normal proto-oncogene. As a result of this conversion, the alteration in the gene contributes to uncontrolled cell growth and cancer initiation (Annenberg Media, n.d.).

For example, *MYC* is a proto-oncogene (normal gene) that codes for a protein transcription factor, c-Myc. The c-Myc protein is a regulator of other genes and binds DNA at specific sites and instructs genes whether or not they should be transcribed into messages for the cell to make other proteins. Mutations in *MYC* convert the proto-oncogene into an oncogene, which is associated with a wide range of cancers, including both solid and hematologic diseases (Dang, 2009). *RAS* is another example of an oncogene that regulates the signaling cascade. Mutations in *RAS* continually activate the signaling pathway, resulting in uncontrolled cell growth. Approximately 30% of cancers, such as myeloid malignancies; myeloid proliferative disorders; and pancreatic, colorectal, lung, and thyroid cancers, are associated with *RAS* gene mutations (Gale, 2003).

Tumor suppressor genes are normal genes that slow down cell growth and division. Any malfunction of the tumor suppressor gene may result in cells not being able to stop growing or dividing, leading to tumor growth. To illustrate this point, consider the oncogene as a gas pedal that is stuck to the floor, producing uncontrolled cell growth. Tumor suppressor genes act like the brake pedal. Malfunctioning of the tumor suppressor gene is like having a brake pedal that does not function as it should, and cells continue to grow and divide.

In normal cells, cross talk (communication between various signaling pathways) is a normal process that occurs to maintain various cell functions. In cancer cells, cross talk between signal transduction pathways can affect disease progression, metastatic potential, and resistance to treatment. Many tumors have changes in signal transduction pathways, or the communication tree within the cell that mediates cell proliferation, survival, energy utilization, cell death, and many other functions. This allows cells to continue to replicate more times than normal cells. For example, conventional chemotherapy or radiation therapy can contribute to cancer cells' resistance to treatment by creating cell signals that allow the cells to avert normal apoptosis (Rixe & Fojo, 2007).

Identifying Targets

Targeted agents interact with specific cellular pathways on which cancer cells depend such as growth, proliferation, angiogenesis, and apoptosis (Ma & Adjei, 2009). Targets can be located on the outside or inside of a cancer cell. The most common targets on the outside of the cell are receptors that help to relay chemical messages. Many of the targets on the inside of the cell are enzymes that help to speed up chemical reactions in the body. The identification of a signaling pathway critical to cancer pathogenesis or progression provides a host of potential therapeutic targets through the following processes (Sharkey & Goldenberg, 2006; Wood, 2002).

- Activating apoptotic signals that cause cell death
- Disrupting communication among cancer cells
- Stimulating downregulation of overexpressed proteins to uphold cell growth and cause cell death
- Stimulating cytokines, which attract other cytotoxic cells, like infections in which cytokines trigger an immune response
- Inhibiting multiple proteins to disrupt signaling pathways at the extracellular and intracellular levels

MECHANISMS FOR TARGETED INTERVENTION

Advances in technology have resulted in a variety of strategies that can be used against cancer-specific targets, including monoclonal antibodies (MoAbs), small-molecule protein kinase inhibitors, cancer vaccines and immunotherapy, **antisense oligonucleotides**, and RNA interference (RNAi) (Ma & Adjei, 2009).

Monoclonal Antibodies

MoAbs are antibodies produced in the laboratory that target tumor-specific antigens mostly located on the cell membrane. Similar to all antibodies, they are attracted to bind with specific antigens. All MoAb drugs end in -mab (e.g., trastuzumab). MoAbs vary, but all have a specific target and are produced using a specific source, which is identified by the drug name suffix: pure mouse is labeled -momab; part mouse but mostly human is labeled -ximab; very small part mouse and mostly human is labeled -zumab; and all human is labeled -umab (Held-Warmkessel, 2008). MoAbs can be used individually to disrupt cell signaling by binding with cell receptors, used to help to stimulate the immune system, or used to help to target the delivery of other therapeutic modalities such as chemotherapy, biologic therapies, and radioactive materials more precisely to the cancer by inhibiting or promoting signals (see Figure 10-5). Also, evidence suggests that some MoAbs may have a synergistic effect with certain chemotherapeutic agents when used in combination (Berdeja, 2003).

Small-Molecule Protein Kinase Inhibitors

Receptor tyrosine kinases are growth factor receptors located on the cell surface (Gschwind, Fischer, & Ulrich, 2004). The human epidermal growth factor receptor (HER) family includes epidermal growth factor receptor (EGFR [ERBB1]), HER2/neu (ERBB2), HER3 (ERBB3), and HER4 (ERBB4), all of which are related structurally (Ma & Adjei, 2009). Receptor tyrosine kinases that have been mutated are involved in many different cancers, and EGFR has been shown to be a central point for several signaling pathways that influence cell proliferation, differentiation, motility, survival, adhesion, and repair (Gschwind et al.; Ma & Adjei). Inhibitors of the HER family of re-

FIGURE 10-5 MONOCLONAL ANTIBODIES

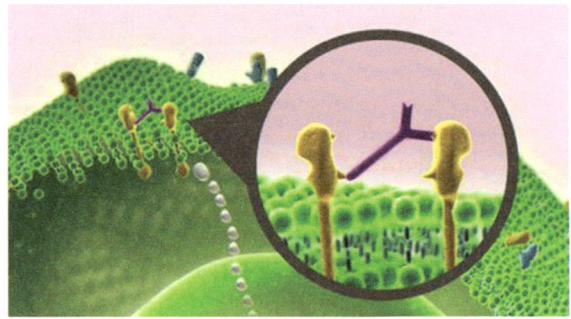

First, antibodies can work outside the cell by preventing signaling molecules and receptors from interacting with each other.

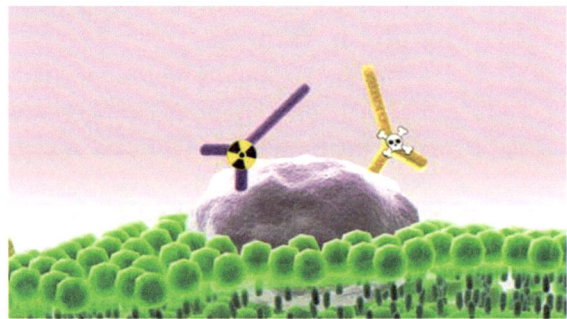

Second, they also can be used as delivery vehicles, guiding radioactive molecules or toxins to the cancer cells.

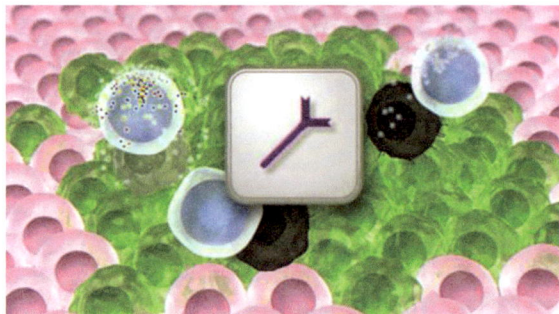

Third, antibodies attached to a cell can trigger an immune response that destroys the cell.

Note. From *Advances in Targeted Therapies Tutorial,* by National Cancer Institute, n.d. Retrieved December 4, 2009, from http://www.cancer.gov/cancertopics/understandingcancer/targetedtherapies/htmlcourse/page2.

ceptors rapidly have demonstrated efficacy against several different malignancies and are used widely in clinical settings.

Cancer Vaccines and Immunotherapy

In contrast to other types of targeted therapies, this therapeutic approach uses the same concepts as those used in the prevention of viral diseases, inducing the host to generate an immune response—in this case, against their cancer (Rosenberg, Yang, & Restifo, 2004) (see Figure 10-6). Unfortunately, response rates from cancer vaccines alone remain low, so focus has turned to the immune T cells that are the critical component of generating an immune response. Current evidence supports three criteria needed for destroying established cancers, including (Rosenberg et al.)

- Adequate number of immune T cells that can recognize tumor antigens
- The ability of the immune T cells to travel to and infiltrate the cancer
- The immune T cells must be capable of activating mechanisms that can destroy the cancer.

Current cancer vaccine research includes a focus on refining ways to develop antigen-specific immune T cells and maximize tumor infiltration, as well as research on the use of vaccines in combination with other adjuvant therapies that can enhance the immune response.

Antisense Oligonucleotides

Antisense oligonucleotides refer to the introduction and binding of short, modified DNA or RNA strands to messenger RNA in order to modify the protein that is being synthesized (Kushner & Silverman, 2000). A variety of genes and proteins are targeted in clinical trials using this approach, including *c-raf*, *bcl-2*, and *TP53*, all of which are involved in a variety of malignancies (Kushner & Silverman).

RNA Interference

Underlying the use of small, interfering ribonucleic acids is the goal of silencing a specific gene (Gewirtz, 2007). For more background on RNA, refer to Chapter 2. RNAi refers to the use of double-stranded RNA targeting a precise sequence of messenger RNA for destruction. Although the use of this approach remains in a predominantly research capacity, this very precise targeted approach has considerable promise (Gewirtz). For more information about this research see Chapter 15.

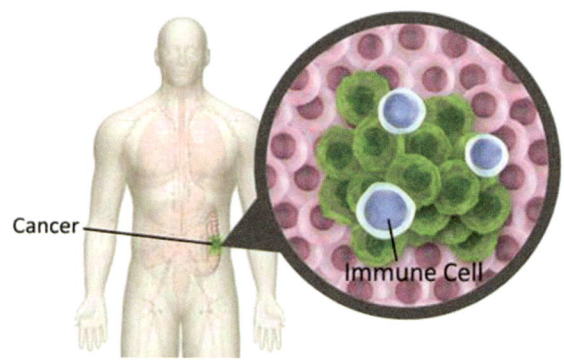

FIGURE 10-6 CANCER VACCINES AND IMMUNOTHERAPY

Unlike other targeted therapies, therapeutic cancer vaccines do not act specifically on pathways in cancer cells. Instead, they act broadly by trying to activate the body's immune system to make it recognize and attack cancer cells.

Note. From *Advances in Targeted Therapies Tutorial*, by National Cancer Institute, n.d. Retrieved December 4, 2009, from http://www.cancer.gov/cancertopics/understandingcancer/targetedtherapies/htmlcourse/page2#d.

APPLYING TARGETED THERAPIES TO SIGNALING PATHWAYS IN CANCER

This section will provide a closer look at specific applications of targeted therapies, highlighting some clinically approved agents. See Table 10-1 for a more extensive list of the U.S. Food and Drug Administration (FDA)-approved targeted therapies.

TABLE 10-1 U.S. Food and Drug Administration–Approved Targeted Therapies for Cancer and Toxicity Profiles

Therapeutic Agent	Target	Cellular Domain	Type of Therapy	Cancer Types	Route	Side Effect Profile
Bevacizumab	Angiogenic pathway	Extracellular	Monoclonal antibody, angiogenesis inhibitor	Colorectal cancer, non-small cell lung cancer	IV	Gastrointestinal (GI) perforation, wound healing complications, hemorrhage, hypertension, epistaxis, proteinuria
Bortezomib	Intracellular proteasomes	Intracellular	Proteasome inhibitor	Multiple myeloma, mantle cell lymphoma	IV	Peripheral neuropathy, neutropenia, thrombocytopenia, asthenic conditions, hypotension, infiltrative pulmonary disease, tumor lysis syndrome
Cetuximab	EGFR	Extracellular	Monoclonal antibody, EGFR inhibitor	Colorectal cancer, head and neck cancer	IV	Hypersensitivity reactions, dermatologic toxicity, radiation dermatitis, cardiopulmonary arrest, interstitial lung disease, sepsis, hypomagnesemia
Dasatinib	Multiple tyrosine kinases	Intracellular	Kinase inhibitor	Chronic myeloid leukemia (CML)	PO	Fluid retention, dermatologic toxicity, diarrhea, headache, fatigue
Erlotinib	ERBB1	Intracellular	Tyrosine kinase inhibitor	Non-small cell lung cancer, pancreatic cancer	PO	Interstitial lung disease, rash, diarrhea
Gefitinib	ERBB1	Intracellular	Enzyme inhibitor	Non-small cell lung cancer (compassionate use only)	PO	Interstitial lung disease, diarrhea, dermatologic toxicity
Ibritumomab	CD20 antigen	Extracellular	Radiolabeled monoclonal antibody	Non-Hodgkin lymphoma	IV	Infusion reactions, cytopenias, cutaneous and mucocutaneous reactions, secondary leukemia and melodysplastic syndrome
Imatinib	Bcr-abl tyrosine kinase and KIT	Intracellular	Enzyme inhibitor	CML, gastrointestinal stromal tumor (GIST)	PO	Fluid retention, cytopenias, congestive heart failure, left ventricular dysfunction, hepatotoxicity, bullous dermatologic reactions, GI perforation

(Continued on next page)

TABLE 10-1 U.S. Food and Drug Administration–Approved Targeted Therapies for Cancer and Toxicity Profiles *(Continued)*

Therapeutic Agent	Target	Cellular Domain	Type of Therapy	Cancer Types	Route	Side Effect Profile
Lapatinib	ERBB1 and ERBB2	Intracellular	Kinase inhibitor	HER2+ Breast cancer	PO	Changes in left ventricular ejection fraction, interstitial lung disease, pneumonitis, prolongation of the QT interval, diarrhea, palmar-plantar erythrodysesthesia, nausea, vomiting, fatigue
Nilotinib	Bcr-abl tyrosine kinase	Intracellular	Enzyme inhibitor	CML	PO	Myelosuppression, prolongation of the QT interval, hepatic impairment, electrolyte imbalances
Panitumumab	ERBB1	Extracellular	EGFR inhibitor	Colorectal cancer	IV	Dermatologic, mucosal and ocular toxicities, infusion reactions, diarrhea, pulmonary toxicity
Rituximab	CD20 antigen	Extracellular	Monoclonal antibody	Non-Hodgkin lymphoma rheumatoid arthritis	IV	Infusion-related reactions, tumor lysis syndrome, mucocutaneous reactions, progressive multifocal leukoencephalopathy
Sorafenib	VEGFR-2 VEGFR-3 PDGFR-β	Intracellular	Angiogenesis inhibitor, enzyme inhibitor	Renal cell carcinoma, unresectable hepatocellular carcinoma	PO	Cardiac ischemia/infarction, bleeding, hypertension, hand-foot skin reaction and rash, GI perforation, wound healing complications
Sunitinib	VEGFR PDGFR KIT FLT3	Intracellular	Enzyme inhibitor	GIST, renal cell carcinoma	PO	Left ventricular ejection fraction decline, prolongation of the QT interval, hypertension, hemorrhagic events, hypothyroidism
Temsirolimus	mTOR	Extracellular	mTOR inhibitor	Renal cell carcinoma	IV	Hypersensitivity reactions, hyperglycemia, hyperlipidemia, interstitial lung disease, GI perforation, abnormal wound healing, anemia, thrombocytopenia, renal failure, dermatologic toxicities, mucositis
Tositumomab	CD20 antigen	Extracellular	Radiolabeled monoclonal antibody	Follicular lymphoma	IV	Hypersensitivity reactions, prolonged cytopenias, secondary malignancies, hypothyroidism, infectious events
Trastuzumab	HER2	Extracellular	Monoclonal antibody	Breast cancer	IV	Left ventricular dysfunction, congestive heart failure, myelosuppression with exacerbation of chemotherapy-induced neutropenia

Note. Based on information from Thomson Healthcare, n.d.

Angiogenesis Inhibition

Anticancer drugs that virtually starve tumors of their blood supply are showing promise in a variety of solid malignancies. These targeted agents block the action of a substance released by tumors called vascular endothelial growth factor, or VEGF. VEGF binds to certain cells to stimulate new blood vessel formation. The three distinct VEGF receptors (VEGFRs) are VEGFR-1, VEGFR-2, and VEGFR-3, all of which contribute to tumor angiogenesis. Angiogenesis refers to the ability of a tumor to release vascular growth factors in order to create a blood supply sufficient for tumor growth (Duda, Batchelor, Willett, & Jain, 2007). The results are inhibition of apoptosis, stimulation of mitosis, and an increase in motility in endothelial cells, preparing for generation of new blood vessels. A number of human tumors secrete VEGF. Blood vessels generated by tumors that secrete VEGF tend to be immature and leaky as compared to normal blood vessels. As a result, unlike mature blood vessels, tumor cells often require continued production of VEGF in order to survive (Duda et al.; Kerbel & Folkman, 2002).

Anti-VEGF agents have multiple effects on angiogenesis, tumor growth, and other types of therapy, including
- Limiting the blood supply to the tumor, causing small blood vessels within the tumor to die
- Blocking new blood vessel formation in the tumor
- Normalizing the vascular structure of the tumor, which may facilitate the delivery of chemotherapy (Duda et al., 2007; Kerbel & Folkman, 2002).

The VEGF pathway potentially can be inhibited in a number of ways (see Figure 10-7). Production of VEGF can be stimulated by a number of biologic signals; therefore, attempting to inhibit VEGF production is not feasible, because blocking only one of those signals will not cease VEGF production. It is possible to prevent receptor activation once VEGF has bound to a receptor. However, because VEGF binds to two different receptors, inhibiting both types of receptors may prove challenging. Finally, VEGF itself can be deactivated. Two strategies that have been employed are soluble VEGFRs, which bind any ligands that interact with VEGFR-1 and VEGFR-2; and antibodies to specifically inhibit VEGF itself (Free Patents Online, n.d.; Kay, 2006). An example is bevacizumab (Avastin®, Genentech, Inc.).

Bevacizumab

Bevacizumab is a recombinant humanized MoAb against the VEGF molecule, first approved in February 2004

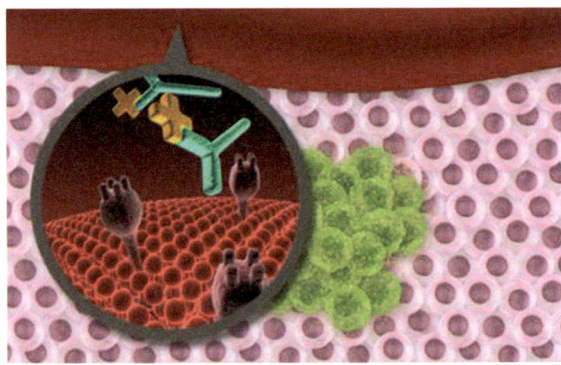

FIGURE 10-7   EXAMPLE OF BEVACIZUMAB

When a patient is given bevacizumab, this monoclonal antibody binds to VEGF and keeps it away from receptors on the surface of endothelial cells. Existing blood vessels no longer receive a signal for increased blood flow, so new blood vessels are not formed. This prevents the tumor from continuing to grow.

Note. From *Advances in Targeted Therapies Tutorial,* by National Cancer Institute, n.d. Retrieved December 4, 2009, from http://www.cancer.gov/cancertopics/understandingcancer/targetedtherapies/htmlcourse/page3#d.

as first-line treatment for patients with metastatic carcinoma of the colon and rectum in combination with standard chemotherapy (Hurwitz & Saini, 2006). Newer treatment indications include metastatic breast cancer, non-small cell lung cancer, and glioblastoma. Research is ongoing to test this agent in other malignancies, including renal, pancreatic, and ovarian cancers (Shih & Lindley, 2006).

Bevacizumab recognizes all forms of VEGF and binds to the VEGF ligand with high affinity. Bevacizumab interrupts the process of angiogenesis by preventing VEGF from binding to its receptors, thereby inhibiting all functions of the VEGF receptor, such as VEGF activity on vascular endothelial cells and VEGF activity on non-endothelial cells (see Figure 10-8). Anti-VEGF therapies were originally thought to impair oxygen and nutrient delivery to the tumor. However, current evidence demonstrates that these agents also can block the growth of abnormal blood vessels by normalizing the tumor vasculature (Duda et al., 2007; Kay, 2006). Overexpression of VEGF is associated with disorganized and dysfunctional vasculature that can lead to cardiovascular events or bleeding problems.

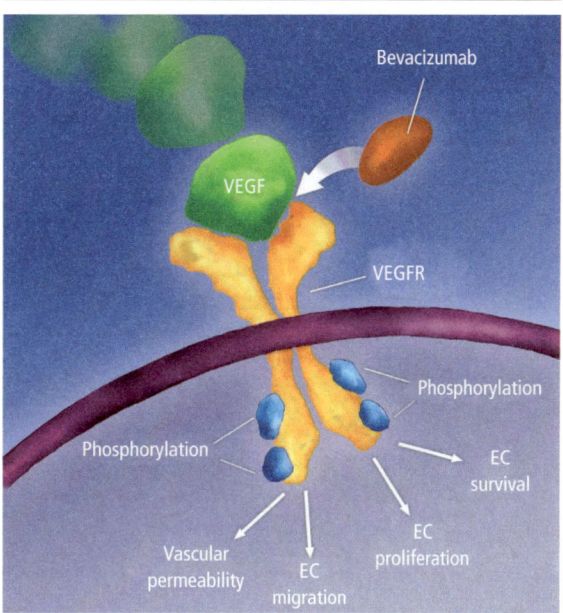

FIGURE 10-8 TARGETS FOR ANGIOGENESIS INHIBITION

Angiogenic agents work by blocking matrix metalloproteinases (MMPs), which degrade the basement membrane and permit tumor cell invasion (1) angiogenic activators, such as VEGF (2), or endothelial cells (EC) work directly (3) or indirectly (4) through the EC-specific integrin/survival signaling).

Note. Image courtesy of IMER. Used with permission.

Tyrosine Kinase Inhibitors

Another targeted therapy milestone occurred in early 2000 with the arrival of imatinib (Gleevec®, Novartis Oncology) for the treatment of chronic myeloid leukemia (CML). CML is a myeloproliferative disorder associated with the translocation t(9;22)(q 34; q11), commonly referred to as the Philadelphia chromosome (Ph). The outcome of the translocation is the presence of the *BCR-ABL* fusion gene (Druker, 2008). For more information on translocations, see Chapter 2. This genetic translocation causes the formation of an active tyrosine kinase. The deregulation as a consequence of this major genetic mutation results in the development of CML. Imatinib competitively inhibits the inactive configuration of the bcr-abl protein tyrosine kinase by blocking the adenosine triphosphate binding site and thereby preventing a conformational switch to the active form (Deininger & Druker, 2003; Druker). Therefore, targeted therapy in CML is aimed at blocking the action of the bcr-abl pathway.

The EGFR part of the tyrosine kinase group of growth factor receptors binds several epidermal growth factor (EGF) signaling molecules (see Figure 10-9). EGF stimulates the proliferation of many epithelial cells. In addition to proliferation, the EGF pathway is implicated in the control of cell differentiation, growth, and survival. The binding of EGF causes the EGF-EGFR complex to dimerize (two receptors join together), which precipitates the autophosphorylation of intracellular tyrosine residues of the receptor. This phosphorylation attracts cytoplasmic proteins containing specific sequences of amino acids called binding domains. This binding precipitates the transduction of the signal along several paths to initiate different responses of the cell. EGFR is highly expressed by many tumors, such as bladder, lung, gastric, breast, brain, head and neck, cervical, ovarian, and

FIGURE 10-9 THE EPIDERMAL GROWTH FACTOR RECEPTOR PATHWAY

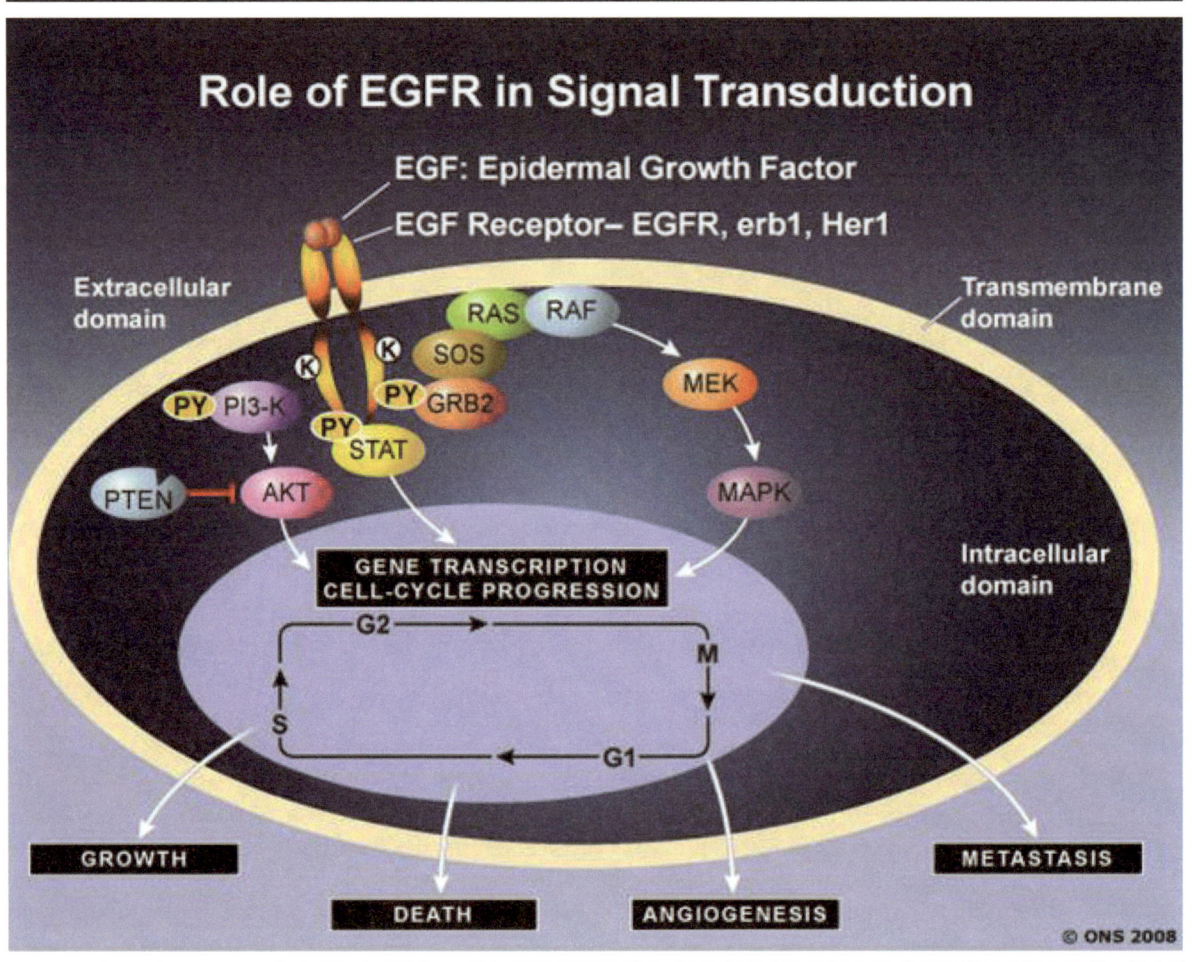

Note. From *Targeted Therapy: Closing in on Cancer* [CD-ROM], by T. Knoop, C. Lemoine, A. Goodrich, and W. Honeycutt. Copyright 2008 by Oncology Nursing Society. Reprinted with permission.

endometrial. Overexpression of EGFR is associated with poor prognostic features. Therapies that inhibit the EGFR signaling pathway have been an attractive target site for drug development and have proven to be an effective target in the treatment of solid tumors (Ma & Adjei, 2009).

Cetuximab

Cetuximab (Erbitux®, Bristol-Myers Squibb Co.) is a MoAb that targets EGFR. It is a highly chimeric (made from mouse and human proteins) MoAb that binds to EGFR and blocks the ability of EGF to initiate receptor activation and signaling of the tumor. This blocking results in an inhibition of tumor growth by interfering with the effects of EGFR activation, including tumor invasion and metastases, cell repair, and the stimulation of VEGF production leading to angiogenesis. The FDA approved cetuximab in February 2004 for treating EGFR-expressing, metastatic colorectal carcinoma in patients who failed treatment with irinotecan-based chemotherapy (Gschwind et al., 2004). Overexpression of EGFR is measured by immunohistochemistry. Cetuximab also has been FDA approved as a single therapy for patients with EGFR+ recurrent metastatic colorectal cancer who cannot tolerate irinotecan therapy (Martinelli, De Palma, Orditura, De Vita, & Ciardiello, 2009).

Erlotinib

Erlotinib (Tarceva®, Genentech, Inc.) is a small-molecule HER1/EGFR tyrosine kinase inhibitor. Erlotinib selectively and reversibly inhibits phosphorylation of the EGFR tyrosine kinase without inducing EGFR internalization or degradation. Inhibition of EGFR downstream signaling by erlotinib exerts antitumor activity through the inhibition of proliferation and tumor angiogenesis through the induction of apoptosis, thereby representing a novel approach to the treatment of solid tumors (Smith, 2005). Erlotinib is one of several anticancer drugs that targets EGFR. The FDA approved erlotinib in November 2004 as monotherapy for the treatment of locally advanced or metastatic non-small cell lung cancer after failure of a minimum of one prior chemotherapy regimen (Hann & Brahmer, 2007). In November 2005, the FDA approved erlotinib in combination with gemcitabine chemotherapy for the treatment of locally advanced, inoperable, or metastatic pancreatic cancer in patients who had not received previous chemotherapy. Erlotinib became the first new approved therapy for pancreatic cancer in nine years (Kelley & Ko, 2008).

TOXICITIES OF TARGETED THERAPIES

Table 10-1 provides an overview of many of the FDA-approved targeted cancer therapies and their most frequent toxicity profile. Therapies may be used either as monotherapy or in combination with other anticancer agents, such as chemotherapy and radiation. Targeted therapies are very costly; even patients with insurance coverage may be required to cover the costs of some agents.

Although targeted therapies are known to exert a less toxic side effect profile, targeted agents come with their own unique set of side effects, often differing from those seen with chemotherapy and radiation. The majority of the side effects experienced by patients undergoing targeted therapies are well tolerated and manageable if a proactive approach is instituted by the healthcare team. Given that the targeted therapies are still emerging, specific protocols, algorithms, and standardized guidelines are still evolving. More detailed information about targeted therapy toxicity management can be found in the Oncology Nursing Society's *Chemotherapy and Biotherapy Guidelines and Recommendations for Practice* (Polovich, Whitford, & Olsen, 2009).

Drug Interactions

Many of these agents are metabolized via the CYP450 enzyme system (refer to Chapter 9 for a detailed discussion of pharmacogenetics). Various foods, including grapefruit (Stump, Mayo, & Blum, 2006), and non-cancer medications can influence drug absorption, metabolism, and distribution in the body (vanSchaik, 2008).

Dermatologic Toxicities

Dermatologic reactions are one of the most prevalent side effects seen with the targeted therapies, mainly the small-molecule inhibitors and MoAbs. The dermatologic toxicities are mostly associated with EGFR inhibitors, occurring on average, in more than 50% of patients who receive treatment (Agero et al., 2006) (see Table 10-2). The tolerability profile of EGFR inhibitors is affected by a unique group of skin, hair, and nail reactions that have a significant potential to disrupt the optimal dosing of these agents, leading to detrimental effects on quality of life and tumor response (Duvic, 2008; Eaby, Culkin, & Lacouture, 2006; Rhee, Oishi, Garey, & Kim, 2005; Robert et al., 2005). The mechanism by which EGFR inhibitors affect skin toxicities is unclear, but interference with the follicular and interfollicular epidermal growth signaling pathway is thought to be involved (Duvic). Medications that result in the inhibition of EGFR are thought to alter keratinocyte proliferation, differentiation, migration, and attachment, which may explain the rash formation and dry skin (xerosis) (Woodworth et al., 2005). In the basal and suprabasal layers of normal skin, expression of phosphorylated EGFR and mitogen-activated protein kinase (MAPK) are present. However, when an EGFR inhibitor is used in treatment, phosphorylated EGFR is absent and MAPK expression is reduced (Lynch et al., 2007).

Microscopically, the skin rash is characterized by various inflammatory changes. The changes that occur early in treatment include infiltration of T lymphocytes around the upper part of the hair follicle (Morse & Calarese, 2006). This infiltration precedes the manifestation of inflammation of and around the hair follicles (perifolliculitis and superficial folliculitis) caused by rupturing of follicles. Changes in skin integrity are thought to be a direct result of signaling pathway intrusion (Busam et al., 2001; Hidalgo et al., 2001).

Some evidence links the appearance of rash to drug efficacy. This relationship is still undergoing investigation with the EGFR inhibitors, as the most common linkage evaluated is that seen with erlotinib. Erlotinib has demonstrated a relationship between rash

TABLE 10-2. Spectrum of Dermatologic Reactions to Epidermal Growth Factor Receptor Inhibitors

Adverse Event	Description	Frequency	Time Course
Rash (papulopustular)	Monomorphous, erythematous, maculopapular, follicular, or pustular lesions that may be associated with pruritus and tenderness	60%–80%	Onset: weeks 1–3 of treatment Maximum: weeks 3–5 of treatment Resolution: within four weeks of treatment cessation, but may wax and wane, and may improve spontaneously without treatment cessation
Paronychia and fissuring	Painful periungual granulation-type or friable pyogenic granuloma-like changes associated with erythema, swelling, and fissuring of lateral nail folds and distal finger tufts	6%–12%	Onset: after two to four months of treatment
Hair changes	Alopecia and curlier, finer, and more brittle hair on scalp and extremities; also trichomegaly and curling of the eyelashes and eyebrows and hypertrichosis of the face	5%–6%	Variable onset: after 7–10 weeks to many months
Dry skin	Diffuse fine scaling	4%–35%	Occurs after appearance of rash
Hypersensitivity reactions	Flushing, urticaria, and anaphylaxis	2%–3%	Most often occurs on the first day of initial dosing
Mucositis	Mild to moderate mucositis, stomatitis, aphthous ulcers	2%–36%	Onset during treatment, not related to dose or schedule; resolution without specific measures

Note. From "Epidermal Growth Factor Receptor Inhibitor–Associated Cutaneous Toxicities: An Evolving Paradigm in Clinical Management," by T.J. Lynch, Jr., E.S. Kim, B. Eaby, J. Garey, D.P. West, and M.E. Lacouture, 2007, *Oncologist, 12*(5), p. 614. Copyright 2007 by AlphaMed Press. Reprinted with permission.

severity and treatment response (Lynch et al., 2007). However, practitioners cannot assume that EGFR inhibitors are ineffective in patients who do not develop rash, as clinical trials continue to evolve surrounding dose escalation and target rash response in select patients.

Although skin rashes are common side effects of chemotherapy, the rashes seen as a side effect of EGFR inhibitors are more severe (Viele, 2005). Typically, the rash presents as erythematous, discolored papulopustules on the face, neck, and upper torso on 50% of the body. The rash usually appears in the first two weeks of therapy, is mild to moderate, and may be preceded by or accompanied by xerosis (dry skin) and pruritus (Esper, Gale, & Muehlbauer, 2007). Other skin changes include scalp rash, acral erythema (painful symmetrical erythematous areas on the palms and soles), subungual splinter hemorrhages (lines under the nail bed), hair and skin depigmentation and alopecia, paronychia (inflammation of the nail folds), and trichomegaly (long, curly, rigid eyelashes) (Esper et al.). These skin alterations have the potential to adversely affect quality of life if not managed proactively.

Diarrhea

Diarrhea is another common side effect of the EGFR inhibitors, as EGFR is expressed in the intestinal mucosa. This toxicity may be elevated when combination regimens are used and include chemotherapy agents that are already known to cause diarrhea as a side effect (e.g., irinotecan, 5-FU).

The underlying mechanism of drug-induced diarrhea remains undetermined. One possible explanation could be from the occurrence of secretory diarrhea, which is related to excessive chloride secretion and deficient sodium absorption. Normally, the colon's sodium absorption and chloride secretion is triggered by the intracellular messengers like cyclic adenosine monophosphate (refered to as AMP) and intracellular calcium. EGFR frequently is overexpressed in normal gastrointestinal mucosa and is a negative regulator of chloride secretion (Loriot et al., 2008). EGFR inhibitors, therefore, could block this regulation loop and thereby induce secretory diarrhea (Loriot et al.).

Diarrhea is a dose-limiting toxicity known to be associated with EGFR inhibitors such as erlotinib and gefitinib in clinical trials (Loriot et al., 2008). This type of diarrhea is characteristically watery without blood or mucus and usually occurs in the initial three weeks of therapy. Diarrhea is also a common side effect of panitumumab and cetuximab.

Hypertension

Hypertension is a common side effect of the current antiangiogenic agents, including bevacizumab, sorafenib, and sunitinib. Although the exact mechanism is not clearly understood, factors may involve VEGF blocking and the angiogenesis pathway (Veronese et al., 2006). Several factors are theorized to contribute to this side effect, including alterations in endothelial nitric oxide synthase and changes in the microvascular system (Bhargava, 2009). Anti-VEGF therapies oppose these effects, causing vasoconstriction, which increases blood pressure, thereby causing hypertension or worsening existing hypertension (Ignoffo, 2004). Patients do not need to have a previous diagnosis of hypertension to be considered at risk. The onset of hypertension can occur gradually or become apparent during each cycle. Close monitoring of patients' blood pressure throughout therapy is essential to recognizing and controlling trends in blood pressure elevations, especially in individuals with a history of hypertension.

Hemorrhage and Gastrointestinal Perforation

An increased risk of bleeding has been noted with the targeted therapies, mainly those with antiangiogenic properties, including bevacizumab, sunitinib, and sorafenib. Two distinct patterns of bleeding have been noted in patients who receive bevacizumab: minor hemorrhage and serious fatal hemorrhagic events (Shih & Lindley, 2006). The VEGF actions are thought to be mediated by nitric oxide, which regulates vascular tone, blood pressure, and platelet aggregation (Ignoffo, 2004). This interference of the vascular protective effect of VEGF, which results in a coagulopathy, has been proposed as the cause for thromboembolism. In summary, severe or fatal hemorrhages, including hemoptysis, gastrointestinal bleeding, hematemesis, central nervous system hemorrhage, epistaxis, and vaginal bleeding, can occur.

Gastrointestinal perforation is another adverse effect seen with targeted antiangiogenic agents. The underlying basis for perforation remains uncertain, but influence of VEGF on the vascular endothelium may play a role, and the inhibition of VEGF may result in a destabilization of the vascular endothelium (Shih & Lindley, 2006).

Interstitial Lung Disease

An infrequent but serious adverse effect of the EGF tyrosine kinase inhibitors is the development of interstitial lung disease. This term has been used to capture a variety of chronic lung complications. When a person has this disease, the lung is affected in three ways: (a) the lung tissue is damaged in some known or unknown way; (b) the walls of the air sacs in the lung become inflamed; and (c) scarring (fibrosis) begins in the interstitium (tissue between the air sacs), and the lung becomes stiff (Yoneda, Hardin, Gandara, & Shelton, 2006). Although a comprehensive understanding of interstitial lung disease is still unclear, this toxicity appears to be drug-induced. One proposed theory suggests that inhibition of EGFR signaling alters the repair of pulmonary injury, thus worsening the problem, especially in patients with prior pulmonary disease (Ando et al., 2006).

Signs of interstitial lung disease often are subtle in nature and may resemble other pulmonary etiology, including pneumonia, upper respiratory infection, and bronchitis. A biopsy of lung tissue usually is required to determine a definitive diagnosis; this is usually obtained through a bronchoscopy. Erlotinib and gefitinib are the main agents that cause interstitial lung disease.

Hypersensitivity and Infusion Reactions

MoAbs have been linked strongly to hypersensitivity and infusion reactions. These reactions can range from mild (rash) to severe (anaphylaxis) and are common with agents such as cetuximab, rituximab, panitumumab, and bevacizumab. The mechanism associated with infusion reactions to MoAbs is unclear but is unlikely to be a type 1 IgE-mediated hypersensitivity reaction. Theories suggest that infusion reactions to chimeric and humanized MoAbs may be the result of their ability to elicit human antichimeric antibodies (HACAs) and human anti-human antibodies (HAHAs) (Lenz, 2007).

Although different possible underlying mechanisms can cause hypersensitivity and infusion reactions, the clinical picture surrounding this phenomenon can range from mild to moderate reactions, including flushing, rash, fever, rigors, and chills, to more severe reactions associated with cardiac dysfunction, anaphylaxis, bronchospasm, hypotension requiring treatment, and other symptoms (Lenz, 2007).

Cognitive Alterations

Mood changes are a common side effect of immunotherapy agents. Current evidence supports that the activation of inflammation may contribute to the development of behavioral alterations commonly experienced by patients with cancer, including depression, fatigue, impaired sleep, and cognitive dysfunction (Miller, Ancoli-Israel, Bower, Capuron, & Irwin, 2008). Biotherapy with agents such as interferon-α and interleukin-2 may increase depression (Cuaron, 2001). With chronic administration, some patients exhibit symptoms of major depression that include significant decrease in appetite and weight loss (Cuaron).

The development of depression and other cognitive alterations is a complex process with many cytokine pathways involved in the onset of these symptoms. The mechanisms by which cytokines stimulate behavior change appear to be associated with changes in the metabolism of critical neurotransmitters that play a role in behavior, including serotonin, norepinephrine, and dopamine (Miller et al., 2008). This complex interplay between the brain and the immune system prompts nurses to be aware of the potential for cognitive changes in patients receiving such therapy from start to completion of treatment.

FUTURE DIRECTION OF TARGETED THERAPIES

The targeted therapies described in this chapter represent just the beginning of the plethora of novel targeted agents on the horizon in the cancer clinical research pipeline. As the understanding of the underlying biologic mechanisms of cancer continues to be illuminated, the complex network of cell signaling pathways will continue to form the basis for new targets for the design of potential therapy (Ma & Adjei, 2009). New pathways and targets for therapy are being or already have been developed and many are actively undergoing clinical investigation, including (Ma & Adjei)

- Receptor kinases
  - Hepatocyte growth factor and the cMet pathway
  - Insulin-like growth factor receptor pathway
- Intracellular signaling kinases
  - Src
  - PI3K/Akt/mTOR pathway
  - Mitogen-activated protein kinase pathway
- Tumor vasculature
  - Hypoxia-inducible factors
- Vascular disrupting agents
  - Tubular destabilizers
  - Flavonoids
- Epigenetic modulators
  - DNA methyltransferase inhibitors
  - Histone deacetylase inhibitors
- Integrins
- Heat shock protein
- Ubiquitin-proteasome system
- Direct apoptosis enhancers
  - Tumor necrosis factor–related apoptosis-inducing ligand
  - Survivin
- PARP inhibitors
- Mitotic kinase inhibitors
  - Kinesin spindle protein.

Although the mainstay of cancer care will likely remain surgery, chemotherapy, and radiation for years to come, targeted agents have found their place in limiting dose toxicity while extending the lives of many patients with cancer. The future of the targeted therapy approach holds promise, but questions still remain related to possible unidentified secondary long-term side effects, identification of methods to overcome drug resistance, the timing of introduction of such agents into the armamentarium of cancer therapy, and the role of tumor profiling. Other challenges are in developing effective delivery vehicles for these agents, the long-term management of patients who receive this type of targeted treatment because drug therapy with such agents may be a lifelong strategy, and the cost of such agents initially and long term.

SUMMARY

The advent of targeted therapies has resulted from an increased understanding of the molecular mechanisms of the miscommunication that occurs during the cancer process, with a focus on disarming the pathways and signaling that result in rapid growth and proliferation, vascular networking, and the development of metastasis. As the knowledge continues to expand, new targets and their inhibitors will continue to be identified (Hait & Hambley, 2009). In addition, this improved understanding is expected to lead to predictive biomarkers, companion diagnostic tests to optimize therapeutic decision making, and elucidating the mechanisms of drug resistance with ultimate strategies to overcome this obstacle (Hait & Hambley).

REFERENCES

Agero, A.L., Dusza, S.W., Benvenuto-Andrade, C., Busam, K.J., Myskowski, P., & Halpern, A.C. (2006). Dermatologic side effects associated with the epidermal growth factor receptor inhibitors. *Journal of the American Academy of Dermatology, 55*(4), 657–670.

Ando, M., Okamoto, I., Yamamoto, N., Takeda, K., Tamura, K., Seto, T., et al. (2006). Predictive responses for interstitial lung disease, antitumor response, and survival in non-small cell lung cancer patients treated with gefitinib. *Journal of Clinical Oncology, 24*(16), 2459–2556.

Annenberg Media. (n.d.). *Rediscovering biology online textbook. Unit 8: Cell biology and cancer.* Retrieved November 17, 2009, from http://www.learner.org/courses/biology/textbook/cancer/cancer_3.html

Battiato, L.A., & Wheeler, V.S. (2005). Biologic and targeted therapy. In C.H. Yarbro, M.H. Frogge, & M. Goodman (Eds.), *Cancer nursing: Principles and practice* (6th ed., pp. 510–558). Sudbury, MA: Jones and Bartlett.

Berdeja, J.G. (2003). Immunotherapy of lymphoma: Update and review of the literature. *Current Opinion in Oncology, 15*(5), 363–370.

Bhargava, P. (2009). VEGF kinase inhibitors: How do they cause hypertension? *American Journal of Physiology: Regulatory, Integrative and Comparative Physiology, 297*(1), R1–R5.

Busam, K.J., Capodieci, P., Motzer, R., Kiehn, T., Phelan, D., & Halpern, A.C. (2001). Cutaneous side-effects in cancer patients treated with the antiepidermal growth factor receptor antibody C225. *British Journal of Dermatology, 144*(6), 1169–1176.

Consensus Panel on Genetic/Genomic Nursing Competencies. (2009). *Essentials of genetic and genomic nursing: Competencies, curricula guidelines, and outcome indicators* (2nd ed.). Silver Spring, MD: American Nurses Association.

Cuaron, L. (2001). Anorexia as a side effect of biotherapy. In P. Trahan-Rieger (Ed.), *Biotherapy: A comprehensive review* (2nd ed., pp. 579–604). Sudbury, MA: Jones and Bartlett.

Dang, C.V. (2009). MYC, microRNAs and glutamine addiction in cancers. *Cell Cycle, 8*(20), 3243–3245.

Deininger, M., & Druker, B.J. (2003). Specific targeted therapy of chronic myelogenous leukemia with imatinib. *Pharmacological Reviews, 55*(3), 401–423.

Druker, B.J. (2008). Translation of the Philadelphia chromosome into therapy for CML. *Blood, 112*(13), 4808–4817.

Duda, D.G., Batchelor, T.T., Willett, C.G., & Jain, R.K. (2007). VEGF-targeted cancer therapy strategies: Current progress, hurdles and future prospects. *Trends in Molecular Medicine, 13*(6), 223–230.

Duvic, M. (2008). EGFR inhibitor-associated acneform folliculitis: Assessment and management. *American Journal of Clinical Dermatology, 9*(5), 285–294.

Eaby, B., Culkin, A., & Lacouture, M.E. (2006). An interdisciplinary consensus on managing skin reactions associated with human epidermal growth factor receptor inhibitors. *Clinical Journal of Oncology Nursing, 12*(2), 283–290.

Esper, P., Gale, D., & Muehlbauer, P. (2007). What kind of rash is it? Deciphering the dermatologic toxicities of biologic and targeted therapies. *Clinical Journal of Oncology Nursing, 11*(5), 659–666.

Free Patents Online. (n.d.). *Azulene compounds.* Retrieved August 18, 2009, from http://www.freepatentsonline.com/y2008/0125590.html

Gale, D.M. (2003). Molecular targets in cancer therapy. *Seminars in Oncology Nursing, 19*(3), 193–205.

Gemmill, R., & Idell, C.S. (2003). Biological advances for new treatment approaches. *Seminars in Oncology Nursing, 19*(3), 162–168.

Gewirtz, A.M. (2007). On future's doorstep: RNA interference and the pharmacopeia of tomorrow. *Journal of Clinical Investigation, 117*(12), 3612–3614.

Gschwind, A., Fischer, O.M., & Ulrich, A. (2004). The discovery of receptor tyrosine kinases: Targets for cancer therapy. *Nature Reviews Cancer, 4*(5), 361–370.

Hait, W.N., & Hambley, T.W. (2009). Targeted cancer therapeutics. *Cancer Research, 69*(4), 1263–1267.

Hann, C.L., & Brahmer, J.R. (2007). Who should receive epidermal growth factor receptor inhibitors for non-small cell lung cancer and when? *Current Treatment Options in Oncology, 8*(1), 28–37.

Held-Warmkessel, J. (2008). Targeted cancer therapies: These "smart weapons" hit cancer in novel ways. *Nursing, 38*(9), 26–32.

Hidalgo, M., Siu, L.L., Nemunaitis, J., Rizzo, J., Hammond, L.A., Takimoto, C., et al. (2001). Phase I and pharmacologic study of OSI-774, an epidermal growth factor receptor tyrosine kinase inhibitor, in patients with advanced solid malignancies. *Journal of Clinical Oncology, 19*(13), 3267–3279.

Hurwitz, J., & Saini, S. (2006). Bevacizumab in the treatment of metastatic colorectal cancer: Safety profile and management of adverse events. *Seminars in Oncology, 33*(5, Suppl. 10), S26–S34.

Ignoffo, R.J. (2004). Overview of bevacizumab: A new cancer therapeutic strategy targeting vascular endothelial growth factor. *American Journal of Health-System Pharmacy, 61*(21, Suppl. 5), S21–S26.

Jordan, V.C. (2009). A century of deciphering the control mechanisms of sex steroid action in breast and prostate cancer: The origins of targeted therapy and chemoprevention. *Cancer Research, 69*(4), 1243–1254.

Kay, P. (2006). Targeted therapies: A nursing perspective. *Seminars in Oncology Nursing, 22*(1, Suppl. 1), 1–4.

Kelley, R.K., & Ko, A.H. (2008). Erlotinib in the treatment of advanced pancreatic cancer. *Biologics: Targets and Therapy, 2*(1), 83–95.

Kerbel, R., & Folkman, J. (2002). Clinical translation of angiogenesis inhibitors. *Nature Reviews Cancer, 2*(10), 727–739.

Kushner, D.M., & Silverman, R.H. (2000). Antisense cancer therapy: The state of the science. *Current Oncology Reports, 2*(1), 23–30.

Lenz, H.J. (2007). Management and preparedness for infusion and hypersensitivity reactions. *Oncologist, 12*(5), 601–609.

Loriot, Y., Perlemuter, G., Malka, D., Penault-Llorca, F., Boige, V., Deutsch, E., et al. (2008). Drug insight: Gastrointestinal and hepatic adverse effects of molecular-targeted agents in cancer therapy. *Nature Clinical Practice Oncology, 5*(5), 268–278.

Lynch, T.J., Jr., Kim, E.S., Eaby, B., Garey, J., West, D.P., & Lacouture, M.E. (2007). Epidermal growth factor receptor inhibitor–associated cutaneous toxicities: An evolving paradigm in clinical management. *Oncologist, 12*(5), 610–621.

Ma, W.W., & Adjei, A.A. (2009). Novel agents on the horizon for cancer therapy. *CA: A Cancer Journal for Clinicians, 59*(2), 111–137.

Martinelli, E., De Palma, R., Orditura, M., De Vita, F., & Ciardiello, F. (2009). Anti-epidermal growth factor receptor monoclonal antibodies in cancer therapy. *Clinical and Experimental Immunology, 158*(1), 1–9.

Miller, A.H., Ancoli-Israel, S., Bower, J.E., Capuron, L., & Irwin, M.R. (2008). Neuroendocrine-Immune mechanisms of behavioral comorbidities in patients with cancer. *Journal of Clinical Oncology, 26*(6), 971–982.

Morse, L., & Calarese, P. (2006). EGFR-targeted therapy and related skin toxicity. *Seminars in Oncology Nursing, 22*(3), 152–162.

Polovich, M., Whitford, J.M., & Olsen, M. (Eds.). (2009). *Chemotherapy and biotherapy guidelines and recommendations for practice* (3rd ed.). Pittsburgh, PA: Oncology Nursing Society.

Remer, S.E. (2009). Targeted therapy agents. In S. Newton, M. Hickey, & J. Marrs (Eds.), *Mosby's oncology nursing advisor: A comprehensive guide to clinical practice* (pp. 298–313). St. Louis, MO: Elsevier Mosby.

Rhee, J., Oishi, K., Garey, J., & Kim, E. (2005). Management of rash and other toxicities in patients treated with epidermal growth factor receptor-targeted agents. *Clinical Colorectal Cancer, 5*(Suppl. 2), S101–S106.

Rixe, O., & Fojo, T. (2007). Is cell death a critical end point for anticancer therapies or is cytostasis sufficient? *Clinical Cancer Research, 13*(24), 7280–7287.

Robert, C., Soria, J.C., Spatz, A., Le Cesne, A., Malka, D., Pautier, P., et al. (2005). Cutaneous side-effects of kinase inhibitors and blocking antibodies. *Lancet Oncology, 6*(7), 491–500.

Rosenberg, S.A., Yang, J.C., & Restifo, N.P. (2004). Cancer immunotherapy: Moving beyond current vaccines. *Nature Medicine, 10*(9), 909–915.

Sengupta, S., & Jordan, V.C. (2008). Selective estrogen modulators as an anticancer tool: Mechanisms of efficiency and resistance. *Advances in Experimental Medicine and Biology, 630,* 206–219.

Sharkey, R.M., & Goldenberg, D.M. (2006). Targeted therapy of cancer: New prospects for antibodies and immunoconjugates. *CA: A Cancer Journal for Clinicians, 56*(4), 226–243.

Shih, T., & Lindley, C. (2006). Bevacizumab: An angiogenesis inhibitor for the treatment of solid malignancies. *Clinical Therapeutics, 28*(11), 1780–1802.

Smith, J. (2005). Erlotinib: Small-molecule targeted therapy in the treatment of non-small-cell lung cancer. *Clinical Therapeutics, 27*(10), 1513–1534.

Stump, A.L., Mayo, T., & Blum, A. (2006). Management of grapefruit-drug interactions. *American Family Physician, 74*(4), 605–608.

Thomson Healthcare. (n.d.). *MICROMEDEX healthcare series.* Retrieved December 9, 2009, from http://www.thomsonhc.com/home/dispatch

vanSchaik, R.H. (2008). CYP450 pharmacogenetics for personalizing cancer therapy. *Drug Resistance Updates, 11*(3), 77–98.

Veronese, M.L., Mosenkis, A., Flaherty, K.T., Gallagher, M., Stevenson, J.P., Townsend, R.R., et al. (2006). Mechanisms of hypertension associated with BAY 43–9006. *Journal of Clinical Oncology, 24*(9), 1363–1369.

Viele, C.S. (2005). Keys to unlock cancer: Targeted therapy. *Oncology Nursing Forum, 32*(5), 935–940.

Wood, L.S. (2002). Rationale for EGFR as a target for cancer therapy. *Seminars in Oncology Nursing, 16*(Suppl. 4), 3–10.

Woodworth, C.D., Michael, E., Marker, D., Allen, S., Smith, L., & Nees, M. (2005). Inhibition of the epidermal growth factor receptor increases expression of genes that stimulate inflammation, apoptosis, and cell attachment. *Molecular Cancer Therapeutics, 4*(4), 650–658.

Wujcik, D. (2006). EGFR as a target: Rationale for therapy. *Seminars in Oncology Nursing, 22*(1), 5–9.

Yoneda, K.Y., Hardin, K.A., Gandara, D.R., & Shelton, D.K. (2006). Interstitial lung disease associated with epidermal growth factor tyrosine kinase inhibitor therapy in non-small cell lung carcinoma. *Clinical Lung Cancer, 8*(Suppl. 1), S3–S35.

SECTION IV

Ethical, Legal, and Social Issues of Genetics and Genomics

CHAPTER 11 HANDLING GENETIC AND GENOMIC INFORMATION RESPONSIBLY

CHAPTER 12 MULTICULTURAL CONSIDERATIONS IN PROVIDING GENETIC AND GENOMIC CANCER CARE

CHAPTER 11

Handling Genetic and Genomic Information Responsibly

Dale Halsey Lea, MPH, RN, CGC, FAAN

Professional Responsibilities Domain:
- Recognize when one's own attitudes and values related to genetic and genomic science may affect care provided to clients
- Advocate for clients' access to desired genetic and genomic services and resources including support groups
- Advocate for the rights of all clients for autonomous, informed genetic and genomic–related decision making and voluntary action

Professional Practice Domain:
- Identification—Defines issues that undermine the rights of all clients for autonomous, informed genetic and genomic–related decision making and voluntary action

(Consensus Panel on Genetic/Genomic Nursing Competencies, 2009)

INTRODUCTION

Oncology nursing practice is expanding to include genetics and genomics across the cancer care continuum (Calzone, Lea, & Masny, 2006). As noted in the *Essentials of Genetic and Genomic Nursing: Competencies, Curricula Guidelines, and Outcome Indicators*, genetic and genomic information and technology will be applied along the pathways of prevention, screening, diagnostics, prognostics, selection of treatment, and monitoring of treatment effectiveness (Consensus Panel on Genetic/Genomic Nursing Competencies, 2009). Genetic and genomic discoveries resulting from the Human Genome Project and current research efforts building on this foundational science are paving the way for new cancer screening, prevention, interventions, and therapies that can be tailored to each individual. These discoveries also are creating potential ethical dilemmas for individuals and their families (see Figure 11-1).

Predictive genetic testing for hereditary breast/ovarian cancer became available to individuals and families in the mid-1990s. Since that time, predictive genetic testing has become available for many other cancers. Human genome discoveries paved the way for a new class of cancer drugs and treatments based on the genetic testing and analysis of individual cancers and tumors to determine a specific and effective treatment. Examples include the treatment of chronic myeloid leukemia (CML) with imatinib (Gleevec®, Novartis Oncology) in those patients who carry a specific chromosomal rearrangement called the Philadelphia chromosome (Ph+), in which segments of chromosomes 9 and 22 are rearranged and fused together to create the abnormal protein in CML. Imatinib treatment shuts off the abnormal protein in patients with CML (National Cancer Institute [NCI], 2001). Another example of gene-based cancer treatment is that of treating breast cancer with trastuzumab (Herceptin®, Genentech Biotechnology) in those patients who test positive for the *HER2* gene (Hortobagyi, 2005). A more detailed discussion of targeted cancer therapy can be found in Chapter 10.

The individualized approach to cancer treatment is rapidly expanding to all aspects of cancer care, including the identification of individuals at risk before disease occurs, diagnosis, and the characterization of the aggressiveness of the cancer using gene expression (Calzone et al., 2006). All of these advances hold great promise for cancer prevention, diagnosis, treatment, and management, but the potential for misuse also exists. Thus, the ethical, social, and legal implications of genetics and genomics are important for oncology nurses to know.

FIGURE 11-1 ETHICAL ISSUES IN GENOMIC HEALTH CARE

- Privacy and confidentiality of genetic and genomic information
- Right to accept or refuse genetic and genomic interventions
- Potential insurance or employment discrimination when gene status is known
- Pre-implantation genetic diagnosis and prenatal diagnosis of late-onset genetic conditions
- Just and fair access to and use of genetic interventions
- Genetic susceptibility testing in children

This new era of healthcare—personalized medicine—requires that oncology nurses in every role and at all levels of education and practice become knowledgeable about the expanding use of genetic and genomic information and technologies in cancer care. Acquiring this knowledge foundation is the first step in considering and applying ethical, social, and legal principles to nursing practice and the care of patients and families throughout the cancer care continuum, and in handling genetic and genomic information responsibly (Calzone et al., 2006; Williams, Skirton, & Masny, 2006).

This chapter considers the use of ethical principles founded on the American Nurses Association (ANA, 2001) code of ethics and the *Essentials of Genetic and Genomic Nursing: Competencies, Curricula Guidelines, and Outcome Indicators* (Consensus Panel on Genetic/Genomic Nursing Competencies, 2009) to guide oncology nurses in applying genetic and genomic knowledge responsibly to patient care. For example, oncology nurses will rely on these ethical principles throughout the cancer care continuum when providing patient education, ensuring informed decision making and consent, advocating for confidentiality and privacy with regard to genetic and genomic information and test results, and helping clients and families to understand the complex issues involved in genetic and genomic detection, interventions, and therapeutics. Figures 11-2 and 11-3 present the guiding principles of the code of ethics for nurses and the identified professional responsibilities from Oncology Nursing Society (ONS).

This chapter also addresses emerging ethical issues in genetics and genomics for all nurses and healthcare professionals including direct-to-consumer genetic testing, pre-implantation genetic diagnosis (PGD)—testing early embryos for a genetic condition before implantation—and prenatal genetic testing for adult-onset genetic disorders, as well as oversight of genetic testing, cancer predisposition genetic testing in children, stem cell research, and human cloning. National resources to help oncology nurses to maintain a current knowledge base in genetic and genomic developments and client resources are presented in this chapter.

ETHICAL CONSIDERATIONS OF GENETIC AND GENOMIC INFORMATION

Genetic and genomic–related ethical issues that challenge oncology nurses in all levels of practice include privacy, confidentiality, access to and justice in health care, and in-

FIGURE 11-2. ONCOLOGY NURSING PRACTICE ACTIVITIES IN GENETIC AND GENOMIC HEALTH CARE THAT SUPPORT RESPONSIBLE HANDLING OF GENETIC AND GENOMIC INFORMATION

- Participate as a member of the healthcare team in offering information about genetic and genomic topics and interventions.
- Offer written and Web-based information about genetic and genomic topics and interventions.
- Participate in client and family education by reinforcing genetic and genomic information.
- Participate in the informed decision-making process by ensuring that clients have adequate and accurate information.
- Discuss with clients the relevance and importance of sharing genetic and genomic information with family members at risk.
- Maintain privacy and confidentiality of genetic information collected and recorded in the medical record.
  - Advocate, through education and participation with the healthcare team, against discrimination resulting from genetic testing and genetic information.
  - Help clients to understand and assimilate the complex issues involved in genetic and genomic interventions.
  - Be knowledgeable about local genetics resources for clients and for nursing professionals.
- Work within institutions and support equal access to genetic and genomic health care.
- Advocate, through education of clients and other oncology nurses, for equal access to and payment for genetic and genomic healthcare services.
- Make clients and other oncology nurses aware of the newly passed Genetic Information Nondiscrimination Act (GINA) that prevents insurance and employment discrimination based on a person's genetic information.
- Participate in social policy development with regard to genetic and genomic health care.

Note. Based on information from Consensus Panel on Genetic/Genomic Nursing Competencies, 2009; Oncology Nursing Society, 2000; Rieger, 2001.

FIGURE 11-3. IMPORTANT ETHICAL PRINCIPLES THAT GUIDE NURSES IN ETHICAL ANALYSIS

Respect for Persons—The obligation to respect the capacities and differences in human beings and to act in accordance with this obligation.

Respect for Autonomy—The most important principle to consider in resolving an ethical dilemma: the freedom to choose; an obligation to respect the self-determined (autonomous) choices and actions of individuals. Moral decision making requires individuals who are able to judge circumstances independently, make choices based on actions freely chosen, and who are not constrained in their reasoning process.

Beneficence—The obligation to maximize benefits, minimize risks, and promote the welfare of others; the focus of the practitioner is on positive benefits and doing good.

Nonmaleficence—The obligation to never do harm to clients, either intentionally or unintentionally.

Confidentiality—The obligation to protect and not disclose personal information provided to the nurse in confidence by another.

Privacy—The right to have control over one's own body, thoughts, and actions.

Equity—The obligation to be fair in the distribution of social goods such as health care or in respect for people's rights; the right to be treated equally regardless of race, sex, socioeconomic status, etc.

Veracity (truthfulness)—The obligation to provide truthful information and not to intentionally deceive or mislead individuals.

Note. Based on information from Dahnke & Dreher, 2006.

formed health decisions. Although these ethical issues are not new, their application to clinical practice that integrates genetics and genomics presents additional and unique ethical dimensions requiring nursing attention (Giarelli, Lea, Jones, & Lewis, 2006). Nurses in all levels of practice will now be participating in aspects and applications of genetics and genomics throughout the cancer care continuum. Figure 11-4 outlines some of the ethical issues that may arise at each phase of the continuum.

FIGURE 11-4 ETHICAL ISSUES IN GENETICS AND GENOMICS ACROSS THE CANCER CARE CONTINUUM

Conception to Initiation—Nurses help to identify families at risk for inherited cancers, conduct clinical assessment for history of health problems that increase risk for cancer, and develop a risk-management plan.
Ethical Issues:
1. Collection of family history and ensuring privacy and confidentiality of family history information, particularly when family history is collected and stored in electronic medical records.
2. In collecting family history, nurses may be presented with a ethical dilemma related to privacy and confidentiality of the family history and genetic information when a family member chooses not to share the genetic health information with other family members.

Initiation to Diagnosis—Nurses help to identify high-risk populations, detect genetic markers, screen body tissues and fluids for genetic mutations predictive of cancer, and test tumors for genetic characteristics suggestive of prognosis.
Ethical Issues:
1. Ensuring informed consent for genetic testing that predicts cancer is an important ethical concern for nurses.
2. Cost of genetic testing—An individual's health insurance may not pay for the testing for diagnosis and prognosis. For example, Medicare does not cover genetic testing in those individuals who are older than 65 years and affected with a disease such as cancer. Individuals may not have health insurance or the financial means to pay for a genetic test.

Treatment/Prognosis—Nurses care for patients who are being diagnosed with specific malignancies. The malignancies are characterized; prognosis predicted; effective treatments, including gene-based treatments are selected; and new therapeutic modalities designed and used.
Ethical Issues:
1. As oncology care moves forward toward individualized cancer therapies, nurses may face inequities in care, for example, patients who are part of a small group that would benefit from a targeted therapy. Drug companies may be reluctant to research and manufacture drugs that will only benefit a few patients. Oncology nurses will need to consider how they will advocate for these patients.
2. Treatment involving genetic testing of tumors and gene-based treatment options may be very costly with some patients able to afford the care and others not. Oncology nurses will need to consider how they will present treatment options and potential costs to their patients.

Disease Progression to End of Life—Nurses will be involved with monitoring disease progression; providing gene-based therapeutics; and effective pain management interventions.
Ethical Issue:
Increasingly, pain management interventions and dosages will become gene-based (i.e., pharmacogenomics). Nurses will need guidance on issues of evidence-based practice and the clinical validity and utility of these treatments. This raises the ethical issue of beneficence for nursing consideration.

Note. Based on information from Calzone et al., 2006; Lea, 2008.

Ethical Principles, Theories, and Framework Used in Ethical Decision Making

Ethics is a branch of moral philosophy that focuses on values related to human conduct and teaches individuals how to choose what is good or right and why. Ethics requires that healthcare professionals use an analytical approach and previous experiences to respond to questions such as: Is the person performing the act meeting his or her duties and obligations? Are the motives of the person virtuous (Beauchamp & Childress, 2001)? Bioethics refers to the application of ethical theory and concepts to biology, medicine, and health professions. Ethical dilemmas are problems or situations in which competing rights, values, or goods clash. Ethical analysis is then required to clarify and perhaps solve moral problems (Beauchamp & Childress; Dahnke & Dreher, 2006).

Ethical theories and principles can guide healthcare professionals in analyzing and finding solutions to bioethical problems. Ethical theories guide the nurse to organize and justify ethical analysis in different ways, depending upon the nature of the theory. Ethical principles, on the other hand, are general statements that provide reasons for a choice of actions and serve as guides to analyzing and resolving conflicting ethical choices. Ethical principles help to guide healthcare professionals in acting appropriately in a given situation while allowing for interpretation in clinical judgment in specific cases (Beauchamp & Childress, 2001; Lowrey, 2004) (see Figure 11-5).

FIGURE 11-5 ETHICAL PRINCIPLES USED TO RESOLVE AN ETHICAL DILEMMA

- Respect for individuals
- Respect for client autonomy
- Beneficence
- Nonmaleficence
- Justice

In addition to ethical theories and principles, nurses also can use an ethical assessment framework as a means to evaluate an ethical issue and to support the process of ethical decision making. An ethical assessment framework outlines the skills that can assist nurses in developing expertise in ethical decision making and serves as a model for addressing genetics and genomics ethical issues in clinical practice (Cassells, Jenkins, Lea, Calzone, & Johnson, 2003). The ethical assessment framework involves four phases: assessment of the concern or issue that may be an ethical problem, a plan of action based on the assessment, implementation of the plan, and evaluation of the plan of action. During the assessment phase, the nurse gathers all of the relevant facts about the potential problem, determines whether the problem poses an ethical dilemma, and proposes actions or options to resolve the ethical dilemma. This includes identifying and using relevant interdisciplinary resources such as an ethics committee, consultants, administrators, clergy, ethicists, lawyers, colleagues, and literature. An ethically justified plan of action or option is chosen from those that are identified and is then implemented. The nurse then evaluates the selected action or option taken, looking at short- and long-term outcomes. Figure 11-6 outlines in detail the steps that can be used to identify, analyze, and evaluate ethical conflicts, issues, and uncertainties. This framework is based upon the nurse's knowledge of ethical principles, theories, and ethical decision making.

An ethical assessment framework will help oncology nurses to assess clinical situations that present moral or ethical dilemmas. It also will enable each oncology nurse to act with integrity as he or she supports and educates clients, families, and the public to deal responsibly with the complex ethical issues related to genetic and genomic interventions and services (Dahnke & Dreher, 2006; Dugas, 2005).

Respect for persons is the ethical foundation that directs all of nursing care. Four ethical principles based on respect for people generally are accepted as being central guides to bioethical decision making: respect for autonomy, nonmaleficence, beneficence, and justice (Beauchamp & Childress, 2001). Additional principles that are important for nurses to consider when providing genetic and genomic–related health care are confidentiality, privacy, and equity. These principles offer guidance to nurses when engaged in ethical analyses of relevant questions related to genomic health care (ANA, 2001) (see Figure 11-3).

Moral reasoning is the thought process that occurs when one recognizes an ethical dilemma and reacts to it. It is the decision-making process through which a healthcare profes-

---

FIGURE 11-6 ETHICAL ASSESSMENT FRAMEWORK (EAF) FOR CLINICAL PRACTICE

Assessment
1. Identify the concern or issue that may be an ethical problem: uneasiness, uncertainties, and conflicts.
2. Gather relevant facts about the problem(s):
   Medical data: Objective and subjective data.
   Contextual data: Circumstances, people involved, their cultural and religious beliefs, institutional policies, state and federal laws.
3. Determine if the problem is an ethical dilemma.
4. Propose actions or options to assist in resolving the ethical dilemma.
5. Apply methods of ethical justification to each action or option to assist in resolving the dilemma: consequentialism (consequences), deontology (duty), principalism (principles), care (relationships), casuistry (cases), virtue (character).
6. Identify and clarify values, rights, and duties of client, self, and significant persons associated with the dilemma.
7. Apply relevant guidelines from nursing and professional codes of ethics.
8. Identify and use relevant interdisciplinary resources: Ethics Committee, consultants, administrators, clergy, ethicists, lawyers, colleagues, literature, etc.
9. Prioritize the identified actions or options to assist in resolving the dilemma.

Plan of Action
10. Select an ethically justified action or option from those identified.

Implementation
11. Act upon or support the action or option selected.

Evaluation
12. Evaluate the selected action or option taken: short- and long-term outcomes.

Note. © 1998. Ethical Assessment Framework (EAF). Ethical Assessment Skills Survey Instrument (including EAF): Judith M. Cassells, RN, DNSc, and Mary C. Silva, RN, PhD, 1990; revised: EAF/11 Steps in Nursing Process: Cassells, J.M., Johnson, E., & Littlejohn, J., 1996; revised: EAF/12 Steps with Definitions: Cassells, J.M., & Gaul, A.L., 1998. Reprinted with permission.

sional chooses among his or her values and principles to come to a decision as to the appropriate response or behavior to an ethical dilemma (Dahnke & Dreher, 2006).

Recognition of Personal Attitudes and How Values Affect Others' Decisions

The first step in providing genetic and genomic information and in supporting clients' decisions is to recognize one's own values and how they influence the communication of genetic and genomic information (Consensus Panel on Genetic/Genomic Nursing Competencies, 2009). Although it may not be possible to completely hide one's own values and beliefs, nurses, in providing genetic and genomic information, need to be able to maintain sufficient self-awareness to minimize the perception of favoring one decision or intervention over another. This includes discussing genetic and genomic information and interventions in a balanced manner, offering all the information that a client needs to make an informed health decision, assisting the client in considering available health options and potential consequences of each within the context of the client's experiences and circumstances, and supporting the decision that the client ultimately makes (Consensus Panel on Genetic/Genomic Nursing Competencies, 2009). For example, the oncology nurse who believes that all clients who have a significant risk for breast cancer should have predisposition genetic testing brings this belief to the interaction with clients. If he or she is not aware of how this belief may influence the provision of information, the belief may be translated as a value judgment to a client who chooses not to have the testing, and the client may feel unsupported in the choice (see Figure 11-7).

Consider the difference between these two nurses' approaches to describing *BRCA1* gene susceptibility testing to a client and family at increased risk.

FIGURE 11-7 EXAMPLES OF PERSONAL BIASES THAT INTERFERE WITH CLIENT AUTONOMY

- Genetic diseases are caused by "bad genes" and should be eliminated.
- People who have genetic conditions are "different."
- All clients at high risk for inherited genetic conditions are obligated to have testing to find out their status.
- Parents should make the decision to have their children tested for susceptibility to late-onset genetic disorders.

Nurse A says, "This testing has its risks, though. Even if you get a negative result, you can feel guilty, and that would be hard for you because your other family members tested positive. If I were you, I would think twice before you decide to have it." Nurse B: "Making a decision to have or not to have genetic testing may take time and consideration of a number of issues, and I am here to help you to discuss this process. What kinds of questions or thoughts have you had so far?" The first nurse makes assumptions, uses value-laden words such as "risk" and "guilty," interjects her own opinion, and gives advice (e.g., "I would think twice"). The second nurse opens the discussion by making it clear to the client that decision making is a personal process and focuses the discussion on the client. This approach offers the client an opportunity to consider his or her thoughts and options with the knowledge that the nurse is present to provide information and support the client's personal decision.

As noted in the *Essentials of Genetic and Genomic Nursing: Competencies, Curricula Guidelines, and Outcome Indicators* (Consensus Panel on Genetic/Genomic Nursing Competencies, 2009), nurses need to maintain awareness of their personal values and beliefs, and recognize when these values and beliefs related to genetics and genomics may affect the care they provide to clients. Nurses need to remain objective in clinical situations where an advantage to one option over another is not clear. Examples of this situation include decisions related to genetic testing for cancer predisposition and other late-onset conditions, PGD and prenatal diagnosis of cancer predisposition or other conditions, and **gene therapy**. In situations for which interventions are clearly beneficial, such as familial adenomatous polyposis (FAP), however, nurses can be most informative by offering guidelines and recommendations for genetic testing. FAP is a type of colorectal cancer related to hereditary mutations in the *APC* gene, a critical regulator of ß-catenin. Carriers of a gene for FAP can now be detected early and offered aggressive screening and, if needed, prophylactic colectomy (NCI, 2009). In either of these situations, it is essential that nurses achieve sufficient awareness of their own values and biases so that they can allow open and supportive communication with clients and families who are making difficult genetic and genomic–related decisions.

FACILITATING AUTONOMOUS DECISION MAKING

The decision to participate in any genetic or genomic intervention should be the client's own, made after consideration of the risks, benefits, and limitations and of his or her values and beliefs. This perspective incorporates the principle of respect for autonomy of the individual and acknowledges that people have a right to make personal decisions about their own beliefs and property. Respect for autonomy requires that nurses who are involved in a client's decision to undergo a particular genetic or genomic intervention provide sufficient information about the benefits, risks, limitations, and possible outcomes to allow clients to make an informed, independent, and voluntary decision about whether to participate. When nurses provide adequate information in the appropriate educational and cultural context, they allow the client to make free, unpressured decisions about the intervention and demonstrate respect for the client's autonomy. This approach to ensuring informed consent is known as **non-directive counseling** (Weil, 2003) and is most appropriate when a client is considering predisposition, PGD, or prenatal diagnosis for adult-onset cancers. In these situations, nurses should ensure that the client has received adequate counseling and provided fully informed consent (ANA, 2001; Consensus Panel on Genetic/Genomic Nursing Competencies, 2009; Skirton, Patch, & Williams, 2005). Figure 11-8 outlines the central issues included in the informed consent process.

As gene-based therapies have expanded and become more effective in individualizing cancer treatment, a more directive approach to providing information to patients has become accepted as appropriate, as long as the patient is fully informed and makes an autonomous decision. As an example, *HER2* is an epidermal growth factor that is overexpressed in 15%–30% of newly diagnosed breast cancers and is associated with more aggressive breast cancer and poorer prognosis. The American Society of Clinical Oncology (ASCO, 2007) recommends that *HER2* expression and amplification should be evaluated in every patient who has primary invasive breast cancer either at the time of diagnosis or at the time of recurrence. Testing patients with breast cancer for *HER2* will help to guide selection of trastuzumab for treatment of breast cancer in adjuvant or metastatic disease settings (Harris et al., 2007). Understanding the potential impact of genomic test results is key to informed decision making.

FIGURE 11-8 INFORMED CONSENT

Central Issues Discussed
- Purpose of the genetic or genomic intervention
- Reason for offering the intervention
- Type and nature of genetic condition being tested for or treated
- Accuracy of genetic or genomic intervention
- Benefits of participating
- Associated risks, including unexpected results
- Acknowledgment of the right to refuse the intervention at any point in the treatment process
- Other available therapeutic options
- Available treatment and intervention options
- Further decision making that may be needed upon receipt of genetic or genomic information
- Consent to store and use genetic/genomic information for further research purposes
- Availability of additional counseling and support services

Factors That Can Influence the Informed Consent Process
- Coercion by family members and others
- Economic factors such as being uninsured
- Having cancer and being at end of life
- Age, especially older adults
- Being traumatized
- Being imprisoned

Note. Based on information from Giarelli et al., 2006; Jenkins & Lea, 2005.

PRINCIPLES OF BENEFICENCE AND NONMALEFICENCE

Beneficence and nonmaleficence are two fundamental and interconnected principles of nursing ethics that are based upon respect for persons and serve to guide nurses in providing patient care. *Beneficence* refers to the nurse's duty to promote good and maximize the benefits of whatever intervention is being considered. *Nonmaleficence* is based on the nurse's duty to do no harm—that is, to minimize risks (Dahnke & Dreher, 2006) (see Figure 11-9).

To promote good and minimize risks in genomic health care, nurses must be knowledgeable about the risks, benefits, and consequences of genetic and genomic interventions and be able to support and discuss these fully with clients to ensure that they make informed health decisions. The oncology nurse who is aware of the various facets of predisposition genetic testing for breast cancer, for example, and who articulates these to the client in a manner that helps the client to further his or her interests acts with beneficence and nonmaleficence. The nurse who, on the other hand, recommends a particular course of action to the client that does not support the client's wishes or actions is behaving in a manner that may result in harming the client in the long run. As genetics and genomics technologies and applications to cancer prevention, screening, diagnosis, and treatment increase, oncology nurses will need to become well informed and knowledgeable about these new approaches to cancer care so that they can continue to provide the most beneficial and least harmful care.

FIGURE 11-9 PROMOTING BENEFICENCE AND NONMALEFICENCE

- Evaluate self and motives in genetic- and genomic-based health care.
- Promote respect for clients and their health decisions.
- Support clients on the basis of what is "good" for them according to their beliefs, values, and decisions.
- Maximize benefits of genetic and genomic interventions being considered.

RECOGNITION OF ETHNOCULTURAL DIFFERENCES

Clients' family and ethnocultural backgrounds, that is, their ethnic backgrounds and the associated cultural and social influences, may have an impact on their perceptions of genetic and genomic information and interventions, including how they accept information and explanations about the genetic and genomic basis of disease, prevention, and therapeutic intervention options (Gettig & Bhatia, 2009). Furthermore, as Calzone et al. (2006) noted, an important question facing our society is to what extent, if any, genetic traits, conditions, or predispositions should provide a basis for determining access to certain societal goods, such as insurance and employment. A potential exists for genetic and genomic screening and testing to promote or increase discrimination. Concern has been raised that genetic and genomic technology will be available only to the affluent. Stigmatization of groups is an ethical issue when genetic and genomic testing reveals alterations that are more prevalent in minority ethnic populations. For example, specific gene mutations in the *BRCA1* and *BRCA2* genes have been identified as more common in the Ashkenazi Jewish population. Another example pertains to potential discrimination with drug development. Currently, pharmaceutical companies develop medications that can be broadly used. Genetic variations that are found in particular ethnic or racial groups may discourage drug development for small subgroups when the development costs may outweigh the financial return (Lipton, 2003).

Practices specific to certain ethnic groups' beliefs and aspirations surrounding health and reproduction may have an impact on the client's or family's approach to genomic health care and decision making. In some cultures, for example, the cause of a genetic condition may be attributed to magic or divine intervention. Identifying these kinds of cultural, ethnic, and religious influences on a client's perceptions of health and illness helps the nurse to provide appropriate education about the implications of genetics and genomics (Consensus Panel on Genetic/Genomic Nursing Competencies, 2009) (see Figure 11-10).

FIGURE 11-10 ETHNOCULTURAL BELIEFS THAT MAY INFLUENCE PERCEPTIONS OF GENOMIC HEALTH CARE

- Health is the absence of clinical symptoms.
- Health and disease are determined by the will of God.
- Needles take away valuable body fluids and should be avoided.
- The spiritual leader makes all decisions about health care in a community.
- Genes are a part of God's mystery and should not be known.

Clients' family experiences influence their reception and understanding of genetic and genomic information, decision making, and adaptation to their current situation. Family members may have very different reactions to the identification of an inherited predisposition to cancer in the family. Likewise, individual reactions to the prospect of genetic interventions such as genetic susceptibility testing may differ among family members, depending upon whether the family has been newly identified as carrying a susceptibility gene mutation or has been followed for the condition over years (Jenkins & Lea, 2005). A person who has grown up with a sibling who has neurofibromatosis, for example, brings all of those experiences to a prenatal counseling session. As another example, a young woman whose mother died from breast cancer at the same age as the young woman may view the potential burden of the disease as significant and wish to pursue predisposition testing for hereditary breast cancer risk with a greater sense of urgency than a woman whose mother has survived breast cancer for 10 years and is currently healthy (Skirton et al., 2005).

Nurses can incorporate awareness of the impact of ethnocultural and family background when inquiring about the family's genetic history. Given the opportunity, many clients are willing to discuss their experiences and beliefs as a member of a family with a genetic disorder (Jenkins & Lea, 2005). Knowledge of this information helps nurses to provide culturally sensitive and appropriate genetic and genomic information. Including family and significant others in genetic and genomic–related health decisions can help to improve the communication of genetic and genomic health information (Consensus Panel on Genetic/Genomic Nursing Competencies, 2009).

PRIVACY AND CONFIDENTIALITY

Privacy and confidentiality with regard to genetic information are significant issues for nursing consideration. *Privacy*, as defined in ANA's code for nurses (2001), is a person's right to be left alone and free of unwanted intrusions. Privacy as related to genetic and genomic information refers to the individual's right to have control over personal information. The client is considered to have ownership of the information and to have ultimate authority over its disclosure. Informed consent must be obtained from the client prior to the disclosure of information to others, including family members, and information gathered for one purpose may not be used for another purpose without additional informed consent from the client (Skirton et al., 2005).

Nurses have a central role in maintaining client privacy, and this is especially true with regard to genetic and genomic information. Oncology nurses at all levels of practice are involved in obtaining family history information and participating in physical examinations, which often provide genetic and genomic information about clients and families that is then recorded in the client's medical record. Nurses are entrusted with genetic and genomic information that most clients consider to be very private. Oncology nurses have an obligation to promote the integrity, accuracy, and confidential use of the genetic and genomic information that they collect and record. According to the ANA's code for nurses (2001), nurses are obligated to safeguard the clients' right to privacy by judiciously protecting information of a confidential nature. *Confidentiality* is defined as the obligation of one person to another to keep information entrusted in the context of the special relationship in confidence (Dahnke & Dreher, 2006). Nurses have a duty to uphold confidentiality of client information by protecting clients' control over personal information.

Genetic and genomic information about a client, similar to other medical information, is handled as confidential and should not be shared with others without the client's consent. Genetic and genomic information, however, has unique characteristics that distinguish it from other medical information. This information, for example, can provide knowledge about future health risks. Clients who have undergone genetic susceptibility testing for cancer may face difficulties maintaining privacy of this personal medical information about their future health when questioned by an insurance company or prospective employer. Nurses can protect the client's desire for privacy of such information by ensuring that the client always gives written consent to release sensitive material about genetic test results and other genetic data to any third party (ANA, 2001) (see Figure 11-11).

Another consideration is that genetic tests may produce unexpected results, such as revealing misidentified paternity of a child. Such potential consequences should be discussed with individuals and families who are undergoing linkage analysis for a hereditary cancer and families participating in family studies during the informed consent process prior to testing. As another example of unexpected genetic results, microsatellite instability (MSI) testing on colon cancer tumors may reveal that the individual may be a carrier of a germ line gene mutation (gene mutation present in all cells of the body) that has been inherited and can be passed along to that person's children (Hampel et al., 2005). It is therefore important to inform clients who are undergoing this type of screening of this possible outcome and that if found to be MSI positive, they may be referred for genetic testing.

Genetic information also may reveal information about other family members' risk. For example, a client who has a confirmed diagnosis of a gene mutation that puts him or her at higher risk for breast cancer may feel pressure from family members to share this information with the family but may not wish to do so. This presents an ethical dilemma for the nurse who supports client confidentiality and yet wishes to support and promote the health of other family members at risk (Loud et al., 2006). In this situation, the ethical conflict is between

FIGURE 11-11 PRIVACY AND CONFIDENTIALITY: NURSING RESPONSIBILITIES

- Obtain written informed consent from all clients to release genetic and genomic information to any party, including family.
- Advocate for clients to obtain information, before testing or treatment, regarding the use of stored DNA samples.
- Encourage clients to make decisions about sharing appropriate genetic and genomic information with family and relatives.

the nurse and healthcare provider's ethical obligations to respect the privacy of the patient's genetic information versus the potential for harm to family members who will not know their risk, and the potential liabilities resulting from the healthcare providers' failure to notify at-risk relatives. The potential liability includes the failure to warn family members about hereditary disease risk. This has already resulted in several lawsuits against physicians in the United States (Offit, Groeger, Turner, Wadsworth, & Weiser, 2004). The duty of confidentiality needs to be explored with the healthcare team, including medical ethicists, to protect innocent family members from harm (Lowrey, 2004).

Oncology nurses can encourage and support but not coerce clients in making decisions about sharing appropriate genetic and genomic information with relatives, explaining that by sharing this personal information, the client demonstrates respect and caring for others and allows the family members to potentially improve their health outcomes and avoid harm (Jenkins & Lea, 2005; Offit et al., 2004).

Clinical genetics and genomics will be an increasingly important aspect of personalized health care. In addition, use of electronic health records (EHRs) is expanding to manage complex medical information, including a person's genetic and genomic information. It is anticipated that including genetic and genomic information in EHRs will help to inform healthcare providers about a person's family health history, particular disease risk, the appropriate drug dosage to avoid adverse effects, and the selection of effective and appropriate treatment. However, the availability of this information in EHRs raises important ethical issues with regard to privacy and confidentiality and the security of genetic and genomic information. Policies are needed that will protect the information with regard to access and use. The U.S. Department of Health and Human Services recently has developed the Personalized Health Care Initiative to provide leadership in the design of policy interventions that will assist with the introduction of personalized medicine into clinical practice. The Secretary's Advisory Committee on Genetics, Health, and Society; the National Committee on Vital and Health Statistics; and the American Health Information Community are working with the initiative to consider the issues that relate to the inclusion of genetic and genomic test information in EHRs and proper protection and disclosure of this information (McGuire et al., 2008).

CLIENT ADVOCACY

Client advocacy is a long-standing nursing ethic that, like autonomy, beneficence, and nonmaleficence, is founded upon the principle of justice. In the advocate role, oncology nurses ensure that patients are treated equitably (Lowrey, 2004). This includes supporting the client's right to be given accurate genetic and genomic information, to have access to interventions and treatments, and to fair use of this information. At the most basic level, this means that nurses are knowledgeable about resources and ensure that clients have access to the most up-to-date information and interventions.

Oncology nurses can help clients to locate genetic and genomic services so that they can receive appropriate interventions, including predisposition and diagnostic genetic testing. This may require that the nurse advocate for the client and family by working with the client's insurance company to facilitate medical reimbursement, or if the client and family are without financial support, to help them to obtain alternative resources. Advocacy on the part of all oncology nurses includes participation in developing and promoting social policies that support equal access to genetic and genomic information and services (Dugas, 2005).

Advocating for nondiscrimination is another important nursing function. Genetic and genomic information has the potential to lead to discrimination by others, including healthcare providers. The code for nurses stipulates that the nurse will provide care with respect for human dignity and the uniqueness of the client. Nursing care is unrestricted by consideration of social or economic status, personal attributes, or the nature of the health problem. Nursing care is delivered without prejudicial behavior (ANA, 2001). When advocating for nondiscrimination, all healthcare professionals need to be aware of their own values, beliefs, and biases, as previously discussed. Professionals who are aware of their own biases will be less likely to act upon these biases in dealing with clients. Recognition of the continuous need for values clarification is an ongoing challenge for all oncology nurses that will help them to successfully advocate against discriminatory behavior toward clients and families with genetic concerns (ANA).

Identifying Potentially Discriminatory Situations

Oncology nurses, as advocates, can help clients to recognize situations in which discrimination might occur. For example, clients should be informed in advance of participating in genetic and genomic evaluation, testing, or treatment that an insurance company may deny reimbursement or coverage in the future. Until recently, this knowledge has led some clients and families to pay for genetic interventions on their own, outside of their insurance company, so that they will not be denied coverage in the future.

In 2008, a major breakthrough in protecting Americans from genetic discrimination took place. On May 21, 2008, a federal law called the Genetic Information Nondiscrimination Act (GINA) was signed into law. GINA prohibits health insurers and employers from discriminating against an individual based on his or her genetic information. The regulations interpreting the law were drafted and became available in May 2009. The health insurance provisions also became effective in May 2009, and the employment provisions took effect in November 2009. GINA prohibits group and individual health insurers from using a person's genetic information in determining eligibility or premiums and prohibits an insurer from requiring that a person undergo a genetic test. GINA also prohibits employers from using a person's genetic information in making employment decisions such as hiring, firing, job assignments, or any other terms of employment. It also prohibits employers from requesting, requiring, or purchasing genetic information about a person or his or her family members. It is important for nurses to know that GINA does not mandate coverage for any particular test or treatment, nor does it prohibit medical underwriting based on current health status. GINA also does not cover life, disability, or long-term care insurance (Hudson, Holohan, & Collins, 2008).

Active duty military personnel represent an exception to the described protections against employment and insurance discrimination based on genetic information. GINA and other state and federal protections against discrimination based on genetic information do not extend to genetic testing of active duty military personnel or genetic information obtained from active duty military personnel (Hudson et al., 2008). At this point, the military is able to routinely take genetic information such as family history and genetic testing results from service members into account when making assignments, terminating or promoting individuals in the military, and deciding disability healthcare benefits. The military uses genetic testing to obtain medical information that will help to protect military personnel from harmful duty or other exposures that could worsen the health problem. For example, high altitudes and extreme exertion can trigger symptoms in people who have sickle-cell anemia. Knowing who is susceptible to such conditions can help the military to prevent disruption of duty and potential injury. However, genetic test results, such as *BRCA1* and *BRCA2* mutation status, also could have an influence on military eligibility for new assignments and promotions. Additionally, active duty military personnel who have less than eight years of active duty service have the risk that if they become disabled and must go before the medical board to establish benefit eligibility, the results of a predisposition genetic test could be considered a preexisting condition that affects their benefits (Genetics and Public Policy Center, 2008).

Education as Advocacy

Educating clients, organizations, and the public about the application of molecular genetics and genomics to health care is a major way for all nurses to advocate for equal and just use of genetic and genomic information. Because genomics is a relatively new field, healthcare professionals need to educate themselves about the ethical genetic and genomic health issues and the potential for inequity in access to and unjust use of genetic and genomic information and technologies. Professionals who are well versed in these and other issues related to genetic and genomic health care can educate or provide for the education of clients, the public, and those working for organizations or institutions who may be engaged in making genetic-related healthcare decisions (Consensus Panel on Genetic/Genomic Nursing Competencies, 2009). For example, oncology nurses may advocate for clients by clarifying the nature of an inherited cancer syndrome to a school or community nurse in an effort to ensure that these healthcare professionals have sufficient knowledge about the nature of the condition to develop appropriate healthcare plans.

EMERGING ETHICAL ISSUES FOR ONCOLOGY NURSES

Ethical issues facing oncology nurses are increasing as the applications of genetic and genomic technologies expand. The complete mapping and sequencing of the human genome has opened doors for new research approaches that scan human genomes for genes that cause common, complex disorders such as diabetes, stroke, and cancer. These studies, called genome-wide association (GWA) studies, have the ability to detect common variants that contribute to large or small increases in disease risk in an individual. As improvements occur in the cost and utility of GWA study results, health professionals will be able to use these tools to provide clients with individualized information about their risks of developing certain diseases. This information will help health professionals to tailor prevention and early intervention efforts to each person's unique genetic makeup. Research studies currently are under way to look at the interest level of young adults in having testing for eight common diseases including lung cancer, colon cancer, and malignant melanoma, and how people who decide to take the tests respond to knowing their risks, and interpret and use the results in making their own healthcare decisions in the future (National Human Genome Research Institute [NHGRI], 2009). See Chapter 7 for more detailed information (see Figure 11-12).

FIGURE 11-12 EMERGING ETHICAL ISSUES FOR NURSES

- Fair use of genetic and genomic interventions
- Equal access to genetic and genomic health care
- Potential for misuse of genetic and genomic information (e.g., eugenics, cloning of humans)
- Potential for fragmented care of individuals and families with genetic conditions

Direct-to-Consumer Genetic Testing

Many for-profit companies, such as 23andMe (www.23andme.com) and Navigenics (www.navigenics.com), offer genetic testing for common, complex diseases. This is called direct-to-consumer (DTC) genetic testing. Individuals can send in a cheek swab of their DNA and receive the results directly from the company, usually without the involvement of a healthcare provider or the benefits of counseling. The increasing availability of DTC raises many questions about the reliability of the test results, consumers' abilities to interpret the test results, and whether healthcare providers are prepared to interpret and use the information to improve patient care (American College of Medical Genetics, 2008; Eaton, 2003; Genetics Home Reference, 2009; Williams-Jones, 2003).

A 2008 survey by Cogent Research of members of the general public revealed that more than half of those surveyed indicated they were ready to make healthcare decisions and choices based on genetic test results, such as increasing the frequency of check-ups after receiving results of genetic tests. Three-fourths of survey respondents, however, identified potential concerns about having genetic testing, including the risk that their genetic information might be used against them by third parties. These individuals were not aware of the recent passage of GINA. The survey also found that the cost of the genetic tests would prohibit respondents from having the testing and that they would be less likely to have a DTC genetic test if their insurance company did not cover it (Cogent Research, 2008).

Healthcare providers, including oncology nurses, have a significant role to play in advising their clients and the general public about the availability of genetic testing. However, to date, healthcare providers have had a small role in consumers' decisions about accessing DTC genetic tests. In the Cogent Survey, only 4% of respondents said that they had ever discussed genetic testing with their healthcare provider. On the other hand, 88% of those surveyed said they would talk with their doctor about their genetic test results if the tests indicated they were at risk for a specific disease (Cogent Research, 2008).

The Cogent survey results showed a paradox of results. On the one hand, the survey showed that consumers are aware of and are becoming excited about the new genetic testing services and technology and feel more empowered about managing their health. On the other hand, it showed that the public and the professionals have little understanding about when and how the genetic information can be used and what they should do with the results of a genetic test (Cogent Research, 2008).

The American Society of Human Genetics (ASHG) issued a position statement regarding a number of concerns about DTC, including (Hudson, Javitt, Burke, Byers, & ASHG Social Issues Committee, 2007):

- Consumers may not receive adequate counseling either before or after the genetic testing.
- The quality of the testing may be poor because of a lack of adequate analytic or clinical validity.
- The claims made about DTC may be exaggerated or unsupported by scientific evidence.

The ASHG position statement recommends that the DTC companies promote transparency and permit both providers and consumers to make informed decisions about DTC by providing "all relevant information about offered tests in a readily accessible and understandable manner" (Hudson et al., 2007, p. 636).

Pre-implantation Genetic Diagnosis and Prenatal Diagnosis

The increasing availability of genetic testing and improving survival of young adults with hereditary cancers are opening new doors to the use of genetic tests to guide reproductive choices. Prenatal diagnosis to identify fetuses that carry a hereditary cancer mutation has been available to couples for some time. More recently, PGD has become available to couples with a hereditary cancer risk to guide the selection of embryos for implantation. To date, PGD and prenatal diagnosis have been performed for common cancer predisposition syndromes to colon, breast, and ovarian cancer as well as many of the dominantly inherited cancer predisposition syndromes (Offit, Sagi, & Hurley, 2006). Another ethical consideration is the cost of and reimbursement for PGD. PGD is expensive and is reimbursed by healthcare systems in only a few countries, and in the United States is covered only in cases of infertility. The ethical concern here is that PGD may be available only to those who can afford it, raising "the specter of genetic selection according to economic means" (Offit, Kohut, et al., 2006, p. 4780). Ethical acceptance of assisted reproductive technologies like PGD for adult-onset disorders such as cancer predisposition syndromes is being further discussed and defined to inform the responsible use of these technologies to decrease the burden of heritable cancers (Offit, Sagi, et al., 2006).

Another use of PGD is its use to identify human leukocyte antigen (HLA)-matched siblings for children who are born with bone marrow disorders and who are in need of stem cell transplantation (e.g., Fanconi anemia, a rare disorder that is associated with an increased risk for leukemia). The use of PGD in couples who have had children with autosomal recessive cancer syndromes has resulted in an unaffected, HLA-matched brother and a subsequent successful transplantation with umbilical cord blood (Verlinsky, Rechitsky, Schoolcraft, Strom, & Kuliev, 2001). PGD for HLA-matched siblings also has been used by couples who have had children affected with acute lymphoid leukemia, acute myeloid leukemia, and Blackfan-Diamond syndrome with successful birth outcomes (Verlinsky et al., 2004). PGD has been performed in families who have concern about having children with an autosomal dominant inherited risk such as familial adenomatous polyposis and neurofibromatosis types 1 and 2 (Rechitsky et al., 2002; Verlinsky et al., 2002). These expanding applications of the use of PGD require oncologists, oncology nurses, and healthcare practitioners to increase their knowledge and awareness of PGD as a reproductive option for patients who have hereditary cancers (Offit, Kohut, et al., 2006).

Oversight of Genetic Testing

The expanding number of genetic tests and their applications in the care of people with cancer and other common and rare diseases raise important questions about the validity and clinical utility of the tests. The Centers for Disease Control and Prevention (CDC) sponsors a program called ACCE (Analytic Validity, Clinical Validity, Clinical Utility, and Associated Ethical, Legal, and Social Implications) that serves as a model process for evaluating the data on genetic tests as they become available. The ACCE project involves a process of collection, evaluation, interpretation, and reporting data on genetic testing for disorders that have a genetic component. The outcomes of this process provide policy makers with access to current and reliable information for decision making about the value of using a genetic test. The ethical, legal, and social issues are considered at each step of the process and include questions regarding (a) stigmatization, discrimination, privacy and confidentiality, and personal family issues; (b) legal issues regarding consent, ownership of data, patents, licensing, obligation to disclose, and reporting requirements; and (c) safeguards that have been described and whether these are in place and effective (CDC, 2009). Attention to the clinical utility of genetic tests is of great value as an important step in not causing harm to patients because they often are eager to pursue a new genetic test or treatment as soon as it is announced and before its utility and safety have been established.

Cancer Predisposition Testing in Children

Genetic testing of children for cancer susceptibility is another pressing ethical issue that healthcare providers face today (Monsen, 2009). Children are involved as informed or uninformed observers of their parent's or family's participation in predisposition testing and potentially as being tested themselves. Their involvement raises questions about communication of complex, abstract medical information to children and also about the ethics of having parents make decisions about such testing for an adult-onset disease before the child has reached adulthood. Making a decision as a parent to have a child tested may eliminate that child's right as an adult to make an independent decision about whether or not to have genetic testing. As noted in the final report of the Task Force on Genetic Testing, difficulties in living with the uncertain health status of the child does not negate the child's right to make an independent decision regarding genetic testing in adulthood (Holtzman & Watson, 1997). Older children may be able to be more involved in the decision-making process; however, children could be vulnerable to the fears and anxieties that can be associated with genetic testing. This decision also may influence their future opportunities to obtain health, life, disability, and long-term care insurance and can create familial and psychological issues.

Several practice guidelines for genetic testing of minors have been written by the genetics community and medical and pediatric professional associations. Most of these recommendations advise against presymptomatic genetic testing of children for adult-onset disorders (Borry, Stultiens, Nys, Cassiman, & Dierickx, 2006). The current justification for presymptomatic genetic testing of children is when an immediate health benefit would be missed if the testing were not done or was delayed. ASCO has developed a policy statement regarding genetic testing for cancer susceptibility that includes a section on special issues to consider in testing children for cancer susceptibility (ASCO, 2003; Robson et al., 2010). In the policy statement, ASCO recommended that the decision to offer genetic testing to children who potentially are affected take into consideration the availability of evidence-based risk-reduction strategies as well as the probability of malignancy development during childhood. The policy also recommended that parents have the right to decide for or against genetic testing when risk-reduction strategies are available or the cancer usually develops in childhood. Furthermore, the policy indicated that genetic testing must be delayed in the absence of increased risk of childhood malignancy until the person is at a sufficient age to make an informed decision about whether to have such genetic tests (ASCO, 2003; Robson et al., 2010).

Examples of cancer syndromes where predisposition genetic testing of children has been used based on the benefits of early treatment include FAP, multiple endocrine neoplasia, and neurofibromatosis. ASCO further advised that clinical cancer genetics professionals serve as advocates for the best interests of the child.

Stem Cell Research

The promise of stem cell research for science and advances in health care is creating excitement. However, the application of human stem cells to develop new therapies also is creating controversy (Giarelli et al., 2006). Sources of human pluripotent stem cells include early-stage embryos created in excess of clinical need in an in-vitro fertilization clinic. Other sources of stem cells include fetal tissue and adult stem cells, called somatic stem cells. Many people do not support embryonic stem cell research because of the need for the destruction of an embryo. The National Institutes of Health has developed a Web site (http://stemcells.nih.gov/info/basics/basics4.asp) with stem cell information and guidelines regarding the current clinical use of both embryonic and adult stem cells (National Institutes of Health, 2009).

Human Cloning

The idea of cloning humans to create the "perfect" person or to eliminate certain genetic traits that are considered undesirable is another emerging ethical issue for nursing consideration (Giarelli et al., 2006). Oncology nurses will need to maintain a current knowledge base regarding these emerging technologies and associated ethical issues to be able to responsibly respond to personal, client, and family questions. NHGRI (http://www.genome.gov/10004765) has summarized information about cloning for healthcare providers that will assist oncology nurses and other healthcare professionals in maintaining current knowledge about cloning (NHGRI, 2006).

MAINTAINING A CURRENT KNOWLEDGE BASE IN GENETIC AND GENOMIC DEVELOPMENTS

The need for oncology nurses to participate in ongoing education in genetics and genomics in the clinical setting, professional schools, the community, and social policy realms cannot be overemphasized. All nurses need to be knowledgeable about where and how to access relevant genetic and genomic information so that they can promote competent nursing practice within the framework of genetic and genomic advances (Williams et al., 2006).

National Resources

NHGRI has set aside approximately 5% of its budget for the Ethical, Legal, and Social Implications (ELSI) Program. The goal of this project is to identify and clarify the initial responses to the emerging issues raised by the Human Genome Project and current genome research. The ELSI Program supports research projects, conferences, working groups, fellowships, and other initiatives that focus on issues such as privacy and confidentiality, insurance and employment discrimination, quality control of genetic testing procedures, and public education. Oncology nurses can obtain valuable information about the Human Genome Project and current research initiatives for themselves and for clients via the NHGRI Web site (www.genome.gov/Research). This information will facilitate nurses to be active participants in discussions of the ethical, legal, and social considerations and to influence the provision of quality genetic and genomic health care.

Other national agencies, such as the National Coalition for Health Professional Education in Genetics (NCHPEG), a national coalition developed by several federal agencies, professional and private organizations, consumers, and industry, have worked to develop a coordinated and systematic genetic educational effort, including the development of *Core Competencies in Genetics for Health Professionals* (NCHPEG, 2007). NCHPEG was one of the stakeholders that endorsed the *Essentials of Genetic and Genomic Nursing: Competencies, Curricula Guidelines, and Outcome Indicators* for all nurses (Consensus Panel on Genetic/Genomic Nursing Competencies, 2009). Attention to ethical issues is an important component of these educational endeavors to ensure competency of nurses. Through these efforts, new ways to integrate genetic and genomic information and ethical decision making into clinical nursing practice are being developed that will support oncology nursing practice.

Professional Societies

Several key professional genetics and nursing societies can serve as educational and professional resources to oncology nurses when facing difficult ethical dilemmas. Societies such as the International Society of Nurses in Genetics (ISONG), a recognized group of nursing experts in genetics, offers opportunities to nurses for genetic and genomic education. Through ISONG's Web site, oncology nurses can take advantage of opportunities to have dialogue with genetics nurse specialists and to gain access to a genetics and genomics resource center, including a nursing literature database (www.isong.org/resources/index.cfm#). ONS also has taken steps to develop genetic and genomic resources for oncology nurses. For example, in recognition of the relevance and importance of genetics and genomics to oncology nursing practice, ONS created the Cancer Genetics Special Interest Group, which has more than 90 members who provide cancer genetic counseling services across the country (Rieger, 2001). ONS also has collaborated with ISONG in a number of educational activities to enhance educational goals and opportunities for oncology nurses. Other professional societies that may offer valuable information and educational opportunities to oncology nurses are ASHG (www.ashg.org), and the National Society of Genetic Counselors (www.nsgc.org). Figure 11-13 provides a listing of genetic, genomic, and ethical information resources for nurses.

Client and Public Resources

Knowing how and when to access current genetic and genomic resources will help oncology nurses to responsibly address the increasing demand from clients for genetic and

FIGURE 11-13 ONLINE GENETIC, GENOMIC, AND ETHICAL INFORMATION RESOURCES FOR NURSES

American Society of Human Genetics (www.ashg.org): The primary professional organization for human geneticists in the United States. Informs health professionals, legislators, health policy makers, and the general public about all aspects of human genetics.

Coalition for Genetic Fairness (www.geneticfairness.org/about.html): The Coalition for Genetic Fairness was founded in 2000 to address the growing concern surrounding the misuse of genetic information in insurance and employment decisions.

Evaluation of Genomic Applications in Practice and Prevention (EGAPP) (www.cdc.gov/genomics/gtesting/EGAPP/about.htm): A pilot project initiated by the Centers for Disease Control and Prevention's National Office of Public Health Genomics in 2004 to establish and evaluate a systematic, evidence-based process for assessing genetic tests and other applications of genomic technology in transition from research to clinical and public health practice.

Genetic Alliance (www.geneticalliance.org): A coalition of more than 600 advocacy organizations serving 25 million people affected by 1,000 conditions. The organization works to transform leadership in the genetics community to build capacity in advocacy organizations and to educate policy makers by leveraging the voices of individuals and families. Genetic Alliance increases the capacity of genetic advocacy organizations to achieve their missions and leverages the voices of millions of individuals and families living with genetic conditions.

Genetics and Public Policy Center at Johns Hopkins University (www.DNAPolicy.org): The Center helps policy leaders, decision makers, and the general public better understand the growing field of genetics and genomics and its application to health care.

Genetics Education Center, University of Kansas Medical Center (www.kumc.edu/gec/prof/geneelsi.html): Information on the ethical, legal, and social issues of the Human Genome Project.

International Society of Nurses in Genetics (ISONG) (www.isong.org): ISONG, the International Society of Nurses in Genetics, is a global nursing specialty organization dedicated to fostering the scientific and professional growth of nurses in human genetics and genomics worldwide.

National Cancer Institute (www.cancer.gov): The National Cancer Institute coordinates the National Cancer Program, which conducts and supports research, training, health information dissemination, and other programs with respect to the cause, diagnosis, prevention, and treatment of cancer, rehabilitation from cancer, and the continuing care of patients with cancer and their families.

National Human Genome Research Institute (NHGRI) (www.genome.gov): NHGRI supports the development of resources and technology that will accelerate genome research and its application to human health. A critical part of the NHGRI mission continues to be the study of the ethical, legal, and social implications of genome research. NHGRI also supports the training of investigators and the dissemination of genome information to the public and to health professionals.

National Reference Center for Bioethics Literature (http://bioethics.georgetown.edu/nirehg): A collection of books, articles, and other publications concerned with biomedical issues, including the Human Genome Project and genetic testing.

Oncology Nursing Society (ONS) (www.ons.org): ONS is a professional organization of more than 35,000 RNs and other healthcare providers dedicated to excellence in patient care, education, research, and administration in oncology nursing.

Secretary's Advisory Committee on Genetics, Health, and Society (SACGHS) (http://oba.od.nih.gov/SACGHS/sacghs_home.html): SACGHS provides policy advice to the Department of Health and Human Services on the broad array of complex medical, ethical, legal, and social issues raised by the development and use of genetic technologies.

genomic information. Clients and the public are anxious to receive correct and appropriate genetic and genomic information. Oncology nurses need to know how to locate genetic and genomic information and resources that may be useful to answer their clients' questions and concerns. Support groups for clients with genetic conditions are one important resource. These can be identified through a number of voluntary and national organizations (see Figure 11-14).

FIGURE 11-14 GENETIC AND GENOMIC RESOURCES FOR PATIENTS AND FAMILIES

Genomics and Your Health (www.cdc.gov/genomics/public/index.htm): The Centers for Disease Control and Prevention has created a new Web site for the public that includes easy-to-understand information about the exciting and emerging field of genomics.

Genetic Alliance (www.geneticalliance.org): The Genetic Alliance is a coalition of more than 600 advocacy organizations serving 25 million people affected by 1,000 conditions.

Genetic Centers, Clinics and Departments (www.kumc.edu/gec/prof/genecntr.html): This Web site, sponsored by the National Society of Genetic Counselors, provides information about how and where to locate genetics professionals and clinics.

Genetic and Rare Diseases Information Center (GARD) (http://rarediseases.info.nih.gov/GARD): GARD employs experienced information specialists to answer questions in English and Spanish from the general public, including patients and their families, healthcare professionals, and biomedical researchers. It was established by the National Human Genome Research Institute and the Office of Rare Diseases Research.

Genetics Home Reference (http://ghr.nlm.nih.gov): The Genetics Home Reference provides consumer-friendly information about genetic conditions, basic genetics topics and concepts, and the effects of genetic variations on human health.

Genetics and Genomics for Patients and the Public (www.genome.gov/19016903): The National Human Genome Research Institute has created genetic and genomic health information on its Web site. The information presented covers everything from detailed information about genetic disorders, background on genetic and genomic science, the new science of pharmacogenomics, tools to create a family health history, and a list of online health resources.

National Cancer Institute (www.cancer.gov): The National Cancer Institute has created Web pages for the general public, patients, and health professionals on a wide range of topics as well as comprehensive descriptions of its research programs and clinical trials.

Office of Rare Diseases Research (ORDR) (http://rarediseases.info.nih.gov): ORDR at the National Institutes of Health (NIH) coordinates research and information on rare diseases for the NIH and for the rare diseases community, and provides information for patients and their families with rare diseases and about NIH- and ORDR-sponsored biomedical research and scientific conferences.

SUMMARY

The nursing profession faces the challenge of assuring the public that nurses are competent in understanding and using genetic and genomic information. Oncology nurses can increase their knowledge and understanding of genetics and genomics and their applications to oncology health care so that they can provide quality and personalized care. Enhanced knowledge of genetics and genomics and related ethical, social, and legal issues supports oncology nurses' abilities to translate this new knowledge in an effective way to support clients, families, and communities.

REFERENCES

American College of Medical Genetics. (2008). *ACMG statement on direct-to-consumer genetic testing*. Retrieved August 19, 2008, from http://www.acmg.net/StaticContent/StaticPages/DTC_Statement.pdf

American Nurses Association. (2001). *Code for nurses with interpretive statements*. Kansas City, MO: Author.

American Society of Clinical Oncology. (2003). American Society of Clinical Oncology policy statement update: Genetic testing for cancer susceptibility. *Journal of Clinical Oncology, 21*(12), 2397–2406.

American Society of Clinical Oncology. (2007). Guideline summary: American Society of Clinical Oncology/College of American Pathologists guideline recommendations for human epidermal growth factor receptor HER2 testing in breast cancer. *Journal of Oncology Practice, 3*(1), 48–50.

Beauchamp, T.L., & Childress, J.F. (2001). *Principles of biomedical ethics* (5th ed.). New York: Oxford University Press.

Borry, P., Stultiens, L., Nys, H., Cassiman, J.J., & Dierickx, K. (2006). Presymptomatic and predictive genetic testing in minors: A systematic review of guidelines and position papers. *Clinical Genetics, 70*(5), 364–381.

Calzone, K.A., Lea, D.H., & Masny, A. (2006). Non-Hodgkin's lymphoma as an exemplar of the effects of genetics and genomics. *Journal of Nursing Scholarship, 38*(4), 335–343.

Cassells, J.M., Jenkins, J., Lea, D.H., Calzone, K., & Johnson, E. (2003). An ethical assessment framework for addressing global issues in clinical practice. *Oncology Nursing Forum, 30*(3), 383–390.

Centers for Disease Control and Prevention. (2009, July). *Genomic translation: ACCE model process for evaluating genetic tests.* Retrieved October 22, 2009, from http://www.cdc.gov/genomics/gtesting/ACCE/index.htm

Cogent Research. (2008). *4th annual Cogent Research genomics attitudes and trends: Consumer 2008.* Retrieved October 5, 2008, from http://www.cogentresearch.com/products/CGAT_Brochure.pdf

Consensus Panel on Genetic/Genomic Nursing Competencies. (2009). *Essentials of genetic and genomic nursing: Competencies, curricula guidelines, and outcome indicators* (2nd ed.). Silver Spring, MD: American Nurses Association.

Dahnke, M., & Dreher, M. (2006). Defining ethics and applying the theories. In V.D. Lachman (Ed.), *Applied ethics in nursing* (pp. 3–13). New York: Springer.

Dugas, R. (2005). Nursing and genetics: Applying the American Nurses Association's Code of Ethics. *Journal of Professional Nursing, 21*(2), 103–113.

Eaton, L. (2003). Commission warns against selling genetic tests direct to the public. *BMJ, 326*(7393), 781.

Genetics Home Reference. (2009, October). *What is direct-to-consumer genetic testing?* Retrieved October 21, 2009, from http://ghr.nlm.nih.gov/handbook/testing/directtoconsumer

Genetics and Public Policy Center. (2008, December). *About GINA.* Retrieved March 9, 2009, from http://www.dnapolicy.org/gina/gina.html

Gettig, E.A., & Bhatia, T. (2009). Hinduism and Sikhism: Genetic counseling aspects. In R.B. Monsen (Ed.), *Genetics and ethics in health care: New questions in the age of genomic health* (pp. 109–128). Silver Spring, MD: American Nurses Association.

Giarelli, E., Lea, D.H., Jones, S.L., & Lewis, J.A. (2006). Genetic technology: The frontiers of nursing ethics. In V.D. Lachman (Ed.), *Applied ethics in nursing* (pp. 61–80). New York: Springer.

Hampel, H., Frankel, W.L., Martin, E., Arnold, M., Khanduja, K., Kuebler, P., et al. (2005). Screening for the Lynch syndrome (hereditary nonpolyposis colorectal cancer). *New England Journal of Medicine, 352*(18), 1851–1860.

Harris, L., Fritsche, H., Mennel, R., Norton, L., Ravdin, P., Taube, S., et al. (2007). American Society of Clinical Oncology 2007 update of recommendations for the use of tumor markers in breast cancer. *Journal of Clinical Oncology, 25*(33), 5287–5312.

Holtzman, N.A., & Watson, M.S. (Eds.). (1997). *Final report of the Task Force on Genetic Testing.* Retrieved on March 15, 2010, from http://www.genome.gov/10001733

Hortobagyi, G.N. (2005). Trastuzumab in the treatment of breast cancer. *New England Journal of Medicine, 353*(16), 1734–1736.

Hudson, K., Javitt, G., Burke, W., Byers, P., & ASHG Social Issues Committee. (2007). ASHG statement on direct-to-consumer genetic testing in the United States. *American Journal of Human Genetics, 81*(3), 635–637.

Hudson, K.L., Holohan, M.K., & Collins, F.S. (2008). Keeping pace with the times—the Genetic Information Nondiscrimination Act of 2008. *New England Journal of Medicine, 358*(25), 2661–2663.

Jenkins, J.F., & Lea, D.H. (2005). *Nursing care in the genomic era: A case-based approach.* Sudbury, MA: Jones and Bartlett.

Lea, D.H. (2008, January). Genetic and genomic healthcare: Ethical issues of importance to nurses. *Online Journal of Issues in Nursing, 13*(1), Manuscript 4. Retrieved October 22, 2009, from http://www.nursingworld.org/MainMenuCategories/ANAMarketplace/ANAPeriodicals/OJIN/TableofContents/vol132008/No1Jan08/GeneticandGenomicHealthcare.aspx

Lipton, P. (2003). Pharmacogenetics: ethical issues. *Pharmacogenomics Journal, 3*(1), 14–16.

Loud, J.T., Weissman, N.E., Peters, J.A., Giusti, R.M., Wilfond, B.S., Burke, W., et al. (2006). Deliberate deceit of family members: A challenge to providers of clinical genetics services. *Journal of Clinical Oncology, 24*(10), 1643–1646.

Lowrey, K.M. (2004). Legal and ethical issues in cancer genetics nursing. *Seminars in Oncology Nursing, 20*(3), 203–208.

McGuire, A.L., Fisher, R., Cusenza, P., Hudson, K., Rothstein, M.A., McGraw, D., et al. (2008). Confidentiality, privacy, and security of genetic and genomic test information in electronic health records: Points to consider. *Genetics in Medicine, 30*(7), 495–499.

Monsen, R.B. (Ed.). (2009). *Genetics and ethics in health care: New questions in the age of genomic health.* Silver Spring, MD: American Nurses Association.

National Cancer Institute. (2001, May). *Gleevec: Questions and answers.* Retrieved August 12, 2008, from http://www.cancer.gov/cancertopics/factsheet/gleevecqa

National Cancer Institute. (2009, October). *Genetics of colorectal cancer.* Retrieved November 12, 2009, from http://www.cancer.gov/cancertopics/pdq/genetics/colorectal/HealthProfessional/page2

National Coalition for Health Professional Education in Genetics. (2007). *Core competencies in genetics for health professionals* (3rd ed.). Retrieved August 20, 2008, from http://www.nchpeg.org/core/corecomps-3rd_ed_aug07.pdf

National Human Genome Research Institute. (2006, April). *Cloning/embryonic stem cells.* Retrieved November 12, 2009, from http://www.genome.gov/10004765

National Human Genome Research Institute. (2009, July 15). *Study to probe how healthy younger adults make use of genetic tests.* Retrieved November 12, 2009, from http://www.genome.gov/25521052

National Institutes of Health. (2009, April). *Stem cell basics.* Retrieved November 12, 2009, from http://stemcells.nih.gov/info/basics/basics4.asp

Offit, K., Groeger, E., Turner, S., Wadsworth, E.A., & Weiser, M.A. (2004). The "duty to warn" a patient's family members about hereditary disease risks. *JAMA, 292*(12), 1469–1473.

Offit, K., Kohut, K., Clagett, B., Wadsworth, E.A., Lafaro, K.J., Cummings, S., et al. (2006). Cancer genetic testing and assisted reproduction. *Journal of Clinical Oncology, 24*(29), 4775–4782.

Offit, K., Sagi, M., & Hurley, K. (2006). Preimplantation genetic diagnosis for cancer syndromes: A new challenge for preventive medicine. *JAMA, 296*(22), 2727–2730.

Oncology Nursing Society. (2000). Cancer predisposition genetic testing and risk assessment counseling. *Oncology Nursing Forum, 27*(9), 1349.

Rechitsky, S., Verlinsky, O., Chistokhina, A., Sharapova, T., Ozen, S., Masciangelo, C., et al. (2002). Preimplantation genetic diagnosis for cancer predisposition. *Reproductive Biomedicine Online, 5*(2), 148–155.

Rieger, P.T. (2001, August). *Commentary on genetic education of health professionals.* Paper presented on behalf of Oncology Nursing Society at the meeting of the Secretary's Advisory Committee on Genetic Testing, Washington, DC.

Robson, M.E. Storm, C.D., Weitzel, J., Wollins, D.S., Offit, K., & American Society of Clinical Oncology. (2010). American Society of Clinical Oncology policy statement update: Genetic and genomic testing for cancer susceptibility. *Journal of Clinical Oncology, 28*(5), 893–901.

Skirton, H., Patch, C., & Williams, J. (2005). *Applied genetics in healthcare: A handbook for specialist practitioners.* New York: Taylor and Francis.

Verlinsky, Y., Rechitsky, S., Schoolcraft, W., Strom, C., & Kuliev, A. (2001). Preimplantation diagnosis for Fanconi anemia combined with HLA matching. *JAMA, 285*(24), 3130–3133.

Verlinsky, Y., Rechitsky, S., Sharpova, T., Morris, R., Taranissi, M., & Kuliev, A. (2004). Preimplantation HLS testing. *JAMA, 291*(17), 2079–2085.

Verlinsky, Y., Rechitsky, S., Verlinsky, O., Chistokhina, A. Sharapova, T., Masciangelo, C., et al. (2002). Preimplantation diagnosis for neurofibromatosis. *Reproductive BioMedicine Online, 4*(3), 218–222.

Weil, J. (2003). Psychosocial genetic counseling in the post-nondirective era: A point of view. *Journal of Genetic Counseling, 12*(3), 199–211.

Williams, J.K., Skirton, H., & Masny, A. (2006). Ethics, policy, and educational issues in genetic testing. *Journal of Nursing Scholarship, 38*(2), 119–125.

Williams-Jones, B. (2003). Where there's a Web, there's a way: Commercial genetic testing and the internet. *Community Genetics, 6*(1), 46–57.

CHAPTER 12
Multicultural Considerations in Providing Genetic and Genomic Cancer Care

Bernice L. Coleman, PhD, ACNP-BC, FAHA, and Walter Brown, PhD

Professional Practice Domain:
- Demonstrate in practice the importance of tailoring genetic and genomic information and services to clients based on their culture, religion, knowledge level, literacy, and preferred language

Professional Responsibilities Domain:
- Identification—Identify ethical, ethnic/ancestral, cultural, religious, legal, fiscal, and societal issues related to genetic and genomic information and technologies

(Consensus Panel on Genetic/Genomic Nursing Competencies, 2009)

INTRODUCTION

A paramount challenge to oncology nurses, every bit as dramatic as the mapping of the human genome, is the changing paradigm of clients seeking or requiring services. The explosion of genetic and genomic knowledge and technology converging with ethnic demographic shifts in the U.S. population and anticipated increases in health disparities has created a perfect storm for the emergence of the need for nurses to consider multicultural perspectives when providing cancer care that incorporates genetic and genomic information. As the scientific knowledge expands, consideration of human genetic variation in correlation with health status will contribute to the improved understanding of currently unrecognized inherited host factors that influence screening, diagnosis, and treatment outcomes for all populations and all ethnic groups. It is important for nurses to understand all of the factors that alter cancer survival outcomes, including genetic factors (Albain, Unger, Crowley, Coltman, & Hershman, 2009).

The provision of care that includes genetic and genomic information for clients with or at risk for rare and common complex diseases such as cancer, diabetes, heart disease, and asthma is practiced at the crossroads of all the biopsychosocial dimensions that make up the client, his or her family, and supporters. Beyond the medical mechanisms actuating common diseases, age, physical comorbidities, gender, spiritual tradition, culture, race, and ethnicity are all examples of other client domains that affect health and disease assessment, treatment, and clinical outcomes. Incorporating these additional client domains augments the efficacy and efficiency of all aspects of care.

Several factors influence the delivery of genetic and genomic services to diverse groups. One challenge influencing the successful utilization of genetics and genomics in clinical care is that of genetic health literacy (Green, 2003). Genetic health literacy is the extent to which individuals are able to negotiate the complex healthcare system and access and make health decisions regarding the emerging care options that integrate genetic and genomic information and services (American Public Health Association, 2009). Consideration of how to explain complex information to the client and then how that client interprets the information and communicates to family and significant others is important. This will facilitate the ability of the healthcare system and the workforce to competently address the needs of every client regardless of race, ethnicity, culture, or language proficiency (Betancourt, Green, Carrillo, & Park, 2005).

A person's genetic makeup interacts with physical and social environments and thus is influenced by one's race, ethnicity, geographic setting, culture, lifestyle, and behaviors. As concepts and variables, *culture*, *race*, and *ethnicity* often are used interchangeably in biomedical literature, and for this reason they remain ill defined (Sankar, Cho, & Mountain, 2007). This chapter will define key multicultural considerations in cancer nursing in the context of delivering genetic and genomic care to individuals, families, and communities. Increasing knowledge of the prevalence and implications of human genetic variation has the potential to change the prevailing paradigms of human health and identity with major implications for culturally competent nursing care (Albain et al., 2009). This chapter will recommend strategies for achieving multicultural competence and end with guidance as to further research needed to ensure the success of this important aspect of cancer nursing.

MULTICULTURAL CONSIDERATIONS IN THE DELIVERY OF GENETIC AND GENOMIC CANCER NURSING CARE

Operationally Defining Culture, Race, and Ethnicity

Culture is a generationally transmitted set of behaviors, beliefs, and understandings, including language, history, religion, and world view (Lipson, Dibble, & Minarik, 2000). Cultural differences in world view and communication styles may particularly affect client perceptions of the nurse as supportive and empathic. Nurses often accept mainstream American cultural patterns and the culture of nursing without thought, following the "myth of sameness" characterized by Bernard and Goodyear (1992). In other words, "what I do is what everyone else does." Regardless of apparent sameness, issues will arise in nurse-client multicultural interactions at some point.

Embedded in the multicultural interaction between the nurse and the client is an understanding of racial difference. Betancourt and Lopez (1993) define race in terms of physical characteristics that are permanent features. These characteristics include skin color, hair texture, and facial appearance (Landrine & Klonoff, 1996). Race frequently is used as a proxy for culture and ethnicity. The construct of race as biology, however, is of limited value. Racial designations were formed without the benefit of current understanding of genetics and do not reflect the broad spectrum of biologic characteristics within and between groups. With current genetic and genomic understanding, knowledge of race alone is insufficient to explain the health status or the clinical picture of a client (Royal & Dunston, 2004). However, race as a social construct may provide some indication as to the psychosocial environment of the client and may be an indicator of social exploitation, privilege, victimization, or membership within a particular ethnic group.

Ethnicity, on the other hand, relates to a shared geographic origin, nationality, language, values, and beliefs (Betancourt & Lopez, 1993). Genealogic linkages, childhood locale, and other social-shaping factors such as language influence one's ethnic identity (Alvidrez, Azocar, & Miranda, 1996). The genetically determined phenotype of race is tied to ethnicity because of the clustering of racial groups within migratory patterns. These same patterns are responsible for significant racial dispersals. Consequently, within any ethnic classification, multiple subgroups and cultural diversity are present. The concept of ethnicity may provide a more fixed, homogeneous, and reliable understanding of an individual's cultural experience. This concept still is limited in that it may not capture the complexity, vitality, and multifaceted nature of any individual ethnic minority experience.

Ethnicity itself is not homogeneous. In specific ethnic populations, genetic differences are inherited from the populations of origin. For example, this means that Latinos may have inherited a mix of European, Native American, and African ancestry. This intermixing of a population of origin with other races or ethnic background is called *admixture* (Burchard et al., 2003). African Americans may have a mix of European, East African, West African, or Caribbean African ancestry. A new method called genome-wide admixture mapping is using ancestry-informative markers to help to determine the origin of chromosomal regions in admixed individuals. This admixture mapping potentially will help in the identification of genetic risk factors, **complex traits**, and disease showing prevalence among populations (Mao et al., 2007). For example, some data show that the high rate of diabetes, obesity, and cardiovascular disease in older adult Puerto Ricans living in the United States cannot be solely explained by poverty, healthcare access, urban environments, and health behaviors. Genetic variation associated with that specific admixture may contribute to disease (Lai et al., 2009). Additionally, variation in drug metabolism and effectiveness may be influenced by genetic admixture (Suarez-Kurtz & Pena, 2006).

A judgment of this fusion of biology and culture determines one's ethnicity. Personal identification with a particular ethnic group is a common aspect of self-development. Such information can be helpful to oncology nurses as a background context in which to begin to assess the multicultural impact of genetic and genomic information, family history, and illness.

Ethnicity and Disease

With the explication of the Human Genome Project (*Human Genome Project Information*, 2008; Venter et al., 2001) and the ongoing human variation investigation (International HapMap Consortium, 2003; Sabeti et al., 2007), identification of genetic contributions to rare and common complex diseases including cancer and the potential to influence individualized treatment strategies remains a hopeful outcome to current research (Royal & Dunston, 2004). The challenge remains in understanding the value of individual ethnic group differences as one applies evidence-based risk reduction, screening, and treatment plans to alleviate ethnic disparities. Of the three billion base pairs in the human haploid genome, any two people will differ by only two or three million base pairs, or 0.1% (Jorde & Wooding, 2004; Keita et al., 2004; Mountain & Risch, 2004). Jorde and Wooding completed a human genetic analysis that confirmed geographical variation consistent with historical gene patterns and flow of humans. These findings suggest that ethnicity could be a surrogate for group affiliation. However, caution must be taken in the use of ethnicity in that manner.

Variation is greater within ethnic groups, not between ethnic groups. Some, but not all, researchers argue that self-identified race offers no benefit in genetic research (Burchard et al., 2003; Cooper, Kaufman, & Ward, 2003). These investigators see race as a social construct having little to do with biology, but more to do with the interaction of ethnicity, culture, and environment (Keita et al., 2004). Clients' self-reported ethnicity as a general category may, in itself, be an indicator of the interaction, albeit imperfect, of genes and environment. However, where the benefit of this information may offer a contribution to oncology nurses is in delving deeper into the individual's genetic and genomic profile as it relates to the genetic contribution to a specific disease. For example, three specific *BRCA* gene mutations occur at a greater prevalence in the Ashkenazi Jewish population (Struewing et al., 1997; Warner et al., 1999). Mutations in *BRCA1* or *BRCA2* increase the risk for breast and ovarian cancer. Members of Ashkenazi Jewish families are at higher risk for breast cancer than the general population, which now, in part, has been found to be associated with an inherited predisposition to breast cancer secondary to *BRCA* mutations. This discovery was made possible because of a genetic founder effect, where a gene mutation is observed more frequently in a population group founded by a small ancestral group or a group that was once geographically or culturally isolated (Behar et al., 2008). Exploring the incidence or presence of an individual's specific candidate gene or cluster of genes that may show predisposition to diseases in groups from a geographic area offers one of the most powerful tools in the prevention and management of ethnic health disparities.

Certainly, the cancer statistical data lend support for ethnic disparities in cancer (National Cancer Institute[NCI], 2008). For example, prostate cancer is the most common cancer among American men. One of the important risk factors that have been identified for prostate cancer is ethnicity. African American men are more likely to be diagnosed with prostate cancer at advanced stages and more than twice as likely to die from complications than Caucasian men (NCI, 2009). On the other hand, Asian Americans and Hispanics are less likely than non-Hispanic Caucasians to develop prostate cancer. In 2008, three genomic research studies identified 11 new DNA changes (called genetic variants) associated with an increased risk for prostate cancer. A theory is that inheriting some of these variants may explain the disproportionate number of young African American men who have prostate cancer. These studies are contributing to a further understanding of prostate cancer risk linked to multiple genetic variants (Lea, Feero, & Jenkins, 2008; NCI, 2009; National Human Genome Research Institute [NHGRI], 2009a). For example, vitamin D has been reported to be associated with the aggressiveness of prostate cancer disease (Ahn et al., 2008). Building on this knowledge, research indicates that a genetic variant of the vitamin D receptor found only in African Americans may explain differing degrees of risk among ethnic groups such as the increased risk of advanced prostate cancer (Cicek, Liu, Schumacher, Casey, & Witte, 2006; Roff & Wilson, 2008).

WHY ARE MULTICULTURAL CONSIDERATIONS IMPORTANT FOR ONCOLOGY NURSES?

Magnitude of the Problem

The change in the number of people affected by cancer including incidence, prevalence, and morbidity in the U.S. population is related to shifts in the ethnic population (American

Cancer Society, 2009; NCI Surveillance, Epidemiology, and End Results Program, n.d.), as well as prevalence and morbidity because of common complex diseases. By sheer numbers, the U.S. Census Bureau predicts that by the year 2050, Hispanics and African Americans alone will make up more than one-third of the total U.S. population. The number of non-Hispanic Caucasians is predicted to fall to a low of 50% of the U.S. population (U.S. Census Bureau, 2004). These data derived from the U.S. Census Bureau are from self-reported information on race and ethnicity. Both race and ethnicity as categories in the U.S. Census database are used interchangeably. Five racial categories—White, Black or African American, American Indian or Alaska Native, Asian, and Native Hawaiian or Other Pacific Islander—were defined by the U.S. Office of Management and Budget (OMB). Two changes made to the 2000 census-taking process were the addition of a sixth race category, "some other race," and the allowance for responders to report their race alone or as any combined race category provided (U.S. Census Bureau). The crucial impact of the projected ethnic change in the U.S. composition suggests that a health disparity burden of a personal, financial, and national nature is anticipated.

The National Institutes of Health (NIH) defines health disparities as "differences in the incidence, prevalence, mortality, and burden of disease and other adverse health condition that exist among specific population groups in the United States" (NCI Center to Reduce Cancer Health Disparities, 2009, para. 1). Such declaration was given further protection through legal definition under the Minority Health and Health Disparities Research Act 2000, which also established the National Center on Minority Health and Health Disparities (NCMHD). This center promotes minority health and leads, coordinates, supports, and assesses the NIH effort to reduce and ultimately eliminate health disparities (see www.ncmhd.nih.gov).

NHGRI, in recognition of the need to further define and understand health disparities, developed the *Five-Year Strategic Plan for Reducing Health Disparities*. NHGRI submitted the five-year plan to the NCMHD in November 2001 for the NIH Comprehensive Strategic Plan and Budget to Reduce and Ultimately Eliminate Health Disparities (NHGRI, 2001). Building on this foundation, one of the top areas of emphasis in the NHGRI 2004–2008 strategic plan is research "to study the genetic factors contributing to diseases that disproportionately affect populations affected by health disparities" (NHGRI, n.d., p. 5). Research has been initiated to look at risk factors for common diseases such as diabetes and prostate cancer and the genetic, environmental, behavioral, and social factors involved. NHGRI is working with the NIH Office of Behavioral and Social Science Research to look into strategies for studying the interaction among the genetic, social, and behavioral factors in health. NHGRI also is helping to develop the research capacity in minority institutions to conduct research that uses the tools and information that have become available as a result of the Human Genome Project (NHGRI, n.d.).

ETHNICITY AND SOCIOPOLITICAL FACTORS

Keep in mind that culturally and ethnically distinct populations may not all be minorities, as illustrated by the increased prevalence of *BRCA* mutations in those of Ashkenazi Jewish heritage discussed previously. The Centers for Disease Control and Prevention Office of Minority Health and Health Disparities (2009) has recognized health disparities occurring in populations categorized "by gender, race or ethnicity, education or income, disability, geographic location, or sexual orientation" (para. 1). Ethnic health disparities in the incidence and prevalence of common complex diseases including cancer also are influenced by sociopolitical factors (Lai et al., 2009). These include discrimination, trust of healthcare providers, stress, and environmental factors (see Table 12-1).

Discrimination

A concern is that people with identified genetic predispositions may be discriminated against by employers and health and life insurance companies. The historical unethical research misconduct in the Tuskegee experiments illustrates the reason for minority populations' concerns about the potential for misuse of this information. The Tuskegee nontherapeutic experiment followed African American men to determine the natural progression of untreated syphilis over 40 years. The men were never provided adequate treatment for their disease, resulting in a legacy of mistrust among African Americans toward government

TABLE 12-1 Influential Factors of Health Disparities With Genetic and Genomic Contributions

Factor	Issues	Actions
1. Social class	Socioeconomic stressors	a. Eliminate barriers and ensure access to appropriate care and resources (e.g., genetic testing). b. Determine healthcare system effectiveness for provision of genetic-based care for all populations.
2. Discrimination	Fear that insurers or employers may utilize genetic information against them (e.g., increased fees, limited job options)	a. Inform clients of currently available safeguards for privacy and utilization of genetic information. b. Influence policy and actions that protect against the misuse of genetic information.
3. Knowledge	An array of environmental, behavioral, and spiritual beliefs influence one's understanding of health and illness. Personal theories of disease causation may conflict with utilization of genetic risk information.	a. Inform all clients of relevance and availability of genetic care and services as appropriate. b. Ensure effective communication and translation of complex information. c. Treat each person as an individual; avoid stereotyping. d. Recognize that religiosity and spirituality may influence uptake of genetic services.
4. Trust of healthcare providers	Mistrust of medical establishments	a. Acknowledge the past. b. Provide open and honest communication about known benefits and risks with any care options. c. Respect client preferences for interventions.
5. Stressors	The struggle to adapt to the wishes of those with perceived power is a common tension.	a. Be cognizant of and accommodate values and beliefs. b. Assess psychological and attitudinal factors influencing decisions. c. Provide supportive resources when indicated.
6. Environment	Potential for high-risk exposures is increased for those living in suboptimal conditions.	a. Recognize sites of increased disease prevalence in minority populations. b. Assess factors that may influence personal, family, and population risk for cancer.

health agencies (Washington, 2006). As a result, it is not hard to comprehend the sensitivity of ascribing genetic disease differences to ethnic populations and the concern about use of genetic information to discriminate against ethnic minorities.

Despite the newness of the area of genetic testing, discrimination has been documented (Williams, Sarata, & Redhead, 2007). Some investigators have found that perceived and actual racial discrimination is a risk factor for diseases such as cancer (Taylor et al., 2007). For example, Taylor reported that women who reported discrimination were 48% more likely to develop breast cancer than women who denied being victims of discrimination. Bias and discrimination are seen as chronic stressors, a variable shown to weaken physical health in general, and potentially contributing to cancer development and treatment response (Oliver & Muntaner, 2005; Simon & Petrucelli, 2009; Taylor et al.).

Although federal and state statutes prohibit such discrimination, some people fear that this advancing knowledge will only be used to benefit certain races or ethnic groups (Braff et al., 2008). For example, race-based tailored therapy may never reach those who might benefit the most from such treatment because of the cost of bringing such treatments to the marketplace. A concern is that the challenge of accessing adequate representation of multiple populations for research that determines the value of integrating such complex scientific and social constructs will be difficult because of historical and ongoing fear.

Trust

African American cultural messages generally engender a mistrust of the medical assistance provided by mainstream medical institutions as well as biomedical research. This stems from a variety of factors, such as the widespread use of slaves for medical experimentation, the involuntary government-sanctioned sterilization of African Americans during the 20th century, and the participation of medical establishments in separate and unequal health care from reconstruction to the present day (Dula, 1994; Dula, Royal, & Secundy, 2003; Halbert, Armstrong, Gandy, & Shaker, 2006; Washington, 2006). Native Americans are another underserved ethnic group with concerns about use and misuse of genetic research on human beings. Such concerns include privacy rights, property rights, informed consent, and use of biologic materials (Tsosie, 2007). For example, the Havasupai Tribe in Arizona sued Arizona State University for a breach in a research agreement for the study of diabetes (*Havasupai Tribe v. Arizona State University*, 2004; *Tilousi v. Arizona State University*, 2004). The allegation of unauthorized use of genetic resources and data, including research into the frequency of mental health disorders, resulted in litigation and further mistrust by the tribe whose norms, values, and agreements were not respected.

The dawn of the genomic era brings heightened concerns, particularly for the underserved populations, regarding the misuse or access of an individual's genetic information. On May 21, 2008, a historic law, the Genetic Information Nondiscrimination Act, known as GINA, was signed into law by President George W. Bush. The law makes it illegal for employers or insurers to discriminate against a person based on his or her genetic information (see Genetics and Public Policy Center, www.dnapolicy.org/gina). For more information about GINA, see Chapter 11. Additional information is available in an article by Braff et al. (2009) about the patchwork of American legal, regulatory, and legislative protections regarding personalized medicine. Genetic and healthcare professionals must understand these protections when studying the implications of ethical, legal, and social issues surrounding the availability of genetic and genomic information. Applying this knowledge will promote trust from health disparity populations, as well as the general public, both now and in the future.

Stressors

Underserved minority ethnic groups experience intense and qualitatively different stressors than are typically present within the mainstream culture. Social adjustment to the dominant culture is not an optional activity. Quality of life and even life itself requires adaptations despite internal reluctance or the magnitude of the challenge to change. Each generation may experience this stress differently, but the struggle to adapt is a common one. This type of pressure is referred to as *acculturative stress*, a tension often felt by immigrants who must adjust to leaving their place of birth and simultaneously adapt to new and sometimes radically different ways of behaving (Caplan, 2007; Finch, Hummer, Bohdan, & Vega, 2001; Vadaparampil, Wideroff, Breen, & Trapido, 2006). The stress is aggravated by the pull of the familial values, taboos, and customs and the dictates of the new ways, sometimes diametrically opposed to one another. This often is compounded by socioeconomic stress felt because of limited financial resources and diminished social standing.

Environmental Health

The environmental health status of ethnic minority communities is a major source of health problems in general and contributes to the risk for common complex diseases, including cancer (Olden & White, 2005). High-risk exposures for cancer include indoor and outdoor air pollution, industrial pollution as an occupational hazard, lead poisoning, and pollutants in drinking water, all of which have major implications for those living in suboptimal conditions (Schneider, 2002). People of color consistently face exposure levels that represent significant threats to health. Recent scientific investigations have begun to demonstrate connections between genetics and social environments (Payne, Royal, & Kardia, 2007). Differences in metabolism and detoxification enzyme levels because of genetic variation in populations have been identified. European populations with low enzyme activity associated with polymorphisms were more sensitive to industrial toxins, resulting in a higher incidence of bladder cancer (Thier et al., 2003). This type of inquiry has implications for genetic and genomic assessment, counseling, and intervention. Furthermore, known links between genetic polymorphisms, the environment, and common complex disease incidences will have particular implications for ethnic populations. Health practitioners will need to consider metabolic and detoxification pathways related to environmental exposures in diagnosing and treating a variety of common complex health conditions that have a genetic component affecting all clients.

MULTICULTURAL ASPECTS OF DELIVERY OF GENETIC AND GENOMIC SERVICES

Ethnicity and Families

The use of family history assessment to identify genetic risk factors and to construct pedigree-based assessment plans for individuals remains one of the fundamental nursing tools.

The ethnic background of individual clients can influence the validity and availability of information given, simply because of the way cultures view family and personal information. For example, in the Hispanic community, factors such as language, cultural beliefs, and family values may affect participation in cancer genetic counseling and testing. Some Native American tribes prohibit the discussion of individuals who are deceased, making the collection of family history data for accurate risk assessment difficult (Vadaparampil, Wey, & Kinney, 2004). Offspring resulting from sexual relationships between genetically close individuals may result in a higher phenotypic expression of deleterious recessive genes. Patrilineal consanguinity in traditional Muslim families may result in inbreeding and influence the potential for reproductive risks. Consideration of attitudes and beliefs about health, disease, family, and spiritual matters will influence healthcare choices (Berka et al., 2009). For example, the practice of arranged marriages within orthodox Muslim families influences their reproductive risks based on the family assessment. Assessment for patrilineal consanguinity is needed when assessing family history in individuals of orthodox Muslim heritage, as this variable can complicate the analysis of family information if intrafamilial relationships are not fully understood.

How groups perceive the concept of family affects taking a family history, and the role of family members influences to whom and how information is given. The definition of *family* differs greatly between ethnic groups. The mainstream American (Anglo) definition centers on the nuclear family, whereas African American families focus on a much wider set of connections of kin and community to constitute family. Many Chinese cultures include ancestors and descendants in their concept of family (Lee & Mock, 2005). Certain traits have been described as typical for families of one or another ethnic group. For example, in Hispanic cultures it may be important to adhere to traditional male-female roles. African Americans often are described as more accepting of an informal kinship network with the social relationship being just as important as the biologic relationship. They tend to have more flexibility in family roles than many other groups. This necessitates that the clinician verify when taking and documenting the family history if they are reporting on a kinship or blood relative. The clinician could acknowledge the broad support of non-blood relatives and then ask for clarification of those who are only the blood relatives to create an accurate picture of the biologic family and their risks. Family caregivers are important sources of health information, including when communicating family information or risk. It is important for the nurse to assess who gives and receives the information in the family and how well they comprehend information provided. Considering client and family health literacy guides how the nurse can best access and provide information to benefit the whole family (Bevan & Pecchioni, 2008).

Cultures differ in their attitudes about group boundaries. As mentioned, African Americans tend to have flexible boundaries between the family and the surrounding community, so that informal adoption is a familiar and customary practice. Exploration of family history for some African Americans may be met with some degree of reluctance. The culture views relationships as family. Thus, a less than biologic relationship may be viewed as diminished in value if exposed as a non-biologic relationship. These concerns may prevent germane forthcoming information or threaten a known relationship that has no biologic link. Vogel et al. (2007) reported that they were successful in obtaining 225 genetic histories for a sample population of African Americans over a one-year period. However, 50% of all initially interested subjects were lost to follow-up and did not participate. By way of contrast, Anglo American mainstream culture draws much clearer boundaries between insiders and outsiders. Each group will relate to nurses and other healthcare clinicians in a way that often mirrors its cultural attitudes.

Both African American and Hispanic groups place high importance on spiritual values. In Hispanic cultures, family loyalty and respect, especially for older members of the family, are cherished concepts. People are appreciated more for their character than for their career success. Chinese families often stress agreement and interdependence in relationships, respect for one's place in the line of ancestry, and avoiding shame. Food is an important symbol used for purposes beyond physical nutrition to aid in meeting emotional and spiritual needs. Although the traits of underserved ethnic groups often have been identified, it is important to note that each group has several subgroups within it with varying and sometimes contradictory values and beliefs that need to be considered when receiving care that integrates genetic and genomic information (Lee & Mock, 2005).

Ethnicity and Language

Linguistic and cultural language differences are present in groups, and health literacy problems are considered one of the biggest barriers to preventive health options, screening, and treatment decisions (Nutbeam, 2000). Health literacy has been well documented as a factor in health practices and treatment decisions (Bennett et al., 1998). The National Library of Medicine describes *health literacy* as "the degree to which individuals have the capacity to obtain, process, and understand basic health information and services needed to make appropriate decisions" (Selden, Zorn, Ratzan, & Parker, 2000, p. vi). Genetic literacy is an added dimension to health literacy and language comprehension. The general public has a poor understanding of cancer concepts (Lanie et al., 2004). Exploring the public understanding of basic genetic concepts indicates a limited understanding of genetic terminology and misconceptions about basic genetic concepts and terms. A bit of a twist in this is that healthcare providers are not literate in genetics either, so this poses an even greater challenge in how professionals communicate something that they do not understand.

Recognizing the influence of one's ethnic culture allows for the appreciation of cultural differences in attitudes toward many American mainstream values. For example, nurses rely on "talk" as the chief tool to provide services to clients. However, cultures vary in the importance each places on verbal communications. In Anglo American mainstream culture, words are used as tools to achieve goals. Conversation beyond utility often is seen as superfluous, "wordy," or rambling. In Chinese culture, families often reject the notion that blunt and exhaustive verbal communication is the preferred way to communicate important ideas. Various Hispanic cultures stress nonverbal communication. Respect is communicated by lack of eye contact with authority figures seen as experts or of a higher social class (Lipson et al., 1996). Nurses cognizant of the style and variation within various cultures understand how this may influence the method utilized to obtain family history information and communicate genetic and genomic information. Nurses take these potential differences into account when making an assessment, considering carefully their own biases and the values of their clients.

EDUCATION

Similar to healthcare professionals' efforts to educate diverse populations about cancer risk management–related behaviors, such as mammography or colonoscopy, genetic counselors' and nurses' efforts to impart information related to genetic testing may integrate temporal orientation (e.g., living more in the present and not having an orientation toward the future) into their approaches for individuals of African and African Caribbean descent. Edwards et al. (2008) recommended that awareness of temporal orientation as a factor in testing decisions may help to increase healthcare providers' sensitivity to the sociocultural context within which individuals make such decisions. Similarly, structured decision aids designed to facilitate genetic testing decisions also potentially could be strengthened by taking into account the sociocultural context. For example, Baty, Kinney, and Ellis (2002) developed and evaluated culturally sensitive education materials to communicate *BRCA1* genetic health information to African Americans. This type of communication aid illustrated the development and presentation of messages and materials that acknowledged variability in communication of targeted materials for women and the potential impact this has on health-related behaviors and decisions.

CONSENT

Individuals have the right to consent to or decline genetic testing. Mandatory testing is a fundamental breach of the most intimate privacy known. Unlike, for example, fingerprinting, knowledge of one's genetic profile reveals information about one's relatives as well. Even when voluntary, clients need understandable information to make informed autonomous choices. Some decline genetic testing because of a wish not to know their family history or risk status. This reluctance is often the result of a fear of stigmatization, discrimination by employers or insurance companies, the impact of knowledge on family relations, or the desire to avoid psychological distress (Suther & Kiros, 2009).

The clinical perspective on informed consent is to ensure that the consent is voluntary and that the client is aware and supportive of the need for the test and services provided. Prior to obtaining consent, the client needs to be aware of the research purpose, process, positive and negative implications, costs, confidentiality, and expected outcomes of any interventions (NHGRI, 2009b). The process of consent then necessitates that clients are asked if they have any additional questions or need to consult with anyone before consenting. Some individuals and minority groups may be unwilling to sign a written consent based on political or a personal history of the misuse of such documents. Such issues have become critically important issues to address by genome-wide association researchers and genome sequencers to ensure that data obtained from the NIH Genome-Wide Association Studies data repository are used in a manner consistent with the informed consent initially provided by research participants (NIH Office of Extramural Research, 2007). Nurses may be involved in ensuring adequate understanding by the client's and the client's family and addressing any remaining concerns that are expressed by potential research participants.

COMMUNITY HEALING MODELS

Health providers can benefit from an increased awareness and understanding of the different health beliefs and treatments of their clients. This task may be even more sensitive when the use of genetic and genomic information for risk management is the goal rather than treatment. At-risk individuals who are not symptomatic may feel stereotyped by assumptions of risk. Thus, they may feel offended by assertions that greater care should be considered in diet, drug-seeking, or alcohol consumption (McBride, Lipkus, Jolly, & Lyna, 2005). Of great consideration is the need for culturally sensitive communications specific to the target group of focus (Baty et al., 2002; Lara, Gamboa, Kahramanian, Morales, & Baustisa, 2005).

Fundamentally, health care can be conceptualized in a variety of ways, first springing from one's view of the world and the nature of existence. Western medicine emphasizes a separation of the mind and the body. This approach holds firmly to evidence-based understandings and practices. Patients also may be inclined to react to disease and disorders with aggressive techniques and to be relatively tolerant of unwanted side effects. What might be called the popular approach to health care leans heavily on consensus treatments coming from friends with experience with similar ailments and other informal knowledge sources such as advertisements and the popular media. The folk medicine or traditional healing approach stems from cultural traditions with long histories. This approach stresses a holistic understanding of health as a product of the mind, the body, and the spirit (Feldmann, Wienann, Sewer, & Hergenroeder, 2008; Howes & Houghton, 2003).

Many African American, Hispanic, and Asian American clients have a strong religious faith and may bring together the health beliefs of the faith with mainstream medicine and traditional healing. Many people of color, aware of all three paradigms, select a preference or tend to be guided by aspects of each of these approaches. This may result in an open understanding of health and health care. Alternatively, the client may be persuaded to eschew the mainstream Western approach and rely on an alternative treatment strategy at odds with contemporary American understandings. Clinicians often will encounter clients influenced by popular or traditional healthcare views. Treating and communicating with these clients is improved by an attitude of openness to learning and respect and understanding of their perspective. This outlook will facilitate a culturally competent relationship (National Alliance of Hispanic Health, 2000; Paniagua & Taylor, 2008).

A Hispanic tradition encourages the theory that disease is caused by an imbalance between hot and cold. Health is maintained by consuming proper foods and liquids and by avoiding exposure to extreme temperatures. "Cold" diseases include menstrual cramps, pneumonia, and colic. Examples of "hot" diseases or disorders are hypertension, diabetes, and indigestion. "Cold" diseases are treated with "hot" remedies, and vice versa. The goal of treatment is to restore balance. Assisting clients to recognize how genetic and genomic services can restore balance is a goal when explaining the risk and benefits of such services (Kuipers, 1995).

Some Native American cultures profess the belief that healing will result from sacred ceremonies that depend on visions and using plants and objects to symbolize an individual, the treatment, or the illness. Traditional Navajo medicine includes chanting, prayer, dancing, and the use of herbal mixtures. Examples of herbal medicines include echinacea, goldenseal, and burdock. Many Native American tribes rely on the sweat lodge to cure a variety of physical and emotional ills (Schiff & Moore, 2006).

Chinese medicine is a well-established healthcare tradition that uses acupuncture, herbs, and other modalities often in combination with dietary supplements and Western medicine. Clients preferring these or other traditions may be reluctant to acknowledge these health beliefs, expecting the disapproval of Western-based healthcare providers.

Not all people of color hold traditional health beliefs. Some, but not all, members of a cultural group adhere to traditional health beliefs or follow alternative health practices. Traditional beliefs and practices may be more common among people who have had little exposure to modern medicine. Even people with more modern beliefs may feel more comfortable and adhere more closely to recommended Western treatments if primary care providers offer treatment that does not conflict with the client's understanding of wellness.

STEPS TOWARD MULTICULTURAL COMPETENCE

Gaining competency in utilizing multicultural genetic and genomic information sharing will require understanding one's self in the context of appreciating differences in others. Oncology nurses enhance their clinical proficiency by developing *multicultural competence*—a three-pronged domain consisting of culture-specific awareness, knowledge, and skill acquisition (see Figure 12-1 and Table 12-2). Many resources and publications are available to offer fundamental knowledge for providing culturally competent care to individuals, families, and communities from various ethnic, religious, cultural, or social settings (see Figure 12-2). Cultural competency is emerging as an important strategy to assess and address the potential for health disparities.

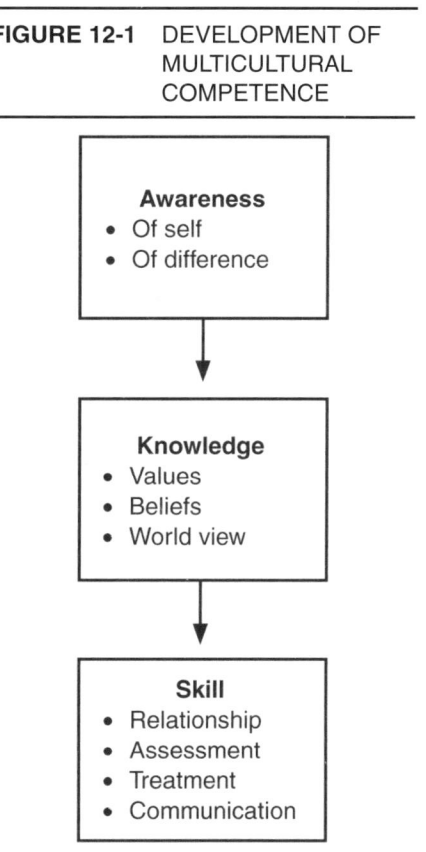

FIGURE 12-1 DEVELOPMENT OF MULTICULTURAL COMPETENCE

RESEARCH IMPLICATIONS

Multicultural competence requires more than personal conviction or motivation, but also requires additional research on issues such as language barriers, genetic literacy, the clinical environment, client and provider control in decision making, and differences in health outcomes preferred by clients and providers. Research attention to the spiritual dimension of culture and its perspective on disease outcomes also is necessary. Investigations such as these may greatly improve the nurse-client-family relationship and the effectiveness of nursing interventions.

TABLE 12-2 Multicultural Considerations in Providing Genetic and Genomic Cancer Care

Recommendation	Considerations
1. Avoid overgeneralization.	Do not stereotype based on race, ethnicity, or socioeconomic status. Ethnic information is only a starting point.
2. Facilitate trust.	Recognize that the fear of exploitation and neglect exists for some groups.
3. Be open to alternative treatment options.	Recognize the values and beliefs of individuals.
4. Recognize that clients of the same race or ethnicity can challenge cultural competency.	Often, as much intracultural difference is present as intercultural difference.
5. Provide culturally appropriate client education materials.	Consider language, style, and materials utilized for communication of complex messages.
6. Be informed about racial and ethnic modifiers of drug response and side effects.	Pharmacologic evidence points to the possibility of dosage adjustments for clients from different groups based on their genetic and genomic makeup.
7. Stay current on emerging advances to expand client benefits.	Advances in ethnic-specific pharmacogenomics, diagnostic, and therapeutic understandings improves the ability to individualize treatment.

FIGURE 12-2 SUGGESTED RESOURCES FOR MULTICULTURAL GENETIC AND GENOMIC COMPETENCE

Awesome Library. (1999, September). *Multicultural toolkit. (Toolkit for cross-cultural collaboration).* Retrieved July 20, 2009, from http://www.awesomelibrary.org/multiculturaltoolkit.html

Bassetti, S. (2002). Culturally relevant genetic counseling: Nurses play a critical role in helping women and families. *AWHONN Lifelines, 6*(3), 254–257.

Dubriwnya, T.N., Batesb, B.R., & Bevan, J.L. (2004). Lay understandings of race: Cultural and genetic definitions. *Community Genetics, 7*(4), 185–195.

National Cancer Institute. (2008, March). *NCI fact sheet: Cancer health disparities.* Retrieved July 20, 2009, from http://www.cancer.gov/cancertopics/factsheet/cancer-health-disparities

Purnell, L.D. (2009). *Guide to culturally competent health care* (2nd ed.). Philadelphia: F.A. Davis.

Salas, A., Carracedo, A., Richards, M., & Macaulay, V. (2005). Charting the ancestry of African Americans. *American Journal of Human Genetics, 77*(4), 676–680.

U.S. Department of Health and Human Services Office of Minority Health. (n.d.). *Think cultural health.* Retrieved July 20, 2009, from https://www.thinkculturalhealth.org

Consideration of the ways that genetic and genomic information influences both the individual and families from specific ethnic and cultural backgrounds needs to occur in conjunction with all research about cancer, including its predisposition, diagnosis, prognosis, and treatment. Scientific research will provide new information about the underpinnings of ethnic origins based on admixture mapping and potential population susceptibility to common disease based on polymorphisms. Exploration of these influences may include the impact of genetics and genomics on the individual and the cultural perception of disease causation and its treatment. Nursing research about the communication of such information within the family or the larger community will help to explore the genetic and genomic component of cultural competence. Knowledge and understanding of the implications of genomic science, services, and care options for all populations has significant gaps. Adequate representation of minority participants or specific population groups in any research can help to ensure adequate access, benefit, and utilizations of this genetic and genomic information in health care (Spruill & Coleman, 2009).

SUMMARY

Culturally competent nursing genetic and genomic healthcare practice rests on a foundation of honest self-awareness and knowledge of the interaction of resources and risk factors associated with biologic predispositions affecting health. The impact of genetic and genomic information on ethnicity may include issues such as

- The current deficit in the scientific understanding of ethnic-based genetic differences
- Ethnic differences in common disease risk, including cancer, that is related to obesity, lower socioeconomic status, and cultural lifestyles
- The impact of the legacy of research exploitation on ethnic cooperation with clinical regimens
- The effect of culture-based health beliefs at variance with mainstream health assumptions
- Psychosocial differences in locus of control, healthy paranoia, or racial identity.

Culture plays a key role in one's ability to influence behavior in a client. Nurses cannot afford to let cultural barriers limit their ability to meet the needs of their clients or reduce clients' opportunity to benefit from genetic and genomic services. Targeting primary care providers in underserved areas for education may reduce access barriers to competently provide genetic and genomic cancer care. By deepening their understanding of culture, nurses can strengthen the promise of high-quality primary health care that is accessible, effective, and cost efficient for all clients. The ability to manage the dynamics of ethnic differences to ensure improved care and outcomes is essential to the role of oncology nurses.

REFERENCES

Ahn, J., Peters, U., Albanes, D., Purdue, M.P., Abnet, C.C., Chatterjee, N., et al. (2008). Serum vitamin D concentration and prostate cancer risk: A nested case-control study. *Journal of the National Cancer Institute, 100*(11), 796–804.

Albain, K., Unger, J.M., Crowley, J.J., Coltman, C.A., Jr., & Hershman, D.L. (2009). Racial disparities in cancer survival among randomized clinical trials patients of the Southwest Oncology Group. *Journal of the National Cancer Institute, 101*(14), 984–992.

Alvidrez, J., Azocar, F., & Miranda, J. (1996). Demystifying the concept of ethnicity for psychotherapy researchers. *Journal of Consulting and Clinical Psychology, 64*(5), 903–908.

American Cancer Society. (2009). *Cancer facts and figures 2009.* Retrieved June 30, 2009, from http://www.cancer.org/docroot/STT/stt_0_2008.asp?sitearea=STT&level=1

American Public Health Association. (2009, February). *Proposed policy: Genetic health literacy, cultural competence, public and professional education.* Retrieved July 14, 2009, from http://www.apha.org/NR/rdonlyres/23876234-5DB9-4080-A526-8642C2588B43/0/A2ProposedPolicyGeneticLiteracy2.pdf

Baty, B.J., Kinney, A.Y., & Ellis, S.M. (2002). Developing culturally sensitive cancer genetics communication aids for African Americans. *American Journal of Medical Genetics, 118A*(2), 146–155.

Behar, D., Metspalu, E., Kivisild, T., Rosset, S., Tzur, S., Hadid, Y., et al. (2008). Counting the founders: The matrilineal genetic ancestry of the Jewish Diaspora. *PLoS ONE, 3*(4), e2062. Retrieved December 17, 2009, from http://www.plosone.org/article/info%3Adoi%2F10.1371%2Fjournal.pone.0002062

Bennett, C.L., Ferreira, M.R., Davis, T.C., Kaplan, J., Weinberger, M., Kuzel, T., et al. (1998). Relation between literacy, race, and stage of presentation among low-income patients with prostate cancer. *Journal of Clinical Oncology, 16*(9), 3101–3104.

Berka, N., Vaughn, T., Headings, V., Harrison, B., Murray, R., Ampy, F., et al. (2009). Attitudes of Muslims regarding the new genetics: Testing, treatment, and technology. In R.B. Monsen (Ed.), *Genetics and ethics in health care: New questions in the age of genomic health* (pp. 149–163). Silver Spring, MD: American Nurses Association.

Bernard, J., & Goodyear, R.K. (1992). *Fundamentals of clinical supervision.* Needham Heights, MA: Allyn and Bacon.

Betancourt, H., & Lopez, S. (1993). The study of culture, ethnicity and race in American psychology. *American Psychologist, 48*(6), 629–637.

Betancourt, J.R., Green, A.R., Carrillo, J.E., & Park, E.R. (2005). Cultural competence and health care disparities: Key perspectives and trends. *Health Affairs, 24*(2), 499–505.

Bevan, J.L., & Pecchioni, L.L. (2008). Understanding the impact of family caregiver cancer literacy on patient health outcomes. *Patient Education and Counseling, 71*(3), 356–364.

Braff, J.P., Chatterjee, B., Hochman, M., Kelton, T., Kennington, J., Kolavala, C., et al. (2008). Patient-tailored medicine. Part 1: The impact of race and genetics on medicine. *Journal of Health and Life Sciences Law, 2*(1), 5–36.

Braff, J.P., Chatterjee, B., Hochman, M., Kennington, J., Kolavala, C., Layman, K., et al. (2009). Patient-tailored medicine. Part 2: Personalized medicine and the legal landscape. *Journal of Health and Life Sciences Law, 2*(2), 1–3, 5–43.

Burchard, E.G., Ziv, E., Coyle, N., Gomez, S.L., Tang, H., Karter, A.J., et al. (2003). The importance of race and ethnic background in biomedical research and clinical practice. *New England Journal of Medicine, 348*(12), 1170–1175.

Caplan, S. (2007). Latinos, acculturation, and acculturation stress: A dimensional concept analysis. *Policy, Politics and Nursing Practice, 8*(2), 93–106.

Centers for Disease Control and Prevention Office of Minority Health and Health Disparities. (2009, March). *Eliminating racial and ethnic health disparities.* Retrieved October 23, 2009, from http://www.cdc.gov/omhd/About/disparities.htm

Cicek, M., Liu, X., Schumacher, F., Casey, G., & Witte, J. (2006). Vitamin D receptor genotype/haplotype and prostate cancer risk. *Cancer Epidemiology, Biomarkers and Prevention, 15*(12), 2549–2552.

Consensus Panel on Genetic/Genomic Nursing Competencies. (2009). *Essentials of genetic and genomic nursing: Competencies, curricula guidelines, and outcome indicators* (2nd ed.). Silver Spring, MD: American Nurses Association.

Cooper, R.S., Kaufman, J.S., & Ward, R. (2003). Race and genomics. *New England Journal of Medicine, 348*(12), 1166–1170.

Dula, A. (1994). African American suspicion of healthcare system is justified: What do we do about it? *Cambridge Quality Healthcare Ethics, 3*(3), 347–357.

Dula, A., Royal, C., & Secundy, M.G. (2003). The ethical and social implications of exploring African American genealogies. *Developing World Bioethics, 3*(2), 133–141.

Edwards, T.A., Thompson, H.S., Kwate, N.O., Brown, K., McGovern, M.M., Forman, A., et al. (2008). Association between temporal orientation and attitudes about BRCA1/2 testing among women of African descent with family histories of breast cancer. *Patient Education and Counseling, 72*(2), 276–282.

Feldmann, J., Wienann, C., Sewer, L., & Hergenroeder, A., (2008). Folk and traditional medicine use in a subset of Hispanic adolescents. *International Journal of Adolescent Medicine and Health, 20*(1), 41–51.

Finch, B., Hummer, R.A., Bohdan, K., & Vega, W.A. (2001). The role of discrimination and acculturation stress in the physical health of Mexican-origin adults. *Hispanic Journal of Behavioral Science, 23*(4), 399–429.

Green, S. (2003). The genomic era: What must public health do? *Virtual Mentor, 5*(11). Retrieved July 14, 2009, from http://virtualmentor.ama-assn.org/2003/11/gene1-0311.html

Halbert, C.H., Armstrong, K., Gandy, O.H., Jr., & Shaker, L. (2006). Racial differences in trust in healthcare providers. *Archives of Internal Medicine, 166*(8), 896–901.

Havasupai Tribe v. Arizona State University. CV 20040146, AZ Superior Court, Coconino County (2004).

Howes, M., & Houghton, P. (2003). Plants used in Chinese and Indian traditional medicine for improvement of memory and cognitive function. *Pharmacology, Biochemistry, and Behavior, 75*(3), 513–527.

Human Genome Project Information. (2008). Retrieved June 30, 2009, from http://www.ornl.gov/sci/techresources/Human_Genome/elsi/elsi.shtml

International HapMap Consortium. (2003). The International HapMap Project. *Nature, 426*(6968), 789–796.

Jorde, L.B., & Wooding, S.P. (2004). Genetic variation, classification and "race." *Nature Genetics, 36*(Suppl. 11), S28–S33.

Keita, S.O., Kittles, R.A., Royal, C.D., Bonney, G.E., Furbert-Harris, P., Dunston, G.M., et al. (2004). Conceptualizing human variation. *Nature Genetics, 36*(Suppl. 11), S17–S20.

Kuipers, J. (1995). Mexican Americans. In J.N. Giger & R.E. Davidhizar (Eds.), *Transcultural nursing: Assessment and intervention* (2nd ed., pp. 205–236). St. Louis, MO: Mosby.

Lai, C.Q., Tucker, K.L., Choudhry, S., Parnell, L.D., Mattei, J., García-Bailo, B., et al. (2009). Population admixture associated with disease prevalence in the Boston Puerto Rican health study. *Human Genetics, 125*(2), 199–209.

Landrine, H., & Klonoff, E.A. (1996). *African American acculturation: Deconstructing race and reviving culture.* Thousand Oaks, CA: Sage.

Lanie, A., Jayaratne, T., Sheldon, J., Kardia, S., Anderson, E., Feldbaum, M., et al. (2004). Exploring the public understanding of basic genetic concepts. *Journal of Genetic Counseling, 13*(4), 305–320.

Lara, M., Gamboa, C., Kahramanian, M., Morales, L., & Baustisa, D. (2005). Acculturation and Latinos health in the United States: A review of the literature and sociopolitical context. *Annual Review of Public Health, 26*, 367–397.

Lea, D., Feero, W., & Jenkins, J. (2008). Genetic research sheds light on common complex disorders. *American Nurse Today, 3*(12), 24–25.

Lee, E., & Mock, M.R. (2005). Chinese families. In M. McGoldrick, J. Giordano, & N. Garcia-Preto (Eds.), *Ethnicity and family therapy* (3rd ed., pp. 302–318). New York: Guilford Press.

Lipson, J., Dibble, S.L., & Minarik, P.A. (2000). *Culture and nursing care: A pocket guide.* San Francisco: UCSF Nursing Press.

Mao, X., Bigham, A.W., Mei, R., Gutierrez, G., Weiss, K.M., Brutsaert, T.D., et al. (2007). A genome-wide admixture mapping panel for Hispanic/Latino populations. *American Journal of Human Genetics, 80*(6), 1171–1178.

McBride, C.M., Lipkus, I.M., Jolly, D., & Lyna, P. (2005). Interest in testing for genetic susceptibility to lung cancer among black college students "at risk" of becoming cigarette smokers. *Cancer Epidemiology, Biomarkers and Prevention, 14*(12), 2978–2981.

Mountain, J.L., & Risch, N. (2004). Assessing genetic contributions to phenotypic differences among "racial" and "ethnic" groups. *Nature Genetics, 36*(Suppl. 11), S48–S53.

National Alliance of Hispanic Health. (2000). *Quality health services for Hispanics: The cultural competency component* (Vol. No. 99-21). Washington, DC: U.S. Department of Health and Human Services.

National Cancer Institute. (2008, March). *Cancer health disparities.* Retrieved June 30, 2009, from http://www.cancer.gov/cancertopics/factsheet/cancer-health-disparities

National Cancer Institute. (2009, October). *Genetics of prostate cancer (PDQ®).* Retrieved October 26, 2009, from http://www.cancer.gov/cancertopics/pdq/genetics/prostate/HealthProfessional

National Cancer Institute Center to Reduce Cancer Health Disparities. (2009, August). *Health disparities defined.* Retrieved August 31, 2009, from http://crchd.cancer.gov/disparities/defined.html

National Cancer Institute Surveillance, Epidemiology, and End Results Program. (n.d.). *SEER stat fact sheets: Incidence and mortality.* Retrieved June 30, 2009, from http://www.seer.cancer.gov/statfacts/html/all.html

National Human Genome Research Institute. (2001). *National Human Genome Research Institute five-year strategic plan for reducing health disparities.* Retrieved June 29, 2009, from http://www.genome.gov/10001492

National Human Genome Research Institute. (2009a, January). *Genome-wide association studies.* Retrieved June 29, 2009, from http://www.genome.gov/20019523

National Human Genome Research Institute. (2009b, July). *Informed consent for genomics research.* Retrieved October 27, 2009, from http://www.genome.gov/27026588

National Human Genome Research Institute. (n.d.). *NIH health disparities strategic plan fiscal years 2004–2008.* Retrieved June 29, 2009, from http://www.genome.gov/Pages/Research/DER/DERReportsPublications/NHGRIHealthDisparitiesPlan.pdf

National Institutes of Health Office of Extramural Research. (2007, December). *Genome-wide association studies (GWAS)—Frequently asked questions.* Retrieved October 27, 2009, from http://grants.nih.gov/grants/gwas/GWAS_faq.htm

Nutbeam, D. (2000). Health literacy as public health goal. *Health Promotion International, 15*(3), 259–267.

Olden, K., & White, S.L. (2005). Health-related disparities: Influence of environmental factors. *Medical Clinics of North America, 89*(4), 721–738.

Oliver, M., & Muntaner, C. (2005). Researching health inequities among African Americans: The imperative to understand social class. *International Journal of Health Services, 35*(3), 485–498.

Paniagua, C.T., & Taylor, R.E. (2008). The cultural lens of genomics. *Online Journal of Issues in Nursing, 13*(1). Retrieved October 27, 2009, from http://www.nursingworld.org/MainMenuCategories/ANAMarketplace/ANAPeriodicals/OJIN/TableofContents/vol132008/No1Jan08/CulturalLens.aspx

Payne, P.W., Jr., Royal, C., & Kardia, S.L. (2007). Genetic and social environment interactions and their impact on health policy. *Journal of the American Academy of Orthopaedic Surgeons, 15*(Suppl. 1), S95–S98.

Roff, A., & Wilson, R.T. (2008). A novel SNP in a vitamin D response element of the CYP24A1 promoter reduces protein binding, transactivation, and gene expression. *Journal of Steroid Biochemistry and Molecular Biology, 112*(1–3), 47–54.

Royal, C.D., & Dunston, G.M. (2004). Changing the paradigm from "race" to human genome variation. *Nature Genetics, 36*(Suppl. 11), S5–S7.

Sabeti, P.C., Varilly, P., Fry, B., Lohmueller, J., Hostetter, E., Cotsapas, C., et al. (2007). Genome-wide detection and characterization of positive selection in human populations. *Nature, 449*(7164), 913–919.

Sankar, P., Cho, M.K., & Mountain, J. (2007). Race and ethnicity in genetic research. *American Journal of Medical Genetics, 143A*(9), 961–970.

Schiff, J., & Moore, K. (2006). The impact of the sweat lodge ceremony on dimensions of well-being. *American Indian and Alaska Native Mental Health Research, 13*(3), 48–69.

Schneider, K. (2002). *Counseling about cancer: Strategies for genetic counselors* (2nd ed.). New York: Wiley-Liss.

Selden, C.R., Zorn, M., Ratzan, S., & Parker, R.M. (Eds.). (2000). *Current bibliographies in medicine: Health literacy.* Bethesda, MD: National Institutes of Health National Library of Medicine. Retrieved October 27, 2009, from http://www.nlm.nih.gov/archive//20061214/pubs/cbm/hliteracy.pdf

Simon, M., & Petrucelli, N. (2009). Hereditary breast and ovarian cancer syndrome: The impact of race on uptake of genetic counseling and testing. *Methods in Molecular Biology, 471*, 487–500.

Spruill, I., & Coleman, B. (2009). African American perspectives on genetics and ethics. In R.B. Monsen (Ed.), *Genetics and ethics in health care: New questions in the age of genomic health* (pp. 213–233). Silver Spring, MD: American Nurses Association.

Struewing, J., Hartge, P., Wacholder, S., Baker, S.M., Berlin, M., McAdams, M., et al. (1997). The risk of cancer associated with specific mutations of BRCA1 and BRCA2 among Ashkenazi Jews. *New England Journal of Medicine, 336*(20), 1401–1408.

Suarez-Kurtz, G., & Pena, S.D. (2006). Pharmacogenomics in the Americas: The impact of genetic admixture. *Current Drug Targets, 7*(12), 1649–1658.

Suther, S., & Kiros, G.-E. (2009). Barriers to the use of genetic testing: A study of racial and ethnic disparities. *Genetics in Medicine, 11*(9), 655–662.

Taylor, T.R., Williams, C.D., Makambi, K.H., Mouton, C., Harrell, J.P., Cozier, Y., et al. (2007). Racial discrimination and breast cancer incidence in U.S. Black women: The Black Women's Health Study. *American Journal of Epidemiology, 166*(1), 46–54.

Thier, R., Brüning, T., Roos, P.H., Rihs, H.P., Golka, K., Ko, Y., et al. (2003). Markers of genetic susceptibility in human environmental hygiene and toxicology: The role of selected CYP, NAT, and GST genes. *International Journal of Hygiene and Environmental Health, 206*(3), 149–171.

Tilousi v. Arizona State University. CV-20040115, AZ Superior Court, Coconino County (2004).

Tsosie, R. (2007). Cultural challenges to biotechnology: Native American genetic resources and the concept of cultural harm. *Journal of Law, Medicine, and Ethics, 35*(3), 396–411.

U.S. Census Bureau. (2004). *Projected population of the United States, by race and Hispanic origin: 2000 to 2050.* Retrieved December 7, 2009, from http://www.census.gov/population/www/projections/usinterimproj/natprojtab01a.pdf

Vadaparampil, S.T., Wey, J.P., & Kinney, A.Y. (2004). Psychosocial aspects of genetic counseling and testing. *Seminars in Oncology Nursing, 20*(3), 186–195.

Vadaparampil, S.T., Wideroff, L., Breen, N., & Trapido, E. (2006). The impact of acculturation on awareness of genetic testing for increased cancer risk among Hispanics in the year 2000 National Health Interview Survey. *Cancer Epidemiology, Biomarkers and Prevention, 15*(4), 618–623.

Venter, J.C., Adams, M.D., Myers, E.W., Li, P.W., Mural, R.J., Sutton, G.G., et al. (2001). The sequence of the human genome. *Science, 291*(5507), 1304–1351.

Vogel, K.J., Murthy, V.S., Dudley, B., Grubs, R.E., Gettig, E., Ford, A., et al. (2007). The use of family health histories to address health disparities in an African American community. *Health Promotion Practice, 8*(4), 350–357.

Warner, E., Foulkes, W., Goodwin, P., Meschino, W., Blondal, J., Paterson, C., et al. (1999). Prevalence and penetrance of BRCA1 and BRCA2 gene mutations in unselected Ashkenazi Jewish women with breast cancer. *Journal of the National Cancer Institute, 91*(14), 1241–1247.

Washington, H. (2006). *Medical apartheid.* New York: Doubleday.

Williams, E.D., Sarata, A.K., & Redhead, C.S. (2007). *Genetic discrimination: Overview of the issue and proposed legislation.* Washington, DC: Congressional Research Service. Retrieved March 7, 2007, from http://digitalcommons.ilr.cornell.edu/cgi/viewcontent.cgi?article=1028&context=crs

SECTION V

Professional Practice Issues

CHAPTER 13 GENETIC/GENOMIC COMPETENCIES AND RECOMMENDATIONS FOR EDUCATION

CHAPTER 14 ENSURING COMPETENCE: NURSING CREDENTIALING IN CANCER GENETICS

CHAPTER 15 RESEARCH: MAKING A DIFFERENCE IN PRACTICE

CHAPTER 13

Genetic/Genomic Competencies and Recommendations for Education

Lorraine Frazier, PhD, RN, MS, FAHA, FAAN, Kathleen A. Calzone, MSN, RN, APNG, FAAN, and Jean Jenkins, PhD, RN, FAAN

> **Professional Responsibilities Domain:**
> - Examine competency of practice on a regular basis, identifying areas of strength as well as areas in which professional development related to genetics and genomics would be beneficial (Consensus Panel on Genetic/Genomic Nursing Competencies, 2009)

INTRODUCTION

Genetic and genomic information is rapidly moving to include the primary care community, where nurses play a major role in the provision of genetic and genomic services. Oncology nurses across the healthcare spectrum can no longer practice without a foundational understanding of genetics and genomics as contributing factors in the process of cancer risk, occurrence, and response to interventions. The current environment of discovery in genetic and genomic science is occurring at lightning speed. Dramatic advances are published daily that are moving the healthcare provider community to be able to translate these discoveries into practice. Steps to incorporate genetic and genomic discoveries into practice include deciding what services are essential to include in clinical care, how to design such services, what information is needed by the consumer to make informed decisions, and what social issues need to be considered (e.g., privacy, reimbursement). Nurses can provide leadership in the dialogue about such decisions if adequately informed. This chapter presents guidance about cancer genetic and genomic education for all oncology nurses, at every level of practice regardless of academic preparation and including nursing students. Whether the education is provided in an academic or practice setting, the following content provides a framework for assessing personal and professional oncology nursing education and competency. Potential questions useful for contemplation include
- What do nurses already know about genetics and genomics?
- Are all nurses the target for genetic and genomic education?
- What is important to include in academic and continuing education programs about genetic and genomic information and services?

WHAT DO NURSES ALREADY KNOW ABOUT GENETICS AND GENOMICS?

Recognition of the importance of genetic and genomic information for nurses continues to be limited (Jenkins, Grady, & Collins, 2005). Reports indicate that the genetics content in basic nursing curricula is sparse and that little has changed in the intervening years (Cohen, 1979; Hetteberg, Prows, Deets, Monsen, & Kenner, 1999; Monsen, 1984; Scanlon & Fibison, 1995). As of the latter part of 2005, only 30% of academic nursing programs had included curriculum content on genetics (Prows, Calzone, & Jenkins, 2006). As a result, most practicing nurses' genetic and genomic knowledge remains sparse; the majority of new graduates also have a limited knowledge base in this area. This is especially concerning in the practice of oncology, where genetics and genomics have permeated all aspects of cancer care. Table 13-1 identifies gaps in the translation of genetics and genomics knowledge into practice.

Table 13-1. Gaps in the Translation of Genetics and Genomics Knowledge to Clinical Practice

Category	Components
Outcomes: Better understanding of the outcomes of genomic-based interventions for common chronic diseases such as cancer is needed.	• Psychological • Behavioral • Clinical
Consumer information needs: Consumers have inconsistent understanding and interest in genetic services such as genetic testing. The possibility of adverse consequences is a concern.	• Knowledge, attitudes, and beliefs • Intention to seek genetic services • Participation in genetic services
Delivery of genetic services: The workforce feels underprepared to integrate genomics into clinical care. Few successful models for integration currently exist.	• Existing services and workforce • Integrating genetics into primary care practice
Barriers to integration of genetic services: Health professionals' perceived lack of knowledge about genetics and genomics affects ability to counsel, interpret, or refer patients as appropriate.	• Health professionals' knowledge, attitudes, beliefs, and abilities • Lack of oversight of genetic testing • Privacy and discrimination concerns

Note. Based on information from Scheuner et al., 2008.

A study that assessed practicing oncology nurses' knowledge, practice, and educational needs regarding cancer genetics found that the oncology nurses surveyed viewed cancer genetics as important to their specialty practice (Peterson, Rieger, Marani, deMoor, & Gritz, 2001). Almost half (48%) of respondents indicated that patients or family members had inquired about cancer genetic counseling or testing during the previous year. However, knowledge deficits existed at all levels of practice. Additionally, Calzone, Lea, and Masny (2006) affirmed that genetic and genomic education for all oncology nurses is crucial to ensure competency in the knowledge and skills necessary to safely care for patients with cancer whose care is and will be influenced by genetics and genomics.

ARE ALL NURSES THE TARGET FOR EDUCATION?

As of March 2004, 2,915,309 nurses were licensed to practice as an RN in the United States, of which 2,421,351 were employed in nursing (Health Resources Services Administration, 2007). In addition, comparison with prior surveys conducted in 2000 and 1980 demonstrated that the average age of the RN continues to rise. In the 2004 survey, less than 27% of RNs were younger than 40 years old. These nurses have not had genetics, and certainly not genomics, included in their academic training. Even now, genetic and genomic content is not consistently incorporated into entry-level nursing programs or National Council licensure examinations (Prows, Glass, Nicol, Skirton, & Williams, 2005). Furthermore, the challenge is accentuated because practicing nurses have varied education, specialization, work settings, and responsibilities (Feetham, Thomson, & Hinshaw, 2005). A major concern is that training opportunities, albeit increasing, are limited for nurses who want to improve their understanding of genetics and genomics. All these factors make it difficult for most nurses today to apply leading-edge genetic and genomic concepts as part of holistic patient care. Similar data on this gap are demonstrated for medicine and other health professionals (Harvey et al., 2007; Trinidad et al., 2008).

An oncology nurse may not immediately recognize the fact that an understanding of genetics and genomics is important to his or her professional role as a healthcare provider. Cancer nurses, more than any other specialty, are affected the most by advances in genetic and genomic technology (Calzone et al., 2006). The emerging genetic and genomic technologies are elucidating the underlying molecular pathways that lead to cancer. Increasingly, these discoveries are becoming part of routine options for care, including inherited predisposition genetic testing, genomic tumor profiling, use of genetic and genomic markers as therapeutic indicators, and individualization of targeted therapies. As more individuals are seeking advice about genetic testing and other applications of the evolving science of genetics and genomics, oncology nurses already are integrating genetic and genomic information into oncology nursing practice across the entire healthcare continuum.

EDUCATION RECOMMENDATIONS FOR ONCOLOGY NURSES

Oncology Nursing Society (ONS, 2006b) has supported the integration of genetic and genomic information into curricula at all levels of nursing education. Oncology nurses with a subspecialty in genetics and genomics who practice at both the general and advanced practice levels must have educational preparation in the principles of human genetics; genomics; the scope of genetic and genomic information; and the ethical, legal, and social implications of the use of genetic and genomic information in cancer care (International Society of Nurses in Genetics [ISONG], 2007; ONS, 2006b).

What Do All Nurses Need to Know?

Oncology is one of the first specialties where basic genetic and genomic science discoveries already are changing options for clinical care. Whether it is identifying a family at risk for cancer secondary to a hereditary cancer syndrome or using genetically targeted therapies, the oncology nurse has a responsibility to optimize health outcomes through the clinical application of cancer genetic and genomic information. A landmark consensus document delineating genetic core competencies of knowledge, skill, and attitudes of all health professionals was published by the National Coalition for Health Professional Education in Genetics (2000, 2007). This document has been a resource for the development of discipline-specific genetic and genomic competencies, including nursing (Centers for Disease Control and Prevention, 2001; Jenkins & Calzone, 2007).

Professional Organizations' Contributions to Educational Recommendations and Competencies

ONS has recently joined with 48 other professional nursing organizations in endorsing the *Essentials of Genetic and Genomic Nursing: Competencies, Curricula Guidelines, and Outcome Indicators* (Consensus Panel on Genetic/Genomic Nursing Competencies, 2009). These competencies outline the goal of such educational preparation for all nurses regardless of clinical specialty, role, or academic preparation (Jenkins & Calzone, 2007). This essential competency document was created through an extensive consensus process that encouraged review, comment, discussion, and reflection by experts, the nursing community, and key stakeholders. The competencies reflect the *minimal* amount of genetic and genomic competency expected by every nurse. The goal of the essential competency document is to guide educators, regulators, and practicing nurses in becoming prepared to deliver competent genetic and genomic–focused nursing care. Visit www.genome.gov/17517037 for more information about the essential competencies and the list of endorsing organizations. Table 13-2 provides a listing of the specific competencies.

All oncology nurses need a basic foundation in genetics and genomics (Calzone et al., 2006). Only with such a foundation can nurses expand their specialty knowledge to include cancer-specific applications. The essential competencies provide the foundation upon which specialty organizations can build education programs that individualize content to respond to their specialty's specific needs. Oncology nursing is an example of a specialty in need of an expanded curriculum. All oncology nurses need to know when to refer patients to a genetic specialist, recognize and apply new genetic and genomic technology and therapeutics, and promote responsible handling of genetic and genomic information. These expectations necessitate education that includes genetic and genomic concepts so that the general oncology nurse is competent to meet today's oncology healthcare needs. Several education programs have been developed for oncology nurses. More information about continuing education and academic educational programs can be found in Chapter 16.

Peterson et al. (2001) proposed a targeted specialty educational approach for practicing oncology nurses based on survey results. A study of 656 oncology nurses' knowledge of basic genetics, cancer biology, cancer genetics, and cell biology identified suggested content areas that should be included in training. Those surveyed were most knowledgeable about cancer biology but had deficits in the areas of cell biology, basic genetics, and cancer genetics. This study found a significant need for cancer genetics education for those who worked in nursing staff positions, those with a bachelor's degree or less, and those who had not had cancer genetics continuing education.

Genetic and genomic knowledge is especially critical for advanced practice oncology nurses (APONs) already in clinical practice because of their leadership role. Graduate program faculty are beginning to incorporate genetic and genomic courses and distance learning strategies, and offer other resources throughout the curriculum to prepare master's students to assume greater leadership roles in meeting the demands of genomics-based health care (Maradiegue, Edwards, Seibert, Macri, & Sitzer, 2005; Prows et al., 2005; Seibert, Edwards, & Maradiegue, 2007).

TABLE 13-2 Essential Nursing Competencies in Genetics and Genomics

Domain	Competencies
Professional responsibilities	All registered nurses are expected to engage in professional role activities that are consistent with *Nursing: Scope and Standards of Practice*, 2004, American Nurses Association. In addition, competent nursing practice now requires the incorporation of genetic and genomic knowledge and skills in order to: • Recognize when one's own attitudes and values related to genetic and genomic science may affect care provided to clients. • Advocate for clients' access to desired genetic and genomic services and resources including support groups. • Examine competency of practice on a regular basis, identifying areas of strength, as well as areas in which professional development related to genetics and genomics would be beneficial. • Incorporate genetic and genomic technologies and information into registered nurse practice. • Demonstrate in practice the importance of tailoring genetic and genomic information and services to clients based on their culture, religion, knowledge level, literacy, and preferred language. • Advocate for the rights of all clients for autonomous, informed genetic and genomic-related decision-making and voluntary action.
Professional practice	Nursing assessment: Applying and integrating genetic and genomic knowledge The registered nurse: • Demonstrates an understanding of the relationship of genetics and genomics to health, prevention, screening, diagnostics, prognostics, selection of treatment, and monitoring of treatment effectiveness. • Demonstrates ability to elicit a minimum of three-generation family health history. • Constructs a pedigree from collected family history information using standardized symbols and terminology. • Collects personal, health, and developmental histories that consider genetic, environmental, and genomic influences and risks. • Conducts comprehensive health and physical assessments, which incorporate knowledge about genetic, environmental, and genomic influences and risk factors. • Critically analyzes the history and physical assessment findings for genetic, environmental, and genomic influences and risk factors. • Assesses clients' knowledge, perceptions, and responses to genetic and genomic information. • Develops a plan of care that incorporates genetic and genomic assessment information. Identification The registered nurse: • Identifies clients who may benefit from specific genetic and genomic information and/or services based on assessment data. • Identifies credible, accurate, appropriate, and current genetic and genomic information, resources, services, and/or technologies specific to given clients. • Identifies ethical, ethnic/ancestral, cultural, religious, legal, fiscal, and societal issues related to genetic and genomic information and technologies. • Defines issues that undermine the rights of all clients for autonomous, informed genetic and genomic-related decision-making and voluntary action. Referral activities The registered nurse: • Facilitates referrals for specialized genetic and genomic services for clients as needed.

(Continued on next page)

Domain	Competencies

Professional practice *(cont.)*	**Provision of education, care, and support**
	The registered nurse:
	• Provides clients with interpretation of selective genetic and genomic information or services.
	• Provides clients with credible, accurate, appropriate, and current genetic and genomic information, resources, services, and technologies that facilitate decision-making.
	• Uses health promotion and disease prevention practices to:
	  – Consider genetic and genomic influences on personal and environmental risk factors.
	  – Incorporate knowledge of genetic and/or genomic risk factors (e.g., a client with a genetic predisposition for high cholesterol who can benefit from a change in lifestyle that will decrease the likelihood that the genetic risk will be expressed).
	• Uses genetic and genomic-based interventions and information to improve clients' outcomes.
	• Collaborates with healthcare providers in providing genetic and genomic healthcare.
	• Collaborates with insurance providers and payers to facilitate reimbursement for genetic and genomic healthcare services.
	• Performs interventions and treatments appropriate to clients' genetic and genomic healthcare needs.
	• Evaluates impact and effectiveness of genetic and genomic technology, information, interventions, and treatments on clients' outcome.

Note. From "Establishing the Essential Nursing Competencies for Genetics and Genomics," by J. Jenkins and K.A. Calzone, 2007, *Journal of Nursing Scholarship, 39*(1), p. 13. Copyright 2007 by Blackwell Publishing. Reprinted with permission.

The essential competencies apply to APONs; however, they have additional theoretical knowledge in all aspects of cancer care (Lynch, Cope, & Murphy-Ende, 2001). Therefore, to practice at this level, APONs need to be competent in cancer genetics and genomics beyond that which the competencies specify (Calzone & Masny, 2004; Maradiegue et al., 2005). In 2002, skills, attitudes, and competencies for cancer genetics were defined for APONs (Calzone, Jenkins, & Masny, 2002).

ONS consistently offers continuing nursing education in genetics and genomics at its annual Congress and Institutes of Learning conferences. ONS also offers the Genetics Online Education Series (http://onsopcontent.ons.org/education/Genetics/index.shtml), which provides a basic primer in cancer genetics, as well as a CD-ROM on genetics and cancer clinical applications.

Education Recommendations for Oncology Nurses With a Subspecialty in Genetics

Oncology nurses with specialized education in genetics obtained through an academic program or via continuing education are assuming responsibilities similar to oncologists with specialized training or genetic counselors in offering cancer care. Such responsibilities include cancer genetic counseling, comprehensive risk assessment, planning for genetic testing based on empirical evidence of a cancer predisposition syndrome and differential, and providing risk-reduction recommendations. The position of ONS is that cancer predisposition genetic testing and risk assessment counseling requires informed consent and must include pre- and post-test counseling by qualified individuals such as advanced practice nurse in genetics (ONS, 2006a). However, the ISONG (2007) standards of practice apply to nurses at both the basic and advanced levels. The ISONG standards of care require advanced genetics education that prepares the nurse to identify individuals who may benefit from genetic services, obtain comprehensive family and health history information, construct and interpret family pedigrees, ensure informed consent, implement interventions (e.g., genetic testing), provide results, monitor for effects, and provide follow-up care to genetic services offered to individuals and their families. The Genetic Nursing Credentialing Commission awards credentials at both the basic and advanced level. A more detailed discussion of credentialing can be found in Chapter 14.

EXEMPLARS

Integrating Essential Nursing Competences and Curricula Guidelines for Genetics and Genomics Into Nursing Practice

The Mayo Clinic's Nursing Genomics Program in Rochester, MN, was awarded the Magnet® prize from the American Nurses Credentialing Center in 2006 for its efforts in developing a diverse and extensive plan for nursing education about genomics. This prestigious designation given to a select group of nursing programs (http://nursecredentialing.org/magnet/index.html) was based on the efforts of Beth Pestka and her colleagues that focused on communication to nurses about the relevance and importance of genomics nursing competency (Pestka & Brown, 2004). Strategies used at the Mayo Clinic included interactive presentations and discussions with the nursing leadership, newsletter articles, an extensive genomics nursing course, and poster presentations. A list of genomic resources was provided to staff on the organization's intranet site. Incorporation of genomic education into new nurse orientation and nursing specialty curricula was achieved, and support for staff to attend continuing education conferences with a genetic/genomic focus was made available. A nursing genomics interest group was established, which provided leadership in the creative efforts involved with extensive staff nurse educational activities. These multifaceted activities have been effective in raising the awareness of Mayo Clinic nurses about the importance of genetics and genomics to their nursing practice.

Integrating Essential Nursing Competences and Curricula Guidelines for Genetics and Genomics Into Nursing Education Programs

Curricula in cancer genetics have been built on the basic nursing core curriculum recommendations found in the *Essentials of Genetic and Genomic Nursing: Competencies, Curricula Guidelines, and Outcome Indicators* (Consensus Panel on Genetic/Genomic Nursing Competencies, 2009). The competencies were built around the domains of professional responsibilities and professional practice. The essential competencies are intended to guide nurse educators in designing and implementing programs that help students, learners, and practicing nurses to learn these genetic and genomic competencies. The use of competencies that are designed to enable the nurse to deliver nursing care with a genetic and genomic focus helps to incorporate a genetic and genomic perspective into nursing practice (Jenkins & Calzone, 2007).

The University of Texas, Houston used the nursing competencies in the development of a doctorate of nursing practice course in genetics. The course description is available at the University of Texas Health Science Center at Houston School of Nursing Web site at http://son.uth.tmc.edu and also on the Southern Region Educational Board Electronic Campus. Using the competencies as a basis for the course enabled the development of objectives focused on professional responsibilities (knowledge) and resulting professional practice (application). The competencies are particularly useful in designing courses that focus on clinical practice. The students are expected to show mastery of the information through the development of a detailed case study that will include all of the components of the course. As a result of using the nursing competencies, the course content focuses on the clinical application of genetics and genomics that clinicians most likely will encounter in practice.

The nursing literature offers some resources that discuss the specific educational needs of oncology nurses. The *Journal of Nursing Scholarship* published peer-reviewed articles over a period of two years that summarized the evidence that genetics and genomics science was beginning to transform healthcare services and illustrated the impact of these transformations on nursing practice. In addition, as of this writing, few schools of nursing offer graduate-level nursing options in genetics, although the number is growing. See Chapter 16 for a listing of these academic resources.

All oncology nurses with appropriate education and experience can provide comprehensive care that integrates genetic and genomic information and services. Oncology nursing practice that integrates genetic and genomic information includes all levels of practice—nurses at the general level, APONs, and APONs with specialty training in genetics (ONS, 2006b). Outlining the recommended competencies for each level is only the beginning step in ensuring that comprehensive care includes the translation of basic genetic and genomic research discoveries into appropriate and effective care of all consumers. Now the work begins. Nurses can provide leadership that ensures that significant changes occur in the design of educational preparation and healthcare service delivery. Only then can clinical outcomes across the cancer continuum be enhanced, making a difference for all patients with cancer and their families.

SUMMARY

Oncology nurses find themselves in the midst of new knowledge and interventions regarding the molecular biology of cancer. The identification and sequencing of human genes that play roles in the initiation, promotion, and progression of malignancies are having a major impact on diagnosis for individuals at risk for inheriting mutated cancer-susceptibility genes as well as all people with cancer. As more is learned about how these genes are expressed and how their protein products function, genetic and genomic knowledge will continue to be applied in cancer care across the entire healthcare continuum. Oncology nurses in particular need to recognize a new paradigm, one in which genetics and genomics move from a tangential concept to a central underpinning of nursing practice (Calzone et al., 2006; Feetham et al., 2005). Furthermore, oncology nurses in clinical practice and in education need to be proactive in articulating the necessity to incorporate genetics and genomics into undergraduate and graduate courses, with the ultimate goal of enhancing oncology nursing practice and establishing oncology nurses as leaders in the area of cancer genetics and genomics.

Many nurses question the introduction of genetic and genomic information: "Why do I need to know about genetics? I'm an *oncology* nurse." Patient care is the main justification for oncology nurses to become knowledgeable about genetics and genomics. Genetic and genomic–based oncology knowledge and tools promise the ability to individually treat each person most effectively, resulting in improved healthcare outcomes. Expertise in genetics and genomics definitely is needed to facilitate the clinical application of genomic knowledge by all healthcare disciplines. Only with training and an appreciation of the clinical importance of moving the benefits of genomic discoveries into patient care can the healthcare system infrastructure be redesigned to efficiently integrate genetics and genomics into all services provided resulting in improved health (Guttmacher, Porteous, & McInerney, 2007).

Opportunities and challenges will be encountered by clinicians, organizations, and patients as professionals move forward in realizing the potential benefits of genomics in clinical practice. Scheuner, Sieverding, and Shekelle (2008) synthesized available information on attempts to integrate genetic and genomic knowledge of common chronic conditions into clinical practice and identified many gaps that will need to be addressed. Oncology nurses have an opportunity to be part of the solution to these emerging issues.

If not proactive in designing care models that use knowledgeable nurses in the delivery of genomic services for cancer care, consumers may take the decision into their own hands. Already, direct consumer advertising about genetic testing is appearing (Geransar & Einsiedel, 2008). Healthcare providers must gain sufficient expertise to answer consumers' questions, which are driven by Internet and media information (Taylor, Alman, & Manchester, 2001). For healthcare providers, learning and understanding new tests, new terminology, and new ways of doing business will be constant. Recognition of factors influencing client decisions about preventive care and health promotion must be the focus of ongoing research. Through better understanding of the psychological and physical consequences of genetic information, factors influencing client decisions can be addressed proactively (Broadstock, Michie, & Marteau, 2000).

Ongoing advances in the understanding of genetic and genomic changes that predict cancer risk, treatment response, and prognosis continue to expand options in cancer care. Simultaneously, these scientific advances create new concerns as new genetic and genomic technology revolutionizes human capabilities. New capabilities and technologies, such as genetic targeted therapy, genetic engineering, gene therapy, cloning, and DNA chips, are transforming health care. Oncology nurses who have a clear understanding of the value of genetic and genomic technologies can take the lead in introducing potential lifesaving changes across the cancer continuum. These nurse leaders will be able to head off problems and expand ethical discussion regarding genetics and genomics in oncology practice.

REFERENCES

Broadstock, M., Michie, S., & Marteau, T. (2000). Psychological consequences of predictive genetic testing: A systematic review. *European Journal of Human Genetics, 8*(10), 731–738.

Calzone, K.A., Jenkins, J., & Masny, A. (2002). Core competencies in cancer genetics for advanced practice oncology nurses. *Oncology Nursing Forum, 29*(9), 1327–1333.

Calzone, K.A., Lea, D.H., & Masny, A. (2006). Non-Hodgkin's lymphoma as an exemplar of the effects of genetics and genomics. *Journal of Nursing Scholarship, 38*(4), 335–343.

Calzone, K.A., & Masny, A. (2004). Genetics and the evolving role of the oncology nurse. *Seminars in Oncology Nursing, 20*(3), 178–185.

Centers for Disease Control and Prevention. (2001). *Genomic translation: Genomic workforce competencies, 2001.* Retrieved October 28, 2009, from http://www.cdc.gov/genomics/training/competencies/comps.htm

Cohen, F. (1979). Genetic knowledge possessed by American nurses and nursing students. *Journal of Advanced Nursing, 4*(5), 493–501.

Consensus Panel on Genetic/Genomic Nursing Competencies. (2009). *Essentials of genetic and genomic nursing: Competencies, curricula guidelines, and outcome indicators* (2nd ed.). Silver Spring, MD: American Nurses Association.

Feetham, S., Thomson, E.J., & Hinshaw, A.S. (2005). Genomics for health and society: A framework for nursing leadership. *Journal of Nursing Scholarship, 37*(2), 102–110.

Geransar, R., & Einsiedel, E. (2008). Evaluating online direct-to-consumer marketing of genetic tests: Informed choices or buyer beware? *Genetic Testing, 12*(1), 13–24.

Guttmacher, A.E., Porteous, M.E., & McInerney, J.D. (2007). Educating health-care professionals about genetics and genomics. *Nature Reviews Genetics, 8*(2), 151–157.

Harvey, E.K., Fogel, C.E., Peyrot, M., Christensen, K.D., Terry, S.F., & McInerney, J.D. (2007). Providers' knowledge of genetics: A survey of 5,915 individuals and families with genetic conditions. *Genetics in Medicine, 9*(5), 259–267.

Health Resources Services Administration. (2007). *The registered nurse population: Findings from the March 2004 National Sample Survey of Registered Nurses.* Bethesda, MD: U.S. Department of Health and Human Services. Retrieved May 12, 2008, from ftp://ftp.hrsa.gov/bhpr/workforce/0306rnss.pdf

Hetteberg, C.G., Prows, C.A., Deets, C., Monsen, R.B., & Kenner, C.A. (1999). Survey of genetics content in basic nursing preparatory programs in the United States. *Nursing Outlook, 47*(4), 168–180.

International Society of Nurses in Genetics. (2007). *Genetics/genomics nursing: Scope and standards of practice.* Silver Spring, MD: American Nurses Association.

Jenkins, J., & Calzone, K.A. (2007). Establishing the essential nursing competencies for genetics and genomics. *Journal of Nursing Scholarship, 39*(1), 10–16.

Jenkins, J., Grady, P., & Collins, F.S. (2005). Nurses and the genomic revolution. *Journal of Nursing Scholarship, 37*(2), 98–101.

Lynch, M.P., Cope, D.G., & Murphy-Ende, K. (2001). Advanced practice issues: Results of the ONS Advanced Practice Nursing survey. *Oncology Nursing Forum, 28*(10), 1521–1530.

Maradiegue, A., Edwards, Q.T., Seibert, D., Macri, C., & Sitzer, L. (2005). Knowledge, perceptions, and attitudes of advanced practice nursing students regarding medical genetics. *Journal of the American Academy of Nurse Practitioners, 17*(11), 472–479.

Monsen, R. (1984). Genetics in basic nursing program curricula: A national survey. *Maternal-Child Nursing Journal, 13*(3), 177–185.

National Coalition for Health Professional Education in Genetics. (2000). *Core competencies in genetics essential for all health-care professionals.* Retrieved April 4, 2008, from http://www.nchpeg.org

National Coalition for Health Professional Education in Genetics. (2007). *Core competencies in genetics for health professionals* (3rd ed.). Retrieved April 4, 2008, from http://www.nchpeg.org/core/Core_Comps_English_2007.pdf

Oncology Nursing Society. (2006a). *Cancer predisposition genetic testing and risk assessment counseling* [Position statement]. Retrieved April 4, 2008, from http://www.ons.org/Publications/Positions/Predisposition

Oncology Nursing Society. (2006b). *The role of the oncology nurse in cancer genetic counseling* [Position statement]. Retrieved April 4, 2008, from http://www.ons.org/Publications/Positions/GeneticCounseling

Pestka, E.L., & Brown, J.K. (2004). Genomics education for nurses in practice. *Journal for Nurses in Staff Development, 20*(3), 145–149.

Peterson, S.K., Rieger, P.T., Marani, S.K., deMoor, C., & Gritz, E.R. (2001). Oncology nurses' knowledge, practice, and educational needs regarding cancer genetics. *American Journal of Medical Genetics, 98*(1), 3–12.

Prows, C., Calzone, K., & Jenkins, J. (2006, September). *Genetics content in nursing curriculum.* Paper presented at the National Coalition for Health Professional Education in Genetics, Bethesda, MD.

Prows, C.A., Glass, M., Nicol, M.J., Skirton, H., & Williams, J. (2005). Genomics in nursing education. *Journal of Nursing Scholarship, 37*(3), 196–202.

Scanlon, C., & Fibison, W. (1995). *Managing genetic information: Implications for nursing education.* Washington, DC: American Nurses Association.

Scheuner, M.T., Sieverding, P., & Shekelle, P.G. (2008). Delivery of genomic medicine for common chronic adult diseases: A systematic review. *JAMA, 299*(11), 1320–1334.

Seibert, D., Edwards, Q., & Maradiegue, A. (2007). Integrating genetics into advanced practice nursing curriculum: Strategies for success. *Community Genetics, 10*(1), 45–51.

Taylor, M., Alman, A., & Manchester, D. (2001). Use of the Internet by patients and their families to obtain genetics-related information. *Mayo Clinical Proceedings, 76*(8), 772–776.

Trinidad, S., Fryer-Edwards, K., Crest, A., Kyler, P., Lloyd-Puryear, M., & Burke, W. (2008). Educational needs in genetic medicine: Primary care perspectives. *Community Genetics, 11*(3), 160–165.

CHAPTER 14

Ensuring Competence: Nursing Credentialing in Cancer Genetics

Rita Black Monsen, DSN, MPH, RN, FAAN

Professional Responsibilities Domain:
- Examine competency of practice on a regular basis, indentifying areas of strength as well as areas in which professional development related to genetics and genomics would be beneficial (Consensus Panel on Genetic/Genomic Nursing Competencies, 2009)

INTRODUCTION

Nurses, particularly oncology nurses, must possess a basic knowledge of genetics and genomics. In 2004, two nurses from the National Institutes of Health were instrumental in developing a consensus process among representative nursing leaders in practice, education, and research for essential competencies for all nurses in genetics and genomics (Jenkins & Calzone, 2007). This effort resulted in competencies to guide the education of the nation's nursing workforce to implement genetic and genomic information into clinical practice and has been endorsed by nearly 50 nursing and related organizations. Indeed, Jenkins and Calzone noted, "When synthesizing the emerging evidence, genetics and genomics redefines traditional health and illness approaches, and genomics has become the central science for all health professionals in the 21st century" (p. 10).

However, the majority of nurses at all levels of educational preparation have had minimal instruction in genetics and genomics. Surveys in the 1990s showed that a majority of practicing nurses were not knowledgeable (Scanlon & Fibison, 1995) and that nursing education offered only a modicum of instruction in genetics and genomics (Hetteberg, Prows, Deets, Monsen, & Kenner, 1999). A decade later, less than one-third of nursing program curricula included a genetics or genomic thread (Edwards, Maradiegue, Seibert, Macri, & Sitzer, 2006; Prows, Calzone, & Jenkins, 2006).

A survey among Oncology Nursing Society (ONS) members conducted in the late 1990s found that nurses in cancer care felt they needed to improve their knowledge of genetics, and although half had received patient questions about cancer genetics, only slightly more than one-third knew of referral resources, and 26% actually had made referrals for assistance (Peterson, Rieger, Marani, deMoor, & Gritz, 2001). Although educators have made strong efforts toward the incorporation of genetics and genomics into nursing curricula, nurses still are limited in their realization that this area of science is important for their knowledge base (Pfeil & Luo, 2005).

Across the nation, nurses are taking advantage of continuing education venues to increase genetics and genomics knowledge that can be applied in practice. Online courses and print media have proliferated in genetics content, particularly in the area of cancer genetics. On the national level, ONS has been instrumental in providing short courses and presentations on specific topics in genetics and genomics to advance the knowledge bases of nurses in clinical oncology. (Resources for courses, online programs, and printed materials are available at the ONS Web site, www.ons.org.) A number of other organizations and journals in nursing have turned their attention to providing instructional programming and materials for nurses to build their knowledge of genetics and better equip themselves to respond to patients and families with genetic concerns. For online links, visit the National Coalition for Health Professional Education in Genetics Web site at www.nchpeg.org.

In a position statement on the role of the oncology nurse in cancer genetic counseling, ONS (2006b) stated that oncology nurses possess the skills to and are well suited to assume expanded roles in cancer genetics and genetic counseling. The position specifies that appropriate education and experience are prerequisites to providing comprehensive care in the area of cancer genetics and meeting the needs of the increased number of individuals requiring cancer genetic risk counseling. How are nurses motivated to learn something that basic training did not emphasize, is not perceived to be relevant to current practice, and is scientifically challenging? Because most nurses have not had formal training in human genetics, how can a nurse practicing at the advanced level in cancer genetics demonstrate competence in the field of genetics? How can the public and other professionals feel confident in oncology nurses' knowledge and expertise in this emerging field?

One method of ensuring specialty knowledge is through credentialing. This chapter will explore issues related to the credentialing of oncology nurses and nurses in genetics. The discussion will be limited to licensure and certification. Methods of ensuring competence will be summarized briefly, and the chapter will end with strategic suggestions for the future.

THE SIGNIFICANCE OF CREDENTIALING TO CLINICAL PRACTICE

Credentialing is the process whereby an authorized body affirms that an individual warrants credit or confidence (Merriam-Webster, 2009b). *Licensure,* one form of credentialing, is the process of granting authority to act; and in the context of nursing practice, it is the legal permission to perform the duties of the professional nurse in a particular jurisdiction. Licensure at the registered and practical nurse levels occurs after achievement of required preparation (approved nursing education program) and successful performance on the required licensure examination. Advanced practice nursing is licensed by the individual states, and many state boards require a minimum of a master's degree in nursing with certification in a specific area of specialty clinical practice. The state boards of nursing regulate nursing practice in the individual states according to boundaries or scope of practice.

The U.S. National Council of State Boards of Nursing (NCSBN, 2006) is a nonprofit organization composed of the state boards of nursing in the 50 states, American Samoa, Guam, the Northern Mariana Islands, and the Virgin Islands. The NCSBN mission is protection of the public, and it pursues this mission by ensuring safety of nursing practice. NCSBN conducts meticulous surveys and job analyses of the practice of registered and practical nursing to prepare two of its major products, the NCLEX-RN and NCLEX-PN licensure examinations.

Another form of credentialing is *certification*, which is the process whereby an authority attests to the truth of a statement or to the fact that a person or group meets a standard (Merriam-Webster, 2009a). In nursing, certification occurs after achievement of licensure, completion of the required education and clinical practice, and demonstration of competence in a given clinical area or specialty. As in nursing education, organizations that provide certification are governed by professional peers and seek accreditation by the appropriate body to demonstrate that their credential is conducted with integrity according to national educational and professional standards. Certifying bodies also seek respect by health professional organizations and consumer groups nationwide. The American Board of Nursing Specialties (ABNS) aims to set and maintain standards of professional specialty nursing certification and to increase consumers' awareness of the meaning and value of specialty nursing certification. The National Commission for Certifying Agencies (NCCA) is part of the National Organization for Competency Assurance (NOCA) and accredits certifying agencies in several industries to ensure the "health, welfare, and safety of the public" (NOCA, n.d.). The Oncology Nursing Certification Corporation (ONCC), which provides certification for nurses in clinical oncology, is accredited by NCCA and ABNS. The Genetic Nursing Credentialing Commission (GNCC) currently is cooperating with the American Nurses Credentialing Commission (also accredited by NCCA and ABNS) for further development of its certifications (see section on certification of nurses in genetics later in this chapter).

Nursing certification assures employers, payers, and the public that an individual has mastered a body of knowledge in a particular specialty. The principal advantage of certification is that it provides an additional measure of professional qualifications beyond licensure. Nursing certification validates that the nurse meets high standards of care by measuring the competencies expected in a specialized practice area. Nurses usually seek certification to advance their careers, achieve professional recognition, and gain personal satisfaction. Certification is a tangible acknowledgment of professional achievement in nursing.

Since 1997, the NCSBN has cooperated with the American Nurses Association; representatives of nursing specialty organizations, education, and certification; and the two nursing education accreditation agencies to develop a consensus model for advanced practice registered nurse (APRN) licensure and regulation (NCSBN, 2008). This model is being considered for adoption at the national level now and, if supported, will later be considered by the individual state boards for implementation. The model delineates APRN practice into four roles: certified nurse practitioner, clinical nurse specialist, certified nurse-midwife, and certified nurse anesthetist. The four roles are to be prepared and certified at the master's level for six population foci: family, adult-gerontology, neonatal, pediatrics, women's health/gender-related, and psychiatric/mental health. According to the model, APRNs initially must be certified in one of these four roles, but subsequently can seek specialty certification in an area such as oncology. The model prescribes that all certifications to be recognized for APRN licensure are to be granted through organizations that are accredited by the NCCA and ABNS. This is an important effort to unify the various states with regard to the licensure and regulation of APRNs, largely for assurance of competence and equal standards of nursing care, as well as to address the issues associated with mobility of nurses and interstate and national telehealth resources now proliferating.

Today, consumers can make informed choices about their caregivers and medical facilities (an example is the online service, www.angieslist.com, which provides ratings for physicians and hospitals in the United States). A common marketing strategy for many healthcare provider organizations, including insurance companies and hospitals, is to advertise the qualifications, including certifications, of providers in the various areas of services available. Nurses can be confident that the standards for licensure and certification are designed to ensure public safety and promote high-quality nursing care in all of the healthcare delivery settings in the nation. Nurses stand as colleagues with other providers and advocates for patients and families when they achieve such licensure and certifications that attest to their professional knowledge and abilities.

ESTABLISHMENT OF COMPETENCE

Competence is a central hallmark of a professional nurse. According to a Texas survey of nursing leaders, it consists of one's ability to "think in action, have clarity in decision making, and retrieve information throughout the career trajectory" (Alien et al., 2008, p. 81). Nurses who are certified in a specific area are expected to be knowledgeable about the assessment and diagnosis of problems, apply evidence-based interventions, evaluate their performance, and make appropriate changes in their care. They are receptive to acquiring new information and synthesizing it for the improvement of the health and well-being of the patients and families with whom they practice. Alien et al. noted that professional nurses practice with self-reflection. They are self-confident in collaboration with other health professionals and resources in the practice environment.

All measurements of competence must be psychometrically sound (see Table 14-1). This means that they are valid (i.e., they are a true test or demonstration of the content or behavior they intend to measure) and reliable (i.e., they yield consistent results when used on more than one occasion and among different individuals and groups). In the case of professional competence, they must conform to legal mandates and be legally defensible. Although most testing for competence is based upon examination and observation, a portfolio of evidence submitted by the candidate is recognized by the GNCC (see the section that follows). In the future, new computer technologies are expected to expand simulation testing and open virtual reality applications in health professional education and perhaps licensure and certification.

Measuring continuing competence has been a greater challenge for the various organizations that provide certification. For many forms of certification, continuing education and clinical practice requirements have been used to recognize continuing competence, but unless testing or independent validation of the nurse's performance occurs, the nurse's progress in his or her abilities is not guaranteed. For this reason, several certification organizations, including ONCC, recommend additional achievements such as publications, preceptorships, and volunteer service in a healthcare organization (see the ONCC Web site, www.oncc.org/renewal/oncpro.shtml). In addition, certain categories of nurses who wish to be recerti-

TABLE 14-1 Measurement of Competence

Attribute	Evidence
Knowledge	Written or oral examination, paper or presentation of specific content, computer-based simulation testing
Skill	Observed demonstration, self-report
Attitudes	Observed behavior, self-report of examples of behavior and decision making

fied by ONCC and who do not have the required appropriate education within the required time frame may retake a specific certification examination in addition to completing academic courses and continuing education programs.

CERTIFICATION OF NURSES IN ONCOLOGY

More than 28,800 nurses in oncology are certified through ONCC, one of the most important certification agencies in the United States (ONCC, n.d.). Formed in 1984, ONCC is allied closely with ONS and the Association of Pediatric Hematology/Oncology Nurses. As the trends of an aging public continue, the increasing incidence and prevalence of cancer in society will impel the workforce to prepare and maintain a nursing workforce that is knowledgeable and competent to provide care in a variety of settings. ONCC offers seven certifications: the OCN® (Oncology Certified Nurse), the CPON® (Certified Pediatric Oncology Nurse—renewal only), the CPHON® (Certified Pediatric Hematology/Oncology Nurse), the CBCN® (Certified Breast Care Nurse), the AOCN® (Advanced Oncology Certified Nurse—renewal only), the AOCNP® (Advanced Oncology Certified Nurse Practitioner), and the AOCNS® (Advanced Oncology Certified Clinical Nurse Specialist) (as of 2010). All of these certifications require that candidates be knowledgeable about genetics and genomics as applied in clinical oncology. The CBCN certification will have some content focused on the genetics of breast cancer risk assessment. All of the certifications are based upon role delineation and cover the range of cancer care, including lifestyle and related risk-management measures, detection and diagnostic procedures, therapies and approaches to care, survivor care, and care at the end of life. Nurses with basic-level certifications are expected to be knowledgeable about direct care of patients and families, whereas those in advanced practice roles will have the ability to participate in planning and delivery of diagnoses and therapies, interpretation of findings, care coordination, and advanced evaluation of care effectiveness. All certified nurses are expected to participate in the education of other professionals as well as the public in community venues, including presentation of papers, publication, and preparation of print and online media. ONCC provides many opportunities for the successful completion of its certifications (see www.oncc.org) including test blueprints and resources for study and continuing education. ONS advocates certification for assuring the public that certified nurses in oncology are fully qualified to deliver care and that employers, patients, and families should be aware of the qualifications and strengths of those who are practicing in this field (ONS, 2006a).

CERTIFICATION OF NURSES IN GENETICS

Specialty nurses in genetics focus on patients and families who have or are at risk for having a disease associated with one or more genetic mutations. They typically practice in collaboration with other providers such as physicians, genetic and genomic scientists, genetic counselors, social workers, therapists, nutritionists, and a variety of other allied health personnel. Many are involved in tertiary care settings, public health agencies, academic health sciences centers, and biotechnology companies.

Nurses in this specialty participate in the assessment and genetic diagnosis of the presence of or risk for gene-based illness. They perform genetic-based assessments and provide education, counseling, coordination of care with other healthcare resources in communities, and follow-up of care. Nurses with a baccalaureate degree in nursing may qualify for the GCN (Genetics Clinical Nurse) credential. Advanced practice nurses in genetics (APNG credential) must complete a master's degree in nursing, education in genetics and genomics, and specified clinical practice. They are qualified to interpret diagnostic findings including the family pedigree (an as-accurate-as-possible graphic depiction of at least three generations of a kindred), to project the presence of risk for inheritance of a genetic condition, and to provide genetic counseling (detailed explanation of the disease and its implications for inheritance in a family or kindred). They are expected to provide education in genetics to patients, families, communities, and other health professionals as well as participate in scholarly work, including research and publication.

The International Society of Nurses in Genetics has offered credentialing for the APNG since 2001 through its associated organization, GNCC (www.geneticnurse.org). This credentialing process involves the approval of a portfolio that documents educational requirements and clinical practice experiences. Passing an examination is not part of the GNCC credential. Rather, the nurse must submit the required documents (see Figure 14-1), including a clinical log and four case studies, which demonstrate competency in genetics and genomics. The GNCC portfolio is based upon *Genetics/Genomic Nursing: Scope and Standards of Practice*, published by the American Nurses Association and the International Society of Nurses in Genetics. GNCC and ANCC collaborate in the further development of this credential, a model for recognizing the knowledge, skills, and attitudes of clinicians in specialized nursing practice. This collaboration continues with the goal of making the credentialing process through the portfolio mechanism as credible, standardized, and sound as possible.

FIGURE 14-1 REQUIREMENTS FOR THE ADVANCED PRACTICE NURSE IN GENETICS CREDENTIAL PORTFOLIO

- Application cover form with applicant information, signature, and notary public signature and seal
- Proof of registered nurse license in good standing
- Nonrefundable money order or cashier's check for application fee made out to GNCC, INC.
- Curriculum vitae
- Letter of verification from employer, supervisor, or professional colleague; verifies that applicant has provided care to clients named in Log and/or Case Studies—must be sealed in envelope with signature on flap
- Professional performance verification and evaluation—use GNCC form —must be sealed in envelope with signature on flap
- Three peer reviews—must be sealed in envelope with signature on flap
- Official transcripts in sealed envelopes for all applicable undergraduate and graduate education programs (BSN required; Master's in Nursing or related field required)
- Continuing education certificates and/or proof of attendance at applicable continuing education programs (minimum of 50 contact hours in the past 5 years)
- 50-case log with verification signature of supervisor or professional colleague for log required (use log form); cases within five years of application
- 4 case studies (taken from cases in case log) illustrating clinical practice that reflects the International Society of Nurses in Genetics, Inc. standards of care
- Appendices: Education and other sections (teaching materials, research summaries, abstracts, publications, awards, recognitions, etc.)

Note. From *Genetics Nursing Portfolios: A New Model for Credentialing* (pp. 122–124), by R.B. Monsen (Ed.), 2005, Silver Spring, MD: American Nurses Association and International Society of Nurses in Genetics. Copyright 2005 by American Nurses Association. All rights reserved. Adapted with permission.

GNCC uses the portfolio approach rather than testing because it requires nurses to provide concrete evidence of competence (including case logs and narrative case studies) that conform to the scope and standards of specialized genetics nursing. This approach has demonstrated very strong overall statistical accuracy by its use of neural net technology to examine the evaluation process in scoring portfolio submissions (Holmes, McAlpine, & Russell, 2005). Neural net technology is a form of computer-based mathematical calculation that considers multiple sources of data, such as scores on portfolio components from a number of evaluators, and analyzes their patterns and relationships. It may be used to confirm the reliability of patterns of data rendered over time, such as the scores from several teams of portfolio evaluators (NeuroDimension, Inc., n.d.). The GNCC portfolio acknowledges the competence of the basic and the advanced practice nurse in genetics, but it is not specific to cancer genetics. A large number of nurses in cancer risk assessment have earned the GNCC credential by developing a portfolio related to clinical cancer genetics education and experience.

FUTURE DIRECTIONS IN LICENSURE AND CERTIFICATION

Genetics and genomics information will assume greater importance as healthcare delivery increases its use of gene-based technologies, yet state boards of nursing and nursing accreditation agencies have only begun to direct faculties in basic and graduate education in nursing to include this topic area in curricula. Licensure and certification examinations will have more content in genetics and genomics as job analyses demonstrate that this knowledge is used in the workplace. As healthcare delivery continues to become increasingly specialized, certification of nurses in highly specialized settings will require an appropriate measurement of competence. Technologies in nursing and education will make individualized assessment of competence possible, yet our nation's leaders recognize that a basic threshold for high-quality care must be met in every part of the country. Efforts by the leading nursing organizations and NCSBN to establish a national standard for licensure at the basic and advanced levels are becoming imperative as the public demands and deserves professional practice competence. Patients and the public can feel confident that nurses in oncology will be required and will desire to demonstrate their understanding of the impact of genetics and genomics as central in the risk reduction, appearance, and cure of cancer in the future.

SUMMARY

Discoveries in genetics and genomics are rapidly changing the face of healthcare delivery, and nurses in nearly every area of clinical specialty, especially in oncology, are witnessing the incorporation of gene-based diagnostics and therapeutics in their everyday practices. Licensure and certification are two forms of credentialing that validate the competency of the nurse to practice in today's healthcare settings. Nurses are increasingly realizing that although licensure authorizes professional practice, certification is the mark of distinction in providing high-quality nursing care to the public. Knowledge of genetics and genomics is essential for today's professional nurses both at the basic and advanced practice levels.

Certification from ONCC and GNCC offer opportunities for nurses in specialized oncology and genetic settings to demonstrate their knowledge, skills, and abilities to provide care that meets professional standards of practice.

The author would like to thank Faith Fields, MSN, RN, president of the National Council of State Boards of Nursing and executive director of the Arkansas State Board of Nursing, and her associate, Jackie Murphree, EdD, MNSc, RN, director of advanced practice nursing at the Arkansas State Board of Nursing, for their contribution to this manuscript.

REFERENCES

Alien, P., Lauchner, K., Bridges, R.A., Francis-Johnson, P., McBride, S.G., & Olivarez, A., Jr. (2008). Evaluating continuing competency: A challenge for nursing. *Journal of Continuing Education in Nursing, 39*(2), 81–85.

Consensus Panel on Genetic/Genomic Nursing Competencies. (2009). *Essentials of genetic and genomic nursing: Competencies, curricula guidelines, and outcome indicators* (2nd ed.). Silver Spring, MD: American Nurses Association.

Edwards, T., Maradiegue, A., Seibert, D., Macri, C., & Sitzer, L. (2006). Faculty members' perceptions of medical genetics and its integration into nurse practitioner curricula. *Journal of Nursing Education, 45*(3), 124–130.

Hetteberg, C.G., Prows, C.A., Deets, C., Monsen, R.B., & Kenner, C.A. (1999). Survey of genetics content in basic nursing preparatory programs in the United States. *Nursing Outlook, 47*(4), 168–180.

Holmes, D., McAlpine, R., & Russell, J. (2005). Use of neural net technology to quantify portfolio evaluations. In R.B. Monsen (Ed.), *Genetics nursing portfolios: A new model for credentialing* (pp. 79–90). Silver Spring, MD: American Nurses Association.

Jenkins, J., & Calzone, K. (2007). Establishing the essential nursing competencies for genetics and genomics. *Journal of Nursing Scholarship, 39*(1), 10–16.

Merriam-Webster. (2009a). *Certification.* Retrieved October 29, 2009, from http://www.merriam-webster.com/dictionary/certification

Merriam-Webster. (2009b). *Credential.* Retrieved October 29, 2009, from http://www.merriam-webster.com/dictionary/credential

National Council of State Boards of Nursing. (2006). *Annual report.* Retrieved July 26, 2008, from https://www.ncsbn.org/NCSBN_AnnualReport2006.pdf

National Council of State Boards of Nursing. (2008). *Consensus model for APRN regulation: Licensure, accreditation, certification, and education.* Retrieved July 28, 2008, from https://www.ncsbn.org/Joint_Dialogue_Report_6_18_08.pdf

National Organization for Competency Assurance. (n.d.). *NCCA accreditation.* Retrieved December 21, 2009, from http://www.noca.org/Resources/NOCAAccreditation/tabid/82/Default.aspx

NeuroDimension, Inc. (n.d.). *NeuroSolutions: What is a neural network?* Retrieved December 17, 2009, from http://www.nd.com/neurosolutions/products/ns/whatisNN.html

Oncology Nursing Certification Corporation. (n.d.). *About ONCC.* Retrieved January 19, 2010, from http://www.oncc.org/about

Oncology Nursing Society. (2006a). *Oncology certification for nurses.* Retrieved October 29, 2009, from http://www.ons.org/Publications/Positions/Certification

Oncology Nursing Society. (2006b). *Oncology Nursing Society position on the role of the nurse in cancer genetic counseling.* Retrieved July 11, 2008, from http://www.ons.org/Publications/Positions/GeneticCounseling

Peterson, S.K., Rieger, P.T., Marani, S.K., deMoor, C., & Gritz, E.R. (2001). Oncology nurses' knowledge, practice, and educational needs regarding cancer genetics. *American Journal of Medical Genetics, 98*(1), 3–12.

Pfeil, M., & Luo, C.M. (2005). Genetics knowledge for nurses: Necessity or luxury? *British Journal of Nursing, 14*(21), 1128–1131.

Prows, C., Calzone, K., & Jenkins, J. (2006, February). *Genetics content in the nursing curriculum.* Paper presented at the 9th annual meeting of the National Coalition for Professional Education in Genetics/Genetics on the Web, Bethesda, MD.

Scanlon, C., & Fibison, W. (1995). *Managing genetic information: Implications for nursing education.* Washington, DC: American Nurses Association.

CHAPTER 15

Research: Making a Difference in Practice

Yvette P. Conley, PhD

Professional Practice Domain:
Provision of Education, Care, and Support
- Evaluate impact and effectiveness of genetic and genomic technology, information, interventions, and treatments on clients' outcome

(Consensus Panel on Genetic/Genomic Nursing Competencies, 2009)

INTRODUCTION

Genetic and genomic–based research has had an enormous impact on the field of oncology, from understanding the etiology of cancer to informing practice. The goal of this chapter is not to reiterate the research findings that have informed current practice; those are covered comprehensively throughout the other chapters of this book. The objectives of this chapter are to (a) immerse the reader into the current research environment with the hope that the reader will gain perspective on where the science is from a translational research point of view, (b) introduce the reader to an example of cutting-edge technology that is not in clinical use but has great potential for translation to patients in the future, (c) introduce the reader to selected research initiatives that are under way and are likely to expand the understanding of cancer genomics, and (d) provide the reader with resources that will allow the individual to stay current with research relevant to oncology genomics.

TRANSLATIONAL RESEARCH: NECESSARY TO MAKE A DIFFERENCE IN PRACTICE

The National Cancer Institute (NCI) Translational Research Working Group (TRWG) of the National Cancer Advisory Board described *translational research*: "translational research transforms scientific discoveries arising from laboratory, clinical, or population studies into clinical applications to reduce cancer incidence, morbidity, and mortality" (TRWG, 2007, p. 99). Key to this description is the clinical application. Most research that is funded and conducted never reaches the point of affecting the patient (Contopoulos-Ioannidis, Ntzani, & Ioannidis, 2003; Khoury et al., 2007). However, considerable interest has mounted in moving research into the clinical and public health arenas. A key initiative to advance clinical research is the National Institutes of Health (NIH) Roadmap. The NIH Roadmap grew out of the knowledge that as the understanding of the basic science of disease grows, scientists are learning that many diseases are linked through common biologic pathways and unifying principles and, therefore, potentially could be linked through therapeutic approaches (Zerhouni, 2003). The NIH Roadmap attempts to integrate NIH resources and expertise to accelerate and streamline progress in clinical research and the clinical application of research findings (Zerhouni, 2003). It is exciting to note that the successes associated with the sequencing of the human genome and the advancement of technologies that allow the characterization of the molecular aspects of disease are at the forefront of much of the progress in basic science, as well as represent much potential for advancing clinical science (Zerhouni, 2005).

Translational research from a genomic point of view has been described by Khoury et al. (2007) using phases to organize the continuum of translational research leading to the development of evidence-based practice and the impact on the public's health. Organization using phases is useful when trying to put the continuum of translational genomic research into perspective. Four phases are included in this continuum (see Figure 15-1). The type 1 phase of research (T1) encompasses the research that occurs after a gene is discovered to the point where that gene is related to disease and health application. This would include research such as genetic association studies and test evaluations, as well as phase I and phase II clinical trials (Khoury et al.; Westfall, Mold, & Fagnan, 2007).

The vast majority of genetic and genomic research publications are related to T1 research or research leading to gene discovery and characterization that is necessary prior to T1 research. To facilitate extraction of evidence from the enormous amount of publi-

FIGURE 15-1 THE CONTINUUM OF TRANSLATION RESEARCH IN GENOMIC MEDICINE

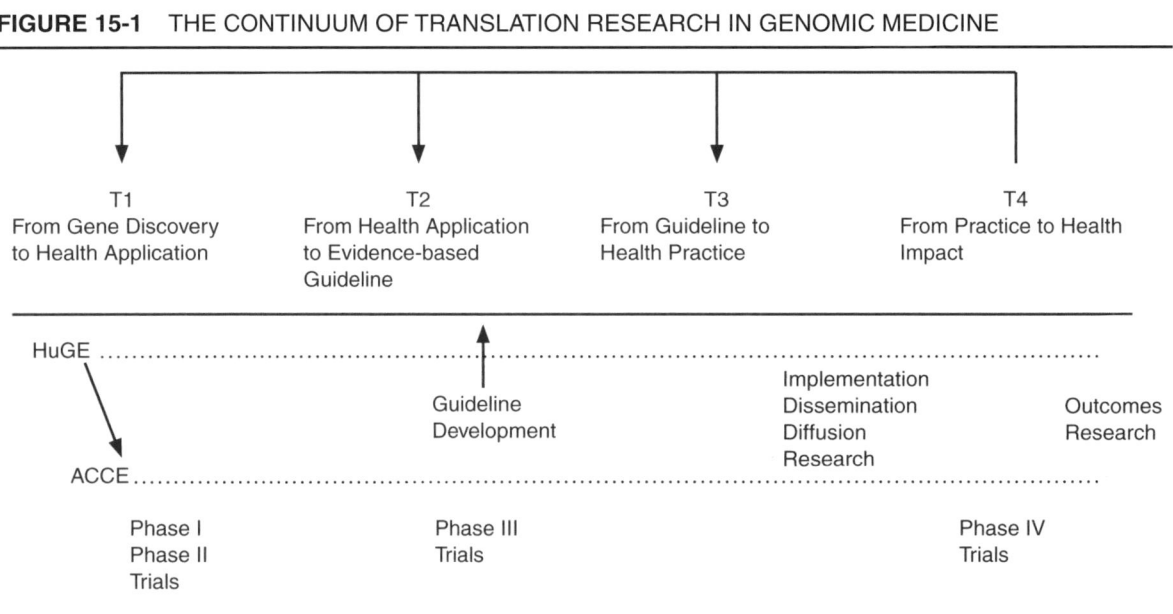

ACCE—analytic validity; clinical validity; clinical utility; ethical, legal, and social issues; HuGE—human genome epidemiology

Note. From "The Continuum of Translation Research in Genomic Medicine: How Can We Accelerate the Appropriate Integration of Human Genome Discoveries Into Health Care and Disease Prevention?" by M.J. Khoury, M. Gwinn, P.W. Yoon, N. Dowling, C.A. Moore, and L. Bradley, 2007, *Genetics in Medicine, 9*(10), p. 667. Copyright 2007 by American College of Medical Genetics. Reprinted with permission.

cations related to research in genomics, the Human Genome Epidemiology (HuGE) published literature database was developed. The criteria for inclusion of articles in this database include being published since October 2000, reporting a study conducted in humans, inclusion of genotype information, and population-based analysis (Lin et al., 2006). Key categories within this database are HuGE review and meta-analysis articles (Yu et al., 2008). These types of articles are vital for evaluating the robustness of research findings for the purpose of moving the research forward toward translation to clinical practice. Access to the HuGE published literature database can be gained through the HuGE Navigator portal at http://hugenavigator.net.

The type 2 phase of research (T2) encompasses the research that occurs from the establishment of health application to the development of evidence-based guidelines. This would include phase III clinical trials and the development of practice guidelines for clinical use, including the development of guidelines for clinical genetic testing (Khoury et al., 2007).

The ACCE model, which stands for analytic validity, clinical validity, clinical utility, and associated ethical, legal, and social implications, is an evaluation process for genetic testing that is sponsored by the Centers for Disease Control and Prevention (see Table 15-1). ACCE is a valuable framework for moving T1 research to T2 research for genetic tests (Haddow & Palomaki, 2004). The evaluation process requires that the clinical disorder and clinical setting for the test be established. Further evaluation includes issues around sensitivity, specificity, prevalence, whether interventions are available, quality assurance, results of pilot trials,

TABLE 15-1   Information About Evaluating Genetic Testing Using the ACCE Process

Evaluation Component	Description
Analytic validity	The focus of this component is on the laboratory-based aspects of the test, and the goal is to define the ability of a test to accurately and reliably measure a genotype of interest. The sensitivity of the test is measured to determine how effectively a mutation or polymorphism is detected. The specificity of the test is measured to determine how effectively the test classifies samples without the mutation or polymorphism. Quality control and robustness of the test also is assessed.
Clinical validity	Involves establishing the ability of the test to detect or predict a phenotype. This involves assessment of the sensitivity (ability to detect the phenotype) and specificity (ability to classify those without the phenotype). Assessment within the context of the phenotype being tested is important. For example, prevalence and penetrance of the phenotype are relevant to this evaluation.
Clinical utility	Involves evaluating the risks and benefits of the test. The risks and benefits are test specific and will vary based on many factors, such as the natural history of the phenotype, how test results may affect clinical management, who is being offered the test, results of pilot studies, cost of the test and any economic benefits of testing, and what education is provided to a patient undergoing testing.
Ethical, legal, and social implications	Involves establishing and evaluating the impediments to the test and safeguards that are in place. Impediments include stigmatization, discrimination, and issues regarding family dynamics. The safeguards that are in place, for example, those involving the education of the patient and protection of confidentiality, and their effectiveness, are important to evaluating the test.

Note. Based on information from Centers for Disease Control and Prevention, 2009.

health risks associated with testing, economic issues from testing, facilities available, education and informed consent issues, monitoring effects of testing, impediments to testing, and safeguards that have been established (Haddow & Palomaki). A list of targeted questions that are used with the ACCE model to evaluate genetic testing along with additional information about the ACCE model can be found at www.cdc.gov/genomics/gtesting/ACCE/index.htm.

The type 3 phase of research (T3) encompasses research that moves the field from evidence-based guidelines to implementation into health practice. This type would include research related to dissemination and implementation of the guidelines, as well as phase IV clinical trials (Khoury et al., 2007). The type 4 phase of research (T4) takes the field from health practice to the level of the population to determine the impact on the health of the population. This type of research would require monitoring the risks and benefits to the population from the established health practices utilizing outcomes-based research. For example, continued epidemiologic and genetic research that will help characterize predisposition to genetic mutations and guide clinical interventions is sponsored by NCI (2009). Currently, research that falls into the T3 and T4 categories is rare (Khoury et al.).

MOLECULAR GENOMIC TUMOR PROFILING FOR BREAST CANCER AS AN EXAMPLE OF MOVING BASIC RESEARCH TOWARD CLINICAL UTILITY

The central dogma of genetics is that DNA is transcribed into messenger RNA (mRNA), which is then translated into protein. The intermediate step of mRNA production offers a window of opportunity to measure how active a gene is in a particular cell type or tissue in a particular situation, also called gene expression. Although a cell may have every gene represented at the DNA level, only the genes necessary at that time are expressed. Gene expression is a dynamic process, meaning that the genes that are expressed and the level of expression of those genes can change over time, depending on the needs of the cell, often in response to its environment. Investigating differences in gene expression in normal versus abnormal cells has been an approach utilized by researchers to try to understand the underlying mechanisms in an abnormal cancer cell. Characterizing the gene expression patterns in breast cancer cells has advanced the understanding of the clinical spectrum of this condition and has resulted in more informed prognoses and treatment decisions.

Three examples of gene expression–based breast cancer tests that are being used in clinical assessment are Oncotype DX® (Genomic Health, Inc.), MammaPrint™ (Agendia), and Theros H/I℠ (bioTheranostics). All of these tests rely on investigating the gene expression pattern of select genes by measuring their RNA levels. Each test focuses on a different number and different group of selected genes (Marchionni et al., 2008). Additional information about gene expression–based tumor profiling can be found in Chapter 8.

Getting to the point where gene expression–based assessment of breast cancer cells is clinically used required basic research to characterize the structure and function of genes, research to identify the genes of interest (T1 research), development of guidelines for clinical genetic testing (T2 research), and implementation of the findings into health practice (T3 research). Currently, clinical trials are attempting to prospectively validate two of these tests in specific breast cancer populations by using data generated from the test to inform treatment assignment and evaluate outcomes (T4 research) (see Figure 15-1). The

Microarray in Node-Negative Disease May Avoid Chemotherapy (MINDACT) trial is enrolling 6,000 patients with node-negative breast cancer who will have their risks assessed using MammaPrint as well as traditional risk assessments. If both assessments indicate a low risk of relapse, that patient does not receive adjuvant chemotherapy. If both assessments indicate a high risk of relapse, adjuvant chemotherapy is proposed for that patient. If discordant results are obtained (estimated to be approximately 35% of enrollees), that patient will be randomized to follow either the traditional risk assessment or the MammaPrint assessment results. A good overview of this trial is provided by Cardoso et al. (2008). Additional information and updates about MINDACT can be found at www.breastinternationalgroup.org/research/TRANSBIG/MINDACT.aspx.

The second trial is the Trial Assigning IndividuaLized Options for Treatment (Rx) (TAILORx) that is enrolling more than 10,000 estrogen receptor and/or progesterone receptor positive, node-negative, *HER2/neu*-negative patients with breast cancer. These patients will have their risks assessed using OncotypeDx. Women with a low recurrence score (less than 10) will receive hormone therapy alone. Those with intermediate recurrence scores (11–25) are randomized to hormone therapy alone or hormone therapy plus chemotherapy. Women with a high recurrence score (greater than or equal to 26) will receive adjuvant chemotherapy and hormone therapy. Paik (2007) provides a good overview of Oncotype DX and this trial, and the NCI Web site (www.cancer.gov/clinicaltrials/digestpage/TAILORx) houses a summary of the TAILORx protocol and provides updates about the project.

RNA INTERFERENCE AS AN EXAMPLE OF CUTTING-EDGE TECHNOLOGIES EXPECTED TO AFFECT PRACTICE

Imagine if the production of a disease-causing protein could be prevented. A potent therapy would be available for many disorders, including certain types of cancer that are caused by the production of an abnormal protein or the overproduction of a protein. RNA interference (RNAi) provides a means of halting protein production that occurs after mRNA is made but prior to the production of protein, resulting in gene silencing because the result is no protein production. RNAi was first characterized in animal cells in 1998 (Fire et al., 1998), and basic research related to RNAi has proliferated ever since. RNAi in mammalian cells occurs by first breaking up double-stranded RNA into shorter pieces called short-interfering RNA (siRNA). The siRNA then interacts with other proteins to form an RNA-inducing silencing complex (RISC). The RISC that is produced will have specificity for mRNA that closely resembles the complex. The RISC then interacts with mRNA that holds a close resemblance to it, and the end result is degradation of that mRNA and hence specific gene silencing (Jackson & Linsley, 2004; Tuschl, Zamore, Lehmann, Bartel, & Sharp, 1999; Zamore, Tuschl, Sharp, & Bartel, 2000). Scientists can capitalize on RNAi for research and development of potential therapeutics by targeting specific mRNAs known to be implicated in disease.

siRNA is usually 21–23 bases of RNA, which is enough RNA sequence for it to have specificity for a particular mRNA (Elbashir et al., 2001); therefore, targeted gene silencing is possible by manufacturing and introducing siRNA for a specific mRNA. A variety of genes involved in the initiation and development of cancer and metastasis could be targeted with this methodology. These include genes related to cell-cycle regulation (e.g., *Rb* and *TP53*), apoptosis (e.g., *BCL2*), cellular senescence (e.g., telomerase), oncogenesis pathways (e.g., *HER2/neu*), and angiogenesis (e.g., *VEGF*) (Pai et al., 2006).

Technologic limitations for moving forward with RNAi-based therapy are very similar to those related to gene therapy, and scientists are working actively toward removing those limitations. Mainly, issues are related to how to deliver the siRNA to the target cells, avoid nonspecific immune stimulation, prevent affecting nontarget genes, and prevent resistance to therapy brought about by changes in target sequences. These limitations as well as potential solutions are reviewed briefly by Pai et al. (2006). Takeshita and Ochiya (2006) provide a review of RNAi-based research in cancer models that addresses the potential for RNAi specifically in the field of oncology.

HIGHLIGHTS OF SELECT RESEARCH INITIATIVES

Resources, technologic advances, and sharing of information among researchers are vital to the future of cancer genomic research. Fortunately, many initiatives are in place to facilitate cancer-related genetic and genomic data acquisition as well as the sharing of this data among investigators.

The Cancer Genetic Markers of Susceptibility (CGEMS) project is coordinated through NCI and focuses on identifying common DNA variants that are associated with risk for prostate and breast cancer using a genome-wide association approach. A detailed description of genome-wide association studies can be found in Chapter 7. CGEMS has the potential to radically enhance the understanding of breast and prostate cancer because they use large, well-phenotyped, population-based studies such as the Nurses' Health Study to conduct data collection. Another very important aspect of the CGEMS project that will drastically facilitate breast and prostate cancer research is that the generated data are made publicly available to researchers to enhance their efforts. Given the scale, type of data generated, and the cohorts utilized for the CGEMS project, it is logical to anticipate that the project will significantly improve the understanding of breast and prostate cancer. To learn more about the CGEMS project, visit http://cgems.cancer.gov.

Genome-wide association studies and multidisciplinary research in epidemiology and genomics are enhanced by applying genomic technologies to existing population and clinical studies. Resources such as PhenX have been created as new population resources for the investigation of genetic and environmental contributions to complex diseases. PhenX will identify up to 20 domains of high research and public health significance and then develop and disseminate 15 standard measures for each domain to the research community. The toolkit of phenotype and exposure measures produced by PhenX will facilitate integrated design and analysis of genome-wide association studies, as well as other genomics- and epidemiology-based studies (National Human Genome Research Institute [NHGRI], 2009).

NCI has initiated the Breast and Colon Cancer Family Registries. The goals for these registries include the development of a better understanding of the genetic factors affecting cancer susceptibility and how environment and lifestyle modification can affect that susceptibility, protection of those with increased susceptibility to develop cancer, and to provide life-prolonging treatment to those found to be genetically susceptible. More information about these registries and other initiatives can be found at http://epi.grants.cancer.gov/CFR.

The Cancer Genome Anatomy Project (CGAP) is focused on characterizing gene expression profiles for the continuum of cancer from normal to preclinical to cancer cells, and to make this data available to researchers. Expression profiling, which provides data related to how actively genes are transcribed (transcriptome) or how actively proteins are generated (proteome), allows a researcher to go beyond the genome and to investigate gene activity. This is important because in cancer, some genes are overexpressed, whereas others are underexpressed. Characterizing these profiles not only could affect the understanding of the mechanisms of cancer but also could highlight therapeutic targets. Expression profiling also allows one to investigate the interaction of the genome and environment, potentially providing important clues on modifiable risks. To stay informed of the efforts of the CGAP, visit http://cgap.nci.nih.gov for information related to the databases available, bioinformatic tools, and recent publications related to the project.

The Encyclopedia of DNA Elements (ENCODE) project is a consortium supported through NHGRI with the main focus of identifying functional elements in the human genome and making this information publicly available. It is interesting to note that only a small portion of the DNA that makes up the human genome is considered functional, meaning that the DNA harbors sequence that codes for proteins, sequences utilized for gene regulation or processing, or sequences required for chromosome replication and maintenance (Pheasant & Mattick, 2007). Additionally, data support that the portion of the human genome that is considered functional, a conservative figure of approximately 5%, is underestimated, and that the figure may exceed 20% (Pheasant & Mattick). Characterizing and cataloging functional elements within the genome could provide genomic sequences important to gene regulation and chromosome stability, highlighting areas for potential therapeutic targets in oncology. Therefore, the ENCODE project may have a large impact on translational cancer research. To learn more and to stay informed of the efforts of the ENCODE project, visit www.genome.gov/10005107.

Development of biomarkers for disease detection, diagnosis, prognosis, and informed treatment selection is necessary to improve early detection and to provide safer individualized therapy options. Biomarkers are defined by the Biomarkers Definitions Working Group as "a characteristic that is objectively measured and evaluated as an indicator of normal biological processes, pathogenic processes, or pharmacologic responses to a therapeutic intervention" (Biomarkers Definitions Working Group, 2001, p. 91). Evaluations of DNA and gene products thus qualify as biomarkers. One resource that has developed through the efforts of public and private enterprise is the Biomarkers Consortium. This consortium was developed in response to the great potential for biomarkers to improve patient health and the relatively few biomarkers that qualified for clinical utility (Zerhouni, Sanders, & von Eschenbach, 2007). The Biomarkers Consortium strives to coordinate efforts that will speed up the identification and validation of biomarkers that support research and clinical practice. Although it is not a funding agency itself, one role of the Biomarkers Consortium is to facilitate the acquisition of funding from appropriate sources for projects that it deems worthy to pursue. To stay informed of the efforts of the Biomarkers Consortium, visit www.biomarkersconsortium.org.

The therapeutic response to drugs and the development of side effects are paramount issues in the treatment of patients with cancer. The variability in therapeutic response and susceptibility to side effects from drugs has a profound influence on clinical outcome; therefore, research to better understand this variability could provide opportunities to individualize the therapeutic management of patients. This is where pharmacogenetic (how genetic makeup affects individual response to medication) research is of value. The Pharmacogenetics Research Network was formed to bring multidisciplinary collaborators together in an attempt to move the science of pharmacogenomics along as well as develop a knowledge base, known as the Pharmacogenetics and Pharmacogenomics Knowledge Base or PharmGKB. This knowledge base is available to all investigators and clinicians and includes information about specific drugs, genes, and variants that have been evaluated. More information and updates about the network and knowledge base can be found at www.nigms.nih.gov/Initiatives/PGRN and www.pharmgkb.org, respectively.

The Cancer Genome Project (CGP) is supported by the Wellcome Trust through the Wellcome Trust Sanger Institute. CGP strives to interrogate the DNA sequences of cancer cells primarily to identify and catalog acquired mutations in somatic cells. The Cancer Genome Atlas, which is supported by NCI and NHGRI, has similar aspirations to catalog genomic sequences of cancer cells. By cataloging these findings, data can accumulate that lead to specific variants or mutations in specific genes associated with specific types of cancer. This is important information that is needed to move toward the development of sensitive and reliable testing for specific cancers. Theoretically, this effort will provide data on commonalities among cancers, potentially informing the development of therapies of broader effect. To stay informed of the efforts of the Cancer Genome Atlas, visit http://cancergenome.nih.gov. For more information about the CGP, visit www.sanger.ac.uk/genetics/CGP, which includes information on the project itself as well as access to the catalog of somatic mutations in cancers, genomic information for commonly used cancer cell lines, and information about copy number variations in cancer cells.

ADDITIONAL TIPS TO STAY CURRENT WITH GENOMIC RESEARCH

Keeping up with new developments in research can be a daunting task. Three resources can greatly facilitate staying current with research literature and genomics in the news and lay press. The first resource is automated updates from PubMed through the National Center for Biotechnology Information. Users can register for this free service at www.pubmed.gov and enter key words for automated literature searches. Results are sent via e-mail in a user-friendly format with clickable citations that link directly to the abstract, and in many cases to the full-text article.

The second resource is from the Office of Public Health Genomics, part of the Centers for Disease Control and Prevention. This resource provides weekly updates via e-mail that cover genomics in the news and scientific literature, as well as new HuGE publications. This is a particularly good resource to stay abreast of genomics in the popular press, which is important given that this is what patients and students are often reading. To register for this free service, visit www.cdc.gov/genomics/update/current.htm.

Third, the Evaluation of Genomic Applications in Practice and Prevention (EGAPP) is an initiative launched in 2004 to support a coordinated, systematic process for evaluating genetic tests and other genomic applications that are in transition from research to clinical and public health practice in the United States. This resource is of value to the nurse because the EGAPP working group provides evidence reports and recommendations for clinical utility, and highlights what is not yet known (e.g., the potential harms of tumor expression profiles on patient decision making). For more information, see www.egappreviews.org/default.htm.

INCORPORATING GENETICS AND GENOMICS INTO ONCOLOGY NURSING RESEARCH

This chapter points out the continuum of research that is necessary for genetic and genomic research to be translated to clinical care. Throughout this continuum, oncology nurse scientists use their expertise and perspectives to move the science forward, allowing for translation to occur at a quicker pace. Many of the issues that need to be addressed and evaluated, for example, those mentioned in reference to the ACCE evaluation process in moving genetic testing to clinical utility, are paramount issues for scientists involved in clinical oncology outcomes.

Essential to translating genomic findings to patients, families, and the general public is the need to evaluate the psychological and behavioral impact of genetic testing and the obtainment of genetic and genomic information to inform evidence-based practice. A dearth of publications addresses these issues, although the application of genetic testing and cancer risk assessment continues to grow. Nurses have contributed significantly to the field of biobehavioral research and have the capacity to continue these contributions in relation to genetic testing and the issues related to knowing the increased risks for cancer or the discovery of a gene mutation that predisposes patients to existing disease.

The initiatives mentioned in this chapter have the common characteristic of moving oncology research forward in a collaborative manner. Oncology nurse scientists are among those collaborators who assist in progression of these initiatives. They also are among those researchers who use the networking, resources, and databases made possible by these initiatives. Oncology nurse scientists can familiarize themselves with the initiatives that are most in alignment with their area of research interest and incorporate those initiatives into their grant proposals, research protocols, and publications. Identifying global genomic-based resources and opportunities for nurse scientists to incorporate genomic concepts into their programs of research was the purpose of a paper by Conley and Tinkle (2007). This paper utilized research themes for the future developed by the National Institute of Nursing Research (NINR) in 2003 as a framework for incorporating genomic research into the research trajectories of nurse scientists. The current NINR strategic plan can be assessed at the NINR Web site (www.ninr.nih.gov). Genomic-based research will be integral to many of the areas of research emphasis outlined in the strategic plan, and NINR is very supportive of genomic-based research and training of nurse scientists in genomics.

SUMMARY

The future looks promising for genetic and genomic investigations to continue to move the field of oncology forward. This promising future is because of the increased focus on translational research, the potential clinical utility of novel therapeutic approaches, the immense improvements in technology for data collection and data analysis, and enhanced access to information and data sharing among researchers. One of the most important aspects of oncology research that will transform practice is that research findings are more organized and readily accessible than ever before. It is impressive that most of the major research initiatives mentioned in this chapter incorporate data sharing among researchers as a part of their mission, which should greatly improve the research process as well as accelerate translation of research findings to the patient. Nurses are encouraged to stay informed of recent research findings relevant to their clinical area and to use evidence-based practices. The research initiatives that are presented and the resources provided in this chapter should assist with this effort and are consolidated and summarized in Table 15-2.

TABLE 15-2 Summary of Research Initiatives and Resources

Initiative/Resource	Brief Description	Web Address
ACCE model for evaluation of genetic testing	This is a model that evaluates genetic tests and is sponsored by the Centers for Disease Control and Prevention. The model includes the evaluation of analytic validity; clinical validity; clinical utility; and associated ethical, legal, and social implications of genetic tests.	www.cdc.gov/genomics/gtesting/ACCE/index.htm
Biomarkers Consortium	The Biomarkers Consortium strives to coordinate efforts that will speed up the identification and validation of biomarkers that support research and clinical practice.	www.biomarkersconsortium.org
Cancer Genetic Markers of Susceptibility (CGEMS) project	CGEMS project focuses on identifying common DNA variants that are associated with risk for prostate and breast cancer using a genome-wide association approach.	http://cgems.cancer.gov
Cancer Genome Anatomy Project (CGAP)	CGAP is focused on characterizing gene expression profiles for the continuum of cancer from normal to preclinical to cancer cells and to make this data available to researchers.	http://cgap.nci.nih.gov
The Cancer Genome Atlas (TCGA)	TCGA catalogs genomic sequences of cancer cells.	http://cancergenome.nih.gov
Cancer Genome Project (CGP)	CGP interrogates the DNA sequences of cancer cells to identify and catalog acquired mutations in somatic cells.	www.sanger.ac.uk/genetics/CGP
Encyclopedia of DNA Elements (ENCODE) Project	ENCODE Project's focus is to identify functional elements in the human genome and to make this information publicly available.	www.genome.gov/10005107

(Continued on next page)

TABLE 15-2 Summary of Research Initiatives and Resources *(Continued)*

Initiative/Resource	Brief Description	Web Address
Evaluation of Genomic Applications in Practice and Prevention (EGAPP)	EGAPP provides evidence-based reviews and recommendations regarding the utilization of genetic testing and other applications in clinical practice.	www.egappreviews.org/default.htm
Genomics and Health Weekly Update from the CDC	Free weekly updates are automatically e-mailed that assist subscribers in staying current about genomics in both the popular press and in scientific publications.	www.cdc.gov/genomics/update/current.htm
Human Genome Epidemiology Navigator Portal	This is a published literature database. The criteria for inclusion in this database include publication dates of October 2000–present, reporting a study conducted in humans, inclusion of genotype information, and the population-based analysis.	http://hugenavigator.net
Microarray in Node-Negative Disease May Avoid Chemotherapy (MINDACT) clinical trial	The MINDACT trial is evaluating the outcome of randomized assignment to adjunct chemotherapy based on results of a gene expression evaluation versus traditional assessment.	www.breastinternationalgroup.org/Research/TRANSBIG/MINDACT.aspx
National Cancer Institute Family Registries	This epidemiology and genetics research home page is used to facilitate breast and colon cancer studies.	http://epi.grants.cancer.gov/CFR
National Institute of Nursing Research (NINR)	The National Institutes of Health is composed of 27 institutes, including NINR. NINR supports and conducts clinical and basic research and research training on health and illness across the lifespan. NINR supports integrating genomics into research and training in genomic-based approaches.	www.ninr.nih.gov
Pharmacogenetics and Pharmacogenomics Knowledge Base (PharmGKB)	PharmGKB includes information about genes, variants, diseases, and drugs that have been investigated from a pharmacogenetic and pharmacogenomic perspective.	www.pharmgkb.org
PhenX Toolkit	PhenX is a toolkit of phenotype and exposure measures for utilization in genome-wide association studies.	www.phenxtoolkit.org
PubMed	PubMed is a literature search and retrieval system available through the U.S. National Library of Medicine.	www.pubmed.gov
TAILORx clinical trial	The Trial Assigning IndividuaLized Options for Treatment (Rx) (TAILORx) trial is evaluating the outcome of randomized assignment to chemotherapy based on results of a gene expression evaluation and risk score assignment.	www.cancer.gov/clinicaltrials/digestpage/TAILORx

REFERENCES

Biomarkers Definitions Working Group. (2001). Biomarkers and surrogate endpoints: Preferred definitions and conceptual framework. *Clinical Pharmacology and Therapeutics, 69*(3), 89–95.

Cardoso, F., Van't Veer, L., Rutgers, E., Loi, S., Mook, S., & Piccart-Gebhart, M.J. (2008). Clinical application of the 70-gene profile: The MINDACT trial. *Journal of Clinical Oncology, 26*(5), 729–735.

Centers for Disease Control and Prevention. (2009, July). *Genomic translation—ACCE: A CDC-sponsored project (2000–2004)*. Retrieved December 17, 2009, from http://www.cdc.gov/genomics/gtesting/ACCE/acce_proj.htm#T

Conley, Y.P., & Tinkle, M.B. (2007). The future of genomic nursing research. *Journal of Nursing Scholarship, 39*(1), 17–24.

Consensus Panel on Genetic/Genomic Nursing Competencies. (2009). *Essentials of genetic and genomic nursing: Competencies, curricula guidelines, and outcome indicators* (2nd ed.). Silver Spring, MD: American Nurses Association.

Contopoulos-Ioannidis, D.G., Ntzani, E., & Ioannidis, J.P. (2003). Translation of highly promising basic science research into clinical applications. *American Journal of Medicine, 114*(6), 477–484.

Elbashir, S.M., Harborth, J., Lendeckel, W., Yalcin, A., Weber, K., & Tuschl, T. (2001). Duplexes of 21-nucleotide RNAs mediate RNA interference in cultured mammalian cells. *Nature, 411*(6836), 494–498.

Fire, A., Xu, S., Montgomery, M.K., Kostas, S.A., Driver, S.E., & Mello, C.C. (1998). Potent and specific genetic interference by double-stranded RNA in Caenorhabditis elegans. *Nature, 391*(6669), 806–811.

Haddow, J.E., & Palomaki, G.E. (2004). ACCE: A model process for evaluating data on emerging genetic tests. In M.J. Khoury, J. Little, & W. Burke (Eds.), *Human genome epidemiology: A scientific foundation for using genetic information to improve health and prevent disease* (pp. 217–233). New York: Oxford University Press.

Jackson, A.L., & Linsley, P.S. (2004). Noise amidst the silence: Off-target effects of siRNAs? *Trends in Genetics, 20*(11), 521–524.

Khoury, M.J., Gwinn, M., Yoon, P.W., Dowling, N., Moore, C.A., & Bradley, L. (2007). The continuum of translation research in genomic medicine: How can we accelerate the appropriate integration of human genome discoveries into health care and disease prevention? *Genetics in Medicine, 9*(10), 665–674.

Lin, B.K., Clyne, M., Walsh, M., Gomez, O., Yu, W., Gwinn, M., et al. (2006). Tracking the epidemiology of human genes in the literature: The HuGE published literature database. *American Journal of Epidemiology, 164*(1), 1–4.

Marchionni, L., Wilson, R.F., Wolff, A.C., Marinopoulos, S., Parmigiani, G., Bass, E.B., et al. (2008). Systematic review: Gene expression profiling assays in early-stage breast cancer. *Annals of Internal Medicine, 148*(5), 358–369.

National Cancer Institute. (2009, October). *Epidemiology and genetics research: Breast and colon cancer family registries*. Retrieved November 5, 2009, from http://epi.grants.cancer.gov/CFR/about_breast_goals.html

National Human Genome Research Institute. (2009, September). *Office of Population Genomics*. Retrieved November 5, 2009, from http://www.genome.gov/19518660

Pai, S.I., Lin, Y.Y., Macaes, B., Meneshian, A., Hung, C.F., & Wu, T.C. (2006). Prospects of RNA interference therapy for cancer. *Gene Therapy, 13*(6), 464–477.

Paik, S. (2007). Development and clinical utility of a 21-gene recurrence score prognostic assay in patients with early breast cancer treated with tamoxifen. *Oncologist, 12*(6), 631–635.

Pheasant, M., & Mattick, J.S. (2007). Raising the estimate of functional human sequences. *Genome Research, 17*(9), 1245–1253.

Takeshita, F., & Ochiya, T. (2006). Therapeutic potential of RNA interference against cancer. *Cancer Science, 97*(8), 689–696.

Translational Research Working Group of the National Cancer Advisory Board. (2007). *Transforming translation—harnessing discovery for patient and public benefit* [No. 07-6239]. Bethesda, MD: U.S. Department of Health and Human Services National Institutes of Health.

Tuschl, T., Zamore, P.D., Lehmann, R., Bartel, D.P., & Sharp, P.A. (1999). Targeted mRNA degradation by double-stranded RNA in vitro. *Genes and Development, 13*(24), 3191–3197.

Westfall, J.M., Mold, J., & Fagnan, L. (2007). Practice-based research—"Blue Highways" on the NIH roadmap. *JAMA, 297*(4), 403–406.

Yu, W., Yesupriya, A., Clyne, M., Wulf, A., Gwinn, M., & Khoury, M.J. (2008). *HuGE Literature Finder. HuGE Navigator*. Retrieved January 2008, from http://www.hugenavigator.net/HuGENavigator/startPagePubLit.do/

Zamore, P.D., Tuschl, T., Sharp, P.A., & Bartel, D.P. (2000). RNAi: Double-stranded RNA directs the ATP-dependent cleavage of mRNA at 21 to 23 nucleotide intervals. *Cell, 101*(1), 25–33.

Zerhouni, E. (2003). Medicine. The NIH Roadmap. *Science, 302*(5642), 63–72.

Zerhouni, E.A. (2005). U.S. biomedical research: Basic, translational, and clinical sciences. *JAMA, 294*(11), 1352–1358.

Zerhouni, E.A., Sanders, C.A., & von Eschenbach, A.C. (2007). The Biomarkers Consortium: Public and private sectors working in partnership to improve the public health. *Oncologist, 12*(3), 250–252.

SECTION VI

Resources

CHAPTER 16 IDENTIFYING APPROPRIATE REFERRALS AND RESOURCES

CHAPTER 16

Identifying Appropriate Referrals and Resources

Susan R.M. Vasquez, BA, and Jean Jenkins, PhD, RN, FAAN

Professional Practice Domain:
Identification
- Identify credible, accurate, appropriate, and current genetic and genomic information, resources, services, and technologies specific to a given client

Referral
- Facilitate referrals for specialized genetic and genomic services for clients as needed

(Consensus Panel on Genetic/Genomic Nursing Competencies, 2009)

INTRODUCTION

Regardless of their specialty area, all nurses need to gain a basic knowledge in genetics and genomics to understand the implications of this burgeoning amount of information (Consensus Panel on Genetic/Genomic Nursing Competencies, 2009). Patients traditionally have looked to nurses to interpret the sometimes complex medical data that they encounter. Now, nurses are educating and interpreting genetic and genomic information about predisposition testing, genetic and genomic markers to identify disease, prognosis and recurrence, and the underlying genetic and genomic mechanisms of targeted therapies. In their role as patient advocate, nurses frequently serve as resources for education, referral, and emotional support. To continue this function, nurses must take advantage of evidence-based resources to enhance their own basic genetic and genomic knowledge; identify resources for clients, families, and their communities; and develop novel ways of incorporating new technologies into comprehensive nursing care.

Web sites published by organizations (see Table 16-1) are valuable resources for nurses who want to enhance their knowledge of genetics and genomics. This chapter will provide resources important for professional networking, continuing education, client education, and clinical reviews that are needed to stay current in this quickly advancing field.

PROFESSIONAL ORGANIZATIONS: RESOURCES FOR NETWORKING AND GENETIC AND GENOMIC INFORMATION

Oncology Nursing Society

One of the most accessible resources for nurses seeking to enhance their understanding of genetic and genomic information in all cancer care often can be overlooked: their own colleagues.

TABLE 16-1   Web Resources for Cancer Genetics and Genomics

Resource	Web Site
Professional Organizations	
American Academy of Family Physicians (AAFP)	www.aafp.org
American Academy of Nursing (AAN)	www.aannet.org
American Board of Medical Genetics (ABMG)	www.abmg.org
American College of Medical Genetics (ACMG)	www.acmg.net
American Medical Association (AMA)	www.ama-assn.org
American Nurses Association (ANA)	www.nursingworld.org
American Society of Clinical Oncology (ASCO)	www.asco.org
American Society of Human Genetics (ASHG)	www.ashg.org
Genetic Nursing Credentialing Commission (GNCC)	www.geneticnurse.org
International Society of Nurses in Genetics (ISONG)	www.isong.org
National Coalition for Health Professional Education in Genetics (NCHPEG)	www.nchpeg.org
National Coalition of Ethnic Minority Nurse Associations (NCEMNA)	www.ncemna.org
National Society of Genetic Counselors, Inc. (NSGC)	www.nsgc.org
Oncology Nursing Society (ONS)	www.ons.org
Continuing Education	
Fox Chase Cancer Center: Personalized Cancer Risk Assessment: Genetics and Genomics for Nursing Practice	www.fccc.edu/nursing/education
Cincinnati Children's Hospital Medical Center: Web-Based Genetics Institute	www.cincinnatichildrens.org/ed/clinical/gpnf/ce/web/default.htm
Cincinnati Children's Hospital Medical Center: Genetics Education Program for Nurses	www.cincinnatichildrens.org/ed/clinical/gpnf/ce/apply-genomics/default.htm
City of Hope Cancer Genetics Career Development Program	www.infosci.coh.org/ccgp
National Institute of Nursing Research (NINR) Summer Genetics Institute	www.ninr.nih.gov/Training/TrainingOpportunities Intramural
Telling Stories: Understanding Real Life Genetics	www.geneticseducation.nhs.uk/tellingstories
The Family as Context in Clinical Genetics Project (FCCGP)	www.nursing.ouhsc.edu/CE/fccg

(Continued on next page)

TABLE 16-1 Web Resources for Cancer Genetics and Genomics *(Continued)*

Resource	Web Site
Clinical Resources	
GeneTests	www.genetests.org
FORCE – Facing Our Risk of Cancer Empowered	www.facingourrisk.org
Genetic Alliance	www.geneticalliance.org
Genetic and Rare Diseases Information Center (GARD)	www.genome.gov/10000409
Human Genome Epidemiology Network (HuGENet™)	www.cdc.gov/genomics/hugenet
INFOGENETICS	www.infogenetics.org
National Cancer Institute (NCI)	www.cancer.gov
Family History Tools and Client Resources	
American Medical Association	www.ama-assn.org/ama/pub/physician-resources/medical-science/genetics-molecular-medicine/family-history.shtml
Centers for Disease Control and Prevention National Office for Public Health Genomics	www.cdc.gov/genomics
Cyrillic	www.cyrillicsoftware.com
Pedigree-Draw	www.pedigree-draw.com
Progeny	www.progeny2000.com
U.S. Surgeon General's Family History Initiative	www.hhs.gov/familyhistory
National Human Genome Research Institute: Genetics and Genomics for Patients and the Public	www.genome.gov/19016903
Genetics Education	
National Cancer Institute: Cancer Library	www.cancer.gov/cancertopics/literature
National Human Genome Research Institute: Genetics and Genomics for Health Professionals	www.genome.gov/27527599
Genetics Legislation, Guidelines, and Policies	
National Human Genome Research Institute: Policy and Ethics	www.genome.gov/PolicyEthics
National Comprehensive Cancer Network	www.nccn.org/professionals/physician_gls/default.asp

(Continued on next page)

TABLE 16-1 Web Resources for Cancer Genetics and Genomics (Continued)

Resource	Web Site
The National Guideline Clearinghouse™ (NGC)	www.guideline.gov/about/about.aspx
NIH Genome Wide Association Studies Policy	www.grants.nih.gov/grants/gwas
Secretary's Advisory Committee on Genetics, Health and Society (SACGHS)	www4.od.nih.gov/oba/sacghs.htm
Thomas—U.S. Congress on the Internet	www.thomas.gov
Research and Funding Opportunities	
Cancer Genome Anatomy Project (CGAP)	http://cgap.nci.nih.gov
The Cancer Genome Atlas (TCGA)	http://cancergenome.nih.gov
Genetic Association Information Network (GAIN)	www.genome.gov/19518664
Genes, Environment and Health Initiative (GEI)	www.genesandenvironment.nih.gov
International Society of Nurses in Genetics (ISONG)	www.isong.org
National Human Genome Research Institute: Ethical, Legal, and Social Implications Program	www.genome.gov/10001618
National Human Genome Research Institute: Genome-Wide Association Studies	www.genome.gov/19518660
National Institute of Nursing Research	www.ninr.nih.gov/ResearchAndFunding

The Oncology Nursing Society (ONS) is at the forefront in setting the highest standards of patient care. Through its annual Congress and Institutes of Learning, ONS strives to present oncology nurses with not only the most current medical and nursing information, but also with guidelines to translate the data into improvements in the clinical setting. ONS is working to ensure that oncology nurses, with their established knowledge surrounding the treatment and supportive care of patients with cancer, assume a vital role in the care of patients that integrates genetic and genomic information. ONS local chapters provide an opportunity for networking within communities, and many sponsor continuing education sessions on cancer genetics.

In 2009, ONS revised two position statements related to genetics: *Cancer Predisposition Genetic Testing and Risk Assessment Counseling* and *The Role of the Oncology Nurse in Cancer Genetic Counseling*. The first of these papers stresses the need for obtaining informed consent and the importance of pre- and post-test counseling by individuals trained not only in the technical aspects of cancer genetics but also in the complex psychosocial, ethical, and legal issues surrounding genetic testing. ONS advocates for research in all areas of cancer genetics, development of educational resources, and regulation of laboratories performing genetic testing.

In delineating the oncology nurse's role in cancer genetics, ONS asserts that oncology nurses ideally are prepared to assume expanded roles in cancer genetics, including genetic-risk assessment and counseling. In clarifying the nurse's role, ONS outlines three levels of practice: the general oncology nurse; the advanced practice oncology nurse; and the advanced practice oncology nurse with specialty training in genetics. For nurses at both general and advanced levels, the Society recommends a foundation in genetic and genomic knowledge provided by nursing school curricula, continuing education, and specialized cancer genetics programs. The Oncology Nursing Certification Corporation (ONCC, 2009), an ONS affiliate, includes genetics as a component of both the general and advanced practice certification examinations.

The ONS Cancer Genetics Special Interest Group (SIG) was founded in 1997 to provide a forum for networking, exchange of information, and discussion of implications for clinical practice. The SIG encourages research in the areas of cancer genetics and cancer risk counseling; supports basic and continuing education in the field; advances the establishment of nursing practice guidelines; and serves as a liaison with other groups, such as the International Society of Nurses in Genetics (ISONG) and the National Society of Genetic Counselors (NSGC). The Cancer Genetics SIG has been instrumental in planning educational sessions at ONS meetings. The SIG's newsletter and Virtual Community (http://cancergenetics.vc.ons.org) keep members informed of new research in the field, activities of other members, legislative developments, journal articles of interest, and relevant developments in the field.

In addition to these avenues for networking, the ONS Web site (www.ons.org) provides easy access to the latest developments in oncology nursing. The Web site details upcoming conferences and continuing education programs and provides information on ONS chapters and SIGs. The site's News section summarizes breaking news from the cancer and general medical communities, lists employment opportunities, and updates information on healthcare legislation. Major cancer centers are described and algorithms for disease management are discussed within the Clinical Practice section. The Research section features discussion forums, resources, and information on grants available to oncology nurses.

The Publications tab on the ONS Web site (www.ons.org/Publications) contains links to the full text of its position statements and access to articles from the *Clinical Journal of Oncology Nursing*, *Oncology Nursing Forum*, and *ONS Connect*. This tab also allows users to connect to the ONS Library and Archives, which maintains a collection of electronic resources, as well as print and audiovisual materials (www.ons.org/Publications/Library).

International Society of Nurses in Genetics

ISONG is a professional association for nurses working in all areas of genetics and genomics. ISONG's purpose is to improve the quality of genetic services provided to patients by enhancing the scientific and professional growth of nurses as they incorporate genetics and genomics into clinical practice, research, and education. ISONG has defined the scope and standards of practice for the specialty, last revised in 2006 (ISONG, 2007). The resulting publication, *Genetics/Genomics Nursing: Scope and Standards of Practice*, was developed in collaboration with the American Nurses Association (ANA). These standards have been used as the foundation for credentialing in genetics by the Genetic Nursing Credentialing Commission (www.geneticnurse.org). ANA published a book titled *Genetics Nursing Portfolios: A New Model for Credentialing* (Monsen, 2005). A second publication edited by Monsen (2009) is titled *Genetics and Ethics in Health Care: New Questions in the Age of Genomic Health*. This book provides nurses with a comprehensive text on ethics and genomics.

As the representative organization for nurses working in all areas of genetics and genomics, ISONG encourages networking among members, genetic and genomic education for all nurses, and nursing research in human genetics and genomics. With the impact of genetic and genomic discoveries on the practice of oncology, many oncology nurses have joined the ranks of ISONG members, and the organization is actively involved in developing educational programs and guidelines for this emerging subspecialty. ISONG's annual conference, often held in conjunction with the meeting of the American Society of Human Genetics (ASHG), offers presentations on a variety of genetic and genomic topics, including cancer. The organization maintains an electronic mailing list that provides members with an excellent means of communicating with colleagues and sharing new developments online. The ISONG Web site (www.isong.org) provides nurses with resources to integrate developments in human genetics and genomics into practice, education, and research activities. The site lists educational programs, employment positions, and links to sites for many other genetic and nursing organizations.

American Academy of Nursing

The mission of the American Academy of Nursing (AAN, 2008) is "to serve the public and the nursing profession by advancing health policy and practice through the generation, synthesis, and dissemination of nursing knowledge." The vision of AAN is to transform healthcare policy and practice through nursing knowledge. The academy is poised to advance nursing practice and education that integrates genetic and genomic information with its Genetics Healthcare Expert Panel, whose members represent the leading experts nationally in genetics and nursing. AAN has supported many initiatives, including ongoing work to sponsor a state-of-the-science meeting focused on genetic and genomic nursing; providing input from the perspective of genetics and genomics for the American Association of Colleges of Nursing Baccalaureate Essentials; delivering public and written testimony at the Secretary's Advisory Council on Genetics, Health, and Society; highlighting genetics and genomics as a component of the Raise the Voice Campaign; establishing a position on global health concerns from the perspective of the American AAN Expert Panel on Genetic Healthcare; and nominating and supporting an expert panel member representing AAN on the Evaluation of Genomic Applications in Practice and Prevention Stakeholder Group sponsored by the National Office of Public Health Genomics at the Centers for Disease Control and Prevention.

American Nurses Association

ANA is another organization that is examining the nurse's responsibility in providing care that integrates genetic and genomic information. ANA's seminal publication *Managing*

Genetic Information: Implications for Nursing Practice reviewed the implications of genetic discoveries for nursing practice, including consideration of the ethical, legal, and social issues involved in obtaining informed consent (Scanlon & Fibison, 1995). This study was initiated to evaluate the baseline status of management of genetic information by nurses and to establish professional and ethical standards for utilizing this information to provide comprehensive patient care. Building on this foundation, ANA, through the work of its House of Delegates and Ethics Advisory Board, has been actively creating and passing resolutions and developing policy statements related to genomics. ANA represents nursing as a member of the Institute of Medicine Roundtable on Translating Genomic-Based Research for Health.

In 2005, ANA partnered with the National Human Genome Research Institute (NHGRI), the National Cancer Institute (NCI), and the Office of Rare Diseases Research at the National Institutes of Health (NIH) to support the development of nursing core competencies in genetics and genomics. A consensus panel of nursing leaders came together at the ANA headquarters to identify, review, and generate a plan to formalize genetics and genomic core competencies for all RNs. The final document, *Essential Nursing Competencies and Curricula Guidelines for Genetics and Genomics,* has been endorsed by 49 representative nursing organizations including ONS, the Genetic Alliance, the March of Dimes, and the National Coalition for Health Professional Education in Genetics (NCHPEG) (Consensus Panel on Genetic/Genomic Nursing Competencies, 2006; Jenkins & Calzone, 2007). In 2006, the consensus panel members and representatives of the endorsing organizations met again to establish a strategic plan for competency implementation. Information from the 2006 meeting is located on the ANA Center for Ethics and Human Rights Web site (www.nursingworld.org/MainMenuCategories/ThePracticeofProfessionalNursing/EthicsStandards/CEHR.aspx). The ANA *Online Journal of Issues in Nursing (OJIN)* published a special issue in 2008 on genetics/genomics nursing (www.nursingworld.org/MainMenuCategories/ANAMarketplace/ANAPeriodicals/OJIN/JournalTopics/FirstGeneticsNowGenomics.aspx).

National Society of Genetic Counselors

Although communication within the nursing profession is important, nurses also must maintain relationships with other disciplines involved in cancer genetics. NSGC, a group of genetic counselors who are professionals specially trained in providing education and counseling to patients with all types of genetic diseases, is actively involved in conducting research, establishing patient care guidelines, and educating its members regarding cancer genetics. Genetic counselors are certified by the American Board of Genetic Counseling (ABGC) or by the American Board of Medical Genetics (ABMG). Certification requirements include a graduate degree in genetic counseling; clinical experience in an ABGC-approved site; a log book of 50 supervised cases; and the successful completion of both general and specialty certification examinations, which are prepared and administered by ABGC. NSGC's Annual Education Conference offers cancer genetics information via practice-based symposia, sponsored speakers, workshops, presented papers, and posters. Nurses may attend the conference as associate members of NSGC or as nonmembers. The conference schedule is available through the NSGC Web site (www.nsgc.org). Nurses can be full members of NSGC if they have a master's or higher level degree, have undergone a broad range of clinical genetics training, and can cite genetic counseling as their primary responsibility. In 2006, NSGC, together with ISONG, released a position statement titled *Provision of Quality Genetic*

Services and Care: Building a Multidisciplinary, Collaborative Approach Among Genetic Nurses and Genetic Counselors (www.nsgc.org/about/position.cfm#isong).

National Coalition for Health Professional Education in Genetics

NCHPEG was established in 1996 by the American Medical Association (AMA), ANA, and NHGRI. NCHPEG is an organization composed of more than 140 diverse health professional organizations, consumer and volunteer groups, government agencies, private industry, managed care organizations, and genetics professional societies committed to promoting health professional education and access to information about advances in human genetics (NCHPEG, n.d.). In 2007, NCHPEG published the third edition of the *Core Competencies in Genetics for Health Professionals*. This report recommends that all health professionals possess certain core competencies in genetics so that they can effectively and responsibly integrate genetics into current clinical practice and education of health professionals (NCHPEG, 2007).

NCHPEG hosts an annual meeting and often provides meeting slides and information on its Web site (www.nchpeg.org). Other educational programs of value are listed on their Web site, including two Web-based programs. One program, Genetics in the Physician Assistant's Practice (http://pa.nchpeg.org), provides an interactive genetics primer, family history exercises, genetic testing information, teaching tools, and links to other resources. Additionally, a set of independent self-paced modules for nurses, Genetics Is Relevant Now, is available at www.nchpeg.org/content.asp?dbsection=basic&dbid=8. The *Genetics Application in Practice* newsletter produced and disseminated by NCHPEG (www.nchpeg.org/content.aspx?sc=products&sub=3) provides clinical examples of the utility of genetic information.

PHYSICIAN GROUPS

Physician groups that are involved in genetics and genomics include the American Society of Clinical Oncology (ASCO), the American College of Medical Genetics (ACMG), ABMG, the American Society of Human Genetics (ASHG), AMA, and the American Academy of Family Physicians (AAFP).

ASCO has developed a curriculum for cancer genetics education. Information about ASCO's curriculum guidelines for cancer genetics and cancer predisposition testing is available on its Web site under ASCO Bookstore-Curriculum Series (https://store.asco.org/public/eCommerce/Orders/product.aspx?categoryId=4&productId=159). ASCO has updated and published its policy paper on predisposition genetic testing, outlining recommendations on cancer risk counseling, indications for testing, informed consent, and management after testing (ASCO, 2003; Robson et al., 2010).

The goal of ACMG is the maintenance of high standards in education, practice, and research. Fellows of ACMG must possess a medical degree or a doctorate. Certified genetic counselors may join as associate members, and other individuals, including nurses, with an interest in medical genetics may join as affiliate members. ACMG is involved in professional and public education and works to increase access to medical genetic services with 1,253 ABMG-certified clinical geneticists. In 2005, ACMG published updated practice guidelines for assessment, counseling, and testing for genetic susceptibility to breast and ovarian cancer (available in the Publications section of www.acmg.net).

In 2007, ACMG published "Indications for Genetic Referral: A Guide for Healthcare Providers" (Pletcher et al., 2007). This guide, based on the work of the ACMG Professional Practice and Guidelines Committee, is designed as an educational resource for healthcare providers to help them to provide quality medical genetic services. The referral lists are divided into prenatal, pediatric, and adult indications.

ABMG is the credentialing group for MDs and PhDs in medical genetics. This agency accredits training programs in the field of human genetics and prepares the certifying examination.

Another genetics professional group, ASHG, aims to unite investigators from the many research areas of human genetics. Its membership includes researchers, physicians, laboratory personnel, genetic counselors, and nurses. ASHG's annual meeting serves as a forum for research findings and education about genetics and genomics. The group assumes an active role in establishing policy regarding standards for genetic research and testing; ASHG's numerous policy papers are available on its Web site (www.ashg.org).

The AMA leadership works together on the most important professional and public health issues that shape the future of medicine. Important to the AMA mission is healthcare advocacy, setting standards, and providing professional resources. For example, AMA has developed physician information about the latest research on genetics and molecular medicine (see www.ama-assn.org/ama/pub/category/1799.html). AMA provides its membership with information about medical genetics, including the basics, genetic testing guidance (e.g., warfarin dosing), utilization of family history with screening questionnaires, and content regarding genetics and policy issues.

AAFP was founded to promote and maintain high-quality standards for family doctors who provide continuing comprehensive health care to the public. The topic of the AAFP's 2005 Annual Clinical Focus was genomics. Materials from the 2005 Annual Clinical Focus can be found on the AAFP Web site (www.aafp.org).

RESOURCES FOR CONTINUING EDUCATION

The rapidly changing nature of genetic and genomic information makes quality publications and continuing education essential for all professionals in the field. The previously described professional groups sponsor ongoing education in genetics and genomics through their annual meetings and Web sites. ISONG presents basic genetics educational sessions prior to the start of its annual fall meeting. Additional organizations also offer short courses in cancer genetics; some are highlighted in the following sections.

Fox Chase Cancer Center

Fox Chase Cancer Center, an NCI-designated Comprehensive Cancer Center in Philadelphia, PA, presents an annual, three-day educational program, Personalized Cancer Risk Assessment: Genetics and Genomics in Nursing Practice. This program covers the basics of cancer genetics and familial cancer; techniques for obtaining medical and family history; familial cancer risk factors; risk-counseling strategies; and the ethical, legal, and social issues associated with genetic risk assessment. Additional information, including upcoming course dates, is available at www.fccc.edu/healthProfessionals/continuingNursingEducation or by calling the Department of Continuing Nursing Education at 215-728-3522.

Cincinnati Children's Hospital Medical Center

Cincinnati Children's Hospital Medical Center hosts a Genetics Education Program for Nurses, which offers both free and fee-based online genetic education courses and modules for all nurses. One of the many courses offered is the 18-week Web-Based Genetics Institute (WBGI). To date, 172 nursing faculty and advanced practice nurses have completed a WBGI course. For more information about WBGI, visit www.cincinnatichildrens.org/ed/clinical/gpnf/ce/web/default.htm.

The Genetics Education Program for Nurses (GEPN) offers a five-week online teacher-facilitated offering, Applying Genomics in Nursing Practice. The target audience for this offering is nurses in practice with little to no previous education in genetics. For more information, visit www.cincinnatichildrens.org/ed/clinical/gpnf/ce/apply-genomics/default.htm.

The GEPN Nursing School Genetics Curriculum Modules consists of 14 Modules and each module contains a set of assignments, answers and instructional resources. For more information, visit www.cincinnatichildrens.org/ed/clinical/gpnf/resources/curriculum/nursing/default.htm.

National Institute of Nursing Research, National Institutes of Health

The National Institute of Nursing Research (NINR) offers an intensive one-month summer training program that provides a foundation in molecular genetics and genomics for use in research and clinical practice. The Summer Genetics Institute (SGI) is designed for nursing faculty, graduate students, and advanced practice nurses. The purpose of SGI is to develop and expand the research capability among graduate students and faculty in schools of nursing, and to develop and expand the basis for clinical practice in genetics and genomics among advanced practice nurses. The program features both classroom and laboratory components, and participants spend one month in residence at NIH in Bethesda, MD. The first SGI was held on the NIH campus in 2000. Since that time, 139 nurses have graduated from the program. To date, they have published more than 100 peer-reviewed papers and presented at numerous national and international conferences. For more information, see www.ninr.nih.gov/Training/TrainingOpportunitiesIntramural.

City of Hope

City of Hope, an NCI-designated Comprehensive Cancer Center in Duarte, CA, offers an interdisciplinary Cancer Genetics Career Development Program for doctoral nurses. The program is designed to train research program leaders and team members for careers focused on cancer genetics and prevention and control research. For all healthcare providers the City of Hope offers an intensive cancer genetics course focused on community cancer genetics and research training. This eight-week Web-based course is followed by five days of interactive cancer genetics workshops held on the City of Hope campus. This course focuses on epidemiology, genetics, and oncology principles relevant to clinical genetics practice.

More information about both the fellowship and the intensive cancer genetics course can be found on the City of Hope Web site at www.infosci.coh.org/ccgp.

Additional Online Resources

Telling Stories: Understanding Real Life Genetics is an online resource that nurses can use for their own education or nursing faculty can use as an instructional resource. This resource (www.geneticseducation.nhs.uk/tellingstories) is offered by the National Genetics Education and Development Centre of the United Kingdom National Health Service. Additional patient examples can be found at the Family as Context in Clinical Genetics Project, a Web-based curriculum consisting of three modules that prepare learners to integrate knowledge of genetics with family, environment, and behavioral, psychosocial, ethical, and legal knowledge. For more information, visit www.nursing.ouhsc.edu/CE/fccg.

CLINICAL RESOURCES: SOURCES FOR PATIENT INFORMATION AND REFERRALS

In their role as patient advocates, nurses frequently serve as referral sources. As cancer genetics moves from the research to the clinical setting, it is essential that nurses know what resources are available for genetic counseling and testing. Several Web sites provide access to information about patient outcomes and resources for patient referral (see Table 16-1).

Human Genome Epidemiology Network

The Human Genome Epidemiology Network (HuGENet™) is a global collaboration of individuals and organizations committed to the assessment of the impact of human genome variation on population health and how genetic and genomic information can be used to improve health and reduce the risk of disease. Materials such as review articles, research papers, systematic reviews, meta-analyses, consensus conferences, editorials, and workshop reports are available at www.cdc.gov/genomics/hugenet/default.htm.

INFOGENETICS

The INFOGENETICS Web site (www.infogenetics.org) is designed to assist care providers in utilizing genetic information in the daily care of patients. The site provides links to constantly changing genetic information and resources such as contacts, clinical trials, and genetic testing resources.

National Cancer Institute, National Institutes of Health

NCI provides both professional and patient resources regarding genetics and genomics. A list of professionals specializing in cancer genetics is available through the NCI Web site (www.cancer.gov/search/geneticsservices). This site enables users to search by geographic location, cancer type (e.g., breast, colon, endocrine), or specific genetic condition (e.g., ataxia telangiectasia). The directory lists names and qualifications of the providers, as well as telephone numbers and e-mail and mailing addresses. Also provided are directions regarding how to register as a qualified provider of cancer genetics information. The Cancer Information Service (CIS), sponsored by NCI, provides information on facilities that offer genetic testing and counseling (http://cis.nci.nih.gov). CIS is a resource for up-to-date, accurate information for clients and families, healthcare professionals, and the general public. The service can be reached toll-free in the United States 9 am–4:30 pm ET Monday through Friday at 800-4CANCER (422-6237). In addition, individuals who are hearing-impaired can access TTY services by calling 800-332-8615.

To spearhead national efforts in cancer genetics clinical research, NCI has established several cancer networks. The Cancer Genetics Network (CGN) is a group of eight U.S. medical research centers. This network encourages collaborative efforts in studying the genetic basis of cancer susceptibility, establishing ways to integrate new findings into clinical practice, and clarifying the associated psychosocial, ethical, legal, and public health issues. Information about ongoing studies and whom to contact is on the CGN Web site (http://epi.grants.cancer.gov/CGN).

The Early Detection Research Network (EDRN) is another NCI network that brings together dozens of institutions to help to accelerate the translation of biomarker information into clinical applications and to evaluate new ways of testing cancer in its earliest stages for cancer risk. Additional information about EDRN, including a progress report, is available at http://edrn.nci.nih.gov/about-edrn.

The Cancer Family Registry Network has been established for families with breast and colon cancer as a comprehensive research resource infrastructure to assist with the implementation of collaborative interdisciplinary research protocols in the genetic epidemiology of cancer. The greater scientific community has access to this large and well-characterized resource for studying factors affecting cancer susceptibility and modification. A list of participating sites and approved projects is available at http://epi.grants.cancer.gov/CFR.

Some NIH studies offer genetic services as part of their protocols. Nurses seeking information about studies open for enrollment and eligibility criteria for participation in such a study may call the Patient Recruitment and Public Liaison Office toll-free at 800-411-1222.

National Society of Genetic Counselors

The NSGC Web site (www.nsgc.org) includes a provider list, accessible by clicking the Find a Counselor link on the home page. This information is categorized according to state and identifies which genetic specialty is available (e.g., cancer genetics, prenatal genetics). The list is updated regularly but may not provide a complete list of genetic counselors involved in cancer genetics, particularly those at university medical centers or other hospitals.

FORCE (Facing Our Risk of Cancer Empowered)

FORCE is a nonprofit organization that provides resources, information, and support for families or individuals who are at high risk for or are genetically predisposed to breast and ovarian cancer. FORCE sponsors an annual conference along with the H. Lee Moffitt Cancer Center and Research Institute at the University of South Florida for clients and healthcare providers. The FORCE Web site (www.facingourrisk.org) also provides support via online support groups and chat lines.

GeneTests

Genetic testing is now performed in commercial and research laboratories across the United States and worldwide. GeneTests, a service funded by the NIH National Library of Medicine, provides a list at www.genetests.org of clinical and research laboratories that conduct testing for inherited disorders. GeneTests also sponsors a genetic clinics directory and provides introductory information about genetic counseling and testing. The GeneClinics section of the site offers disease-specific data, including information about diagnosis, management, and counseling. Educational materials, including genetic tools, are available online.

Genetic Alliance

Genetic Alliance is a nonprofit organization dedicated to helping individuals and families with genetic disorders. The alliance serves as a resource for consumers and professionals seeking information about diseases, access to educational tools, and information about genetic support groups and genetic services. Information is available via phone 202-966-5557, e-mail at info@geneticalliance.org, or through their comprehensive Web site at www.geneticalliance.org. The Web site provides interactive resources such as WikiGenetics and WikiAdvocacy, user-friendly, user-generated, online tools that provide credible resources for all stakeholders in lay language.

Genetic and Rare Diseases Information Center

The Genetic and Rare Diseases Information Center (GARD, http://rarediseases.info.nih.gov/GARD) is the result of collaboration between the NIH Office of Rare Diseases Research (ORDR) and NHGRI. Communication specialists at the Center answer questions about genetics and rare diseases; the questions come from the general public, healthcare professionals, and biomedical researchers. For information, call the center's toll-free number (888-205-2311).

FAMILY HISTORY AND OTHER CLIENT RESOURCES

Several federal and non-federal organizations offer information and tools regarding the use of family history in practice (Guttmacher, Collins, & Carmona, 2004). The Centers for Disease Control and Prevention (CDC) Office of Public Health Genomics (OPHG) Web site (www.cdc.gov/genomics) provides links to a variety of resources, podcasts, articles, and tools focused on both adult and pediatric family history. The Web site also features fact sheets and information on the use of genomics in the public health arena. This site offers a subscription to weekly updates from the Evaluation of Genomic Applications in Practice and Prevention (EGAPP) pilot project. Among many other initiatives, OPHG coordinates the

EGAPP pilot project, whose goals are to establish and evaluate a systematic, evidence-based process for assessing genetic tests and other applications of genomic technology in transition from research to clinical and public health practice. CDC also provides a resource, Genomic Competencies for the Public Health Workforce, at www.cdc.gov/genomics/translation/competencies/index.htm.

Free family history collection tools are available through the U.S. Surgeon General's Family History Initiative (www.hhs.gov/familyhistory) and through AMA (www.ama-assn.org/ama/pub/category/2380.html). The U.S. Surgeon General's Family History Initiative Web site offers information for patients about how to begin collecting family medical history information, PDF versions of a paper-based tool, and an interactive Web-based collection tool that is available in both English and Spanish. The site also offers a resource packet of information for health professionals. AMA offers articles and resources for health professionals, including a sample family history collection form.

A pedigree is often an essential piece of the medical record and one way for health professionals to record family history information. Several companies offer pedigree drawing software for health professionals for a fee. Cyrillic (www.cyrillicsoftware.com) offers pedigree drawing software for healthcare providers as well as links to genetic resources. Pedigree-Draw (www.pedigree-draw.com) is a pedigree drawing software for Macintosh users. Progeny (www.progenygenetics.com) offers genetic data management and pedigree drawing software.

NHGRI provides genetic and genomic information for clients. Genetics and Genomics for Patients and the Public covers information about genetic disorders, background on genetic and genomic science, and pharmacogenomics. This site also has links to the family health history tools described previously and a list of online health resources (www.genome.gov/19016903).

RESOURCES FOR INFORMATION REGARDING GENETICS EDUCATION

With new discoveries in genetics and genomics taking place almost daily, staying abreast of vital information has become increasingly difficult. The Internet, with its ability to be updated almost instantaneously, is an invaluable source of cancer genetics material. In addition to the Web sites of the previously mentioned resources, many other sites offer extensive information about the science of genetics, cancer genetics specifically, and health policy regarding genetics (see Table 16-1).

National Cancer Institute, National Institutes of Health

NCI's Web site (www.cancer.gov) is an excellent starting point as a resource for both healthcare professionals and patients. NCI presents information on all types of cancer, training and funding opportunities, and the latest scientific developments. One of its largest components is Cancer Topics, which contains in-depth information on genetic testing and treatment. The Cancer Topics section Prevention, Genetics, Causes links to a Cancer Genetics gateway that offers a comprehensive guide to cancer genetics. A variety of tools are within this section, such as booklets and a glossary, a cancer genetics overview, disease-specific cancer genetics information (e.g., colon, breast), and an overview of risk assessment and counseling. The Web site also details information on clinical trials, presents abstracts of cancer genetics policy papers, and alerts users to a variety of other Web resources such as PDQ® (Physician Data Query).

PDQ is an online database designed to make the most current, credible, and accurate cancer information available to health professionals and the public. It contains peer-reviewed summaries on cancer treatment, screening, prevention, genetics, complementary and alternative medicine, and supportive care; a registry of cancer clinical trials from around the world; and directories of physicians, professionals who provide genetic services, and organizations that provide cancer care. Most of this information and more specific information about PDQ can be found at www.cancer.gov/cancertopics/pdq.

The Cancer Library (www.cancer.gov/cancertopics/literature) is a bibliographic database of cancer literature—including biomedical journals, proceedings, books, reports, and doctoral theses. Although the site does not provide the full text of articles, it supplies authors, sources, abstracts (when available), and other basic information and is updated monthly. Predesigned searches of articles specific to cancer genetics and familial cancer syndromes also are included.

National Human Genome Research Institute, National Institutes of Health

The NHGRI Web site (www.genome.gov) is another comprehensive source of information. The Genomic Healthcare Branch of NHGRI promotes the effective integration of genomic discoveries into health care and provides up-to-date genetics and genomics information related to patient management, curricular resources, and new NIH and NHGRI research activities, as well as ethical, legal, and social issues on its Web site (www.genome.gov/27527599).

The Ethical, Legal, and Social Implications (ELSI) Research Program of NHGRI (www.genome.gov/10001618) supports research to anticipate and resolve ethical, legal, and social issues arising from genetic and genomic research. The group fosters public and professional education and discussion of these issues. In addition to scientific genetic and genomic data, the NHGRI Web site features information about the Human Genome Project, public policy and grants, off-site resources, and intramural research.

Web-based, interactive education tools and short videos provide an alternative medium for delivering cancer genetic education. As part of the Understanding the Human Genome Project education kit, two documentary videos are available on the NHGRI Web site (www.genome.gov/25019879): *The Human Genome Project—Exploring Our Molecular Selves* and *The Secret of Our Lives*. These videos discuss the Human Genome Project and its effect on the future.

GENETICS LEGISLATION, GUIDELINES, AND POLICIES

Legislation

Nurses need to be aware of current legislative developments regarding genetic testing and services. The U.S. Congress passed federal legislation in 2008 to prohibit insurance and employment discrimination based on genetic information. Some states have already passed similar legislation, and other states have bills pending. National advocacy groups, such as the Genetic Alliance, are active in supporting this legislative agenda and informing healthcare professionals of legal developments. A Congress-sponsored Web site (www.thomas.gov) provides a keyword search of the full text of approved and proposed bills, as well as bill summaries and status reports. The Policy and Program Analysis Branch of the NHGRI's Office of Policy, Communications, and Education actively monitors federal legislation related to genetics, genomics, and personalized medicine. The NHGRI Web site features updated information on congressional testimony and activity and provides a link to a legislative database (www.genome.gov/PolicyEthics).

Guidelines

Because cancer genetics and genomics is an expanding field with an abundance of emerging data and opinions, it is essential that guidelines concerning the use of this information be established. NCI's Statement on Genetic Testing for Cancer Risk outlines factors that should be considered in offering cancer predisposition testing. Other groups—such as ISONG, ASHG, ASCO, ACMG, and NSGC—also have issued policy statements on genetic testing and have included the full text of these positions on their Web sites.

National Comprehensive Cancer Network

The National Comprehensive Cancer Network (NCCN, www.nccn.org) is an alliance of 21 comprehensive cancer centers. The goal of NCCN is to improve the quality and effectiveness of cancer care through the development of resources and information. NCCN offers accredited educational opportunities and tools, including conferences and symposia, continuing medical education–accredited webcasts, CD-ROMs, DVDs, and a published journal. To promote the continuous quality improvement, NCCN develops clinical practice guidelines for use by patients, clinicians, and other healthcare decision makers. The *NCCN Clinical Practice Guidelines in Oncology*™ are developed via an evidence-based review process created by a multidisciplinary panel from NCCN member institutions. The guidelines cover the majority of cancers and have specific recommendations for detection, prevention, and risk reduction for breast and ovarian, colorectal, cervical, and prostate cancers and can be accessed at www.nccn.org/professionals/physician_gls/f_guidelines.asp.

National Guideline Clearinghouse

The National Guideline Clearinghouse (NGC) is a public resource of evidence-based clinical practice guidelines. NGC is an initiative of the Agency for Healthcare Research and Quality of the U.S. Department of Health and Human Services (DHHS). NGC offers syntheses of selected guidelines and expert commentary on issues related to the use of clinical guidelines within the community. Guideline topics can be searched using the NGC Web site at www.guideline.gov.

Policies

The Secretary's Advisory Committee on Genetics, Health, and Society (SACGHS) provides policy advice to DHHS on the broad array of complex medical, ethical, legal, and social issues raised by the development and use of genetic technologies. Reports and correspondence, including SACGHS priorities, coverage and reimbursement, and education and training of health professionals are available on the SACGHS Web site at http://oba.od.nih.gov/SACGHS/sacghs_home.html. Slides and summaries from SACGHS meetings also are provided on this Web site. Nurses have been active as invited members of the SACGHS Committee and have provided testimony on important policy issues.

Genetic association studies explore the connection between specific genes, known as genotype information, and their outward expression, known as phenotype information. Genome-wide association (GWA) studies rely on newly available research tools and technologies to rapidly and cost-effectively analyze genetic differences between people with specific illnesses, such as diabetes or heart disease, compared to healthy individuals. The differences facilitate the identification of genetic risk factors for the development or progression of disease. Several investigators have launched or are planning GWA study initiatives with the expectation that the results will accelerate the development of better diagnostic tools and the design of new, safe, and highly effective treatments. Sensitive topics, such as the Policy for Sharing of Data Obtained in NIH-Supported or Conducted Genome-Wide Association Studies, have needed to be considered in the development of these studies. The policy calls for investigators funded by the NIH for GWA studies to (a) submit de-identified genetic (genotypic and phenotypic) data to a centralized NIH repository and (b) to submit documentation that describes how the investigators will protect the privacy and confidentiality of research participants. For more information, visit http://grants.nih.gov/grants/gwas.

RESEARCH OPPORTUNITIES

Compared to the rapid progress of scientific discoveries in genetics, integration of these findings with the behavioral sciences is progressing slowly. For nurses to assume a significant role in the adequate application of findings in cancer care, they must conduct research regarding the clinical application of bench research. The field of genetics and genomics offers a variety of opportunities for nursing research, from biologic studies to behavioral investigations (Conley & Tinkle, 2007). Of particular importance is the establishment of appropriate models for the education and counseling of patients and families and evaluation of the psychosocial effects of genetic testing. For more information about nursing research, refer to Chapter 15.

NHGRI Ethical, Legal, and Social Implications Research Program Grants

The ELSI Research Program funds and manages research grants and projects at institutions throughout the United States. Detailed information on specific programs and grant application instructions are available on the NHGRI Web site (www.genome.gov/10001618). ELSI also provides long- and short-term support for individual postdoctoral and senior fellowships to scientists seeking training that will enable them to investigate the clinical implications of human genetic research. Information about the research objectives and application procedures for these programs are available on the NINR Web site (www.ninr.nih.gov).

Genome-Wide Association Studies

A GWA study is an approach that involves rapidly scanning markers across the complete sets of DNA or genomes of many people to find genetic variations associated with a particular disease. Once new genetic associations are identified, researchers can use the information to develop better strategies to detect, treat, and prevent the disease. Results from GWA studies are being reported and replicated daily. A catalog of published GWA studies is available at www.genome.gov/26525384.

NIH, the Foundation for the NIH, Pfizer Global Research and Development, and others formed a public-private partnership, the Genetic Association Information Network (GAIN), to fund GWA studies. The initial studies include bipolar disorder, major depression, kidney disease in type 1 diabetes, attention-deficit hyperactivity disorder, schizophrenia, and psoriasis. More information about GAIN can be found at www.genome.gov/19518664.

The Genes, Environment, and Health Initiative is another NIH program that adds a unique component that speeds up the development of environmental exposure technology to produce new tools to study the interaction of genes and the environment. More information about the initiative can be found at www.genesandenvironment.nih.gov.

Cancer-Specific Projects With Funding Opportunities

NCI's Cancer Genome Anatomy Project's (CGAP's) goal is to determine the gene expression profiles of normal, precancer, and cancer cells. By collaborating with scientists worldwide, CGAP seeks to increase its scientific expertise and expand its databases for the benefit of all cancer researchers. For more information, visit http://cgap.nci.nih.gov.

The Cancer Genome Atlas (http://cancergenome.nih.gov/index.asp) is a comprehensive and coordinated effort to accelerate understanding of the molecular basis of cancer through the application of genome analysis technologies, including large-scale genome sequencing.

Funding Opportunities—International Society of Nurses in Genetics

The annual ISONG Nursing Research Grant is offered to support research related to genetic nursing practice or that which contributes to the development of genetic nursing science. Research areas should reflect clinical, professional, and societal issues in genetics that affect health and nursing practice related to genetics. Traditionally, ISONG funds one to two awards per year, $1,500 (maximum), for a period of up to 12 months. The grant award is contingent on the successful peer review of the application by the ISONG Research Committee (see www.isong.org).

Funding Opportunities—National Institute of Nursing Research

NINR supports clinical and basic research and research training on health and illness across the life span. The research focus encompasses health promotion, disease prevention, quality of life, health disparities, and end of life. NINR research opportunities are posted at www.ninr.nih.gov/ResearchAndFunding.

SUMMARY

The ongoing expansion of genetic and genomic information presents new challenges for oncology nurses. Understanding the advances in genetics and genomics and their impact on cancer prevention, diagnosis, and treatment is vital to providing comprehensive client education and care. Nursing professional groups are an excellent resource to aid nurses in processing the growing volume of complex information. Professional organizations of other specialties complement this resource and enhance communication within this multidisciplinary field.

Because of their prominent role in patient care, nurses must familiarize themselves with the increasingly significant impact of genetics and genomics in oncology care; they must possess a comprehensive knowledge of genetics and genomics and understand how to access pertinent information. Nurses need to recognize those individuals who could benefit from a referral to a cancer genetics program and acquaint themselves with available resources for assessment, diagnosis, and selection of individualized interventions.

REFERENCES

American Academy of Nursing. (2008). *About AAN*. Retrieved November 6, 2009, from http://www.aannet.org/i4a/pages/index.cfm?pageID=3284

American Society of Clinical Oncology. (2003). ASCO policy statement update: Genetic testing for cancer susceptibility. *Journal of Clinical Oncology, 21*(12), 2397–2406.

Conley, Y.P., & Tinkle, M.B. (2007). The future of genomic nursing research. *Journal of Nursing Scholarship, 39*(1), 17–24.

Consensus Panel on Genetic/Genomic Nursing Competencies. (2006). *Essential nursing competencies and curricula guidelines for genetics and genomics* (1st ed.). Silver Spring, MD: American Nurses Association.

Consensus Panel on Genetic/Genomic Nursing Competencies. (2009). *Essentials of genetic and genomic nursing: Competencies, curricula guidelines, and outcome indicators* (2nd ed.). Silver Spring, MD: American Nurses Association.

Guttmacher, A.E., Collins, F.S., & Carmona, R.H. (2004). The family history—more important than ever. *New England Journal of Medicine, 351*(22), 2333–2336.

International Society of Nurses in Genetics. (2007). *Statement on the scope and standards of genetics clinical nursing practice*. Washington, DC: American Nurses Publishing.

Jenkins, J., & Calzone, K. (2007). Genomics to health: Establishing the essential nursing competencies for genetics and genomics. *Journal of Nursing Scholarship, 39*(1), 10–16.

Monsen, R.B. (Ed.). (2005). *Genetics nursing portfolios: A new model for credentialing*. Silver Spring, MD: American Nurses Association.

Monsen, R.B. (Ed.). (2009). *Genetics and ethics in health care: New questions in the age of genomic health*. Silver Spring, MD: American Nurses Association.

National Coalition for Health Professional Education in Genetics. (2007). *Core competencies in genetics for health professionals* (3rd ed.). Retrieved November 6, 2009, from http://www.nchpeg.org/core/Core_Comps_English_2007.pdf

National Coalition for Health Professional Education in Genetics. (n.d.). *About*. Retrieved November 6, 2009, from http://www.nchpeg.org/content.aspx?sc=about&sub=1

Oncology Nursing Society. (2009a, March). *Cancer predisposition genetic testing and risk assessment counseling*. Retrieved November 5, 2009, from http://www.ons.org/Publications/Positions/media/ons/docs/positions/cancerpredisposition.pdf

Oncology Nursing Society. (2009b, March). *The role of the oncology nurse in cancer genetic counseling*. Retrieved November 5, 2009, from http://www.ons.org/Publications/Positions/media/ons/docs/positions/cancergenetic.pdf

Oncology Nursing Certification Corporation. (2009). *2010 oncology nursing certification test bulletin*. Retrieved November 6, 2008, from http://www.oncc.org/getcertified/TestInformation/docs/TestBulletin.pdf

Pletcher, B., Toriello, H., Noblin, S., Seaver, L., Driscoll, D., Bennett, R., et al. (2007). Indications for genetic referral: A guide for healthcare providers. *Genetics in Medicine, 9*(6), 385–389.

Robson, M.E., Storm, C.D., Weitzel, J., Wollins, D.S., Offit, K., & American Society of Clinical Oncology. (2010). American Society of Clinical Oncology policy statement update: Genetic and genomic testing for cancer susceptibility. *Journal of Clinical Oncology, 28*(5), 893–901.

Scanlon, C., & Fibison, W. (1995). *Managing genetic information: Implications for nursing practice*. Washington, DC: American Nurses Association.

Glossary

Some of the definitions in this glossary are based on definitions developed by the National Human Genome Research Institute (NHGRI). The editors of this text gratefully acknowledge the contributions of the NHGRI authors and refer the reader to the full version of the NHGRI glossary, which is available on the Internet at www.genome.gov/glossary.cfm.

A

abnormal gene expression. The process by which a gene is abnormally turned on in a cell to make RNA and proteins.

absolute risk. In regard to cancer, the measure of the occurrence of cancer, whether incidence (new cases) or mortality (deaths), in the general population.

accuracy. The degree to which a measurement represents the true value of the characteristic being measured.

adenine (A). One of the four bases in DNA. The others are guanine (G), cytosine (C), and thymine (T). Adenine always pairs with T.

allele. One of the variant forms of a gene at a particular locus, or location, on a chromosome. Different alleles produce variation in inherited characteristics (e.g., hair color, blood type). In an individual, one form of the allele (the dominant one) may be expressed more than another form (the recessive one).

allele frequency. The proportion of chromosomes in the population that carry the allele under consideration.

amino acid. One of 20 different kinds of small molecules that link in long chains to form proteins. Amino acids are often called the building blocks of proteins.

aneuploidy. Abnormal chromosome number.

antisense. Refers to the noncoding strand in double-stranded DNA. The antisense strand serves as the template for mRNA synthesis.

apoptosis. Programmed cell death, the body's normal method of disposing of damaged, unwanted, or unneeded cells.

attributable risk. In regard to cancer, the amount of cancer within a population that could be prevented by altering a risk factor.

autosomal dominant. A pattern of Mendelian inheritance whereby an affected individual possesses one copy of a mutant allele and one normal allele. (In contrast, recessive diseases require that the individual have two copies of the mutant allele.) Individuals with autosomal-dominant diseases have a 50-50 chance of passing the mutant allele (hence, the disorder) to their children. Examples of autosomal-dominant diseases include Huntington's disease, neurofibromatosis, and polycystic kidney disease.

autosome. Any chromosome other than a sex chromosome. Humans have 22 pairs of autosomes.

B

base pair. A set of two bases that form a "rung" of the DNA "ladder." The bases are adenine (A), thymine (T), guanine (G), and cytosine (C). A

DNA nucleotide is made of a molecule of sugar, a molecule of phosphoric acid, and a base. In base pairing, A always pairs with T, and G always pairs with C.

BRCA1, BRCA2. The first breast cancer genes to be identified. Mutated forms of these genes are believed to be responsible for about half the cases of inherited breast cancer, especially those that occur in younger women. Both are tumor suppressor genes.

C

candidate gene. A gene believed to influence expression of complex phenotypes because of known biologic and physiologic properties of its products, or to its location near a region of association or linkage.

cell. The basic unit of any living organism. A cell is a small, watery compartment filled with chemicals and a complete copy of the organism's genome.

chromatid. One of two identical halves of a replicated chromosome. During cell division, the chromosomes first replicate so that each daughter cell receives a complete set of chromosomes. Following DNA replication, the chromosome consists of two identical structures called sister chromatids, which are joined at the centromere.

centromere. A specialized chromosome region to which spindle fibers attach during cell division.

chromosome. One of the threadlike "packages" of genes and other DNA in the nucleus of a cell. Different kinds of organisms have different numbers of chromosomes. Humans have 23 pairs of chromosomes, 46 in all: 44 autosomes and two sex chromosomes. Each parent contributes one chromosome to each pair, so a child gets half his or her chromosomes from the mother and half from the father.

clonal population. A population of cells derived from a single cell and thus expected to be genetically identical. Genetic differences in a clonal population may arise from random spontaneous mutations during growth of the cells.

codon. Three bases, in a DNA or RNA sequence, that specify a single amino acid.

Common Disease, Common Variant hypothesis. The hypothesis that genetic influences on many common diseases will be at least partly attributable to a limited number of allelic variants (one or a few at each major disease locus) that are present in more than 1%–5% of the population.

complementary base pair. Two polynucleotide chains that can base-pair to form a double-stranded molecule. Nucleic acid base sequence that can form a double-stranded structure with another DNA fragment by following base-pairing rules (A pairs with T, and C with G). The complementary sequence to GTAC, for example, is CATG.

complex diseases (or complex traits). Traits that do not follow strict Mendelian inheritance and may be influenced by more than one gene and by the environment.

copy number variant. Stretches of genomic sequence of roughly 1 kb to 3 Mb in size that are deleted or are duplicated in varying numbers.

cytosine (C). One of the four bases in DNA. The others are adenine (A), guanine (G), and thymine (T). C always pairs with G.

D

deletion. A particular kind of mutation: loss of a piece of DNA from a chromosome. Deletion of a gene or part of a gene can lead to a disease or abnormality.

DNA replication. The process by which the DNA double helix unwinds and makes an exact copy of itself.

DNA sequence. The specific order of the bases arranged along one strand of the sugar-phosphate backbone.

dominant. In regard to a gene, a gene that almost always results in a specific physical characteristic (e.g., a disease), even though the patient's genome possesses only one copy. With a dominant gene, the chance of passing the gene (therefore, the disease) to children is 50-50 in each pregnancy.

E

enzyme. A protein that encourages a biochemical reaction, usually speeding it up. Organisms could not function if they had no enzymes.

epidermal growth factor receptor. A protein involved in normal cell growth. It is found on some types of cancer cells. Cancer cells removed from the body may be tested for the presence of human epidermal growth factor receptor to help decide the best type of treatment.

exon. The region of a gene that contains the code for producing the gene's protein. Each exon codes for a specific portion of the complete protein. In some species (including humans), a gene's exons are separated by long regions of DNA that have no apparent function. These regions are called introns or junk DNA.

F

false negative (FN). A test result indicating that the tested person does not have cancer, but he or she actually does have cancer.

false positive (FP). A test result indicating that the tested person has cancer, but he or she does not have cancer.

fibroblast. A type of cell found just underneath the surface of the skin. Fibroblasts are part of the support structure for tissues and organs.

fine mapping. Typing additional variants within an associated region to resolve the genetic locus associated with an outcome from a genomic region to, ideally, the base pair level.

fluorescence in situ hybridization (FISH). A process that involves painting chromosomes or portions of chromosomes with fluorescent molecules. This technique is useful for identifying chromosomal abnormalities and for gene mapping.

G

gene. The functional and physical unit of heredity passed from parent to offspring. Genes are pieces of DNA, and most genes contain the information for making a specific protein.

gene expression. The process by which proteins are made from the instructions encoded in DNA.

gene therapy. An evolving medical procedure, used to treat inherited diseases, that involves replacing, manipulating, or supplementing nonfunctional genes with healthy genes.

genetic code. The instructions in a gene that tell the cell how to make a specific protein. The instructions are sequences of the chemicals adenine (A), thymine (T), guanine (G), and cytosine (C). Each gene's code combines the four chemicals in various ways to spell out three-letter "words" that specify which amino acid is needed at every step in making a protein.

genetic heterogeneity. A single disorder, trait, or pattern of traits caused by different mutations within a gene.

genome. All the DNA contained in an organism or cell, including the chromosomes within the nucleus and the DNA in mitochondria.

genome-wide association study. Any study of genetic variation across the entire human genome designed to identify genetic association with observable traits or the presence or absence of a disease, usually referring to studies with genetic marker density of 100,000 or more to represent a large proportion of variation in the human genome.

genotype. Genetic identity that is not manifested as outward characteristics.

germ cell. Sperm and egg cells and their precursors. Germ cells are haploid and have only one set of chromosomes (23 in all), whereas all other cells have two copies (46 in all).

germ line. Inherited material that comes from eggs or sperm and that offspring inherit.

guanine (G). One of the four bases in DNA. The others are adenine (A), cytosine (C), and thymine (T). G always pairs with C.

H

Hardy-Weinberg equilibrium. Population distribution of two alleles (with frequencies p and q) such that the distribution is stable from generation to generation and genotypes occur at frequencies of p^2, $2pq$, and q^2 for the major allele homozygote, heterozygote, and minor allele homozygote, respectively; violations of HWE in GWA studies typically signify genotyping error.

heterozygous. Possessing two different forms of a particular gene, one inherited from each parent.

histone. A protein that provides structural support to a chromosome. In order for very long DNA molecules to fit into the cell nucleus, they wrap around complexes of histone proteins, giving the chromosome a more compact shape. Some variants of histones are associated with the regulation of gene expression.

homologous recombination repair. A mode of filling a gap in one strand of duplex DNA by retrieving a homologous single strand from another duplex.

homozygous. A genetic condition in which an individual inherits the same alleles for a particular gene from both parents.

Human Genome Project. An international research project to map each human gene and to completely sequence human DNA.

I

incidence. In regard to cancer, the number of cancers that develop in a population during a defined period (e.g., one year).

inherited. Transmitted through genes from parents to offspring.

insertion. A type of chromosomal abnormality in which a DNA sequence is inserted into a gene, disrupting the normal structure and function of that gene.

interaction. Modification of gene-disease associations in the presence of environmental or other genetic factors.

International HapMap Project. Genome-wide database of patterns of common human genetic sequence variation among multiple ancestral population samples.

intron. A portion of a gene that does not code for amino acids. In the cells of plants and animals, most gene sequences are broken up by one or more introns. The parts of the gene sequence that are expressed in the protein are called *exons*, because they are expressed, whereas the parts of the gene sequence that are not expressed in the protein are called *introns*, because they come in between the exons.

K

karyotype. The chromosomal complement of an individual, including all the chromosomes and any abnormalities. The term also refers to a photograph of an individual's chromosomes.

L

linkage. The tendency for genes or segments of DNA closely positioned along a chromosome to segregate together at meiosis and therefore be inherited together.

linkage disequilibrium. Association between two alleles located near each other on a chromosome, such that they are inherited together more frequently than expected by chance.

M

Mendelian error. An inconsistency in genotyping where a child's genotype is not compatible with the genotypes of his or her reported parents.

meiosis. The formation of egg and sperm cells.

messenger ribonucleic acid (mRNA). The template for protein synthesis. Each set of three bases, called codons, specifies a certain protein in the sequence of amino acids that composes the protein. The sequence of a strand of mRNA is based on the sequence of a complementary strand of DNA.

microarray. A new way of studying how large numbers of genes interact with each other and how a cell's regulatory networks control vast batteries of genes simultaneously. The method uses a robot, which precisely applies tiny droplets containing functional DNA to glass slides. Researchers then attach fluorescent labels to DNA from the cell they are studying. The labeled probes are allowed to bind to complementary DNA strands on the slides. The slides are put into a scanning microscope that can measure the brightness of each fluorescent dot; brightness reveals how much of a specific DNA fragment is present, an indicator of how active it is.

microsatellite. A repetitive short sequence of DNA that is used as a genetic marker to track inheritance in families.

minor allele frequency. The proportion of chromosomes in the population that carry the minor (or less common) allele of a polymorphism.

mitosis. The type of cell division that occurs in the replication of somatic cells.

mortality rate. In regard to cancer, the number of people who die of a particular cancer during a defined period.

mutation. A permanent structural alteration in DNA. In most cases, DNA changes either have no effect or cause harm. Occasionally, however, a mutation improves an organism's chance of surviving.

mutator gene. A gene that increases the rate of mutation of one or more other genes; also called *mutator*.

N

nominal significance. A standard of statistical significance that meets a specific threshold (commonly $p < 0.05$) but does not account for having performed many statistical tests.

non-directive counseling. Refers to the nature of the genetic counseling process. According to the principle of non-directiveness, the counselor has the responsibility to provide the client with accurate information about a test or outcome but should remain neutral and not try to influence the decisions made by the client.

nonsense point mutation. A single DNA base substitution resulting in a stop codon.

nucleotide. One of the structural components, or building blocks, of DNA and RNA. A nucleotide consists of a base (one of four chemicals: adenine, thymine, guanine, and cytosine) plus one molecule of sugar and one molecule of phosphoric acid.

nucleotide excision repair. A DNA repair mechanism that recognizes damaged regions based on their abnormal DNA structure as well as their abnormal chemistry, and then excises and replaces them.

nucleus. The central cell structure that houses the chromosomes.

O

odds ratio. Odds of disease in persons carrying the risk variant divided by odds in the persons without it.

oligo. Oligonucleotide.

oligonucleotide. A short sequence synthesized to match a region where a mutation is known to occur and then used as a probe.

oncogene. A gene that is capable of causing the transformation of normal cells into cancer cells.

outcome. A benefit, harm, or cost of screening or testing or a diagnostic evaluation that results from screening or testing.

P

phenotype. The physical characteristics of an organism or the presence of a disease that may or may not be genetic.

ploidy. The status of multiplication of chromosome sets (e.g., aneuploidy, diploidy, haploidy).

polymerase. An enzyme that catalyzes the breakdown of nucleotides to polynucleotides.

polymerase chain reaction (PCR). A fast, inexpensive technique for making an unlimited number of copies of any piece of DNA. Sometimes called molecular photocopying, PCR has had an immense impact on biology and medicine, especially genetic research.

population. In regard to cancer, the number of people in a defined group who are capable of developing cancer. It may refer to the general population or a specific group of people defined by geographic, physical, or social characteristics.

population attributable risk. An estimate of the proportion of disease in a population that is associated with a genetic variant.

population stratification (also population structure). A form of confounding in genetic association studies caused by genetic differences between cases and controls unrelated to disease but because of sampling them from populations of different ancestries.

prevalence. In regard to cancer, the actual number of cancers in a defined population at a given time. Usually expressed as the number of cancers per 100,000 individuals.

primary cancer prevention. Measures to avoid carcinogen exposure and improve health practices. In some cases, primary cancer prevention includes the use of chemopreventive agents or prophylactic surgery.

promoter. The part of a gene that contains the information to turn the gene on or off. The process of transcription is initiated at the promoter.

protein. A large, complex molecule made up of one or more chains of amino acids. Proteins perform a wide variety of activities in the cell.

proto-oncogene. A gene involved in regulating cell growth. When transformed through mutation, a proto-oncogene becomes an oncogene involved in unregulated or uncontrolled cell growth.

p value. The probability of observing an association as extreme as the one reported, assuming the association truly did not exist.

R

recessive. A genetic disorder that appears only in patients who have received two copies of a mutant gene, one from each parent.

reciprocal translocation. When a pair of chromosomes exchange exactly the same length and area of DNA. Results in a shuffling of genes.

recombination. A type of genetic recombination that occurs during meiosis (the formation of egg and sperm cells). Paired chromosomes from the male and female parent align so that similar DNA sequences from the paired chromosomes cross over each other. Crossing over results in a shuffling of genetic material and is an important cause of the genetic variation seen among offspring.

reference SNP (rs) number. Unique identifying number for a SNP from the National Center for Biotechnology Information's dbSNP database.

relative risk (RR). In regard to cancer, a comparison of the incidence of a risk factor or the number of deaths among those with the risk factor compared to those without the risk factor.

ribonucleic acid (RNA). A chemical whose composition is similar to a single strand of DNA. In RNA, however, uracil (U), replaces thymine (T) in the genetic code. RNA delivers DNA's genetic message to the cytoplasm of a cell where proteins are made.

ribosome. Cellular organelle that is the site of protein synthesis.

risk factor. A trait or characteristic associated with a statistically significant increased likelihood of developing a disease.

S

secondary cancer prevention. Identifying people at risk of malignancy and implementing appropriate screening recommendations.

sensitivity. In regard to cancer, the ability of a screening test to detect individuals with cancer. It is calculated by dividing the total number of true positives by the total number of cancer cases.

signal transduction. The process by which a cell responds to substances in its environment. The binding of a substance to a molecule on the surface of a cell causes signals to be passed from one molecule to another inside the cell. These signals can affect many functions of the cell, including cell division and cell death. Cells that have permanent changes in signal transduction molecules may develop into cancer.

single locus. The site of a gene on a chromosome.

single nucleotide polymorphism (SNP). Site within the genome that differs by a single nucleotide base across different individuals.

splicing. The process by which introns, noncoding regions, are excised (spliced) out of the primary messenger RNA transcript and exons (i.e., coding regions) are joined together to generate mature messenger RNA.

somatic cells. All body cells, except the reproductive cells.

specificity. In regard to cancer, the ability of a test to identify individuals who do not have cancer. Specificity is calculated by dividing the total number of true negatives by the sum of the number of true negative and false positive results.

T

tag SNP. A readily-measured SNP that is in strong linkage disequilibrium with multiple other SNPs so that it can serve as a proxy for these SNPs on large-scale genotyping platforms.

telomere. The end of a chromosome. This specialized structure is involved in the replication and stability of linear DNA molecules.

tertiary cancer prevention. Monitoring for and preventing recurrence of a previously diagnosed cancer and screening for second primary cancers.

thymine (T). One of the four bases in DNA. The others are adenine (A), guanine (G), and cytosine (C). T always pairs with A.

TP53. A gene that normally regulates the cell cycle and protects a cell from damage to its genome. Mutations in this gene cause cells to develop cancerous abnormalities.

transcription. The process of transforming information from DNA into a single-stranded RNA molecule.

transforming growth factor-beta. One of the growth factors made by the body that functions to regulate cell division and cell survival. Some growth factors also are produced in the laboratory and used in biologic therapy.

translation. The synthesis of amino acids, which then become proteins, from the mRNA template.

translocation. Breakage and removal of a large segment of DNA from one chromosome, followed by the segment's attachment to a different chromosome.

true negative (TN). A test result indicating that the tested person does not have cancer and, indeed, the person neither has nor develops cancer within a defined period.

true positive (TP). A test result indicating that the tested person has cancer and, indeed, the person does have cancer.

tumor suppressor gene. A protective gene that normally limits the growth of tumors. When a tumor suppressor is mutated, it may fail to keep a cancer from growing. *BRCA1* is a well-known tumor suppressor gene.

U

uracil (U). One of the four bases in RNA. The others are adenine (A), guanine (G), and cytosine (C). Like thymine (T), U always pairs with A.

V

validity. A measure of how well a test measures what it is supposed to measure.

W

wild-type. The normal, as opposed to the mutant, gene or allele.

winner's curse. Tendency for an initial study to report an association that is stronger than its actual effect.

Note. Based on information from Genetics Home Reference. (n.d.). *Glossary.* Retrieved January 19, 2010, from http://ghr.nlm.nih.gov/glossary; Human Genome Project. (n.d.). *Genome glossary.* Retrieved January 19, 2010, from http://www.ornl.gov/sci/techresources/Human_Genome/glossary; Lewin, B. (2008). *Genes IX* (9th ed.). Sudbury, MA: Jones and Bartlett; National Human Genome Research Institute. (n.d.). *Talking glossary of genetic terms.* Retrieved January 19, 2010, from http://www.genome.gov/glossary.cfm; Pearson, T.A., & Manolio, T.A. (2008). How to interpret a genome-wide association study. *JAMA, 299*(11), 1335–1344; U.S. Department of Health and Human Services, U.S. Food and Drug Administration. (2010). *Drugs@FDA glossary of terms.* Retrieved March 17, 2010, from http://www.fda.gov/Drugs/InformationOnDrugs/ucm079436.htm#D.

Index

The letter f after a page number indicates that relevant content appears in a figure; the letter t, in a table.

A

ABL proto-oncogene, 37
abnormal gene expression, 339
absolute risk, 83, 87t, 339
absorption, 201
ACCE model, 259, 307t, 307–308, 314t
acculturative stress, 274
accuracy, of genetic testing, 82, 339
acquired mutations, 26
activator protein-1 (AP-1) activity, 33
acute myeloid leukemia, M3 variant, 212
adenine (A), 16, 17f, 339
adenomas, 26
adenomatous polyposis coli *(APC)* gene, 29t, 35
adenomatous polyps, 56, 62, 90
Adjuvant! Online algorithm, 178t, 186, 188
admixtures, 211
adrenocortical carcinoma, 65–66
Advanced Oncology Certified Clinical Nurse Specialist (AOCNS®), 301
Advanced Oncology Certified Nurse (AOCN®), 301
Advanced Oncology Certified Nurse Practitioner (AOCNP®), 301
Advanced Practice Nurse in Genetics (APNG), 302
Advanced Practice Oncology Nurse (APON), 6, 6f, 8–9, 290, 292, 323
Advanced Practice Oncology Nurse with Genetics Subspecialty, 6, 6f, 9–10, 10t, 292–293, 323
advanced practice registered nurse (APRN), 299
Affymetrix genotyping platform, 161
African American population
 definition of family, 275
 mistrust toward health agencies, 272–274
 prostate cancer in, 270
 spirituality in, 276, 278
alanine, 21f
alcohol consumption, as cancer risk, 58
allele frequencies, 159–160, 339
alleles, 18, 83, 203, 339
ambiguous results, 117f, 119, 147
American Academy of Family Physicians (AAFP), 320t, 326–327
American Academy of Nursing (AAN), 320t, 324
American Board of Genetic Counseling (ABGC), 325
American Board of Medical Genetics (ABMG), 320t, 325–327
American Board of Nursing Specialties (ABNS), 299
American Cancer Society (ACS)
 early detection guidelines, 60t–61t
 incidence/prevalence data, 81–82
American College of Medical Genetics (ACMG), 320t, 326–327
American Medical Association (AMA), 320t–321t, 326–327
 family history tools, 68t, 170
American Nurses Association (ANA), 320t, 324–325
 Center for Ethics and Human Rights, 325
 scope of nursing practice, 4, 299, 302, 324–325
American Society of Clinical Oncology (ASCO), 320t, 326
 breast cancer treatment guidelines, 185
 genetic testing guidelines, 52, 80, 109, 113, 259–260
American Society of Human Genetics (ASHG), 257–258, 262f, 320t, 324, 326
amino acid chains, 23
amino acids, 19f, 20–21, 21f, 22, 25, 339
amino acid sequences, 25
amplification, 37
analytic sensitivity, 82
analytic specificity, 82
analytic validity, 82, 307, 307t
aneuploidy, 37, 339
angiogenesis, 32, 228, 229f

347

aniridia, 56
anonymous markers, 155
anti-oncogenes. *See* tumor suppressor genes
antisense, 339
antisense oligonucleotides, 225
APC (adenomatous polyposis coli) gene, 35–36, 110, 113
apoptosis, 42, 339
arginine, 21*f*
Ashkenazi Jewish population, 72–73, 81, 89*f*, 270
Asian populations, 275–276, 278–279
asparagine, 21*f*
aspartic acid, 21*f*
assessments. *See* cancer genetic risk assessments
Association of Pediatric Hematology/Oncology Nurses, 301
assumed hereditary, 50
ATM gene, 36
attributable risk, 84, 339
autonomy, 247–250, 249*f*
autopsy reports, 71
autosomal dominance, 339
autosomes, 14, 339

B

bar graphs, for risk communication, 94, 95*f*
basal cell nevus syndrome, 54*t*
basal cells, 62
base excision repair, 38
base pairs, 14, 15*f*, 16, 17*f*, 339–340
BCL gene, 42
BCR-ABL fusion gene, 37, 212, 229
beneficence, 247, 250–251, 251*f*
Bethesda criteria, for colorectal cancer, 74, 90, 91*f*
bevacizumab, 226*t*, 228*f*, 228–229, 234–235

bilateral disease, as hallmark of hereditary syndrome, 65
billing, 134–138, 135*t*, 136*f*
bioinformatics, 193–194
biomarkers, 311
Biomarkers Consortium, 311, 314*t*
Biomarkers Definitions Working Group, 311
biotechnical information, 193–194
biotransformation. *See* drug metabolism
birth defects, 56
bleeding, from targeted therapies, 234
body mass index, 57
bortezomib, 226*t*
BRCA1/BRCA2 mutations, 61–64, 86, 110, 340
male carriers of, 72, 83
phenocopy cases in, 118
prediction models for, 87*t*, 89*f*–90*f*
risk assessment tool for, 87*t*
BRCA1 gene, xv, 14, 26, 29*t*, 62, 340
BRCA2 gene, 35, 340
BRCAPRO assessment tool, 87*t*
breast cancer. *See also* hereditary breast/ovarian cancer
genome-wide association studies on, 153*t*–154*t*, 159
incidence of, 82
in males, 72, 83
mortality rates for, 82
screening for, 60*t*
treatment guidelines, 185–188
triple-negative, 62
tumor profiling in, 179–180, 185–190, 210, 308–309
breast magnetic resonance imaging, 60*t*
breast self-examination (BSE), 60*t*
Burkitt lymphoma, 37, 191*f*, 191–192

C

calcium, and polyps formation, 59
cancer development, models of, 13–14, 34
Cancer Genetic Markers of Susceptibility (CGEMS) project, xvi, 310, 314*t*
cancer genetic risk assessment programs (CGRAPs), 129–130
client follow-up in, 145–147
client identification/selection for, 143–144
financial considerations, 133–138, 135*t*, 136*f*–137*f*
intake process in, 54–64, 55*f*, 144
multidisciplinary team for, 131–133, 133*f*
needs assessment for, 130, 131*f*
procedures/policies for, 138–141
program/visit designs for, 142–143, 145, 146*t*
quality assurance in, 147–148
scope of services in, 141
strategic planning committee for, 130–131, 132*t*
cancer genetic risk assessments, 49–50, 80–81
components of, 55*f*, 55–64. *See also* family history; physical examination; psychosocial assessment
environment for, 70
examples of, 72–74, 73*f*–74*f*
limitations of, 71–72, 86
motivation for, 69, 106–107, 110
process of, 70–71
purpose of, 50–52
sequence of, 71

terminology in, 80–84
Cancer Genetics Services Directory, 130, 170
Cancer Genome Anatomy Project (CGAP), xvi, 178, 217, 311, 314*t*, 322*t*
The Cancer Genome Atlas (TCGA), xvi, 193–194, 312, 314*t*, 322*t*, 336
Cancer Genome Project (CGP), 314*t*
Cancer Library, 333
Cancer Molecular Analysis Project, 217
Cancer Predisposition Genetic Testing and Risk Assessment Counseling (ONS), 322
cancer stem cell model, 13–14
cancer stem cells, 14
cancer vaccines, 225, 225*f*
candidate genes, 152, 340
carcinogenesis, xv*f*, 13–14, 34
Carney complex type 1, 69–70
CDH1 gene, 86
cell, 340
cell cycle, 40*f*, 40–42, 41*t*
cell division, 17, 23, 40
cell signaling, 218, 219*f*, 222. *See also* signal transduction
cell surface receptors, 204, 219*f*, 219–221
Centers for Disease Control and Prevention (CDC)
family history resources, 68*t*
Office for Public Health Genomics (OPHG), 170, 312, 315*t*, 321*t*, 331–332
Office of Minority Health and Health Disparities, 271–272
Centers for Medicare and Medicaid Services (CMS), 135*t*, 137

centromeres, 14, 15f–16f, 340
certification, 299, 301–303, 302f, 303. *See also* credentialing
Certified Breast Care Nurse (CBCN®), 301
Certified Pediatric Hematology/Oncology Nurse (CPHON), 301
Certified Pediatric Oncology Nurse (CPON®), 301
cervical cancer, screening for, 60t–61t
cetuximab, 209, 226t, 231, 235
checkpoint genes, 41, 41t
ChemBank Web site, 193
chemoprevention, 210
children
  disclosing family results to, 112–113
  genetic testing of, 113, 259–260
chromatids, 14, 15f–16f, 340
chromosomal abnormalities, 36–37
chromosomal deletions, 25, 25f–26f, 37, 340
chromosomal fragile sites, 36
chromosomal translocations, 36–37, 212, 229, 344–345
chromosomes, 14–18, 15f–17f, 19f–20f, 340
chronic myeloid leukemia (CML), reciprocal translocation in, 36–37, 212, 229, 243
Cincinnati Children's Hospital Medical Center
  Genetics Education Program for Nurses (GEPN), 320t, 328
  Web-Based Genetics Institute (WBGI), 320t, 328
City of Hope, Cancer Genetics Career Development Program, 320t, 328–329

client advocacy, 254–256
clinical breast examination (CBE), 60t
Clinical Journal of Oncology Nursing, 323
Clinical Laboratory Improvement Act (CLIA), 140
clinical trials, 190, 308–309, 315t
clinical utility, 83, 307, 307t
clinical validity, 82–83, 307, 307t
clonal evolution, 27
clonal population, 23, 27, 340
cloning, 260
Coalition for Genetic Fairness, 262f
coding, for medical billing, 135t, 137
codons, 20–21, 21f, 340
cognitive alterations, from targeted therapies, 235–236
cognitive assessment, 69
colonoscopy, 60t
colony-stimulating factor, 33
colorectal cancer
  Bethesda criteria for, 74, 90, 91f
  genetic basis of, 26–28, 27f
  genome-wide association studies on, 154t, 159, 165f
  screening for, 60t
common disease, common variant hypothesis, 151–152, 340
competencies. *See also* credentialing
  establishment of, 300t, 300–301
  in genetics/genomics, 291t–292t, 293–294
complementary base pairs, 16–17, 340
complementary DNA (cDNA), 180–183, 182f–184f
complex diseases/traits, 340
computed tomography colonography, 60t

computer-based genetic counseling, 122
Concise Handbook of Familial Cancer Susceptibility Syndromes, 52, 81, 109
confidentiality, 112, 115–116, 120, 141, 252–254, 253f
continuing education, 287–289, 288t
  examples of, 293–294
  recommendations for, 289–294
  resources for, 320t, 327–328. *See also* credentialing
copy number variants, 161, 340
Core Competencies in Genetics for Health Professionals (NCHPEG), 261, 326
Cowden syndrome, 53t, 88–89
CpG dinucleotide, 28
CpG islands, 28
credentialing, 298, 300t, 300–301, 323–324
  future directions in, 303
  in genetics, 292–293, 301–303, 302f
  in oncology, 301
  types of, 298–300
cross talk, 223
cultural background, 251–252, 252f, 268–269
  assessment of, 63–64
  and beliefs about disease, 98
  and language differences, 276
cultural competence, 279, 279f, 280t, 280f. *See also* multicultural considerations
Current Procedural Terminology (CPT) codes, 135t, 137
cyclin-dependent kinases (CDKs), 41
cyclins, 41
CYP2D6 enzyme, 200

CYP3A enzymes, 202
CYP450 enzymes, 200–204, 203t, 232
  mutations in ethnic groups, 210–211
  nomenclature of, 201–202
Cyrillic (pedigree software), 68t, 321t, 332
cysteine, 21f
cytochrome P450 (CYP450) enzyme family, 200–204, 203t, 232
  mutations in ethnic groups, 210–211
  nomenclature of, 201–202
cytosine (C), 16, 17f, 340

D

dasatinib, 226t
death certificates, 71
deletions, 25, 25f–26f, 37, 340
Department of Energy Genome Glossary, 170
depression, from targeted therapies, 235–236
dermatologic toxicities, from targeted therapies, 232–233, 233t
diarrhea, from targeted therapies, 234
diet, and cancer risk, 57
diffuse large b-cell lymphoma, 191f, 191–192
digital rectal examination (DRE), 61t
dihydropyrimidine dehydrogenase (DPD), 207–208
dimer, 221
dimerization, 219f, 221
Ding mutation, 36
direct-to-consumer (DTC) genetic testing, 140, 257–258
discrimination
  employment, 115–116, 255–256, 272, 333–334
  genetic, 115–116, 255–256, 272, 333–334
  racial, 273

distress, during genetic counseling, 107–108, 111
DNA, 14–18, 15f–17f, 19f–20f, 22f
DNA chips, 212–213
DNA microarrays, 180–184, 181f–184f, 212–213
DNA recombination, 23–24
DNA repair genes, 35–36
DNA repair mechanisms, 38–40
DNA replication, 23, 340
DNA sequencing, 16–17, 212, 340
documentation
  of family history, 71, 114
  of informed consent, 114
dominance, 155, 339–341
double-contrast barium enema, 60t
double helix, 16–17, 17f
double minutes, 37
DPYD gene, 207–208
drug absorption, 201
drug effect, 204
drug excretion, 201, 203
drug metabolism, 201–203, 202f, 203t
  pathways of, 204–205, 205f
dry skin, from targeted therapies, 233, 233t
"duty to warn" laws, 112
dysplastic nevi, 56

E

early detection. *See* screening
economic considerations
  for cancer genetic risk assessment programs, 133–138, 135t, 136f–137f
  with genetic testing, 110–111, 114–116, 188
electronic health records (EHRs), 254
embryonic stem cell research, 260
employment discrimination, 115–116, 255–256, 272, 333–334

Encyclopedia of DNA Elements (ENCODE) project, 311, 314t
endocrine cancer, 54t
endometrial biopsy, 61t
endometrial cancer, screening for, 61t
environmental exposures, 57, 274
enzymes, 200–204, 203t, 206–207, 207f, 210–211, 232, 341
epidermal growth factor (EGF), 33, 230, 230f
epidermal growth factor receptor (EGFR), 32, 209, 230, 230f, 231, 341
epidermal growth factor receptor inhibitors, 209, 211–212, 229–234
epigenetics, 28–29
ERBB2/HER2/neu, 32, 37, 179–180, 224
erlotinib, 209–210, 212, 226t, 231–233
erythroblastic leukemia viral oncogene homolog 2 (HER2/neu/ERBB2), 32, 37, 179–180, 224
Essential Nursing Competencies and Curricula Guidelines for Genetics and Genomics, xvii, 325
Essentials of Genetic and Genomic Nursing, 243–244, 249, 261, 290, 293
estrogen receptors (ERs), in breast cancer, 179, 186, 210
ethical assessment framework (EAF), 247, 248f
ethical issues
  in genomic health care, 243–249, 244f–246f, 256–260, 257f
  personal biases and, 248–249, 249f

resources on, 260–262, 262f–263f
with test results, 120–121, 307, 307t
ethical theories/principles, 247, 247f
ethnic background, 251–252, 252f, 268–270
  in assessment process, 63–64
  and beliefs about disease, 98
  and language differences, 276
  pharmacogenomics and, 210–211
evaluation/management (E/M) services, 138
Evaluation of Genomic Applications in Practice and Prevention (EGAPP) project, xxii, 192, 262f, 312–313, 315t, 331–332
excretion, 201, 203
exercise, assessment of, 57–58
exons, 18, 19f, 341
extensive/effective metabolizers (EMs), 204, 205f

F

Facing Our Risk of Cancer Empowered (FORCE), 321t, 330–331
false negative (FN) results, 163, 341
false positive (FP) results, 157, 163, 341
familial adenomatous polyposis (FAP), 53t, 62, 90, 110
familial cancer susceptibility syndromes, 50–55, 53t–54t. *See also specific syndromes*
familial medullary thyroid cancer, 62
Family as Context in Clinical Genetics Project (FCCGP), 320t, 329

family covenant, for disclosing results, 112
family history, 50–51, 51t, 64f, 64–68
  limitations of, 71–72, 86
  multicultural considerations in, 274–276
  resources on, 331–332
  verification of, 71
family issues, in genetic counseling, 111–112, 117, 120, 122–123
family, multicultural definitions of, 275
family studies, 152–155
fat intake, 57
fecal immunochemical test (FIT), 60t
fecal occult blood test (FOBT), 60t
fiber intake, 57
fibroblast, 341
fibroblast growth factor, 32
financial considerations
  for cancer genetic risk assessment programs, 133–138, 135t, 136f–137f
  with genetic testing, 110–111, 114–116, 188
fine mapping, 155, 166, 341
first-degree relatives, 67
5-fluorouracil (5-FU), 207–208
flexible sigmoidoscopy, 60t
fluorescence in situ hybridization (FISH), 341
follicular lymphoma, 42, 191
follow-up, after genetic testing, 121, 123–124, 145–147
FORCE (Facing Our Risk of Cancer Empowered), 321t, 330–331
formalin-fixed, paraffin-embedded (FFPE) tissue, 185
founder effect, 64, 81, 270
Fox Chase Cancer Center, Personalized Cancer Risk Assessment program, 320t, 327–328
fragile sites, 36
frameshift mutations, 25, 26f

framing, of risk information, 93–94
funding, resources for, 322*t*, 335–336

G

G₁/S checkpoint, 41, 41*t*
G₂ checkpoint, 41*t*
gain-of-function events, 31
gametes. *See* germ cells
Garrod, Archibald, 199
gastrointestinal cancer, 53*t*–54*t*
gastrointestinal perforation, from targeted therapies, 235
gefitinib, 209–212, 226*t*
gene expression, 18–23, 21*f*–22*f*, 308, 341. *See also* tumor profiling
gene products, 21
gene profiling. *See* tumor profiling
General Oncology Nurse (GON), 6*f*, 6–8, 323
General Oncology Nurse with Genetics Subspecialty, 6, 6*f*, 8, 292–293
genes, 17–18, 19*f*, 341
Genes, Environment and Health Initiative (GEI), 322*t*
gene signature tumor profiling. *See* tumor profiling
GeneTests (online resource), 55, 109–110, 135, 135*t*, 170, 321*t*, 331
gene therapy, 341
genetic admixtures, 211
Genetic Alliance, 171, 262*f*–263*f*, 321*t*, 331, 334
Genetic and Rare Diseases Information Center (GARD), 170, 263*f*, 321*t*, 331
Genetic Association Information Network (GAIN), 322*t*
genetic code, 18–21, 19*f*, 341
genetic counseling/education, 104, 109, 119–123.
See also risk communication
delivery options for, 105–106
environment for, 70, 120
model for, 105*f*
nurses' role in, 104–108, 108*f*
psychosocial issues in, 107–108, 108*f*
resources for, 106*t*
genetic discoveries, timeline of, xiv*f*
genetic discrimination, 115–116, 255–256, 272, 333–334
genetic/genomic assessment. *See* cancer genetic risk assessments
genetic heterogeneity, 82, 85–86, 167, 341
Genetic Information Nondiscrimination Act (GINA) (2008), 115, 255, 273
Genetic Nursing Credentialing Commission (GNCC), 293, 299, 302–304, 320*t*, 324
genetic profile, 177. *See also* tumor profiling
Genetics and Ethics in Health Care: New Questions in the Age of Genomic Health, 324
Genetics and Public Policy Center, 140
Genetics Clinical Nurse (GCN), 302
genetics/genomics curricula, 287–294. *See also* continuing education
Genetics/Genomics Nursing: Scope and Standards of Practice, 103–104, 302, 323–324
genetics/genomics specialty, 5–6, 6*f*, 8–10, 10*t*, 292–293, 323. *See also* credentialing
Genetics Home Reference, 170–171, 263*f*
Genetics in Oncology Nursing: Cancer Risk Assessment, xiii, xvii
Genetics Nursing Portfolios: A New Model for Credentialing (ANA), 324
genetic testing, 79
barriers to, 110*f*
of children, 113, 259–260
cost of, 135–136. *See also* economic considerations
direct-to-consumer, 140, 257–258
in family history, 66–67
guidelines for, 52, 109–110
informed decision-making about, 110–113, 249–250, 277
motivation for, 69, 106–107, 110
oversight of, 258–259
results disclosure, 119–123
genetic variants, 270
genome, 341
genome-wide association (GWA) studies, 151, 158*f*, 160–164, 256, 277, 310, 322*t*, 335–336, 341
evolution of, 152–158
future directions in, 167–168
limitations of, 166–167, 169*f*
resources on, 169–171
site-specific results, 153*t*–154*t*, 159–160, 161*t*, 164*f*–165*f*
table of results, 153*t*–154*t*, 163
Genomic Access Program, of Genomic Health, Inc., 188
Genomics and Your Health (Web site), 263*f*
genotypes, 28, 341
genotyping platforms, 160–161. *See also* genome-wide association studies

germ cells, 17, 341
germ line, 341
germ line mutations, 23, 36
glutamic acid, 21*f*
glutamine, 21*f*
glycine, 21*f*
Gorlin syndrome, 54*t*
G proteins, 33
grapefruit juice, 202–203
graphs, for risk communication, 94, 95*f*
growth factor receptors, 30*f*, 32, 219*f*
growth factors, 30*f*, 32–33
guanine (G), 16, 17*f*, 342
guidelines
for breast cancer treatment, 186–188
for genetic testing, 52, 109–110, 321*t*–322*t*, 334
for risk assessment, 80
for screening, 60*t*–61*t*, 90, 123
on testing in children, 113, 259–260

H

hair/nail changes, from targeted therapies, 233*t*
Haldane, J.B.S., 199
haplotype blocks, 151
Hardy-Weinberg equilibrium, 162, 342
healthcare provider taxonomy code, 137
health disparities, 110–111, 255, 271
health history, 55–57
health insurance, 110–111, 114–116, 188. *See also* reimbursement
Health Insurance Portability and Accountability Act (HIPAA) (1996), 115–116
Health Care Provider Taxonomy Code Set, 135*t*, 137
health literacy, 276
hemorrhage, from targeted therapies, 234

HER2/neu/ERBB2, 32, 37, 179–180, 224
hereditary breast/ovarian cancer (HBOC), 53*t*, 72–73, 81, 86
  case study of, 88–89, 89*f*–90*f*
  guidelines for testing, 109–110
  risk assessment tool for, 87*t*
hereditary cancer syndromes, 50, 64, 64*f*, 109–110. *See also* family history; *specific syndromes*
hereditary diffuse gastric cancer, 54*t*, 86
hereditary nonpolyposis colorectal cancer. *See* Lynch syndrome
heterodimerization, 219*f*, 221
heterogeneity, 82, 85–86, 167, 341
heterozygosity, 18, 205, 342
  loss of, 34–35
Hispanic populations, 275–276, 278
histidine, 21*f*
histograms, for risk communication, 94, 97*f*
histones, 14, 15*f*, 342
homodimerization, 219*f*, 221
homologous recombination repair, 39, 342
homozygosity, 18, 34, 204, 342
human cloning, 260
human epidermal growth factor receptor (HER) family, 32, 37, 179–180, 224
human genome, 14, 16–17
Human Genome Epidemiology Network (HuGENet™), 307, 315*t*, 321*t*, 329
Human Genome Project, xiii, 106*t*, 178, 180, 201, 204, 333, 342
human leukocyte antigen (HLA) matching, 258
human papillomavirus (HPV) DNA test, 61*t*

hypermethylation, 28–29, 29*t*
hyperplastic polyps, 62
hypersensitivity reactions, from targeted therapies, 233*t*, 235
hypertension, from targeted therapies, 234
hypoxia, 32

I

ibritumomab, 226*t*
ICD-9 codes, 135*t*, 137
idiosyncratic reactions, 201
Illumina genotyping platform, 161
imatinib, 212, 226*t*, 229, 243
immunohistochemistry (IHC) testing, 63, 91
immunotherapy, 225
incidence, 82, 342
induction, of CYP enzyme system, 202–203, 203*f*
infertility, history of, 56
INFOGENETICS, 321*t*, 329
information management, in cancer genetic risk assessment program, 141
informed consent, 114, 250, 250*f*, 277
infusion reactions, from targeted therapies, 235
inheritance, 342
inherited genetic disorders, 26
inhibition, of CYP enzyme system, 202–203, 203*f*
insertion, 25, 25*f*–26*f*, 342
insurance. *See* health insurance
interaction, 167, 342
intermediate metabolizers (IMs), 205*f*
International Classification of Diseases (ICD), 135*t*, 137
International HapMap Project, 151, 157, 342

International Society of Nurses in Genetics (ISONG), 170, 261, 262*f*, 320*t*, 322*t*, 323–325
  funding opportunities, 336
  scope of nursing practice, 4, 105, 293, 302, 323–324
Internet resources
  for billing/reimbursement, 135*t*
  for genetics/genomics, 320*t*–322*t*
  for molecular genomics technology, 194*t*
  for psychosocial support, 121
interstitial lung disease, from targeted therapies, 235
intracellular signaling cascade, 222
introns, 18, 19*f*, 342
invasiveness gene signature (IGS), 188–189
irinotecan, 206–207, 207*f*
isoenzymes, 204
isoleucine, 21*f*

J

Journal of Nursing Scholarship, 294
justice, 247

K

karyotype, 342
Klinefelter syndrome, 56

L

laboratory selection, for cancer genetic risk assessment program, 140
language differences, 276
lapatinib, 227*t*
laser capture microdissection, 184–185

legislation, resources on, 321*t*–322*t*, 333–334
letters of medical necessity, for genetic testing, 115
leucine, 21*f*
licensure, 290, 303. *See also* credentialing
lifestyle assessment, 57–59
Li-Fraumeni syndrome, 35, 53*t*, 86
ligand binding, 219*f*, 221, 221*f*
ligands, 219*f*, 219–221
line graphs, for risk communication, 94, 95*f*
linkage, 342
linkage disequilibrium, 157, 342
linkage studies, 155–156
long-term outcomes, of screening/genetic testing, 82
loss of heterozygosity, 34–35
lung cancer, 35, 84
  genome-wide association studies on, 154*t*, 164*f*
lymphocytic leukemia, 206
lymphoma, microarrays in, 191*f*, 191–192
Lynch syndrome, 38–39, 53*t*, 63, 65, 73–74, 83, 110
  case study on, 88–90, 91*f*
  founder effect in, 64
lysine, 21*f*

M

MammaPrint™ gene expression assay, 188–190, 308–309
mammography, 60*t*
Managing Genetic Information: Implications for Nursing Practice (ANA), 324–325
matrix metalloproteinases (MMPs), 229*f*
Mayo Clinic, Nursing Genomics Program, 293

Index

MDR1 gene, 208
media, risk information in, 98–99
medical history, 56
Medicare, 136
medullary thyroid cancer, 65–66, 113
meiosis, 17, 23, 342
melanoma, 54t, 56, 59, 87t
Melanoma Risk Assessment Tool, 87t
membrane-associated guanine nucleotide-binding proteins (G proteins), 33
menarche, age at, 56
Mendel, Gregor, xiii
Mendelian errors, 162, 342
Mendelian inheritance, 50, 51t, 52, 152
menopause, age at, 56
messenger ribonucleic acid (mRNA), 18, 19f, 22, 22f, 180, 308, 342–343
metabolism, 201–203, 202f, 203t
  pathways of, 204–205, 205f
methotrexate, 202, 208
methylation, 28–29, 29t
methylenetetrahydrofolate reductase (MTHFR), 208
microarray analysis, 180–190, 181f–184f, 343. *See also* tumor profiling
  current work in, 190–192, 191f, 212–213
  future directions in, 192–194
  limitations of, 185
  techniques in, 185–190
Microarray In Node-negative Disease may Avoid ChemoTherapy (MINDACT) study, 190, 309, 315t
microRNAs (miRNAs), 31–32
microsatellite DNA sequences, 38
microsatellite instability (MSI), 38–39, 63, 91
microsatellite instability high (MSI-H) cells, 63, 74
microsatellites, 63, 343
military personnel, genetic information and, 255–256
Million Women Study, 57
MINDACT study, 190, 309, 315t
minor allele frequencies, 162, 343
mismatch repair, 38–39
missense point mutations, 20f, 24, 25t, 26f
mistrust, 272–274
mitogen-activated protein kinases (MAPKs), 33, 232
mitosis, 17, 40, 343
MLH1 mutation, 83, 87t, 90
models of cancer development, 13–14, 34
molecular profiling. *See* tumor profiling
molecular signature. *See* tumor profiling
monoclonal antibodies (MoAbs), 209, 212, 223–224, 224f, 226t, 228–229, 231
  side effects of, 226t–227t, 235
monomers, 219f, 221
mood changes, from targeted therapies, 235–236
mortality rate, 82, 343
MRE11 mutation, 36
MSH2 mutation, 83, 87t, 90
MTS1 gene, 35
mucositis, from targeted therapies, 233t
multicultural competence, 279, 279f, 280t, 280f
multicultural considerations, 251–252, 252f, 268–279
multidisciplinary team, for cancer genetic risk assessment program, 131–133, 133f
multiple endocrine neoplasia type 1/2 (MEN1/MEN2), 54t, 62, 113
multistage sampling design, 159, 160f
Muslim populations, 275
mutations, 18, 20f, 23, 343
  acquired, 26
  causes of, 23, 24f
  frameshift, 25, 26f
  germ line, 23
  missense, 20f, 24, 25t, 26f
  nonsense, 24, 25t, 26f, 343
  point, 23–24, 25t, 26f
  and signal transduction, 222–223
  silent, 20f–21f, 24, 25t
  types of, 21f, 23–25, 25t, 26f
mutator genes, 35–36, 343
MYC oncogene, 37, 222
MYH-associated polyposis, 53t, 110

N

NAME (nevi, atrial myxoma, myxoid neurofibroma, and ephelides), 69–70
National Cancer Institute (NCI), 262f–263f, 321t, 325, 329–330, 332–333
  Breast and Colon Cancer Family Registries, 310, 315t
  Cancer Genome Anatomy Project (CGAP), 193, 194t, 336
  cancer prevalence data from, 81
  Center for Bioinformatics (NCICB), 193, 194t
  genetic education resources, 106t
  genetic testing guidelines, 109
  Initiative for Chemical Genetics (ICG), xvi, 193, 194t
  Office of Cancer Genomics, xvi, 192
  risk model resources, 86–87
  Statement on Genetic Testing for Cancer Risk, 334
  Translational Research Working Group (TRWG), 305
National Center for Biotechnology Information (NCBI), 135, 171, 193, 194t, 200, 312
National Center on Minority Health and Health Disparities (NCMHD), 271
National Coalition for Health Professional Education in Genetics (NCHPEG), 170, 261, 289, 298, 320t, 326
National Coalition of Ethnic Minority Nurse Associations (NCEMNA), 320t
National Commission for Certifying Agencies (NCCA), 299
National Comprehensive Cancer Network (NCCN), 80, 110, 123, 178t, 186, 321t, 334
National Council of State Boards of Nursing (NCSBN), 298, 303
National Guideline Clearinghouse (NGC), 123, 170, 322t, 334
National Human Genome Research Institute (NHGRI), 193, 262f, 325, 331, 333
  Ethical, Legal, and Social Implications (ELSI) Program, 115, 260–261, 322t, 333, 335
  Genetics and Genomics for Patients and the Public, 263f, 321t, 332
  Genome-Wide Association Studies, 322t

on health disparities, 271
Office of Population Genomics, 169–170
on patient advocacy, 121
Policy and Ethics, 321*t*
National Institute of Nursing Research (NINR), 313, 315*t*, 322*t*, 328, 335
funding opportunities, 336
Summer Genetics Institute (SGI), 320*t*
National Institutes of Health (NIH), 332–333
Genome Wide Association Studies Policy, 322*t*
on health disparities, 271
Office of Rare Diseases Research (ORDR), 263*f*, 325, 331
Patient Recruitment Office, 330
Roadmap, 305–306
Summer Genetics Institute (SGI), 328
National Organization for Competency Assurance (NOCA), 299
National Plan and Provider Enumeration System, 135*t*
National Provider Identifier (NPI), 135*t*, 137–138
National Reference Center for Bioethics Literature, 262*f*
National Society of Genetic Counselors, Inc. (NSGC), 130, 135, 170, 320*t*, 323, 325–326, 330
Native American populations, 273, 275, 278
NBS1 (Nijmegen breakage syndrome 1 and non-Hodgkin lymphoma) gene, 36, 86
NCCN Clinical Practice Guidelines in Oncology™, 90, 321*t*, 334

NCLEX examinations, 298
needs assessment, for cancer genetic risk assessment program, 130, 131*f*
negative results in absence of known mutation, 117*f*, 118–119
neoangiogenesis, 32, 228, 229*f*
neural net technology, 303
neurofibromatosis *(NF1)* gene, 35
nevi, atrial myxoma, myxoid neurofibroma, and ephelides (NAME), 69–70
NF1/NF2 genes, 35
Nijmegen breakage syndrome, 36, 86
nilotinib, 227*t*
nominal significance, 343
non-directive counseling, 250, 343
non-Hodgkin lymphoma, 36, 42
nonhomologous end joining (NHEJ), 39
nonmaleficence, 247, 250–251, 251*f*
nonrandom aneuploidy, 37
nonreceptor tyrosine kinases, 33
nonsense point mutations, 24, 25*t*, 26*f*, 343
non-small cell lung cancer, 35
nonverbal communication, 276
nuclear receptors, 204
nucleotide excision repair, 39, 343
nucleotides, 16, 343
nucleus, 343
Nurse Practice Acts, 4

O

obesity, as cancer risk, 57–58
odds ratios, 159, 343
olaparib, xxi
oligonucleotides, 225, 343
oncogenes, 31–33, 222, 343
classifications of, 31–34

Oncology Certified Nurse (OCN®), 301
Oncology Nursing Certification Corporation (ONCC), 299–301, 304
Oncology Nursing Forum, 323
Oncology Nursing Society (ONS), 262*f*, 319–323, 320*t*
Cancer Genetics Special Interest Group (SIG), 261, 323
on genetics/genomics curricula, 289–290
Genetics Online Education Series, 292
genetics position statements, 322
scope of nursing practice, 4, 105, 292–293, 297–301
Oncotype DX tumor expression profile, for breast cancer, 185–188, 187*f*–188*f*, 189–190, 308–309
Online Journal of Issues in Nursing (OJIN) (ANA), 325
Online Mendelian Inheritance in Man (OMIM®), 52, 170
online resources
for billing/reimbursement, 135*t*
for genetics/genomics, 320*t*–322*t*
for molecular genomics technology, 194*t*
for psychosocial support, 121
ONS Connect, 323
outcomes, of screening/genetic testing, 82, 343
ovarian cancer, 63

P

pancreatic cancer, 54*t*
panitumumab, 227*t*, 235
Pap test, 60*t*–61*t*

paraganglioma, 65–66
p arm, of chromosome, 14, 16*f*
paronychia, from targeted therapies, 233*t*
pathology reports, 59–63, 71
patient assessments. *See* cancer genetic risk assessments
Pedigree Assessment Tool, 87*t*
Pedigree-Draw, 68*t*, 321*t*, 332
pedigrees, 50, 67, 67*f*–68*f*, 70
examples, 73*f*–74*f*, 89*f*
tools/resources for, 68*t*, 321*t*, 332
penetrance, 83, 98
Pestka, Beth, 293
Peutz-Jeghers syndrome, 53*t*–54*t*, 62
P-glycoprotein (PGP), 208
pharmacodynamics, 201, 203–204
pharmacogenetics, 199, 201, 311–312
Pharmacogenetics and Pharmacogenomics Knowledge Base (PharmGKB), 211, 312, 315*t*
Pharmacogenetics Research Network, 312
pharmacogenomics
advances in, 212–213
definition of, 199, 201
history of, 199–200
in oncology, 205–212
pharmacokinetics, 201–203, 202*f*–203*f*, 203*t*
PharmGKB, 211, 312, 315*t*
phenocopy, 118
phenotypes, 28, 61–62, 343
PhenX toolkit, 310, 315*t*
phenylalanine, 21*f*, 24
pheochromocytoma, 65–66
Philadelphia chromosome, 37, 212, 229, 243
phone disclosure sessions, 120–122, 145–146
phosphorylation, 219*f*, 221–222, 230
physical activity, assessment of, 57–58

Index   355

physical examination, 53*t*–54*t*, 69–70
Physician Data Query (PDQ®), 333
physician groups, 320*t*–321*t*, 324–327
pictorial elements, in risk communication, 94, 95*f*–97*f*
pie charts, for risk communication, 94, 96*f*
platelet-derived growth factor, 32
ploidy, 344
point mutations, 23–24, 25*t*, 26*f*
policies
  on genetic testing in children, 113
  resources on, 321*t*–322*t*, 334–335
poly adenosine diphosphate-ribose polymerase (PARP) inhibitors, 62
polymerase chain reaction (PCR), 180, 183–185, 344
polymerases, 22, 344
polymorphisms, 18, 20*f*, 23, 38. *See also* single nucleotide polymorphisms
polyps
  adenomatous, 56, 62, 90
  hyperplastic, 62
poor metabolizers (MMs), 204, 205*f*, 211
population, 81, 344
population attributable risk, 344
population stratification/structure, 155–156, 344
portfolio approach, to credentialing, 302*f*, 303, 324
preauthorization, for genetic testing, 115, 135–136
precursor lesions, 62
Prediction of Mutations in *MLH1* and *MSH2* (PREMM1,2) model, 87*t*
pre-implantation genetic diagnosis (PGD), 244, 258
PREMM1,2 (Prediction of Mutations in *MLH1* and *MSH2*) model, 87*t*
prenatal diagnosis, 258
prevalence, 81–82, 344
primary cancer prevention, 81, 344
prior probability, 88
privacy concerns, 112, 252–254, 253*f*
proband, 89, 91, 91*f*
Progeny, 68*t*, 321*t*, 332
Program for the Assessment of Clinical Cancer Tests, 193
programmed cell death, 42, 339
proline, 21*f*
promoter, 344
prostate cancer
  ethnicity and, 270
  genome-wide association studies on, 153*t*, 159–160, 161*t*
  hereditary, 54*t*, 86
  screening for, 61*t*
prostate-specific antigen (PSA) testing, 61*t*
proteins, 17, 19*f*, 20–21, 22*f*, 344
protein synthesis, 20–21, 22*f*
protein translation, 19*f*, 21*f*–22*f*, 22–23, 345
proteomics, xx
proto-oncogenes, 29–31, 30*f*, 222, 344
Provision of Quality Genetic Services and Care (NSGC/ISONG), 325–326
pruritus, from targeted therapies, 233
psychosocial assessment, 68–69
psychosocial issues, in genetic counseling, 97–98, 107–108, 108*f*–112, 117–119
psychosocial support, after testing, 121
PTEN gene, 89

PubMed, 312, 315*t*
purine bases, 16
putative hereditary, 50
p values, 159, 344
pyrimidine bases, 16

Q

q arm, of chromosome, 14, 16*f*
quality assurance, 147–148
questionnaire, in assessment process, 70

R

racial background, 268–269. *See also* ethnic background
racial discrimination, 273
RAF1 kinase, 33
random aneuploidy, 37
random hit model, of cancer development, 13
rare cancers, 65–66
rash, from targeted therapies, 232–233, 233*t*
ras oncogenes, 33, 222
ratios, relative risk expressed as, 84
RB1 gene, 26, 29*t*, 34
real-time polymerase chain reaction (RT-PCR) technique, 180, 185
rearranged during transfection *(RET)* gene, 31, 113
receptors, 204, 219*f*, 219–221
receptor tyrosine kinases, 224
recessive genes, 155, 344
reciprocal translocations, 36, 229, 344
recombination, 23–24, 344
reference SNP (rs) number, 159, 344
reimbursement, 134–138, 135*t*, 136*f*. *See also* economic considerations
relative risk (RR), 83–84, 162, 344

religious beliefs, assessment of, 63–64. *See also* spirituality
replication
  of DNA, 23, 340
  of genome-wide association studies, 163
reproductive history, 56
research. *See also* clinical trials; genome-wide association studies
  resources for, 322*t*, 335–336
  staying current with, 312–313
  translational, 305–312, 314*t*–315*t*
respect for persons, 247
RET gene, 31, 113
retinoblastoma, 26, 34, 65–66
retinoic acid receptor-alpha (RAR-alpha), 212
reverse transcriptase polymerase chain reaction, 183–184
ribonucleic acid (RNA), 21, 344
ribosomes, 22, 22*f*, 344
risk. *See also* cancer genetic risk assessments; risk communication; risk prediction models
  absolute, 83, 87*t*, 339
  attributable, 84, 339
  clients' perception of, 83–84, 92–93, 108–109, 276
  relative, 83–84, 162, 344
risk assessment. *See* cancer genetic risk assessments
risk communication, 79–80, 88, 92–98, 109. *See also* genetic counseling/education
  environment for, 70, 120
  long-term impact of, 99
  media role in, 98–99
  psychosocial issues in, 97–98
  visual aids for, 94, 95*f*–97*f*
risk factors, 80, 344

risk ladders, for risk communication, 94, 96f
risk prediction models, 79–80, 84–88, 87t
  case study of, 88–92, 90f–92f
  evaluation/selection of, 85–86
  limitations of, 86
rituximab, 227t, 235
RNA-inducing silencing complex (RISC), 309
RNA interference (RNAi), 225, 309–310
RNA polymerases, 22
The Role of the Oncology Nurse in Cancer Genetic Counseling (ONS), 322
Rotterdam breast cancer prognosis gene signature, 188–189

S

scope of nursing practice, 4–7, 6f, 103–105, 292–293, 297–302, 323–325. *See also* credentialing
screening, 59, 60t–61t, 81–82, 123f, 123–124, 345
secondary cancer prevention, 81, 345. *See also* screening
second-degree relatives, 67
Secretary's Advisory Committee on Genetics, Health and Society (SACGHS), 262f, 322t, 334–335
selective estrogen receptor modulators (SERMs), 218, 219t
sensitivity, 63, 82, 345
serine, 21f
serine threonine kinases, 33
serline, 21f
sex chromosomes, 14
short-interfering RNA (siRNA), 309–310

short-term outcomes, of screening/genetic testing, 82
side effects, 311–312
signals, 219f, 222–223
signal transduction, 29–31, 30f, 32, 218–222, 219f–221f, 345
  mutations and, 222–223
  terminology in, 219f
silent point mutations, 20f–21f, 24, 25t
single-gene disorder, 26
single locus, 345
single nucleotide polymorphisms (SNPs), 18, 23, 151, 156, 200–201, 203, 345. *See also* genome-wide association studies
  in drug-metabolizing enzymes, 206–208
  in drug targets, 209–212
  in drug transporters, 208
site-specific testing, 66
6-mercaptopurine (6-MP), 206
skin cancer, hereditary, 54t
skin rash, from targeted therapies, 232–233, 233t
slow acetylators, 210–211
small intestine cancer, mortality rates for, 82
small-molecule EGFR tyrosine kinase inhibitors, 209–210, 224–225
smoking, as cancer risk, 58, 84
somatic cells, 17, 260, 345
somatic genetic disorders, 26
somatic mutations, 36
sorafenib, 227t, 234
specialization, in genetics/genomics, 5–6, 6f, 8–10, 10t, 292–293, 323. *See also* credentialing
specificity, 82, 345
S-phase checkpoint, 41t
spirituality, 63–64, 276, 278
splicing, 345
sporadic cancers, 26, 50
start codons, 20, 21f

stem cell model, of cancer development, 13–14
stem cell research, 260
St. Gallen International Consensus Conference, 178t, 187–188
stick figures, for risk communication, 94, 96f
stochastic model, of cancer development, 13
stool DNA test, 60t
stop codons, 20, 21f
Strategic Partnering to Evaluate Cancer Signatures, 193
strategic planning committee, for cancer genetic risk assessment program, 130–131, 132t
sun exposure, as cancer risk, 58–59
sunitinib, 227t, 234
supplements, 59
support groups, 121
surgical history, 59–63
Surveillance, Epidemiology, and End Results (SEER) program, 64–65, 81

T

tag SNPs, 157, 345
TAILORx study, 190, 309, 315t
tamoxifen, 61, 179, 186, 210–211, 218
tanning lamps/booths, 58–59
targeted therapies, xxi, 226t–227t, 226–231, 228f
  food/drug interactions with, 232
  future direction of, 236–237
  history of, 218–223
  mechanisms for, 223–225
  rationale for, 217–218
  side effects of, 226t–227t, 231–236
T cells, 225
telemedicine, 120–122, 145–146

telephone disclosure sessions, 120–122, 145–146
Telling Stories: Understanding Real Life Genetics, 320t, 329
telomerase, 14
telomeres, 14, 15f–16f, 345
temporal orientation, 277
temsirolimus, 227t
tertiary cancer prevention, 81, 345
testicular cancer, 56
Therapeutically Applicable Research to Generate Effective Treatments (TARGET) Initiative, xvi
therapeutic response, 311–312
Theros H/ISM gene expression assay, 308
thiopurine methyltransferase (TPMT) enzyme, 206
third-degree relatives, 67
Thomas—U.S. Congress on the Internet, 322t
threonine, 21f
thymine (T), 16, 17f, 345
TNM system, 178t, 178–179
tobacco use, as cancer risk, 58, 84
tositumomab, 227t
toxicogenomics, xxi
TP53 gene, 33, 35, 41–42, 86, 345
transcription, 19f, 21, 22f, 345
transcription factors, 33
transduction pathways. *See* signal transduction
transfer RNA (tRNA), 19f, 22, 22f
transforming growth factor, 33
transforming growth factor-beta (TGF-beta), 32, 345
translation, 19f, 21f–22f, 22–23, 345
translational research, 206f, 305–308. *See also* clinical trials; genome-wide association studies

examples of, 308–312, 314t–315t
staying current with, 312–313
translesion DNA synthesis, 39–40
translocations, 36–37, 212, 229, 344–345
trastuzumab, 227t, 243
Trial Assigning Individualized Options for Treatment (TAILORx) study, 190, 309, 315t
triple-negative breast cancer, 62
true negative (TN) results, 117f, 118, 120, 345
true positive (TP) results, 116–118, 117f, 120, 163, 345
trust, 272–274
tryptophan, 21f
tumorigenesis, 26–28, 41–42
tumor neoangiogenesis, 32, 228, 229f
tumor profiling
 clinical trials on, 190, 308–309, 316t
 current work in, 190–192, 191f, 308–309
 future directions in, 192–194

history of, 178–179
limitations of, 185
purpose of, 177–178
resources on, 194t
techniques of, 180–190
tumor suppressor genes, 28, 34–35, 35f, 36, 223, 345
Turner syndrome, 56
Tuskegee syphilis study, 272–273
"two-hit" model, of cancer development, 34
tyrosine, 21f
tyrosine kinase inhibitors, 229–231
tyrosine kinase receptors, 32
tyrosine kinases, 32–33, 212, 222, 224

U

UDP-glucuronosyltransferase 1A1 (UGT1A1) enzyme, 206–207, 207f
ultrametabolizers (UMs), 205, 205f
ultraviolet (UV) radiation exposure, as cancer risk, 58–59
uncertainty, in genetic testing, 98, 109–110
undescended testicles, 56

uninformative results, 117f, 118–119
uracil (U), 21, 345
U.S. National Council of State Boards of Nursing (NCSBN), 298, 303
U.S. Preventive Services Task Force (USPSTF), 110
U.S. Surgeon General, Family History Initiative, 68t, 171, 321t, 332

V

vaccines, 225, 225f
validity, 82–83, 307, 307t, 346
valine, 21f
variable penetrance, 98
variant of uncertain significance (VUS), 117f, 119, 147
vascular endothelial growth factor (VEGF), 32, 209, 228, 229f
vascular endothelial growth factor receptors (VEGFRs), 228, 229f
Vectibix® targeted therapy, xxi

video conferencing, 121
virtual colonoscopy, 60t
visual aids, in risk communication, 94, 95f–97f
vitamin supplements, 59
vulnerable populations, genetic testing of, 113

W

Web resources
 for billing/reimbursement, 135t
 for genetics/genomics, 320t–322t
 for molecular genomics technology, 194t
 for psychosocial support, 121
weight, and cancer risk, 57–58
wild-type genes, 18, 25t, 346
Wilms tumor, 56, 65–66
winner's curse, 346
World Health Organization, obesity defined by, 57

X

xerosis, from targeted therapies, 233, 233t